Cardiac Surgery Handbook

Cardiac Surgery Handbook

Edited by **Jessica Clan**

FOSTER
ACADEMICS

New Jersey

Published by Foster Academics,
61 Van Reypen Street,
Jersey City, NJ 07306, USA
www.fosteracademics.com

Cardiac Surgery Handbook
Edited by Jessica Clan

International Standard Book Number: 978-1-63242-068-8 (Hardback)

Printed in China.

Contents

	Preface	**IX**
Chapter 1	**Anesthesia in Cardiac Surgery** Meral Kanbak and Filiz Üzümcügil	**1**
Chapter 2	**Anaesthetic Considerations for Congenital Heart Disease Patient** Mohammad Hamid	**43**
Chapter 3	**Data Integration and Management in Cardiac Surgery** Alessandro Taddei, Maurizio Mangione, Paolo Marcheschi and Stefano Dalmiani	**61**
Chapter 4	**Perioperative Organ Protection in Cardiac Surgery** Maria Carmona, Matheus Vane and Luiz Malbouisson	**75**
Chapter 5	**Perioperative Management of Pulmonary Hypertension** Theofani Antoniou and Kassiani Theodoraki	**93**
Chapter 6	**Monitoring Outcomes in Highly Specialised Cardiac Surgery** Thomas Kenny and Martin Ashton-Key	**109**
Chapter 7	**Early Postoperative Care After Cardiac Surgery** Paul M. H. J. Roekaerts and John H. Heijmans	**125**
Chapter 8	**Hemotherapy in Cardiac Surgery** Robert Wagner	**147**

Chapter 9 **Cardiac Surgery and Allogeneic Blood Transfusions** 159
Yavuz M. Bilgin

Chapter 10 **Glycemic Control in Cardiac Surgery** 179
Martín Martínez Rosas, Eduardo Wilfrido Goicoechea-Turcott, Pastor Luna Ortiz, Alberto Salazar and Benito Antón Palma

Chapter 11 **Coagulation Measurement and Optimisation in Cardiac Surgery** 197
Philip Johnson and Andrew Westbrook

Chapter 12 **Heparin Induced Thrombocytopenia: Its Significance in Cardiac Surgical Patient** 229
Marcin Wąsowicz

Chapter 13 **Antiplatelet Drugs in Coronary Artery Disease** 239
Susanne Maria Picker

Chapter 14 **Thyroid Hormone Therapy for the Cardiac Surgical Patient** 265
Aaron M. Ranasinghe and Robert S. Bonser

Chapter 15 **A Pathophysiological Approach to Understanding Pulmonary Hypertension in Cardiac Surgery** 277
Anne Q. N. Nguyen, Alain Deschamps, France Varin, Louis P. Perrault and André Y. Denault

Chapter 16 **The Physiology and the Clinical Significance of Postoperative Hyperlactatemia After Pediatric Cardiac Surgery** 307
Vered Molina-Hazan and Gideon Paret

Chapter 17 **Sticking Up for the Immune System Integrity: Should the Thymus Be Preserved During Cardiac Surgery?** 325
Sara Ferrando-Martínez, M. Ángeles Muñoz-Fernández and Manuel Leal

Chapter 18 **Relationship Between Natriuretic Peptides and Hemodynamic Parameters Following Heart Surgery in Infancy** 341
Andrea Székely, Tamás Breuer and Béla Merkely

Chapter 19 **Amyloidosis and Cardiac Surgery** **355**
Pavel Zacek and Jan Harrer

Chapter 20 **Ivabradine Versus Beta-Blockers in Patients with Conduction Abnormalities or Left Ventricular Dysfunction Undergoing Coronary Artery Bypass Grafting** **365**
Luminita Iliuta and Roxana Enache

Permissions

List of Contributors

Preface

I am honored to present to you this unique book which encompasses the most up-to-date data in the field. I was extremely pleased to get this opportunity of editing the work of experts from across the globe. I have also written papers in this field and researched the various aspects revolving around the progress of the discipline. I have tried to unify my knowledge along with that of stalwarts from every corner of the world, to produce a text which not only benefits the readers but also facilitates the growth of the field.

A descriptive account based on cardiac surgery has been illuminated in this profound book. It primarily focuses on the present perioperative care techniques and advances in novel cardiac surgery technologies. Perioperative techniques and novel technologies in the field of cardiac surgery will continue to enhance the advancements in postoperative results and aid the cardiac surgical society to improve surgical processes. This book will serve as a valuable source of information for senior surgeons, nurses and trainees engaged in the field of cardiac surgery, as well as perfusionists, anesthesiologists, and associated health care workers who are responsible for taking care of patients with heart disease which need surgical therapy. Reputed experts from across the globe have contributed in this insightful book. It will vastly benefit the patients undergoing cardiac surgery in gaining knowledge regarding perioperative care methodologies.

Finally, I would like to thank all the contributing authors for their valuable time and contributions. This book would not have been possible without their efforts. I would also like to thank my friends and family for their constant support.

Editor

Preface

1

Anesthesia in Cardiac Surgery

Meral Kanbak[1] and Filiz Üzümcügil[2]
[1]Hacettepe University School of Medicine, Department of Anesthesiology and Reanimation, Ankara
[2]TCSB Ankara Etlik Zübeyde Hanım Maternity and Women's Health Clinic Teaching and Research Hospital, Department of Anesthesiology and Reanimation, Ankara
Turkey

1. Introduction

The cardiac surgical procedures are increasingly performed each year up to a number >700000 (data in 1997 in US) per year, of which >600000 are coronary artery bypass grafting (CABG) procedures. After 1997, there has been a gradual decrease in CABG procedures as percutaneous coronary interventions (PCI) grow. In 2005, a total of 699000 cardiac surgical procedures were reported, including 469000 surgical coronary revascularization procedures. It is still debated whether CABG procedures will continue to decrease as relative benefits of PCI continue to be evaluated. As the number of aging population increases and risk factors (e.g.,obesity and diabetes) occur, cardiovascular diseases are also estimated to increase; however, it is not clear that changes in life style or advancing medical management will reduce the prevalance and incidence of these diseases. Although the cardiac surgery is not the primary solution, CABG procedures are still the most commonly performed cardiac procedures and it will remain one of the management options (Thys,2009;London et al,2008).
There is an explosive growth in these procedures due to improvements in operative outcomes, inclusion of older and sicker patients for cardiac surgeries and expansion of these surgeries to community hospitals. However, although the physicians develop greater confidence and capacity to perform the procedures, the morbidity, mortality and resource utilization are still higher in the elderly population; especially in octagenarians. Scott et al. (2005) reported longer intensive care unit (ICU) and hospital stay with higher rates of postoperative renal failure and neurologic complications; and Baskett et al. (2005) reported more death and stroke after CABG in octagenarians. As the cardiac surgical procedures grow with an aging population with increased mortality and morbidity, more anesthesiologists become specialized in cardiovascular anesthesiology, practicing cardiac anesthesia excusively in active cardiac surgical centers; changing their focus from anesthetic management of patients with cardiovascular diseases to cardiovascular medicine; medical and surgical management of cardiovascular patients (Thys,2009).

2. Anesthetic management

The primary goal of cardiac surgery is not just a minimally acceptable outcome where the patient survives without life-threatenening complications or persistent clinically manifest

organ dysfunctions or simply hospital survival; but a healthy, productive long-term survivor (Murphy et al,2009).
Anesthetic protocols in cardiac surgery are investigated and analized in terms of their effect on postoperative mortality and incidence of myocardial infarction following cardiac surgery, postoperative cardiac troponin release, need for inotropic support, time on mechanical ventilation, ICU and hospital stay (Landoni et al,2009).

2.1 Preoperative evaluation and premedication

In order to reduce the fear and anxiety of the patient, provide analgesia for painful interventions such as vascular cannulation before anesthetic induction and to provide amnesia to some degree, pharmacological interventions are used. These agents are also supposed to prevent the anginal episodes which are clinically silent preoperatively. Oral, intravenous or intramuscular benzodiazepines are the agents that are most frequently chosen (London et al,2008). Agents and their dosages to be selected depend on the patients' age and physiologic status. High doses are desirable for the patients with coronary artery disease, whereas low doses are more appropriate for patients with valvular diseases whose physiologic status is compansated with enhanced sympathetic tone (Liu et al,2004). However, on arrival to the operating room the patients may receive further medications in case of an inadequate sedation, prior to the interventions that are planned before the induction. The beneficial effects of premedication should also be secured by the proper conditions of the operating room including the temperature and also the verbal interaction with the patient (London et al,2008).

Most popular premedicants

For anxiolysis and amnesia;

- Diazepam oral: 0.1-0.15 mg/kg
- Midazolam intravenous: 1-2 mg

For analgesia;

- Morphine intramuscular: 0.1-0.15 mg/kg
- Fentanyl intravenous: 50-75 μg

The anesthetist has an important role in preoperative administration of cardiovascular medications especially the anti-anginal medications, ensuring that these agents are ordered for morning with sips of water, as the cardiac anesthesiologist is becoming a 'perioperative physician' (London et al,2008).

2.2 Monitoring

On arrival to the operating room, before induction of anesthesia, preoxygenation, monitoring with pulse oximetry, ECG, non-invasive BP and radial artery cannulation for ABP, ECG and also for the high-risk patients central venous catheters and pulmonary artery catheter should be in place (Reich et al,2008).

2.2.1 Electrocardiogram (ECG)

A multi-lead ECG system with a continuous paper writeout and online ST-segment trending system is useful in early diagnosis of myocardial ischemia and detecting arrhythmias. Also a preinduction rhythm strip or frozen on the monitor screen may help to assess the changes intraoperatively (Morgan et al,2002). An angiographically identified areas that are at risk for transmural ischemia can be observed more sensitively by specific placement of the leads

(Reich et al,2008). The electrocoutery may interfere with ECG recordings resulting in difficulty in dysrhythmia analysis in the operating room (Morgan et al,2002).

2.2.2 Arterial blood pressure monitoring (ABP)

The radial artery is used for the CABG procedures to monitor the blood pressure. The cannulation is applied before anesthetic induction in order to observe the hemodynamic response closely (Reich et al,2008). Radial artery cannulation requires the testing of the competancy of ulnar collateral circulation of the hand in case of radial artery thrombosis. This test is the Allen test; however it is not completely reliable. Some centers prefer the non-dominant side for cannulation and some other prefer to use the side opposite to the proposed internal mammarian artery dissection to avoid inaccurate measurements caused by the sternal retractors tenting the subclavian artery. Furthermore, after the period of hypothermia there can be alterations in the measurements from radial artery (lower than aortic pressure with a gradient 10-30 mmHg) which is mainly caused by decreased vascular resistance. Temporarily measuring blood pressure directly from the aorta via a needle or cardioplegia cannula can be an acceptable approach (Morgan et al,2002).

2.2.3 Central venous cannulation

Cardiac surgery is associated with large fluid shifts and need for multiple drug infusions (Morgan et al,2002). In order to measure pressure to regulate volume infusion and for both volume and vasoactive drug administration, central venous catheterization (CVC) has become a routine practice (London et al,2008). CVC is used for measuring the right ventricle (RV) filling pressures giving an estimate for intravascular volume status and RV function. For accurate measurement of the pressures, the catheter tip should be in one of the large thoracic veins or the right atrium. With a short and straight course to the right atrium (RA) assuring RA or superior venous cava (SVC) localization of the catheter tip, internal jugular vein is preferred for the site of this central catheterization (Reich et al,2008).

Following serial measurements to observe the trends is more reliable and safe when compared to individual numbers. Central venous pressure (CVP) is not a direct indicator of left heart filling pressure, but it may provide an estimate for these pressures in patients with good LV function. The catheter can also be used for both indicating the RA pressures and cerebral venous pressure if the tip is in SVC. The increase in CVP may result in a decrease in cerebral perfusion pressure. Occasionally this may be caused by a malposition of the catheter during CPB, which is to be corrected immediately by the surgeon to avoid cerebral edema and poor cerebral perfusion (Reich et al,2008).

CVC may be applied before induction using sedation including small doses of midazolam and fentanyl supplemented by oxygen via a face mask avioiding hypoxia, or after induction of anesthesia. Multi-lumen catheters allow for both fluid administration and drug infusions at the same time (Morgan et al,2002).

2.2.4 Pulmonary artery catheterization (PAC)

The PAC providing various physiologic information has been shown to have little effect on clinical outcome, leading to a lower use currently; decreased 60-80% over the past decade. Although the criteria to use PAC have not been demonstrated clearly, it is recommended to be reserved for high-risk patients, as the patients with multi-system dysfunction are increasingly scheduled for cardiac surgical procedures (Reich et al,2008).

High-risk patients requiring PAC (Reich et al,2008)

1. Significant impairment of ventricular function
   - EF<40%
   - Acute or Chronic congestive heart failure
   - Elevation of left ventricular end-diastolic pressure (LVEDP) on preoperative catheterization
   - Need for preoperative intraaortic balon pump (IABP)
   - Acute or chronic severe mitral regurgitation due to ischemia
   - Ventricular septal defect after myocardial infarction
   - Other mechanical complications
2. High-risk for intraoperative ischemia or difficult revascularization
   - Recent, large myocardial infarction
   - Severe unstable angina
   - Known poor revascularization targets or severe microcirculatory disease
   - Reoperation
   - Catheterization laboratory PCI 'crash'
3. Severe co-morbidities
   - Renal failure (need for dialysis)
   - Severe chronic obstructive pulmonary disease
4. Combined procedures that prolonges the duration of surgery or add significant blood loss (CABG-carotid, other vascular procedures)

PAC provides detailed information with various parameters such as PCWP, PA diastolic pressure and derived parameters, estimating the left ventricular filling pressures-preload more precisely than CVC (Reich et al,2008;Morgan et al,2002). However, there are some limiting factors altering the accuracy of these measurements such as mitral stenosis, LA myxoma, pulmonary venous obstruction, elevated alveolar pressure, decreased left ventricular compliance and aortic insufficiency; which are to be considered during the anesthetic management (Reich et al,2008).

2.2.5 Transesophageal echocardiography

One of the earliest signs of acute myocardial ischemia is diastolic dysfunction followed by systolic segmental wall motion abnormalities which occurs within seconds after acute coronary occlusion. Coronary artery disease is associated with segmental wall motion abnormalities more than ECG changes. However, these wall motion abnormalities are not specific for myocardial ischemia; that they may occur during CABG procedure due to loading conditions altering pre- and afterload, transient motion abnormalities caused by myocardial stunning during the ischemic periods of weaning from CPB and also inotropic agents or elevated catecholamine levels. TEE is recommended for high-risk patients for myocardial ischemia with a category II indication (*TEE may be helpful in improving clinical outcomes*) by ASA. This indication is strenghtened when ECG cannot be used for detection of ischemia in situations such as the existence of LBBB, extensive Q waves or ST-T segment changes on baseline ECG. However, it is weakened when there are wall motion abnormalities due to fibrotic, calcified or aneurysmal myocardium at the baseline (London et al,2008).

Category I indications (*TEE is useful in improving clinical outcomes*) for the usage of TEE includes, suspected thoracal aortic aneurysm-dissection or disruption in unstable patients in the preoperative period; life-threatening hemodynamic disturbance, valve repair, congenital heart surgery, hypertrophic obstructive cardiomyopathy repair, endocarditis, aortic valve function in aortic dissection repair, evaluation of pericardial window procedures intraoperatively and unexplained hemodynamic disturbances in ICU setting. Category II (*TEE may be helpful in improving clinical outcomes)* indications include hemodynamic disturbances, cardiac aneurysm repair, tumour excision, air emboli, intracardiac embolectomy, aortic dissection repair, pericardial surgery and also increased risk of myocardial ischemia. Category III (*TEE is infrequently useful in improving outcomes)* indications include evaluation of myocardial perfusion, coronary artery anatomy, graft patency, repair of non-HOCMs, endocarditis in non-cardiac surgery, monitoring emboli in orthopedic surgeries, repair of thoracic aortic injuries, uncomplicated pericarditis, pleuropulmonary disease, monitoring cardioplegia administration and also placement of IABP, ICD or PA catheters (Roscoe,2007).

2.3 Anesthetic induction

Anesthetic induction of cardiac surgical patients requires titration of drugs in order to avoid any increase in oxygen consumption and decrease in oxygen supply. Titration of induction agents with monitoring of the hemodynamics is more important than the type of the drug chosen (Barnes,2002a). During induction hypertension and tachycardia in patients with normal ventricular function, hypertension and LV hypertrophy should be avoided as well as hypotension and myocardial depression in patients with depressed ventricular function or stenoses. These agents should also provide smooth intubating conditions for those patients. These major concerns of cardiac anesthetic practice can be managed by using small doses of vasopressors for hypotension and by deepening anesthesia or administering β-blockers for the hyperdynamic responses. In terms of intraoperative ischemia, postoperative myocardial infarction or death, there is no single technique superior to others (London et al,2008).

The choice of the anesthetic method depends mainly on left ventricular (LV) function and whether the patient is suitable for early extubation or not. LV function determines the dosages of the anesthetic agents depending on the hemodynamic response of the patient. Early extubation is a desired method in order to reduce the postoperative need for mechanical ventilation resulting in shorter periods of ICU stay, decreasing the cost. There is no single strategy to be recommended for all cardiac surgical patients; hypnotics, opioids and volatile anesthetics are used in different combinations for both the induction and maintenance of anesthesia (London et al,2008).

2.3.1 Thiopental

Thiopental is the sulphur analogue of the oxybarbiturate pentobarbitone. It is used 3-7 mg/kg intravenously for the induction of anesthesia, rapidly entering the CNS and producing unconsciousness within 30 seconds (Peck,2006; Stoelting&Hillier,2006). The dose that is required for induction depends on patients' age (decreasing with age), weight and cardiac output (Stoelting&Hillier,2006). At sufficient plasma concentrations which is most easily maintained by continuous infusion, thiopental produces an isoelectric EEG, contributing to a maximal reduction of cerebral oxygen requirements. At these concentrations inotropic support may be required to maintain adequate cerebral perfusion (Peck,2006). However, thiopental is seldom used as infusion, because of its long context-sensitive half-time leading to a prolonged recovery period (Stoelting&Hillier,2006).

Thiopental causes a dose-dependent reduction in cardiac output, stroke volume and systemic vascular resistance associated with a compansatory tachycardia. At a dose of 5 mg/kg intravenous thiopental causes a transient 10-20 mmHg decrease in blood pressure with a compansatory 15-20 bpm increase in heart rate. A decrease in myocardial contractility may occur, however it has been shown to be a less reduction when it is compared to volatile anesthetics (Stoelting&Hillier,2006).

Along with the induction of anesthesia with barbiturates mild and transient reduction in systemic blood pressure occurs, which mainly depends on the peripheral vasodilation, depression of the medullary vasomotor center and decreased sympathetic outflow. These minimal alterations in blood pressure and cardiac output with barbiturate induction mainly depend on carotid sinus–mediated baroreceptor reflex responses offsetting the effects of vasodilation. This mechanism explains the vulnerability of the hypovolemic patients to the effects of barbiturate induction (Stoelting&Hillier,2006).

The adverse effects including airway resistance, bronchospasm and postoperative nausea and vomiting, have led to a tendency towards the use of propofol, especially depending on its predictable pharmacokinetics and dynamics (London et al,2008).

2.3.2 Propofol

Propofol is an isopropylphenol (2,6 diisopropylphenol), replacing the barbiturates for induction, particularly for operations where rapid awakening is desirable, because of the complete awareness after propofol without any residual CNS effects (Peck,2006;Stoelting&Hillier,2006). The major advantage of using propofol as a part of the anesthetic protocol is the early extubation leading to reduced costs by shortening the LOS in ICU (D'Attelis et al,1997; Myeles et al,1997).

In healthy adults the induction dose of propofol is 1.5-2.5 mg/kg intravenous, with a 25-50 % reduction to be used in elderly patients, with 2-6 μg/ml blood level producing unconsciousness depending on combined medications and age, and 1-1.5 μg/ml blood level resulting in awakening (Stoelting&Hillier,2006).

Propofol decreases systemic blood pressure with corresponding changes in cardiac output and systemic vascular resistance. The blood pressure effects may be overt in hypovolemic patients, elderly patients and also patients with coronary artery disease compromising the left ventricle. Adequate hydration is often recommended to offset this effect of propofol. Unlike the effect of thiopental on blood pressure compansated by the increase in heart rate, propofol does not change heart rate. Furthermore, bradycardia and asystoli may also occur most probably because of the reduction in sympathetic outflow more than parasympathetic. It has been shown not to have any effect on sinoatrial or atrioventricular node in normal patients and patients with WPW syndrome allowing the usage of this drug for ablation procedures (Stoelting&Hillier,2006).

2.3.3 Etomidate

Etomidate is an imidazole derivative and an ester, which is used as an alternative to propofol and thiopental for induction of anesthesia, at a dose of 0.2-0.4 mg/kg intravenously, especially in patients with unstable hemodynamics, because of its least cardiovascular disturbance when compared to other agents (Peck,2006).

After induction, involuntary myoclonic movements can occur, which can be attenuated by using opioids. Awakening after a single dose is more rapid than barbiturates, however duration of action prolongs with intermittently increased dosage or continuous infusion.

The main limiting factor of usage is the depression of adrenocortical function (Stoelting&Hillier,2006).
The peripheral vascular resistance may fall slightly but there occurs no change in myocardial oxygen supply, contactility, stroke volume, cardiac output and blood pressure. In a dose-dependent manner, especially at the concentrations more than in clinical practice, etomidate may result in cardiac depression (Peck,2006;Stoelting&Hillier,2006).

2.3.4 Ketamine

Ketamine is a phencyclidine derivative, which results in a 'dissociative anesthesia' caused by the dissociation between thalamocortical and limbic systems. The dissociative anesthesia mimics a cataleptic state contributing to open eyes with slow nystagmic gaze; that wakefulness may appear to be present. Amnestic and analgesic properties are profound (Peck,2006;Stoelting&Hillier,2006).
Unlike other induction agents, ketamine produces sympathetic nervous system stimulation with a rise in circulating levels of adrenalin and noradrenalin; increasing the heart rate, cardiac output, blood pressure and myocardial oxygen requirements (Peck,2006). These stimulating effects may be blunted by combination of ketamine with benzodiazepines or opioids or inhaled anesthetic agents (Stoelting&Hillier,2006). It does not seem to precipitate arrhythmias (Peck,2006).
Induction doses of ketamine is 1-2 mg/kg intravenously and 2-4 mg/kg intramuscularly, allowing unconciousness within 30-60 seconds and 2-4 minutes, respectively. Awakening or return of consciousness occurs 10-20 minutes after induction, but full consciousness takes 60-90 minutes. Intermittent doses or continuous infusions lead to prolonged emergence times (Stoelting&Hillier,2006).

2.3.5 Midazolam

Midazolam can be used for anesthetic induction with a dose of 0.1-0.2 mg/kg intravenously administered over 30-60 seconds. However, thiopental usually produces 50-100% faster induction when it is compared with midazolam, furthermore awakening from general anesthesia including midazolam induction has been shown to be 1-2.5 times longer than that of thiopental (Stoelting&Hillier,2006) (see also the maintenance of anesthesia).

2.3.6 Neuromuscular blocking agents

All of the available neuromuscular blocking agents (NMBA) have been used for cardiac surgical patients. Pancuronium offsetting the bradycardia effect of high-dose opioids has been the prefered NMBA, however it has also been shown to have potential to produce a tachycardia causing myocardial ischemia during induction. Rocuronium has been compared with pancuronium and reported to provide more adequate conditions especially for fast-track anesthesia due to its less residual blockade and shorter time to extubation. Neuromuscular transmission monitoring is advised especially if fast-track anesthesia is planned (London et al,2008).

2.4 The maintenance of anesthesia

2.4.1 Intravenous anesthetic agents

The anesthesia should be adequate in order to prevent ischemia during incision and sternotomy/sternal spreading; which are the periods of hyperstimulation. Anesthetic dosages and the type of the drugs that are to be used depend on the desire of 'fast-tracking' the patient (Barnes,2002).

High-dose opioid based anesthetic management of the cardiac surgical patients, with more stable hemodynamics providing a long-term mechanical ventilation ensuring the safety of the newly revascularized myocardium, was popular in cardiac anesthetic practice. However the growing interest in fast-track anesthesia and associated intraoperative awareness with high-dose opioid technique limited its usage (London et al,2008;Stoelting&Hillier,2006). As the sickest patients undergoing multi-vessel bypass grafting combined with valve-repair or replacement, repeat operations and other complex procedures such as ventricular septal defect repairs with CABG after acute myocardial infarction require a long duration of surgery, resulting in greater cumulative doses of anesthetic agents leading to a prolonged period of mechanical ventilation; the anesthetic management evolves into a plan including short-acting agents (e.g.sufentanil, propofol, remifentanil), avoiding agents with long half-lives (e.g.midazolam), depending mainly on volatile agents, identifying the adequate candidates and applying a'wait and see' technique for early extubation (London et al,2008).

Combinations of opioids with benzodiazepines especially low doses of midazolam, because of its ease of use, low cost, hemodynamic stability and postoperative amnesia effects, have been used in order to overcome the adverse effects (Stoelting&Hillier,2006). However, some investigators believe that the combination of midazolam and opioids should be abondoned as general anesthetics; because they believe that this combination only provides general amnesia (Vuylteke et al,1996;Russell et al,1993;Absolam et al,2000). Midazolam has been used in combination with propofol and/or inhaled anesthetics, as well as opioids (Stoelting&Hillier,2006;Barr et al,2000;Lehmann et al,2000;Barvais et al,2000).

Remifentanil is a short-acting, esterase-metabolized without any active metabolites, rapid-onset μ-opioid receptor agonist. It provides stable hemodynamics in high-risk cardiac surgical patients. Remifentanil-propofol combination has been proven to be safe with stable hemodynamics, delivering an adequate depth of anesthesia (Lehmann et al,2000).

Sufentanil is a synthetic opioid, that has been used in combination with midazolam, propofol and inhaled anesthetics. Sufentanil combined with propofol has been shown to provide more stable hemodynamics when it is compared with fentanyl-based anesthetic protocols (Howie et al,1991).

Propofol has already been used for maintenance of anesthesia in cardiac surgical patients with reduced left ventricular function or with low cardiac output states in combination with opioids such as fentanyl, remifentanil, sufentanil or alfentanil; providing stable hemodynamics at the recommended doses of 3-8 mg/kg/hour (Philips et al,1993;Sherry et al,1995;Bailey et al,1996). In combination with ketamine propofol provides more stable hemodynamics than its combination with fentanyl (Stoelting&Hillier,2006).

2.4.2 Volatile anesthetic agents

It was commonly believed that the choice of primary anesthetic agent in cardiac anesthesia does not lead to a different outcome (Tritapepe et al,2007). In 1988, Warltier et al. (1988) reported that both halothane and isoflurane applied before ischemia improved left ventricular systolic function; in 1997 Cason et al. first described the term anesthetic preconditioning, by showing protective effect of isoflurane applied shortly before ischemia. Since than numbers of experimental studies revealed the cardioprotective efficacy of volatile anesthetics (Landoni,2009). The first clinical trial that investigates the clinical efficacy of the halogenated anesthetics was in 2002 reporting that sevoflurane preserves global hemodynamic and left ventricular function with a lower postoperative troponin I compared with total intravenous anesthesia (Cason,1997). Desflurane has also been shown to have cardioprotective effect in terms of ICU stay and weaning from mechanical ventilation (De Hert et al,2003). Anesthetic agents were also investigated for the timing of their usage, before or after ischemic episode or continuously during the procedure; sevoflurane has been shown to exert its protective effect more when it is used throughout the whole procedure (DeHert et al,2004).

Despite these beneficial effects, it has also been shown that there is no difference in outcome of the patients with already jeopardized myocardium. The patients without previous unstabil angina or recent myocardial infarction, had lower postoperative mortality after sevoflurane anesthesia (Jakobsen et al,2007). In non-coronary cardiac surgeries, desflurane and sevoflurane have also been shown to reduce troponin I release and result in better outcome in terms of incidence of atrial fibrillation and ICU stay (Landoni et al,2007a;Cromheecke et al,2006). However, volatile anesthetic agents revealed no difference in interventional cardiac procedures (Landoni et al,2009).

The lack of data demonstrating the adverse effects, primarily the coronary steal, of volatile anesthetics, the preconditioning effects of these agents, resulting in a safe and effective fast-tracking for patients especially when number of off-pump coronary revascularization is rising; has led to an anesthetic management mainly based on volatile anesthetics (London et al,2008). Volatile anesthetic agents, in comparison to TIVA, provide reductions in the rates of all major end points of cardiac surgery; reduce the risk of myocardial infarction and all-cause mortality; increasing in-hospital survival, reducing troponin I release, reducing the need for inotropic support, shortening ICU stay, time to hospital discharge and time on mechanical ventilation. These effects are valid for CABG surgery with or without cardiopulmonary bypass (Landoni et al,2009).

A recent meta-analysis the choice of desflurane and sevoflurane results in better outcome in terms of mortality and cardiac morbidity in cardiac surgical patients (Landoni et al,2007b). Although the results are controversial, the most recent American College of Cardiology/ American Heart Association guidelines recommend the usage of volatile anesthetic agents for non-cardiac surgical patients at risk for MI (Fleisher et al,2007).

2.4.2.1 Preconditioning effects of volatile anesthetic agents

Myocardial infarction is one of the most serious perioperative complications, that makes myocardium one of the most important vital organ to be protected from ischemia during cardiac and non-cardiac surgeries (Landoni et al,2009; Lango&Mrozinski et al, 2010). Ischemic insult is an integral part especially of cardiac surgery, that reducing the risk of myocardial infarction has led to researchs and revealed anesthetic management as an important factor in protecting myocardium.

A powerful cardioprotective phenomenon was first described in 1986, as an adaptive response to brief sublethal ischemic episodes that are exerted on myocardium, providing protection against subsequent lethal ischemia. This is called ischemic preconditioning, which is not very easy to apply clinically, because of the risk of worsening the vulnerable myocardium (Landoni et al,2009). Oxygen inflow to the heart is discontinued for short terms before the main ischemic episode in ischemic preconditioning, which has been shown to provide higher levels of ATP in myocardium and lower levels of troponin I after surgery. As reperfusion begins, ischemia will result in rapid changes during the reperfusion period; which is called reperfusion injury contributing to impaired function of endothelium and reduced metabolism of cardiocytes. Reperfusion injury may also be attenuated by ischemic preconditioning by restoring blood flow intermittently through the organ. In order to provide optimum protection, timing becomes important as the intervention should be performed within a few minutes or during the first minute of coronary blood flow restoration (Lango&Mrozinski et al,2010). Since the ischemic preconditioning is difficult to apply in clinical practice, pharmacological preconditioning comes to our way.

In general, the mechanisms of the myocardial protection provided by anesthetic agents may include; an effect like ischemic preconditioning, prevention of excessive calcium influx to the cell, an effect like antioxidants and an effect on the relationship between neutrophil/platelet-endothelium. The signalling throughout the cell during anesthetic preconditioning include protein kinase C (PKC), protein tirozin kinase (PTK), mitogen-activated protein kinases (MAPK), protein kinase-B, mitochodria and ion channels (sarcolemmal and mitochodrial ATP-dependent potassium channels) (Figure 1) (Lorsomradee et al,2008).

In pharmacological preconditioning, activators of protein kinases, agonists of adenosine receptors, scavengers of free radicals, opioids, ethyl alcohol, acetylcholine, bradykinin, angiotensin II, noradrenalin, platelet-activating factor were all used, but most of them can not be used for their protective effects because of their side effects or insufficient data of their clinical efficacy (Lango&Mrozinski,2010). In experimental studies, although the exact mechanism is not known, volatile anesthetic agents, known to have cardiac depressant effects that reduces myocardial oxygen demand, were demostrated to have direct cardioprotective effects that are not related to their anesthetic or hemodynamic effects (Landoni et al,2009).

Anesthetic preconditioning depends on the concentration of the drug and also the duration of administration, it does not depend on ischemic preconditioning and does not need pre-emptive ischemic episodes, furthermore it may have only slight protective effects on the heart that is already exposed to ischemic preconditioning (Landoni et al,2009;Lango&Mrozinski,2010). There are also some factors such as β-blocker usage and perioperative hyperglycemia that may limit the effectiveness of volatile anesthetics. Volatile anesthetic agents can provide their protective effects both before and after ischemia and also during the reperfusion period. In order to achieve maximum cardioprotection in surgeries including ECC, volatile anesthetics should be used before aorta clamping at >1 MAC for longer than 15-30 minutes. Also for the postconditioning effect, to provide adequate concentrations in blood after unclamping, the agents should be initiated several minutes before unclamping via the oxygen-air supply line of ECC and continued for the first 2-5 minutes of reperfusion. The effectiveness of usage during aorta clamping and late reperfusion period has not been clearly demonstrated yet (Lango&Mrozinski,2010). As an analogy to ischemic postconditioning, anestetic postconditioning describes the usage of volatile anesthetic agent after ischemic period contributing to the reperfusion period. This should be done within the first 2 minutes, lenghtening the period does not improve the protective effects (Obal et al, 2003). The protection occurs at two stages; early, lasting for one or 2 hours and late preconditioning, reappearing after 24 hours, lasting up to 72 hours; which means that the protective effect markedly exeeds the drugs elimination time (Landoni et al,2009;Lango&Mrozinski,2010).

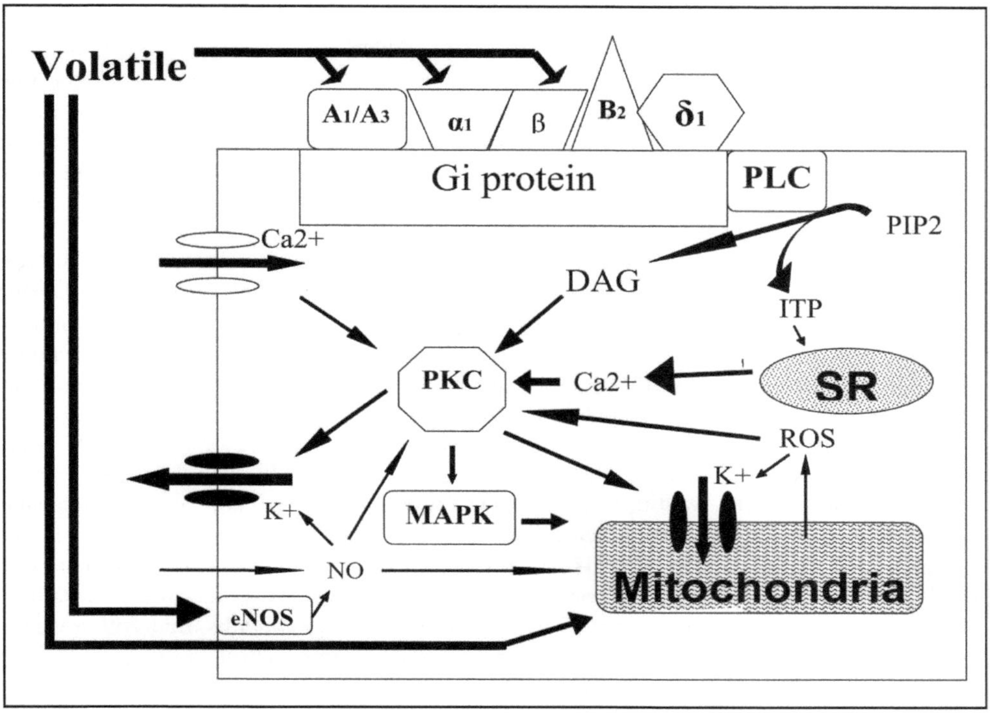

Fig. 1. The cellular mechanism of the preconditioning with volatile anesthetic agents. Volatile anesthetic agents activate phospholipase-C (PLC) and provide opening of the ATP-sensitive potassium channels by stimulating the adrenergic receptors by adenosine A1 and A3 (A1/A3) and activating nitric oxide sythase. (Lorsomradee et al,2008).
B2: bradikinin receptors, Gi protein: Inhibitory guanine nucleotide binding proteins, MAPK: mitogen activated protein kinases, PIP2: phosphotidil inositole bisphosphate, DAG: diacylglycerol, ITP: inositole 1,4,5 triphosphate, NO: nitric oxide, α1: α1-adrenergic receptor, β: β-adrenergic receptor, δ1: opioid receptors, PKC: protein kinase-C, ROS: reactive oxygen species, SR: sarcoplasmic reticulum (Lorsomradee et al,2008).

2.4.3 Fast-track cardiac anesthesia (FTCA)

FTCA contributes to an anesthetic management with a goal of allowing rapid recovery after surgery (Bainbridge&Cheng,2009). Fast-tracking with early extubation (4-8 hours postoperatively) has become the standart of care recently. The patients with normal LV function preoperatively and an uneventful intraoperative course, as long as the hemodynamic stability is ensured, by avoiding high doses of respiratory depressant anesthetics, with adequate rewarming and postoperative analgesia may be candidates for early extubation (London et al,2008).
The two most actively investigated methods in FTCA practice are; intraoperative narcotic that best facilitates FTCA and the pain control during the recovery period. The narcotics examined for their efficacy are fentanyl, remifentanil and sufentanil, which have been found to result in similar times to extubation (Cheng et al,2001;Engoren et al,2001;Mollhoff et al,2001). TEA has been reported to be superior to placebo and spinal

narcotics in terms of pain control (VAS), narcotic consumption, pulmonary complications, dysrhythmias and time to tracheal extubation. However, the risk of epidural hematoma formation limits its usage (Liu et al,2004;Ho et al,2000). A meta-analysis demostrated that PCA in cardiac surgical patients has little benefit whereas NSAIDs provide a reduction in VAS scores and morphine consumption (Bainbridge et al,2006a,2006b). Nurse administered or patient administered narcotics combined with NSAIDs (if there is no contraindication) is the recommended approach for postoperative pain management (Bainbridge &Cheng,2009).
The delay in tracheal extubation may be caused by many factors such as; age, female sex, postoperative bleeding, inotrope use, IABP and atrial arrhythmias (Wong et al,1999). During the operation, the usage of low dosage of narcotics balanced with inhaled agents and/or propofol providing a rapid reversible state facilitates early extubation. The complications associated by inadequate control of temperature, hemodynamics, and/or coagulation may also result in delayed extubation (Bainbridge &Cheng,2009).
The criteria that is suggested for early tracheal extubation includes a stable body temperature of 36-38 C, an arterial pH >7.30, adequate arterial blood gases contributing to PaO_2>70-80 mmHg (Fio_2=0.4-0.5), $PaCO_2$<40-45 mmHg. The patient should be awake, cooperative, alert and able to move all extremities with adequate motor strenght. The hemodynamic parameters should be stable with minimal or no need for inotropes with stable rhythm or good response to pacing. The patient should be spontaneously breathing with minimal respiratory support at a rate of >10-12 and <25-30 breaths/min with a VC>10 ml/kg, a maximal negative inspiratory force>-20 cmH_2O and a chest radiograph without major abnormalities such as atelectasis. Also adequate urine output, stable electrolytes, adequate hemostasis should be achieved (London et al,2008).

2.4.4 Regional anesthesia techniques

Advances in anesthesiology improves outcome after cardiac surgeries by combining the regional anesthesia techniques with general anesthesia. Thoracal epidural anesthesia (TEA) may enhance coronary perfusion, improve myocardial oxygen balance, reduce the incidence of tachyarrhythmias, perioperative myocardial ischemia through sympaticolytic effects; and also by providing superior analgesic effect it facilitates early tracheal extubation and may prevent respiratory complications (Svircevic et al,2011). However, because of the complications especially the epidural hematoma or abcess formation, TEA usage in cardiac surgeries is controversial. Moreover, the chronic use of antiplatelet agents, use of systemic anticoagulation and platelet inhibition for acute therapy of unstable angina and systemic anticoagulation and potential coagulopathy induced by CPB may increase the incidence of these complications (Ho et al,2000;London et al,2008). Also the systemic hypotension caused by intense sympaticolysis may be difficult to correct. The beneficial effects on respiratory system has also been shown to be provided by other strategies; such as spinal anesthesia (Cheng et al,1996; Silbert et al,1998). A meta-analysis by Liu reported that pulmonary complications can also be reduced by spinal anesthesia; as the incidence of hematoma formation is lower after a single spinal injection, this technique can be a choice for cardiac surgical patients at risk for pulmonary complications (Liu et al,2004). Also, modern general anesthetics can also provide other beneficial effects such as earlier extubation. TEA should be used with caution until its benefit-harm profile is clearly demonstrated (Svircevic et al, 2011).

2.4.5 Awareness and recall

The cardiac surgical patients are at increased risk for intraoperative awareness and recall, especially due to intentional avoidance of the cardiodepressant volatile anesthetics in the presence of hemodynamic instability, mostly caused by surgical manipulations of the heart and great vessels, leading to light anesthesia periods. As the volatile anesthetics have been proven to provide preconditioning before CPB, they began to have a major role in cardiac anesthesia protocols reducing the risk of awareness (London et al,2008).

3. Management during cardipulmonary bypass

Cardiac surgical patients are often dehydrated and hypoglycemic on admission for the operation. Rehydrating the patient and administering sufficient glucose increase the heart's ability to tolerate ischemic arrest. Initiation of bypass results in hypotension, requiring vasoactive drugs (e.g. phenylephrine) to maintain coronary perfusion pressure (CPP). Also ventricular distention should be avoided in order to maintain CPP and avoid the reduction in subendocardial oxygen delivery. After initiation of bypass TEE helps for the intravascular volume monitoring. The heart rate should be maintained <80 bpm in patients with ischemic heart disease during the pre-bypass period. For this purpose β-receptor antagonists can be used to provide a reduction in myocardial metabolism and maximize coronary blood flow (London et al,2008).

The sternotomy is the most distressing period, particularly in reoperations, in which there is a higher risk of right ventricular perforation, damage to existing vein grafts and ventricular fibrillation caused by electrocoutery energy transmission through sternal wires; requiring at least 2 units of RBC readily available in the operating room (London et al, 2008)

During dissection of left internal mammarian artery, the operating table should be elevated and rotated to left, while tidal volumes are to be reduced to facilitate surgeon's exposure.

Anticoagulation is provided by administering 300-400 IU/kg heparin and its adequacy is measured by using activated clotting time (ACT) which is desired to be 450-500 seconds. Higher doses of heparin may be required in case of resistance, however resistance can be treated with 1 unit of FFP or recombinant AT III (Kanbak M, 1999;London et al,2008). If anesthesiologist is the one to administer heparin, then the central venous line is the site of injection, whilst many surgeons prefer to give heparin themselves directly into the RA. Before or after anticoagulation, antifibrinolytic therapy may be initiated for bleeding prophylaxis. Aprotinin, being once the most popular agent, has been withdrawn from the market because of the safety concerns including mortality rate, anaphylaxis and renal dysfunction. Tranexamic acid and aminocaproic acid are the major agents that can be used instead of aprotinin (Henry et al,2007;Umscheid et al,2007)(see also bleeding and transfusion).

After heparinization, aortic cannulation is established often using the ascending aorta, following the examination of the cannulation site to be free of disease (London et al,2008;Morgan et al,2002) . In order to minimize the risk of dissection during cannulation systolic blood pressure should be lowered to a lowest safe level of 90-100 mmHg (London et al,2008).

Myocardial preservation involving anterograde or retrograde cardioplegia or both, arrest with high-potassium cardioplegia and hypothermia (systemic, topical and by cardioplegia) is provided by surgeon and perfusionist (London et al,2008). During cardiopulmonary bypass, pump flows, temperature and glucose control, blood gas analysis and management, ventilation strategies will be discussed later in this chapter.

After revascularization, with adequate rewarming (which will be discussed later in this chapter), stable rhythm-preferably sinus-good response to pacing, acceptable levels of pH, calcium, potassium and hematocrit, adequate ventilation with 100% oxygen; CPB is considered to be terminated (Morgan et al,2002). In case of a potential need, inotropes or other vasoactive drugs should be readily available. Heparin is reversed by protamin at 1:1 ratio emprically avoiding rapid injection. The TEE is removed and stomach is aspirated with an orogastric tube. The chest tubes and mediastinal drainages are secured as chest is closed and get ready for transport (London et al,2008).

3.1 Oxygen delivery during CPB

Delivery of oxygen depends on two variables that determine tissue oxygenation; hematocrit values and pump flow rates; that the calculation is: DO_2= pump flow x ((hemoglobin concentration x hemoglobin saturation x 1.36) + (0.003 x arterial oxygen tension)). In the clinical setting, increasing pump flows, increasing hematocrit concentrations (transfusion of PRBCs or use of ultrafiltration for hemoconcentration), or increasing hemoglobin saturation and the amount of dissolved oxygen (increasing the inspired oxygen concentration [F_{IO2}]) can improve delivery of oxygen (Lango&Mrozinski,2010).

Delivery of oxygen during CPB is typically less than that measured in the awake and anesthetized subjects. This is primarily caused by the decrease in the arterial oxygen content that occurs from hemodilution at the onset of bypass. The reduction in the DO_2 is compansated by increasing the oxygen extraction ratio which narrows the safety margin between oxygen supply and demand. At first this compansation maintains oxygen consumption (VO_2) stable (flow independent oxygen consumption), when the maximum extraction ratio is reached VO_2 and tissue oxygenation begin to decrease and lactic acidosis develops (flow dependent oxygen consumption). The critical DO_2 has not been defined, although there are many trials investigating this value; however it is shown that the organs undergoing bypass have hierarchy, that with a low pump flow the DO_2 of the brain is maintained at the expense of other organ systems; kidneys, pancreas, muscle beds. In order to preserve organ functions there should be a critical value to be targeted for DO_2 rather than targeting pump flow rates or a specific hematoctrit value (Lango&Mrozinski, 2010; Ranucci, 2009).

3.1.1 Hemodilution

Hemodilution is used during the CPB to offset the effect of hypothermia on blood viscosity and reduce the need for blood transfusion. However with the decreasing hematocrit level, the oxygen carrying capacity decreases and brain compansates for it by increasing CBF and tissue oxygen extraction; which leads to increased embolic load. Although an optimum level for hematocrit during CPB has not been clearly defined, there is data supporting the reservation of transfusion of blood products for the hemoglobin levels of <6 g/dl during CPB and <7 g/dl after surgery (Ferraris et al,2007). When there is a risk for end-organ ischemia these critical values can be increased by 1-7 gr/dl during CPB. Also it is important to know that the critical values can be altered by the clinical situation of the patient (Grogan et al,2008).

Extreme hemodilution in the elderly should be avoided; a decrease in hematocrit from baseline of 12 percentage points or greater has been shown to be associated with neurocognitive decline (Lombard et al,2010).

Recent guidelines state that heparin-coated bypass circuits (oxygenator alone or the entire circuit) are not unreasonable for blood-conservation (Class IIb, LOE B) (Lango&Mrozinski,2010;Ferraris et al,2007).

Methods to limit the degree of hemodilutional anemia (Lango&Mrozinski,2010)

- Delaying elective surgery to restore red cell mass to normal levels by using iron, erythropoietin
- Limiting the volume of crystalloid administered pre- and post-CPB
- Reducing blood sampling in the perioperative period
- Using retrograde autolog priming of the CPB circuit
- Minimizing tubing size
- Using miniaturized CPB circuits

3.1.2 Intraoperative hemodynamics

Small and microvascular disease could be a leading cause of dementia in up to two thirds of the patients with dementia. The patients who have dementia at baseline have higher incidence of postoperative cognitive dysfunction, that may be caused by their susceptibility to cerebral hypoperfusion (Lombard et al,2010). Even clinically aymptomatic (no dementia) many patients have infarctions and abnormally perfused areas in brain; these patients are also vulnerable to cerebral hypoperfusion as the surgical population ages with structural changes leading to stiffness in their arteries (Tolwani et al,2008). Cerebrovascular disease may then result in oxygen imbalance during surgery. The use of jugular venous bulb monitoring or near infrared spectroscopy (NIRS) revealed oxygen desaturation 27-43% during rewarming period while cerebral metabolic rate increases (Croughwell et al,1994;HL,2005). DWI detects mostly the watershed stroke, which indicate hypoperfusion brain injury that has been shown to be caused by a decrease from baseline mean arterial pressure (MAP) of ≥10 mmHg during CPB (Gottesman et al,2006). Maintaining the pre-CPB cerebral perfusion pressures may be an acceptable approach (Burgers et al,2006). NIRS has been used for the detection of oxygen saturation in order to use interventions such as ensuring adequate CPB flow rate, raising the MAP, ensuring normocarbia, deepening anesthesia, raising FiO_2 and initiating pulsatile CPB flow; and reported to provide lower rates of major organ injury (death, myocardial infarction, stroke) and shorter ICU length of stay (Murkin et al,2007).

Blood pressure during CPB is often kept >50 mmHg, however many trials and retrospective analysis supporting high pressures as a neuroprotection strategy led the institutions to keep the MAP >70 mmHg, especially in elderly; also according to age many centers manipulate this critical value; >70 mmHg for >70 year-old, >80 mmHg for >80 year-old (Grogan et al,2008). Recent investigations report that the lower limit of cerebral autoregulation may be much higher than 50 mmHg, in awake and normotensive adults the lower limit has been demonstrated to be 73-88 mmHg (Murphy et al,2009 as cited in Larsen et al,1994;Waldermar et al,1989;Olsen et al,1995). Noting that most of the cardiac surgical patients are older, hypertensive and have preexisting cerebrovascular diseases, their autoregulatory curve becomes shifted to the right, which requires higher MAPs (>70 mmHg) to reduce the risk of hypoperfusion (Lango&Mrozinski,2010).

Optimum MAP during CPB is affected by many factors, so decision should depend on the individual case. High-risk patients may benefit from higher pressures on bypass (Lango&Mrozinski,2010).

Potential advantages of higher MAPs (Lango&Mrozinski,2010)

- Enhanced tissue perfusion in high risk patients (hypertensive, diabetic, elderly)
- Improved collateral flow to tissues at risk of ischemia
- Allows for higher pump flow rates

Potential advantages of lower MAPs

- Less trauma to blood elements
- Reduction of blood in the surgical field
- Less cardiotomy suction
- Allows usage of smaller venous and arterial cannulae
- Enhanced myocardial protection (reduced collateral coronary blood flow)
- Reduced embolic load to the CNS (reduced pump flow)

Minimally safe pump flow has not been established, however the most commonly used flow rate during bypass is 2.2-2.5 $L.min^{-1}.m^{-2}$ approximating the cardiac index of a normothermic anesthetized patient with normal hematocrit. During hypothermia pump flow rate as low as 1.2 $L.min^{-1}.m^{-2}$ have been reported to have good clinical outcomes. Although there are conflicting results, most studies demonstrated that at pump flow rates of 1.0-2.4 $L.min^{-1}.m^{-2}$, CBF remains constant (Lango&Mrozinski,2010). During severe hemodilutional anemia, increasing pump flows can prevent organ injury, that pump flow may be adapted to hematocrit levels (Ranucci et al,2005). As mentioned before, targeting a critical value for DO_2 is more important than targeting pump flows or a specific hematocrit for preserving organ function (Lango&Mrozinski,2010;Ranucci,2005).

3.2 Temperature control

Hypothermia has been used for decades for cerebral protection. The beneficial effects of hypothermia mainly depend on the two physiologic principles, functional and structural cerebral metabolic need for oxygen that are both reduced by temperature; total cerebral metabolic rate of oxygen ($CMRo_2$) decreases 6-7 % per degree Centigrade reduction; while anesthetic drugs alter only functional $CMRo_2$ (Grigore et al,2009). Thiopental in particular, reduces cerebral metabolic rate required by brain function and synaptic activity, which are achieved during the isoelectric electroencephalographic state. Additional reduction is provided by concomitantly administered hypothermia while preserving CBF-$CMRo_2$ coupling, may also further reduce CBF. Moderate hypothermia without major suppression of neuronal function has been reported to provide better neuroprotection compared with isoelectric doses of barbiturates (Klementavicius et al,1996). Similar effect preserving coupling can be achieved by minimal alveolar concentration (MAC) or sub-MAC doses of volatile anesthetics especially isoflurane. Supramaximal doses uncouple CBF and $CMRo_2$. During profound hypothermia (18-20 C) CBF is disproportionately maintained and is determined more by arterial blood pressure and systemic vascular resistance than by pump flow rates (Grigore et al,2009). Moderate (28 C) and mild hypothermia (32-34 C) was shown to have no difference in terms of cognitive dysfunction, however hyperthermia (especially if the gradient between the temperatures of nasopharyngeal and CPB perfusate is >2C) in the perioperative and postoperative period is clearly associated with neurocognitive decline

(Klementavicius et al,1996). Any potential benefit for cerebral protection of hypothermia can be offset by inappropriate rewarming. More important than the use of hypothermia is avoidance of hyperthermia (Grigore et al,2009). During the rewarming period the returning warmed blood from aortic cannula is in close proximity to cerebral circulation. Also cerebral temperature may be underestimated from the usual monitoring sites (e.g.nasopharynx, esophagus) (Grogan et al,2008). Jugular bulb (JB) is the most reliable site to detect the accurate cerebral temperature, because it receives 99% of the CBF; however it takes time and money with risks associated with placing the device. Nasopharyngeal site and arterial inflow (arterial outlet of membrane oxygenator) temperatures are the closest ones to JB with a gradient of 1-2 C (Grigore et al,2009). Mild hypothermia (32-34 C), slow-rewarming during CPB (maintaining inflow temperature and nasopharyngeal temperature at or below 37 C as the maximum allowable) and avoidance of hyperthermia are the current recommendations (Grigore et al,2009;Grogan et al,2008).

The effects of hypothermia

- Reduction in cerebral metabolism
- Suppression of free radicals
- Inhibition of destructive enzymatic reactions
- Reduction in metabolic requirements in low-flow regions
- Inhibition of the biosynthesis, release and uptake of exitatory nerotransmitters

- Favorable balance between oxygen supply and demand
- Slows the onset of ischemic depolarization
- Decreases the release of ischemic-induced intracellular calcium influx
- Suppresses nicric oxide synthase activity

The effects of hyperthermia

- Increased production of free radicals
- Widening of any cerebral ischemic penumbral zone that developed intraoperatively
- Development or expansion of oxygen supply and demand mismatch
- Increased levels of intracellular acidosis
- Increase in the response of exitatory aminoacid neurotransmitters

3.3 Glucose control

In diabetic patients hyperglycemia may have caused an impaired endothelial function and may attennuate preconditioning. Serum potassium abnormalities should be corrected by glucose and acid-base management. Insulin continuous infusions are recommended for poor glycemic controls, however the possible development of insulin resistance during hypothermic CPB should be considered. Oral hypoglycemic agents; metformin may cause lactic acidosis in patients with low cardiac output state perioperatively, it is to be held several half-lives before the operation and glyburide has been shown to block preconditioning (London et al,2008).

In patients who stays more than 5 days in ICU, aggressive glycemic control was clearly proven to reduce mortality (Van den Berghe et al,2001). Similarly, in a retrospective analysis of cardiac surgical patients a predetermined glucose level (<150 mg/dl) was targeted with a continuous insulin infusion for 3 days postoperatively, had reduced risks of death and deep sternal wound infections (Furnary et al, 2004). There are conflicting results about the association between hyperglycemia and adverse neurological outcome, and yet whether the glycemic control improves neurological outcome is not clear. In diabetic patients hyperglycemia has no influence on cognitive functions and in nondiabetic patients >200 mg/dl glucose level during CPB has been shown to increase the incidence of cognitive dysfunction (Puskas et al,2007). Persistent hyperglycemia (>200 mg/dl) for the 24 hours after stroke, is an independent indicator for the expansion of cerebral infarction (Baird et al,2003). AHA guidelines state that it is reasonable to initiate insulin therapy when glucose level is >140-185 mg/dl (Class IIa, LOE C) after stroke (Adams et al,2007). The NICE SUGAR trial recommends moderate glycemic control compared to intensive control (Finfer et al,2009).

3.4 Blood gas management

Arterial blood gas pressures are monitored during the bypass period in order to measure the adequacy of oxygenation and CO_2 exchange. Hypothermia results in a rightward shift in CO_2 dissociation (increased solubility) leading to alkalemia. There are two measurement and management techniques of arterial blood gases depending on the temperature-dependent solubility of CO_2; pH-stat (temperature corrected) and α-stat (not temperature corrected). During CPB mostly the measurement and management are done without correction. In α-stat management blood is taken from the hypothermic patient and measured at 37 C; the results are uncorrected and the patient remains alkalotic during CPB. In pH-stat management, the measured partial pressures are corrected for the patients temperatures from the published nomograms, CO_2 is added to gas mixture to correct the respiratory alkalosis and low $PaCO_2$. Although there are controversies about the method to be used, pH-stat has been shown to increase the incidence of cerebral injury via obliterating the pressure autoregulation of cerebral blood flow, while α-stat remains to be used in adults preserving pressure autoregulation (Oakes&Mangano,2009).

4. Most common adverse events after cardiac surgery

4.1 Postoperative atrial fibrillation

Postoperative atrial fibrillation (POAF) is the most common atrial arrhythmia after cardiac surgery; its importance has become considerable because of the adverse effects it is associated with; such as congestive heart failure, increased need for intraaortic balloon pump, ventricular arrhythmias, cardiac tamponade, perioperative myocardial infarction, need for permanent pacemaker implantation, infection, increased postoperative bleeding, pneumonia, prolonged mechanical ventilation, increased need for tracheostomy, renal failure, stroke and neurological complications including cognitive dysfunction persisting 6 weeks after surgery , although the role of POAF as a cause of these adverse effects has not been clearly defined (Nair,2010). POAF occurs 30% after isolated CABG, 40% after valve surgery and 50% after combined CABG and valve surgery; mostly between days 2 and 4 (Echahidi et al,2008). The attribution of the mechanisms of atrial fibrillation in general population to POAF is difficult that it is not clear. Multiple factors such as ectopic focal depolarization originating from pulmonary veins and inferior vena cava, redistribution of fluid into vascular compartment causing atrial stretch, inadequate atrial protection during aortic cross-clamping, systemic inflammatory response syndrome thus elevated inflammatory mediators in the cardiac chambers and oxidative stress, excessive sympathetic

and parasympathetic nervous system activity, as well as physical alterations resulting from incisions to atria may cause POAF (Nair,2010; Grogan et al,2008).
Postoperative atrial fibrillation (POAF) as being associated with various adverse events should be assessed preoperatively and measures to prevent this adverse event should be considered before the operation. Most of the anti-arrhythmic agents that is to be used for prevention of POAF have their own side-effects, that prophylactic usage of these agents should be reserved for patients who are at increased risk for developing POAF. Prevention begins with identifying the patients with potential to develop atrial fibrillation after cardiac surgery (Nair,2010).

Risk factors for POAF;

- Valvular heart disease
- Right coronary artery stenosis
- Preoperative digoxin use
- Male gender
- Rheumatic heart disease
- Left ventricular hypertrophy
- Chronic obstructive pulmonary disease
- Diabetes mellitus
- Mild renal dysfunction
- Type of surgery
- Duration of surgery
- Prolonged aortic cross-clamping
- Withdrawal of beta-blockers and/or ACE inhibitors
- Bi-caval venous cannulation (vs single atrial cannula)
- Right superior pulmonary vein cannulation (for left ventricle decompression)
- Cardioplegia
- P wave duration more than 140 ms (Nair, 2010, as cited in Steinberg et al,1993)
- Left atrial appendage area >4 cm^2 and post-CPB left superior pulmonary vein systolic/diastolic velocity ratio <0.5 (combined with >75 years of age; probability is 0.83)(Nair, 2010, as cited in Karthikeyan et al,2009)
- Elevated preoperative BNP/NT-BNP (N-terminal pro-B type natriuretic peptide) (Nair, 2010, as cited in Karthikeyan et al,2009)
- Perioperative use of milrinone causing elevated cyclic AMP levels (Nair,2010,as cited in Fleming et al, 2004)

4.1.1 Prevention of postoperative atrial fibrillation

Pharmacological methods

B-Blockers: The withdrawal of β-blockers is a well known cause for POAF. American Heart Association (AHA), American College of Cardiology (ACC) and European Society of Cardiology recommends usage of β-blockers for prevention of POAF (Class I, LOE A) and give a Class IIb, LOE B indication for sotalol (Fauster et al,2006). In a meta-analysis investigating the effect of sotalol vs the other β-blockers revealed that it is superior to the others in preventing POAF, but although not statistically significant sotalol has major bradycardia and hypotensive effects with a significant incidence of torsade-de-pointes (Mitchell et al,2007).

Amiodarone: Amiodarone can be used oral or intravenous both before and after the surgery for the prophylaxis of POAF. Amiodarone has been shown to be associated with bradycardia and hypotension (Nair,2010). ACC/AHA/ESC give a Class IIa LOE A indication for amiodarone (Fauster et al,2006). American College of Chest Physicians (ACCP) suggests that amiodarone should be an alternative for patients who have contraindication for β-blockers and Canadian Cardiovascular Society also gives a Class IIa recommendation for amiodarone for the patients who have not been on β-blockers for the prevention of POAF (Bradley et al,2005;Mitchell et al,2005).
Calcium-Channel Blockers: Calcium-channel blockers were shown to reduce the incidence of myocardial infarction, ischemia and also tend to reduce mortality. However, these agents exert negative inotropic and negative chronotropic effects which may cause an increase in the incidence of atrioventricular block and low-output syndrome (Nair,2010).
Magnesium: Magnesium deficiency occurs and may persist for at least 4 days after cardiac surgery. Although ACC/AHA/ESC do not recommend the usage of magnesium as prophylaxis for POAF and ACCP is against its usage, CCS gives Class IIa indication for magnesium usage for patients who are not on beta-blocker therapy (Fauster et al,2006; Nair et al,2010). If magnesium therapy is to be used, it should not be limited to the early postoperative period, that the magnesium deficiency may persist for at least 4 days after cardiac surgery (Nair et al,2010).
Other Pharmacological Methods: Digoxin (limited effect) (Mitchell et al,2005), statins (shown to have beneficial effects) (Liakopoulos et al,2009), procainamid (limited usage because of the well-known side effects of Class I antiarrhythmic agents on structural heart diseases) (Nair,2010) and methylprednisolon (beneficial with anti-inflammatory activity but limited usage because of renal adverse side-effects) (Prasongsukarn et al,2005) has been investigated for the prophylaxis of POAF. In patients who have high-risk for the development of AF it is important to continue beta-blockers including the operation day and restart at the earliest postoperative period and as a prophylactic measure to initiate intravenous amiodarone therapy.

Other methods

Since pericardial effusion has been shown to be an important cause for POAF, posterior pericardiotomy allowing drainage to left pleural space has been investigated and shown to reduce the incidence of supraventricular arrhythmias (Nair,2010). Prophylactic atrial pacing has been shown to reduce the development of POAF. Bi-atrial pacing revealed more significant reduction in POAF vs left or right atrial pacing or no pacing (Fan et al, 2000). It has also been shown to be as effective as the pharmacological measures (Crystal et al,2004;Burgers et al,2006).

4.1.2 Treatment of postoperative atrial fibrillation

POAF is a self-terminating but recurrent tachyarrhythmia that usually subsides in 6-8 weeks after cardiac surgery. It should be kept in mind that the adrenergic response in the postoperative period will reduce the effectiveness of any therapy that does not include beta-blokers (Nair,2010). POAF treatment should prevent thromboembolism, control ventricular rate, improve hemodynamics, convert and maintain the sinus rhythm and in-long-term prevent tachycardia-associated cardiomyopathy. The treatment strategy that targets only the rate control may not prevent the adverse effects that are caused by atrial fibrillation. Rhythm control has been shown to be no superior than rate control, however, if the symptoms are not over with rate control only, then rhythm control should also be managed. Rhythm control is recommended for patients who are still symptomatic despite adequate rate control and who cannot achieve an adequate rate control despite therapy. Since it is self-limited, there is no need for long-term therapies for the patients who have normal left ventricular function and restored sinus rhythm. Amiodarone at a maintenance dose for 1 month, up to 3 months maximum, can be used for that kind of patients. Patients with impaired left ventricle function may require longer therapy. ACC/AHA/ECS recommend anticoagulation in addition to rate control (Nair,2010; Fauster et al,2006).

Rate Control: The goal in the control of heart rate is 80-90 beats/min after cardiac surgery, however it should be kept in mind that rate should be titrated in order to achieve a stable hemodynamic profile and myocardial oxygen balance. Beta-blockers and amiodarone are the first-line agents to be used for the treatment of POAF (Class I) (Nair,2010;Mitchell et al,2005). Calcium-channel blockers are the other effective agents to be used; diltiazem has been shown to be better tolerated than verapamil. Although digoxin is recommended for the ventricular rate control in patients with AF and congestive heart failure, without pre-exitation syndromes, has limited efficacy in the postcardiac surgery setting most probably because of the increased sympathetic response after surgery (Nair,2010).

Rhythm Control: Although it is self-limited, frequent recurrence is a rule for POAF. After pharmacotherapy in normal setting and also in the settings of recurrence and refractoriness, pharmacological and/or electrical cardioversion to sinus rhythm is also recommended. Amiodarone is the anti-arrhythmic agent to be used for pharmacological cardioversion, propafenon has been shown to be as effective as amiodarone; procainamid, dronedarone are the agents investigated for efficacy and safety, however they have side-effects and limited efficacy compared to that of amiodarone (Nair,2010).

Electrical Cardioversion: Postoperative atrial fibrillation may cause hemodynamic deterioration, myocardial ischemia, worsening left ventricle function, rapid ventricular response, which requires electrical cardioversion. The adequate waveform and energy level should be chosen; 120-200 j biphasic and 360 j monophasic is the Class IIa, LOE A recommendation (Neumar et al,2010). When it comes to increasing the dose stepwise, it is important to differantiate the 'failure to cardiovert' and 'early re-initiation of AF'. If even a single beat of sinus rhythm does not occur after cardioversion, it is failure to cardiovert, then increasing the delivered energy level, greater pressure on paddles, internal cardioversion and repeating cardioversion after anti-arrhythmic therapy can be tried. However, if it is early re-initiation of AF, additional measures may also end up in the same situation and may be harmful; that initiation of antiarrhythmic therapy (intravenous amiodarone (high ventricle rates) or diltiazem) and correction of the possible contributing factors (e.g. pain, electrolyte imbalance) before the next electrical cardioversion attempt (24-36 hours later) is recommended. If the unstability continues, DC cardioversion should be given after a bolus dose of amiodarone. For the patients who are stable with a low ventricular rate, observation is recommended until 24-48 hours, if AF still continues DC cardioversion may be attempted (Nair,2010). Combining the pharmacological therapy (amiodarone for at least 7 days, if recurrent AF at least 1 month) with electrical cardioversion prevents the recurrence of atrial fibrillation.

As mentioned earlier, anticoagulation is recommended for patients who receive pharmacological and/or electrical tharpies, because in both cardioversion strategies there is 1-7% risk of thromboembolism. Although the applicability of anticoagulation strategy after cardioversion in non-surgical patients (3-4 weeks of anticoagulant therapy before cardioversion in AF more than 48 hours) for cardiac surgical patients is not clear, it is acceptable to use echocardiography especially for left atrial appendage mural thrombus, immediately placing patient on heparin and continue with oral anticoagulants for 3-4 weeks after cardioversion (Echahidi,2008). POAF is well known to increase the incidence of thromboembolism and stroke, but it is also well known that anticoagulation may result in bleeding and cardiac tamponade. Risk-benefit should be considered before anticoagulant therapy is initiated, especially for patients with advanced age, uncontrolled hypertension and history of bleeding.

4.2 Postoperative bleeding and transfusion

One of the most important adverse events after CABG is excessive blood loss, resulting in blood transfusion which increases mortality risk, ischemic morbidity, infections, hospital stay and overall health care costs following CABG (Augoustides et al,2009).
In order to prevent blood loss, it is important to identify the patients with increased risk of bleeding and also the patients who may develop adverse events related to transfusion. Advanced age, low preoperative red cell volume, preoperative usage of antithrombotic and antiplatelet drugs, reoperations, combined procedures, emergency surgery and co-morbidities are the major contributing factors to the risk of bleeding (Augoustides et al,2009). Limiting bleeding and tranfusion after CABG begins with adequate preparation of the operating room and ICU with full institutional support. A guideline to lead a systematic, standardized approach is also an important factor for limiting bleeding and tranfusion (Ferraris&Spiess,2007).
In the preoperative period usage of anticoagulants leads to an increased risk of bleeding, thus if clinically feasible, the anticoagulants should be stopped allowing coagulation system to recover (Augoustides et al,2009). Clopidogrel, a high-intensity platelet blocker, is reasonable to be discontinued for at least 5-7 days before surgery (Ferraris&Spiess,2007). The low-intensity antiplatelet aspirin therapy is recommended to be stopped in elective patients without acute coronary syndromes (Ferraris et al,2002).
In combination with appropriate erythropoietin and iron therapy, donation of 2 units of autologous blood before CABG, significantly reduces allogenic blood transfusions. Kahraman et al. reported that acute intraoperative hemodilution reduces the blood requirements without affecting RBC volume loss and high-volume phlebotomy does not provide any additional benefit (Kahraman et al,1997). Antifibrinolytic agents can be used to limit bleeding and transfusion; tranexamic acid and aminocaproic acid are the major agents that can be used instead of aprotinin, providing a reduction in bleeding and blood transfusion; especially recommended for their usage in the high-risk subgroups (Henry et al, 2007; Umscheid et al, 2007). Desmopressin is reserved for patients who have pletelet dysfunction in the preoperative period and also factor 7a therapy has been shown to be effective in the management of refractory bleeding after CABG (Warren et al,2007).
As it exerts a mechanical pressure on the heart PEEP can be used to limit bleeding and need for transfusion.
Off-pump CABG is a resonable alternative for the prevention of blood loss, however emergent conversion to CABG with CPB increases blood loss and risk of transfusion (Jin et al,2005).
Several parts of CPB circuit have been improved for patient safety. Membrane oxygenators, centrifugal pumps, heparin-coated circuits, minimized low-prime CPB circuits are the recommended types for these parts of the circuit (Augoustides et al,2009).

High-dose heparin therapy preserves coagulation during CPB and also may decrease bleeding and transfusion. The reversal of heparin with protamine may affect bleeding and tranfusion as protamine itself is an anticoagulant. Despite the lack of definitive data, titration and empric low-dose regimen of protamine therapy may both lower the dosage of protamine and reduce bleeding and tranfusion (Jobes et al, 1995; Shore-Lesserson et al, 1998).
Leukofiltration, ultrafiltration or infusion of shed mediastinal blood are other interventions that are addressed in clinical trials (Augoustides et al,2009).
In general, in CPB, it is reasonable to maintain hemoglobin >10 gr/dl in patients who are at risk of non-cardiac end-organ ischemia; and >7 gr/dl in patients who are at risk of critical end-organ injury (Augoustides et al,2009).

4.3 Neurocognitive dysfunction

Adversely affected central nervous system is a well-defined problem following cardiac surgeries especially requiring hypothermic circulatory arrest. However, it is not clear that these neurological problems are related to procedure itself or to the underlying cardiovascular disease. In that point of view Wahrborg et al. found no difference between percutaneous coronary interventions and CABG (Wahrborg et al,2004). The most frequently reported form of brain injury is postoperative neurocognitive decline (POCD), of which recovery is variable, mostly transient, also which may prolong for several years and has no known treatment, leading the search for finding various interventions to reduce this decline (Lombard et al,2010;Grigore et al,2009). The other forms of brain injury such as stroke and encephalopathy have incidences of 1-5.2% and 10% respectively; when compared to POCD the difference is striking; 10-60% at 6 months (Funder et al,2009;Newman et al,2006). Early decline rate is 50-70% within the first week, 30-50% after 6 weeks and 20-40% at 6 months and first year. As mentioned before, multiple factors influence cognitive functions including surgical recovery and analgesic and sedative requirements, that it is difficult to accuse procedures only for the adverse neurocognitive decline. It is well-known that most patients with advanced coronary artery disease already have neurocognitive decline before surgery and have more potential to develop further decline independent of surgery (Lombard et al,2010). Selnes et al (2008) reported that there is a significant late decline in neurocognitive functions after CABG sugeries, however no significant difference compared to non-surgical patients with coronary artery disease. The degree of preexisting vascular disease may influence adverse neurocognitive outcomes after CABG more than expected, as the results of many trials suggest the natural progression of cerebrovascular disease is the main determinant of cognitive decline rather than CABG (Lombard et al,2010;Grogan et al,2008).

The clinical forms of brain injury and their frequencies (Grogan et al, 2008)

- Stroke
  - Low risk patients — $\leq$1%
  - High risk patients — 5%-16%
- Encephalopathy — 8.4%-32%
- Neurocognitive dysfunction
  - Hospital discharge — 40%-75%
  - 1 month after surgery — 12%-30%

In the preoperative period, brain imaging can detect the prior brain infarction, white matter lesions and/or lacunar infarcts that are clinically asymptomatic and also abnormal brain perfusion areas can be detected by SPECT prior to the operation; demonstrating the high-risk patients for the development of POCD.
There are several factors that have been associated with neurological problems such as patient risk factors including aortic atherosclerosis and surgical risk factors including type of surgery, temperature control, glucose control and intraoperative hemodynamics.

4.3.1 Risk factors of neurocognitive dysfunction

Patient Risk Factors; Neuroprotective anesthetic, surgical and perfusion techniques should be the key element in the management of these procedures guided by the identification of the high risk patients in the preoperative period.

Patient risk factors (Lombard et al,2010;Grigore et al,2009)

- Advanced age (>70 yr)
- Non-coronary manifestations of atherosclerosis;
  History of cerebrovascular disease with symptoms or silent infarctions (presence of one or more lacunar infarcts on preoperative magnetic resonance imaging)
  Peripheral vascular disease
- Chronic neurologic illness
- Congestive heart failure
- Fewer years of education
- Limited social support
- Insulin-dependent diabetes mellitus
- Genetic predisposition (minor alleles of C-reactive protein (CRP; 3'UTR 1846C/T), IL-6;-174G/C, platelet glycoprotein IIb/IIIa receptor variants are the candidates requiring further knowledge)(Grogan et al,2008)

Surgical risk factors;

- CPB
- Blood gas management
- Cerebral embolism
- Cell salvage
- Valve surgery
- Temperature control
- Hemodilution
- Oxygen delivery
- Glucose control
- Intraoperative hemodynamics
- Aortic atherosclerosis
- Systemic inflammatory response

4.3.2 Prevention of adverse neurological outcome

CPB; Cerebral hypoperfusion, temperature fluctuations, high incidence of cerebral embolism, inflammatory response, brain swelling and elevated levels of biomarkers of brain injury explains the potential of CABG surgeries for the development of POCD. However, in recent trials the cardiac surgical patients with or without CPB were investigated and no difference was described between them in terms of neurological outcome (Lombard et al,2010; Grigore et al,2009).

Blood gas management; Although there are controversies about the technique to be used during CPB period, α-stat has been shown to preserve pressure autoregulation and recommended for the technique to be used in adults (see also management during CPB).

Cerebral Embolism; Long-term dysfunctions might be mostly related to macroemboli from aortic lesions due to aortic manipulation, rather than gaseous microemboli which is the predominant type of microemboli during bypass period (Wahrborg et al,2004). However, the macroemboli to be a major cause of cognitive dysfunction is unlikely that it has been defined to be more associated with stroke (Bar-Yosef et al,2004). As being the most common type of cerebral emboli detected by transcranial Doppler during CPB are air emboli; in order to increase the rate of absorbtion of intravascular emboli, CO_2 has been used for wound insufflation to replace air in the pericardium, as it is more soluble than air. Although it reduced the number of arterial emboli, it has not been investigated for the brain protection, and also this technique is not without risks (Grogan et al,2008). The imaging techniques improves every year and one of them is the magnetic resonance diffusion-weighted imaging (DWI), which identifies regions of cerebral ischemia with a high sensitivity and specificity differentiating the acute from chronic infarction. 25-50% of patients undergoing cardiac surgery develop new lesions on DWI, however, very few of them show clinically significant infarction. On the other hand there are trials reporting significant correlation between the lesions on DWI and cognitive impairment proving that for the development of cognitive dysfunction, necrosis is not necessary, whereas other trials did not reveal any correlation (Knipp et al,2005;Cook et al,2007). More sensitive imaging techniques such as functional MRI may be used for assessing neurocognitive dysfunction after cardiac surgery.

Cell Salvage; Continuous flow cell saver when compared with conventional cardiotomy suction, may reduce the lipid microemboli (resulting in small arteriolar capillary dilatations) by processing the shed blood a major source of lipid microparticulates, thus reduce the cognitive decline after cardiac surgery (Grogan et al 2008, as cited in Djaiani et al,2007). Simply discarding the pericardial aspirate, when the shed blood is low, is an acceptable choice; and on the other hand using the cell-saver may cause thrombocytopenia and decrease the concentration of coagulation factors leading to bleeding and high rates of transfusion. Thrombocytopenia is a major concern because transfusion of platelets increases the risk of stroke in cardiac surgical patients. The increased requirement for transfusion has been shown by both Rubens et al. (Grogan et al,2008 as cited in Rubens et al,2007) and Djaiani et al. (Grogan et al 2008, as cited in Djaiani et al,2007), although their results in terms of the effects of cell-saver and cardiotomy suction on neurocognitive dysfunction are conflicting.

Valve Surgery; The valve surgeries have an increased incidence of cognitive dysfunction, because of the open heart chambers during the procedure. Furthermore the cognitive dysfunction following valve surgery lasts longer than CPBG surgeries most probably because of the ongoing microemboli (Lombard et al,2010).

Temperature Control; Hypothermia has been the major intervention that is used for cerebral protection. Moderate and mild hypothermia were not dissimilar in terms of POCD, however hyperthermia has been proven clearly to be associated with adverse neurologic outcome. The potential benefit of hypothermia is clearly offset by inappropriate rewarming, which leads to cerebral hyperthermia. Mild hypothermia (32-34 C), slow rewarming, avoiding hyperthermia are the current recommendations (Grigore et al,2009;Grogan et al,2008) (see also management during CPB).

Hypothermic Circulatory Arrest: Moderate or profound hypothermia with periods of circulatory arrest combined with selective anterograde or retrograde brain perfusion periods has become an acceptable technique. Selective anterograde perfusion has been proven to be comparable or better than hypothermic circulatory arrest alone or retrograde perfusion; furthermore it has been reported that shortened period of brain ischemia via selective anterograde perfusion and use of less profound hypothermia is associated with good clinical outcomes (Reich et al,2010).

Hemodilution; In order to avoid the adverse effects of hypothermia on blood viscosity, hemodilution is used, which also reduces blood requirement during cardiac surgery. As hematocrit level decreases, oxygen carrying capacity decreases which in turn increases CBF leading to a high risk of cerebral emboli. Although a definitive recommendation is not available, transfusion of blood products are supported to be reserved for patients with hemoglobin level of <6 gr/dl during CPB and <7 gr/dl after surgery (Ferraris et al,2007) (see also management during CPB).

Oxygen Delivery; Delivery of oxygen during CPB period is less than in awake and anesthetized patients; particularly because of the hemodilution at the onset of bypass reducing the arterial oxygen content. During CPB, delivery of oxygen to the brain is preserved at low pump flow rates at the expense of other organs. A critical DO_2 value should be targeted to preserve organ functions (Murphy et al;2009) (see also management during CPB).

Glucose Control; Moderate glycemic control is recommended instead of tight glycemic control, given a Class IIa, LOE C indication for insulin therapy when the glucose level exceeds 140-185 mg/dl (Adams et al,2007;Finfer et al,2009).

Intraoperative Hemodynamics; The patients with pre-existing cerebrovascular diseases (CVD) are more vulnerable to cerebral hypoperfusion during CPB. Considering the increased age of these patients, most of them already have a symptomatic or asymptomatic CVD, which requires maintenance of pre-CPB cerebral perfusion pressures. MAP>70 mmHg is supported to be the goal especially in the elderly (Grogan et al,2008). Although there is no clear data, pump flow rates of 1-2.4 $L/min/m^2$ have been shown to preserve CBF (Murphy et al,2009).

Aortic Atherosclerosis; As being an important risk factor for the development of cognitive dysfunction, detection of atherosclerosis of the ascending aorta provides risk stratification in the preoperative period that may lead to a decision of 'off-pump' CAB or 'no touch' approach to ascending aorta in order to prevent any adverse neurological outcome. Avoiding ascending aorta manipulations or searching for the atherosclerosis free areas may be beneficial, however after CPB it has been shown that CPB itself (due to sandblasting effect) may result in new mobile lesions on the sites where previously was mild-to-moderate atherosclerosis; at the sites of aortic cannulation and clamping (Reich et al,2010) .

Systemic Inflammatory Response; It is well-known that CPB causes a profound systemic inflammatory response. High baseline level of CRP was found to be associated with greater risk of neurocognitive decline. Cerebral ischemia-reperfusion injury also produces a profound inflammatory response; p-selectin expression on platelets resulting in platelet accumulation, rendering the brain vulnerable to microthrombosis, leading to ischemia (Lombard et al,2010). According to recent guidelines it is not unreasonable to use reduced circuit surface and biocompatible surface-modified circuits which are useful and effective in reducing systemic inflammatory response (Class IIa, LOE B) (Shann et al,2006).

Pharmacological Interventions; One of the methods that is investigated for the prevention of neurological dysfunction after CPB, is pharmacological protection, though remains controversial. It has been reported that the incidence of neurocognitive dysfunction can be lowered by using short-acting anesthetic and analgesic agents, providing a faster recovery from general anesthesia (Chen et al,2001). Shorter emergence times can be achieved by using low blood-gas partition coefficient and rapidly eliminated volatile anesthetics such as sevoflurane and desflurane (Frink et al,1992;Tsai et al,1992). In their preliminary report, Kanbak et al. reported that isoflurane and propofol were similar in terms of neuropsycological test scores and neurological examination after CPB, despite increased levels of S100BP in the propofol group (Kanbak et al,2004). Kanbak et al. also investigated the effects of isoflurane, desflurane and sevoflurane on cognitive function after CABG, comparing them in terms of neurological tests and S100BP levels. Isoflurane has been reported to provide better cognitive outcome (Kanbak et al,2007).

Pexelizumab, lidocaine, magnesium, ketamine, 17β-estradiol, donepezil, aprotinin are the pharmacological agents that are investigated for their efficacy on neurocognitive functions after cardiac surgery, however, all require further evaluation. There are no ideal pharmacological agent for neuroprotection during cardiac surgery (Lombard et al,2010; Grogan et al,2008).

Recommendations to reduce brain injury during cardiac surgery (Grogan et al,2008)

- A membrane oxygenator and an arterial line filter ($\leq$40μM) should be used for CPB (Class I, LOE A)
- Epiaortic ultrasound for detection of atherosclerosis of the ascending aorta (Class I, LOE B)
- Hyperthermia should be avoided during and after CPB (Class I, LOE B)
- A single aortic-cross-clamp tecnique should be used for patients at risk for atheroembolism (Class IIa, LOE B)
- During CPB in adults, α-stat pH management should be considered (Class IIa, LOE A)
- Arterial line temperature during CPB rewarming should be limited to 37 C (Class IIa, LOE B)
- NIRS monitoring should be considered, especially in high-risk patients (Class IIb, LOE B)
- Arterial blood pressure should be maintained At >70 mmHg during CPB in high-risk patients (Class IIb, LOE B)
- Serum glucose should be kept <140 mg/dl with an infusion of insulin (Class IIb, LOE C)
- Transfusion of packed RBC should be considered in high-risk patients when hemoglobin is $\leq$7 gr/dl or higher depending on other patient-specific considerations (Class IIb, LOE C)
- Processing cardiotomy suction aspirate with a cell-saver device as a means for preventing neurocognitive dysfunction (Class indeterminate (LOE A))
- There are no pharmacological neuroprotective agents with proven efficacy in humans (Class indeterminate (LOE B))

4.4 Acute kidney injury (AKI)

Acute kidney injury known to be an independent predictor of mortality in cardiac surgery, has an incidence of 50% by some defnitions, doubling the postoperative and intensive care unit costs (Park et al,2010). The pathophysiologic processes of cardiac-surgery associated AKI (CSA-AKI) were concluded to be; exogenous and endogeneous toxins, metabolic factors, ischemia-reperfusion, neurohormonal activation, inflammation and oxidative stress, which are interrelated and probably synergistic (Garwood,2010).

A common terminology and definition is necessary to determine the high-risk patients for the development of CSA-AKI. The term acute renal injury reflects the entire spectrum of the disease process; from minimal changes in serum creatinin to anuric renal failure, from functional deviations to structural changes and from prerenal azotemia to acute tubular necrosis (Dennen et al,2010). The Second International Cosensus Conference of the Acute Dialysis Quality Initiative (ADQI) group published a classification system for AKI based on the changes in serum creatinin and/or urine output. In this 5-stage classification, first 3 describes the risk, injury and failure for the severity of the AKI based on the changes in serum creatinin, glomerular filtration rate (GFR) and urine output. Last 2 stages describe outcome as loss and end-stage kidney disease, making the acronym RIFLE classification (Bellomo et al,2004). Acute Kıdney Injury Network (AKIN) proposed a modification to this classification and used a time frame of 48 hours in which the AKI has to occur and included lesser degrees of serum creatinin elevation. ADQI subdivided this classification into stages as early (within the first 7 days) and late (occuring between 7 and 30 days after cardiac surgery) (Hoste et al,2008).

In order to prevent cardiac surgery associated acute kidney injury (CSA-AKI) the most important approach is providing adequate renal perfusion throughout the surgery. Although there is no guide for any specific fluid or vasoactive agent to improve renal function, it is important to identify patients who are at increased risk such as patients in volume depletion and have congestive heart failure (Tolwani et al,2008). However it should be kept in mind that pathophysiological events other than changes in RBF are also responsible for development of AKI (Garwood,2010,as cited in Bonventre et al,2004 & Friedewald et al,2004). The patients known to have renal disease are more prone to have systemic acidosis and electrolyte disturbances mainly hyperkalemia, requiring more frequent blood gas and electrolyte sampling. Intraoperatively adequate fluid and medication management should be done for the dialysis patients ensuring that they have a recent dialysis with an adequate serum potassium level (London et al,2008). The ongoing investigations have a goal to define a single or a panel of early biomarkers to prospectively identify the potential for developing AKI after cardiac surgeries (Garwood,2010).

Cardiac surgery patients are particularly at risk of volume-responsive AKI; which is the term used more favorably than prerenal azotemia, emphasizing that despite the reversibility of early stages of AKI, even minor increases above baseline may result in adverse outcomes and any degree of renal insufficiency no matter how small may result in significant clinical consequences even in the absence of complete loss of function (Garwood,2010).

The non-volume responsive AKI also may occur in cardiac surgical patients. Ischemic period which has been clearly defined in experimental models, is also clearly defined to be associated with multiple injurious events in humans during the perioperative period. The key sign is a rapid, progressive and profound decline in GFR, which continue and progress even after return of renal perfusion to baseline (Garwood,2010).

Pathophysiological events other than changes in RBF are also responsible for the development of AKI (Garwood,2010,as cited in Molitoris et al,2004Bonventre et al,2004 & Friedewald et al,2004).
As the AKI is a multifactorial adverse consequence, it is crucial to address these interreacting factors for the prevention and treatment of CSA-AKI. The disease process includes ischemia, endothelial and epithelial dysfunction and tubular injury (Garwood,2010). Despite their limitations and variabilities in the AKI definitions and targeting mostly the prevention rather than treatment, there are many trials investigating the effects of vasodilators-primarily increasing the renal blood flow (dopamine, dopexamine, fenoldopam, angiotensin-converting enzyme inhibitors (ACEI) (captopril, enalaprilat), diltiazem, prostacyclin, nifedipine, PGE-1, sodium nitroprusside, theophylline), interventions inducing natriuresis or diuresis or both (atrial natriuretic peptid, brain natriuretic peptid, urodilatin, diuretic agents (loop diuretics and mannitol), anti-inflammatory agents (N-acetyl cyctein, aspirin, glutathion, corticosteroids, leukodepletion), clonidine, albumin infusion, isotonic saline infusion, insulin therapy, early continous veno-venous hemofiltration and also off vs on-pump technique. Fenoldopam, ACEI, atrial natriuretic peptide (nesiritide), B-natriuretic peptid, urodilatin were associated with reduction in the incidence of CSA-AKI. Off-pump surgical technique and pulsatile flow techniques also were reported to reduce the incidence (Park et al,2010). The recent trials are investigating reactive oxygen molecule scavengers, anti-inflammatory agents and antiapoptotic agents. AKIN also identifies the antiapoptotic agents (e.g.tetracyclines, human recombinant erythropoietin (HrEPO)) as potentially useful for AKI, though further researchs are needed (Garwood,2010).

4.5 Acute lung injury

Impaired pulmonary function is a well-known complication of cardiac surgeries, however it has multiple factors to be related with such as anesthesia, temporary cardiac dysfunction, infused catecolamines, altered mechanics of thoracic cage, duration of mechanical ventilation, neurological, renal and infectious complications rather than a single factor; CPB being the mostly accused. Although it is not possible to perform all the cardiac procedures without CPB, avoiding bypass alone cannot prevent the lung injury completely (Apostolakis et al,2010).
Although there are limited, insufficient data supporting the broad clinical use heparin-coated circuits and miniaturized circuits, minimizing the extracorporeal surface area and being biocompatible and free of any material that activates blood should lower the incidence of lung injury (de Vroege et al,2004). Leucocyte depletion may reduce the entrapment into lung capillaries, that in experimental studies it has been shown to reduce the heart and lung reperfusion injury (Apostolakis et al,2010,as cited in Bando et al,1990). Ultrafiltration and controlled hemodilution reduce interstitial lung edema, improving the lung functions after surgery (Apostolakis et al,2010). Using a controlled cardiac suction device, reducing the time between the contact of shed blood with pericardium and its re-transfusion, becoming activated only when the blood is accumulated in pericardium-minimizing air entrance may also improve lung functions. Furthermore, since the heparin level of pericardial blood is lower than systemic level, topical heparin administration may also diminish the inflammatory reactions contributing to lung injury (Tabuchi et al,1993).
Apnoea during CPB has been shown to be associated with increased incidence of pulmonary dysfunction. The results of clinical trials are conflicting, that some revealed

improvement in lung functions by maintaining ventilation (with or without CPAP) together with pulmonary artery perfusion during CPB, whereas others revealed no difference (Stanley et al,1977;John et al,2008).
The rules of myocardial protection during ischemia and reperfusion, indirectly protect the lungs from several proinflammatory factors produced during the process (Apostolakis et al,2010).

5. Coronary artery bypass grafting without cardiopulmonary bypass

Cardiopulmonary bypass is still the most common technique used for coronary artery bypass grafting procedures. Offpump coronary artery bypass (OPCAB) grafting, being the major improvement in cardiac surgeries, is performed at a rate of 20-30%. Despite the lack of definitive literature, its safety and efficacy in providing improvement in several outcomes have been proven, especially in high-risk patients with co-morbidities associated with higher mortality and morbidity from CPB (e.g. cerebrovascular and renal disease), avoiding the adverse effects of cannulation and CPB including hypothermia, risk of rewarming, coagulation abnormalities, renal impairment, arrhtyhmias, manipulation and cross-clamping of the ascending aorta (which increases the risk of aortic dissection/ neurologic sequelae) and prolonged postoperative ventilation. These procedures shorten the duration of the procedure, lenght of stay in ICU and hospital, and possibly decrease the cost (London et al,2008; Barnes, 2002b).
OP-CAB or minimally invasive direct CAB (MIDCAB) are the alternatives to be used in order to avoid CPB. In these settings the anesthetists encounters more surgeon-induced hemodynamic changes when it is compared to routine CABG; having a major role for anticipating and communicating with the surgeon about the adverse events that occur during surgical manipulation. The operation on the beating heart may be more prone to develop arrhtyhmias because of ischemia, manipulation and reperfusion. Antiarrhtyhmics, asking the surgeon to temporarily stop manipulation and treating severe bradycardia pharmacologically or with epicardial or transvenous pacing are the main strategies. During the exposure of the arteries, the heart is lifted and rotated, when the heart is repositioned venous return will be compromised leading to a decrease in preload reducing the cardiac output. Fluid resuscitation, inotropic medications and peripheral vasoconstrictors may be required. Maintenance of adequate coronary perfusion is provided by the maintenance of the mean blood pressure close to baseline. In OP-CAB for the proximal anastamoses a side-biting C-clamp is placed on the aorta providing that the blood pressure is lowered. Nitroglycerin and nitroprusside can be used for this purpose (Barnes,2002b). With a skilled surgeon, the changes are modest and can be managed by using simply the Trandelenburg position, inotropes and vasoconstrictors, however severe changes associated with acute ischemia, mitral regurgitation or unrecognized right ventricular compression necessiate emergent conversion to CPB (London et al,2008).
A large bore cannulae should be in place, cross-matched blood should be readily available and CPB circuit should be set up with a perfusionist on standby. In MIDCAB method, since the access to the heart is limited, external defibrillator and pacing pads should be ready during the operation (Barnes,2002b). Although there is no definitive type of monitoring described, most observational studies have used extensive monitoring including PAC and TEE. However, as the practice improves, particularly for the low-risk patients the recommended type of monitoring will probably become less sofisticated (London et al,2008).

6. References

Absolam A, Nagels W (2000). Fentanyl and midazolam anesthesia for coronary bypass surgery. *Br J Anaesth* 2000; 85(6):940 Online ISSN:1471-6771 Print ISSN:0007-0912

Adams HPjr; del Zoppo G, Alberts MJ, Bhatt DL, Brass L, Furlan A, Grubb RL, Higashida RT, Jauch EC, Kidwell C, Lyden PD, Morgenstern LB, Qureshi AI, Rosenwasser RH, Scott PA, Wijdicks EF; American Heart Association; American Stroke OnlineISSN:1524-4628 PrintISSN:0039-2499 Association Stroke OnlineISSN:1524-4628 PrintISSN:0039-2499 Council; Clinical Cardiology Council; Cardiovascular Radiology and Intervention Council; Atherosclerotic Peripheral Vascular Disease and Quality of Care Outcomes in Research Interdisciplinary Working Groups (2007). Guidelines for the early management of adults with ischemic Stroke OnlineISSN:1524-4628 PrintISSN:0039-2499: A guideline from the AHA/American Stroke OnlineISSN:1524-4628 PrintISSN:0039-2499 Association, Stroke OnlineISSN:1524-4628 PrintISSN:0039-2499 Council, Clinical Cardiology Council, Cardiovascular Radiology and Intervention Council and the Atherosclerotic Peripheral Vascular Disease and Quality of Care. Outcomes in research ınterdiciplinary working groups; The American academy of Neurology affirms the value of this guideline as an educational tool for neurologists. *Stroke* 2007; 38: 1655-1711 OnlineISSN:1524-4628 PrintISSN:0039-2499

Apostolakis EE; Koletsis EN, Baikoussis NG, Siminelakis SN, Papadopoulos GS (2010). Strategies to prevent intraoperative lung injury during cardiopulmonary bypass. *J of Cardiothoracic surg* 2010; 5:1 ISSN:1749-8090

Augoustides JGT. (2009) Is there a best technique to decrease blood loss and transfusion after coronary artery bypass grafting? *In: Evidence-based practice of Anesthesiology Online ISSN:1528-1175 Print ISSN:0003-3022*. Fleisher LA.pp 411-414, Saunders Elsevier. ISBN 978-1-4160-5996-7. USA

Bailey JM, Mora CT, Shafer SL (1996). Pharmacokinetics of propofol in adult patients undergoing coronary revascularization. The multicenter study of perioperative ischemia research group. *Anesthesiology* 1996; 84: 1288-1297 Online ISSN:1528-1175 Print ISSN:0003-3022

Bainbridge D, Cheng DC, Martin JE, Novick R (2006)a. NSAID-analgesia, pain control and morbidity in cardiothoracic surgery. *Can J Anaesth* 2006; 53: 46-59 Online ISSN:1496-8975 Print ISSN:0832-610X

Bainbridge D, Martin JE, Cheng DC (2006)b. Patient-controlled versus nurse-controlled analgesia after cardiac surgery-a meta-analysis. *Can J Anaesth* 2006; 53: 492-499 Online ISSN:1496-8975 Print ISSN:0832-610X

Bainbridge D, Cheng D.*(2009).Evidence-based practice for fast-track anesthesia-Is it safe? In: Evidence*-based practice of Anesthesiology. Fleisher LA.pp 411-414, Saunders Elsevier. 978-1-4160-5996-7. USA Online ISSN:1528-1175 Print ISSN:0003-3022

Baird TA; Parsons MW, Phash T, Desmond PM, Tress BM, Colman PG, Chambers BR, Davis SM (2006). Persistent postStroke OnlineISSN:1524-4628 PrintISSN:0039-2499 hyperglycemia is independently associated with infarcct expansion and worse clinical outcome. *Stroke* 2003; 34: 2208-2214 OnlineISSN:1524-4628 PrintISSN:0039-2499

Bando K; Pillai R, Cameron DE, Braun JD, Winkelstein JA, Hutchins GM, Reitz BA, Baumgartner WA (1990). Leukocyte depletion ameliorates free radical-mediated lung-injury after CPB. *J Thorac Cardiovasc Surg* 1990; 99: P73-77 Print ISSN: 0022-5223 Online ISSN:1524-0274

Barnes RD. (2002)a. Anesthesia for coronary artery bypass grafting procedures. In: *Anesthesiology Review*, Faust RJ, Cucchiara RF, Rose SH, Spackman TN, Wedel DJ, Wass CT. pp 369-370, Churchill livingstone, ISBN 0-443-06601-9, USA

Barnes RD. (2002)b. Off-pump coronary artery bypass and minimally invasive direct coronary artery bypass. . In: *Anesthesiology Review*, Faust RJ, Cucchiara RF, Rose SH, Spackman TN, Wedel DJ, Wass CT. pp 371-373, Churchill livingstone, ISBN 0-443-06601-9, USA

Barr G; Anderson RE, Samuelsson S, Öwall A, Jacobsson JG (2000). Fentanyl and midazolam anesthesia for coronary bypass surgery: a clinical study of bispectral electroencephalogram analysis, drug concentrations and recall. *Br J Anaesth* 2000; 84:749-52 Online ISSN:1471-6771 Print ISSN:0007-0912

Barvais L; Heitz D, Schmartz D, Maes V, Coussaert E, Contraine F, d'Hollander A (2000). Pharmacokinetic model-driven infusion of sufentanil and midazolam dyring cardiac surgery: Assessment of the prospective predictive accuracy and the quality of anesthesia. *J of Cardiothorac and vasc Anesth* 2000; 14(4): 402-408 ISSN: 1053-0770

Bar-Yosef S; Anders M, Mackensen GB, Ti LK, Mathew JP, Phillips-Bute B, Messier RH, Grocott HP; Neurological Outcome Research Group and CARE Investigators of the Duke Heart Center. (2004). Aortic atheroma burden and cognitive dysfunction after coronary artery bypass grafting surgery. *Ann Thorac Surg* 2004; 78:1556-1562 Online ISSN: 1552-6259 Print ISSN: 0003-4975

Baskett R, Buth K, Ghali W, Norris C, Maas T, Maitland A, Ross D, Forgie R, Hirsch G (2005). Outcomes in octogenerians undergoing coronary artery bypass grafting. *CMAJ* 2005; 172: 1183-6 Online ISSN: 1488-2329 Print ISSN: 0820-3946

Bellomo R; Ronco C, Kellum JA, Ravindra L Mehta, Paul Palevsky the ADQI workgroup (2010) and the ADQI Workgroup. Acute renal failure- Definition, outcome measures, animal models, fluid therapy and information technology needs: The second international consensus conferenceof the Acute Dialysis Quality Initiative (ADQI) Group. *Critical Care* 2004, 8:R204-R212 Available at:http/ccforum.com/content/8/4/R204. ISSN: 1364-8535

Bonventre JV; Zuk A (2004). Ischemic acute renal failure: An inflammatory disease? *Kidney Int.* 2004; 66: 480-85 Print ISSN: 0085-2538. Online ISSN: 1523-1755

Bradley D; Creswell LL, Hague CW, Epstein AE, Prystowsky EN, Daoud EG, American College of Chest Print ISSN: 0012-3692; Online ISSN: 1931-3543 Physicians (2005). Pharmacological prophylaxis.: American college of Chest Print ISSN: 0012-3692; Online ISSN: 1931-3543 physicians guidelines for the prevention and management of postoperative atrial fibrillation after cardiac surgery. *Chest* 2005; 128: 39s-47s Print ISSN: 0012-3692; Online ISSN: 1931-3543

Burgers DC; Kilborn MJ, Keech AC (2006). Interventions for prevention of postoperative atrial fibrillation and its complications after cardiac surgery: a meta-analysis. *Eur Heart J* 2006; 27: 2846-57 Online ISSN 1522-9645 - Print ISSN 0195-668x

Cason BA; Gamperl AK, Slocum RE, Hickey RF (1997). Anesthetic-induced preconditioning: previous administration of isoflurane decreases myocardial infarct size in rabbits. *Anesthesiology* 1997; 87: 1182-90 Online ISSN:1528-1175 Print ISSN:0003-3022

Cheng DC, Newman MF, Duke P, Wong DT, Finegan B, Howie M, Fitch J, Bowdle TA, Hogue C, Hillel Z, Pierce E, Bukenya D (2001). The efficacy and resource utilization of remifentanil and fentanyl in fast-track coronary artery bypass graft surgery: A prospective randomized, double-blinded controlled, multi-center trial. *Anesth Analg* 2001; 92: 1094-1102 Print ISSN: 0003-2999; Online ISSN: 1526-7598

Cheng DC; Karski J, Peniston C, Raveendran G, Asokumar B, Carroll J, David T, Sandler A (1996). Early tracheal extubation after coronary artery bypass graft surgery reduces cost and improves resource use: A prospective randomized, controlled trial. *Anesthesiology* 1996; 85: 1300-10 Online ISSN:1528-1175 Print ISSN:0003-3022

Cook DJ; Huston J 3rd, Trenerry MR, Brown RD Jr, Zehr KJ, Sundt TM 3rd (2007). Postcardiac surgical cognitive impairment in the aged using diffusion-weighted magnetic resonance imaging. *Ann Thorac Surg* 2007; 83: 1389-1395 Online ISSN: 1552-6259 Print ISSN: 0003-4975

Cromheecke S, Pepermans V, Hendrickx E, Lorsomradee S, Ten Broecke PW, Stockman BA, Rodrigus IE, De Hert SG. (2006). Cardioprotective properties of sevoflurane in patients undergoing aortic valve replacement with cardiopulmonary bypass. *Anesth Analg* 2006; 103: 289-96 Print ISSN: 0003-2999; Online ISSN: 1526-7598

Croughwell ND, Newman MF, Blumenthal JA, White WD, Lewis JB, Frasco PE, Smith LR, Thyrum EA, Hurwitz BJ, Leone BJ, (1994). Jugular bulb saturation and cognitive dysfunction after cardiopulmonary bypass. *Ann Thorac Surg.* 1994; 58:1702-1708 Online ISSN: 1552-6259 Print ISSN: 0003-4975

Crystal E; Garfinkle MS, Connolly SS, Ginger TT, Sleik KK, Yusuf SS (2004). Interventions for preventing postoperative atrial fibrillation after coronary artery bypass grafting surgery. *Cochrane Database rev.* 2004; 4: CD003611 ISSN:1469-493X

D'Attelis N; Nicolas-Robin A. Delayance S, Carpentier A, Baron JF. (1997). Early extubation after mitral valve surgery: A target-controlled infusion of propofol and low-dose sufentanil. *J Cardiothorac and vasc Anesth* 1997;11: 467-473 Print ISSN: 1053-0770 Online ISSN:1532-8422

de Vroege R; van Oeveren W, van Klarenbosch J, Stooker W, Huybregts MA, Hack CE, van Barneveld L, Eijsman L, Wildevuur CR (2004). The impact of heparin-coated cardiopulmonary bypass circuits on pulmonary function and the release of inflammatory mediators. *Anesth Analg* 2004; 98: 1586-94 Print ISSN: 0003-2999; Online ISSN: 1526-7598

De Hert SG, ten Broecke PW, Mertens E, Van Sommeren EW, De Blier IG, Stockman BA, Rodrigus IE (2002). Sevoflurane but not propofol preserves myocardial function in coronary surgery patients. *Anesthesiology* 2002; 97: 42-9 Online ISSN:1528-1175 Print ISSN:0003-3022

De Hert SG, Cromheecke, ten Broecke PW, Mertens E, De Blier IG, Stockman BA, Rodrigus IE, Van der Linden PJ (2003). Effects of propofol, desflurane and sevoflurane on recovery of myocardial function after coronary surgery in elderly high risk patients. *Anesthesiology* 2003; 99: 314-323. Online ISSN:1528-1175 Print ISSN:0003-3022

De Hert SG, Van der Linden PJ, Cromheecke S, Meeus R, Nelis A, Van Reeth V, ten Broecke PW, De Blier IG, Stockman BA, Rodrigus IE. (2004). Cardioprotective properties of sevoflurane in patients undergoing coronary surgery with cardiopulmonary bypass are related to the modalities of its administration. *Anesthesiology* Online ISSN:1528-1175 Print ISSN:0003-3022 2004; 101: 299-310

Dennen P, Douglas IS, Anderson, R (2010). Acute kidney injury in the intensive care unit; An update and primer for the intensivist. *Critical Care Med* 2010; 28: 261-275 Print ISSN: 0090-3493. Online ISSN: 1530-0293

Djaiani G; Fedorko L, Borger MA, Green R, Carroll J, Marcon M, Karski J. (2007). Continuous-flow cell saver reduces cognitive decline in elderly patients after coronary artery bypass surgery. *Circulation* 2007; 116: 1888-1895 ISSN 0009-7322

Echahidi N, Pibarot P, O'Hara G, Mathieu P (2008). Mechanisms, prevention and treatment of atrial fibrillation after cardiac surgery. *J Am Coll Cardiol* 2008; 51: 793-801 ISSN: 0735-1097

Engoren M, Luther G, Fenn-Buderer N (2001). A comparison of fentanyl, sufentanil and remifentanil for fast-track cardiac anesthesia. *Anesth Analg* 2001; 93: 859-864 Print ISSN: 0003-2999; Online ISSN: 1526-7598

Fan K; Lee KL, Chiu CS, Lee JW, He GW, Cheung D, Sun MP, Lau CP (2000). Effects of biatrial pacing in prevention of postoperative atrial fibrillation after coronary artery bypass grafting surgery. *Circulation* 2000; 102: 755-60 ISSN 0009-7322

Fauster V; Reyden LE, Cannom DS, Crijns HJ, Curtis AB, Ellenbogen KA, et al (2006). Guidelines for the management of patients with atrial fibrillation. A report of ACC/AHA Task Force on Practice Guidelines and the European Society of Cardiology Commitee for practice guidelines. Developed in colllaboration with the European Heart Rhythm association and the heart rhythm Society. *Circulation* 2006; 114: e 257-354 ISSN 0009-7322

Ferraris VA, Ferraris SP, Joseph O, Wehner P, Mentzer RM Jr (2002): Aspirin and postoperative bleeding after coronary artery bypass grafting. *Ann Surg.* 2002; 235: 820-827 Print ISSN: 0003-4932. Online ISSN: 1528-1140

Ferraris VA; Ferraris SP, Society of Thoracic Surgeons Blood Conservation Guideline Task Force, Ferraris VA, Ferraris SP, Saha SP, Hessel EA 2nd, Haan CK, Royston BD, Bridges CR, Higgins RS, Despotis G, Brown JR; Society of Cardiovascular Anesthesiologists Special Task Force on Blood Transfusion, Spiess BD, Shore-Lesserson L, Stafford-Smith M, Mazer CD, Bennett-Guerrero E, Hill SE, Body S (2007). Society of Thoracic Surgeons and the Society of cardiovascular anesthesiologists Clinical practice guideline. *J Thorac Cardiovasc Surg* 2007; 83: S27-S86 Print ISSN: 0022-5223 Online ISSN:1524-0274

Fleisher LA, Beckman JA, Brown KA, Calkins H, Chaikof E, Fleishman KE, et al (2007). ACC/AHA 2007 guidelines on perioperative cardiovascular evaluation and car efor non-cardiac surgery: Executive summary. A report of the ACC/AHA Task Force on practice guidelines. (Writing comitee to revise the 2002 guidelines on perioperative cardiovascular evaluatşion for non-cardiac surgery). *J Am Coll Cardiol* 2007; 50: 1707-32 ISSN: 0735-1097

Fleming GA; Murray KT, Yu C, Bryne JG, Greelish JP, Petracek MR, et al (2004). Milrinone use is associated with postoperative atrial fibrillation in patients undergoing heart surgery. *Cochrane Database Syst Rev*. 2004; 4: CD003611 ISSN:1469-493X

Friedewald JJ, Rabb H (2004). Inflammatory cells in ischemic acute renal failure. *Kidney Int Print ISSN: 0085-2538. Online ISSN: 1523-1755.* 2004; 66: 486-491

Frink EJ Jr, Malan TP, Atlas M, Dominguez LM, DiNardo JA, Brown BR Jr.(1992). Clinical comparison of sevoflurane and isoflurane in healthy patients. *Anesth Analg* 1992; 74: 241-5 Print ISSN: 0003-2999; Online ISSN: 1526-7598

Funder KS, Steinmetz J, Rasmussen LS (2009). Cognitive dysfunction after cardiovascular surgery. *Minerva Anesthesiol.* 2009; 75: 332 Print ISSN 0375-9393. Online ISSN 1827-1596

Furnary AP, Wu Y, Bookin SO (2004). Effect of hyperglycemia and continuous intravenous infusions on outcomes of cardiac procedures: The portland Diabetic Project. *Endocr Pract* 2004; 10 (suppl2): 21-33 ISSN: 1530-891X

Garwood S (2010). Cardiac surgery associated acute renal ınjury: New paradigms and ınnovative therapies. *J Cardiothorac and vasc Anesth* . 2010; 24(6): 990-1001 Print ISSN: 1053-0770 Online ISSN:1532-8422

Gottesman RF, Sherman PM, Grega MA, Yousem DM, Borowicz LM Jr, Selnes OA, Baumgartner WA, McKhann GM. (2006). Watershed Strokes after cardiac surgery: diagnosis, etiology and outcome. *Stroke* 2006; 37: 2306-2311 OnlineISSN:1524-4628 PrintISSN:0039-2499

Grigore AM; Murray CF, Ramakrishna H, Djaiani G (2009). A core-review of temperature regimens and neuroprotection during CPB: Does rewarming rate matter? *Anesth Analg* 2009; 109: 1741-51 Print ISSN: 0003-2999; Online ISSN: 1526-7598

Grogan K; Stearns J, Hogue CW (2008). Brain protection in cardiac surgery. *Anesthesiol Clin* 2008; 26(3): 521-538 ISSN: 1932-2275

Henry DA, Carless PA, Moxey AJ, O'Connell D, Stokes BJ, McClelland B, Laupacis A, Fergusson D. (2007). Antifibrinolytic use for minimizing perioperative allogenic blood transfusion. *Cochrane Database Syst Rev* 2007; 17: CD 001886 ISSN:1469-493X

HL E (2005). Protective effect of neuromonitoring during cardiac surgery. *Ann NY Acad Sci* 2005; 1053: 12-19 Print ISSN: 0077-8923 Online ISSN:1749-6632

Ho AM; Chung DC, Joynt GM (2000). Neuroaxial blockade and hematoma in cardiac surgery: Estimating the risk of a rare adverse event that has not (yet) occured. *Chest* 2000; 117:551-5 Print ISSN: 0012-3692; Online ISSN: 1931-3543

Hoste EA, Cruz DN, Davenport A, Mehta RL, Piccinni P, Tetta C, Viscovo G, Ronco C (2008). The epidemiology of cardiac surgery-associated acute kidney injury. *Int Artif Organs* 2008; 31: 158-165 Print ISSN:0391-3988 Online ISSN:1724-6040

Howie MB, Smith DF, Reilley TE, McSweeney TD, Silver M, Dasta JF, Reitz J. (1991). Postoperative course after sufentanil or fentanyl anesthesia for coronary artery surgery. *J Cardiothorac and vasc Anesth* 1991; 5: 485-489 Print ISSN: 1053-0770 Online ISSN:1532-8422

Jacobsen CJ, Berg H, Hindsholm KB, Faddy N, Sloth E (2007). The influence of propofol versus sevoflurane anesthesia on outcome in 10535 cardiac surgical procedures. *J Cardiothorac and vasc Anesth* 2007; 21: 672-7 Print ISSN: 1053-0770 Online ISSN:1532-8422

Jin R, Hiratzka LF, Grunkemeier GL, Krause A, Page US (2005). Aborted off-pump coronary artery bypass patients have much worse outcomes than on-pump or successful off-pump patients. *Circulation* ISSN 0009-7322 2005; 112: I332-I337

Jobes DR, Aitken GL, Shaffer GW (1995). Increased accuracy and precision of heparin and protamine dosing reduces blood loss and transfusion in patients undergoing primary cardiac operations. *J Thorac Cardiovasc Surg* 1995; 110; 36-45 Print ISSN: 0022-5223 Online ISSN:1524-0274

John L, Ervine I (2008). A study assessing the potential benefit of continued mechanical ventilation during CPB. *Interactive Cardiovascular and thoracic surgery* 2008; 7: 14-17 Print ISSN: 1569-9293. Online ISSN: 1569-9285

Kahraman S; Altunkaya H, Celebioglu B, Kanbak M, Paşaoglu İ, Erdem K (1997). The effect of acute hemodilution on homologous blood requirements and total estimated red blood cell volume lost. *Acta Anesthesiol Scand.* 1997; 41: 614-617 Print ISSN: 0001-5172. Online ISSN: 1399-6576

Kanbak M(1999): The treatment of heparin resistance with antithrombin III in cardiac surgery. *Can J Anaesth* 1999, 46(6): 581-585 Online ISSN:1496-8975 Print ISSN:0832-610X

Kanbak M, Saricaoglu F, Avci A, Ocal T, Koray Z, Aypar U (2004). Propofol offers no advantage over isoflurane anesthesia for cerebral protection during cardiopulmonary bypass: a preliminary study of S-100B protein levels. *Can J Anaesth* 2004; 51(7): 712-717 Online ISSN:1496-8975 Print ISSN:0832-610X

Kanbak M, Saricaoglu F, Akinci SB, Oc B, Balcı H, Celebioglu B, Aypar U (2007). The effects of isoflurane, sevoflurane and desflurane anesthesia on Neurocognitive outcome after cardiac surgery: A pilot study. *The Heart Surgery Forum* .2007; 10(1) ISSN: 1522-6662

Karthikeyan G, Moncur RA, Levine O, Heels-Ansdell D, Chan MT, Alonso-Coello P, Yusuf S, Sessler D, Villar JC, Berwanger O, McQueen M, Mathew A, Hill S, Gibson S, Berry C, Yeh HM, Devereaux PJ. (2009). Is a preoperative brain natriuretic peptid or N-terminal pro-B-type natriuretic peptide measurement an independent predictor of adverse cardiovascular outcome within 30 days of non-cardiac surgery? A systematic review and meta-analysis of observational studies. *J Am Coll Cardiol* 2009; 54: 1599-606 ISSN: 0735-1097

Klementavicius R, Nemoto EM, Yonas H (1996). The Q10 ratio for basal cerebral metabolic rate of oxygen in rats. *J Neurosurg* 1996; 85: 482-7 Print ISSN: 0268-8697 Online ISSN:1360-046X

Knipp SC, Matatko N, Schlamann M, Wilhelm H, Thielmann M, Forsting M, Diener HC, Jakob H. (2005). Small ischemic brain lesions after cardiac valve replacement detected by diffusion-weighted nagnetic resonance imaging: relation to neurocognitive function. *Eur J Cardiothorac Surg* 2005; 28: 88-96 ISSN: 1010-7940

Landoni G, Biondi-Zoccai GG, Zangrillo A, Bignami E, D'Avolio S, Marchetti C, Calabrò MG, Fochi O, Guarracino F, Tritapepe L, De Hert S, Torri G. (2007)a. Desflurane and sevoflurane in cardiac surgery: A meta-analysis of randomized controlled trials. *J Cardiothorac and vasc Anesth* 2007; 21: 502-11 Print ISSN: 1053-0770 Online ISSN:1532-8422

Landoni G, Calabrò MG, Marchetti C, Bignami E, Scandroglio AM, Dedola E, De Luca M, Tritapepe L, Crescenzi G, Zangrillo A (2007)b. Desflurane versus propofol in patients undergoing mitral valve surgery. *J Cardiothorac and vasc Anesth* 2007; 21: 672-7 Print ISSN: 1053-0770 Online ISSN:1532-8422

Landoni G; Bignami E, Oliviero F, Zangrillo A (2009). Halogenated anesthetics and cardiac protection in cardiac and non-cardiac anesthesia. *Annals of Cardiac Anesthesia* 2009; vol 12:1; 4-9 ISSN:0971-9784

Lango R; Mrozinski P (2010). Clinical importance of anesthetic preconditioning. *Anestezjol Intens Ter* 2010 Oct-Dec; 42 (4) 1206-12 ISSN:0209-1712

Larsen FS; Olsen KS, Hansen BA, Paulson OB, Knudsen GM (1994). Transcranial doppler is valid for determination of the lower limit of cerebral blood flow autoregulation. *Stroke* 1994; 25: 1985-8 Online ISSN:1524-4628 Print ISSN:0039-2499

Lehmann A; Zeitler C, Thaler E, Isgro F, Boldt J (2000). Comparison of two different anesthesia regimens in patients undergoing aortacoronary bypass grafting surgery: Sufentanil-midazolam versus remifentanyl-propofol. *J Cardiothorac and vasc Anesth* 2000; 14(4): 416-420 Print ISSN: 1053-0770 Online ISSN:1532-8422

Liakopoulos OJ, Choi YH, Kuhn EW, Wittwer T, Borys M, Madershahian N, Wassmer G, Wahlers T. (2009). Statins for prevention of Af after cardiac surgery. A systematic literature review. *J Thorac Cardiovasc Surg* 2009; 138: 678-86 Print ISSN: 0022-5223 Online ISSN:1524-0274

Liu SS; Block BM, Wu CL (2004). Effects of perioperative central neuroaxial analgesia on outcome after coronary artery bypass surgery: A meta-analysis. *Anesthesiology* 2004; 101:153-61 Online ISSN:1528-1175 Print ISSN:0003-3022

Lombard FW; Mathew JP (2010). Neurocognitive dysfunction following cardiac surgery. *Semin Cardiothorac Vasc Anesth* . 2010; 14 (2): 102-110 Print ISSN: 1089-2532

London MJ, Mittnacht A, Kaplan JA (2008). Anesthesia for myocardial revascularization. In: *Essentials of Cardiac Anesthesia* Kaplan JA. Pp293-326, Saunders Elsevier, ISBN:978-1-4160-3786-6, China

Lorsomradee S, Cromheecke S, Lorsomradee S, De Hert SG (2008). Cardioprotection with volatile anesthetics in cardiac surgery. *Asian Cardiovasc Thorac Ann* 2008;16:256-64. ISSN: 0218-4923

Mitchell LB (2007). Prophylactic therapy to prevent atrial arrhythmias after cardiac surgery. *Curr Opin Cardiol.* 2007; 22: 18-24 Print ISSN: 0268-4705 Online ISSN: 1531-7080

Mitchell LB, Crystal E, Heilbron B, Page P (2005). Atrial fibrillation following cardiac surgery. *Can J Cardiol.* 2005; 21: 45B-50B Print ISSN: 0828-282X Online ISSN:1916-7075

Molitoris BA; Sutton TA (2004). Endothelial injury and dysfunction: Role in the extension phase of caute renal failure. *Kidney Int.* 2004; 66: 496-99 Print ISSN: 0085-2538. Online ISSN: 1523-1755

Morgan GE, Mikhail MS, Murray MJ (2002) *Clinical Anesthesiology* Mc Graw Hill, ISBN 0-8385-1553-3,USA

Möllhoff T, Herregods L, Moerman A, Blake D, MacAdams C, Demeyere R, Kirnö K, Dybvik T, Shaikh S; Remifentanil Study Group. (2001). Comparative efficacy and safety of remifentanil and fentanyl in fast-track coronary artery bypass graft surgery: A randomized, double-blind study. *Br J Anaesth* 2001; 87: 718-726 Online ISSN:1471-6771 Print ISSN:0007-0912

Murkin JM, Adams SJ, Novick RJ, Quantz M, Bainbridge D, Iglesias I, Cleland A, Schaefer B, Irwin B, Fox S. (2007). Monitoring brain oxygen saturation during coronary artery bypass surgery. A randomized, prospective study. *Anesth Analg* 2007; 104: 51-58 Print ISSN: 0003-2999; Online ISSN: 1526-7598

Murphy GS; Hessel EA, Groom RC (2009). Optimal perfusion during CPB: An evidence-based approach. *Anesth Analg* 2009; 108: 1394-417 Print ISSN: 0003-2999; Online ISSN: 1526-7598

Myles PS, Buckland MR, Weeks AM, Bujor MA, McRae R, Langley M, Moloney JT, Hunt JO, Davis BB. (1997). Hemodynamic effects, myocardial ischemia and timing of tracheal extubation with propofol-based anesthesia for cardiac surgery. *Anesth Analg* 1997; 84:12-19 Print ISSN: 0003-2999; Online ISSN: 1526-7598

Nair SG (2010). Atrial fibrillation after cardiac surgery. *Annals of Cardiac Anesthesia.* 2010; vol 13:3; 196-205 ISSN:0971-9784

Neumar RW, Otto CW, Link MS, Kronick SL, Shuster M, Callaway CW, Kudenchuk PJ; Ornato JP; McNally B; Silvers SM; Passman RS; White RD, Hess EP; Tang W; Davis D; Sinz E; Morrison LJ. Part 8: Adult Advanced Cardiovascular Life Support 2010 American Heart Association Guidelines for Cardiopulmonary Resuscitation and Emergency Cardiovascular Care. *Circulation* 2010; 122 [suppl3]: S729-767 ISSN 0009-7322

Newman MF, Mathew JP, Grocott HP, Mackensen GB, Monk T, Welsh-Bohmer KA, Blumenthal JA, Laskowitz DT, Mark DB. (2006). Central nervous system injury associated with cardiac surgery. *Lancet* 2006; 368:694-703 ISSN: 0140-6736.

NICE-SUGAR Study Investigators, Finfer S, Chittock DR, Su SY, Blair D, Foster D, Dhingra V, Bellomo R, Cook D, Dodek P, Henderson WR, Hébert PC, Heritier S, Heyland DK, McArthur C, McDonald E, Mitchell I, Myburgh JA, Norton R, Potter J, Robinson BG, Ronco JJ. Intensive versus conventional glucose control in critically ill patients. (2009). *N Eng J Med.* 2009; 360: 1283-1297 Online ISSN 1533-4406 Print ISSN 0028-4793

Oakes DA; Mangano CTM (2009). Cardiopulmonary bypass in 2009: Achieving and Circulating best Practices. *Anesth Analg.* 2009; 1368-1369 Print ISSN: 0003-2999; Online ISSN: 1526-7598

Obal D, Scharbatke H, Barthel H, Preckel B, Mullenheim J, Schlack W (2003) Cardioprotection against reperfusion injury is maximal with only two minutes of sevoflurane administrartion in rats. *Can J Anaesth* 2003; 50: 940-945 Online ISSN:1496-8975 Print ISSN:0832-610X

Olsen KS, Svenden LB, Losen FS, Paulson OB (1995). Effect of labetolol on cerebral blood flow, oxygen metabolism and autoregulation in healthy humans. *Br J Anaesth* 1995; 75: 51-4 Online ISSN:1471-6771 Print ISSN:0007-0912

Park M; Coca SG, Nigwekar SU, Garg AX, Garwood S, Parikh CR (2010). Prevention and treatment of acute kidney injury in patients undergoing cardiac surgery: A systematic review. *Am J Nephrol Print* 2010; 31: 408-418 ISSN 0250-8095 OnlineISSN 1421-9670

Peck TE, Hill SA, Williams M (2006). *Pharmacology for Anaesthesia and Intensive care.* Cambridge University Press, ISBN 0-521-68794-2

Phillips AS, McMurray TJ, Mirakhur RK, Gibson FM, Elliott P. (1993). Propofol-fentanyl anesthesia in cardiac surgery: A comparison in patients with good and impaired ventricular function. *Anesthesia* 1993; 48: 661-663 Print ISSN: 0003-2409. Online ISSN: 1365-2044

Prasongsukarn K, Abel JG, Jamieson WR, Cheung A, Russell JA, Walley KR, Lichtenstein SV. (2005). The effect of steroids on the occurence of postoperative atrial fibrillation after coronary artery bypass grafting surgery: a randomized study. *J Thorac Cardiovasc Surg* 2005; 130: 93-8 Print ISSN: 0022-5223 Online ISSN:1524-0274

Puskas F; Grocott HP, White WD, Mathew JP, Newman MF, Bar-yosef S (2007). Intraoperative hyperglycemia and cognitive decline after coronary artery bypass grafting. *Ann Thorac Surg* 2007; 84: 1467-1473 Online ISSN: 1552-6259 Print ISSN: 0003-4975

Ranucci M; Romitti F, Isgro G, Cotza M, Brozzi S, Boncilli A, Ditta A (2005). Oxygen delivery during cardiopulmonary bypass and acute renal failure after coronary operations. *Ann Thorac Surg* 2005; 80: 2213-20 Online ISSN: 1552-6259 Print ISSN: 0003-4975

Reich DL, Mittnacht AL, London MJ, Kaplan JA (2008). Monitoring of the heart and vascular system.In: *Essentials of Cardiac Anesthesias* Kaplan JA. pp167-199, Saunders Elsevier,ISBN 978-1-4160-3786-6, China

Reich DL (2010). Central Nervous system Protection in Cardiac Surgery. *Seminars in Cardiothoracic and Vascular Anesthesia* 2010; 14 (1): 32-37 ISSN: 1089-2532

Roscoe A.2007 *Transoesophageal Echocardiography-study guide and practice* MCQs. Cambridge University Press, ISBN 13 978-0-521-68960-1, UK

Rubens FD, Boodhwani M, Mesana T, Wozny D, Wells G, Nathan HJ; Cardiotomy Investigators. (2007). The cardiotomy trial. A randomized, double blind study to assess the effect of processing of shed blood during cardiopulmonary bypass on tranfusion and neurocognitive function. *Circulation* 2007; 116: I-89-I-197 ISSN 0009-7322

Russell IF (1993). Midazolam-fentanyl; an anesthetic? An investigation using the isolated forearm technique. *Br J Anaesth* 1993; 70: 42-6 Online ISSN:1471-6771 Print ISSN:0007-0912

Scott BH; Seifert FC, Grimson R, Glass PS (2005). Octogenerians undergoing coronary artery bypass graft surgery: resource utilization, postoperative mortallity, and morbidity. *J Cardiothorac and vasc Anesth* 2005; 19: 583-8 Print ISSN: 1053-0770 Online ISSN:1532-8422

Selnes OA, Grega MA, , Bailey MM, Pham LD, Zeger SL, Baumgartner WA, McKhann GM. (2008). Cognition 6 years after surgical or medical therapy for coronary artery disease. *Ann Neurol* 2008; 63: 581-590 *Print ISSN: 0364-5134.Online ISSN: 1531-8249*

Shann KG, LikoskyDS, Murkin JM, Baker RA, Baribeau YR, DeFoe GR, Dickinson TA, Gardner TJ, Grocott HP, O'Connor GT, Rosinski DJ,Sellke FW, Willcox TW (2006). An evidence-based review of the practice of cardiopulmonary bypass in adults: a focus on neurologic injury, glycemic control, hemodilution, and the infalammatory response. *J Thorac Cardiovasc Surg* 2006; 132:283-90 Print ISSN: 0022-5223 Online ISSN:1524-0274

Shann KG; Likosky DS, Murkin JM, Baker RA, Baribeau YR, DeFoe GR, Dickinson TA, Gardner TJ, Grocott HP, O2Connor GT, Rosinski DJ, Sellke FW, Wİllcox TW (2006). An evidence-based review of the practice of cardiopulmonary bypass in adults: a focus on neurologic injury, glycemic control, hemodilution and the inflammatory response. *J Thorac Cardiovasc Surg* 2006; 132: 283-90 Print ISSN: 0022-5223 Online ISSN:1524-0274

Sherry KM, Sartain J, Bell JH, Wilkinson GA (1995). Comparison of the use of a propofol infusion in cardiac surgical patients with normal and low output states. *J Cardiothorac and vasc Anesth* 1995; 9: 368-372 Print ISSN: 1053-0770 Online ISSN:1532-8422

Shore-lesserson L, Reich DL, DePerio M (1998). Heparin and protamine titration do not improve haemostasis in cardiac surgical patients. *Can J Anaesth* 1998; 45: 10-18 Online ISSN:1496-8975 Print ISSN:0832-610X

Silbert BS; Satamaria JD, O'Brian JL, Blyth CM, Kelly WJ, Molnar RR (1998). Early extubation following coronary artery bypass surgery. A propective randomized controlled trial. The Fast-track cardiac care team. *Chest* 1998; 113: 1481-8 Print ISSN: 0012-3692; Online ISSN: 1931-3543

Society of thoracic surgeons blood conservation guideline task force: Ferraris VA, Ferraris SP, Saha SP, et al. ;The society of cardiovascular anesthesiologists special task force on blood transfusion; Spies BD, Shore-Lesserson L, Stafford-Smith M, et al (2007). Perioperative blood transfusion and blood conservation in cardiac surgery: The Society of thoracic surgeons and the society of cardiovascular anesthesiologists clinical practice guideline. *Ann Thorac Surg* 2007; S27-S86 Online ISSN: 1552-6259 Print ISSN: 0003-4975

Stanley TH, Liu WS, Gentry S (1977). Effects of ventilatory techniques during CPB on post-bypass and postoperative pulmmonary compliance and shunt. *Anesthesiology* 1977; 46: 391-5 Online ISSN:1528-1175 Print ISSN:0003-3022

Steinberg JS; Zelenkofske S, Wong SC, Gelernt M, Sciacca R, Menchavez E (1993). Value of the P-wave signal avaraged ECG for predicting atrial fibrillation after cardiac surgery. *Circulation* 1993; 88:2618-22 ISSN 0009-7322

Stoelting RK, Hillier SC (2006). *Pharmacology and Physiology in anesthetic practice.* Lippincott Williams and Wilkins, ISBN-13-978-0-7817-5469-9,ISBN-10-0-7817-5469-0, China

Svircevic V; van Dijk D, Nierich AP, Passier MP, Kalkman CJ, van der Heijden JMGG, Bax L (2011). Meta-analysis of thoracic epidural anesthesia versus general anesthesia for cardiac surgery. *Anesthesiology Online ISSN:1528-1175 Print* 2011; 114:271-82 ISSN:0003-3022

Tabuchi N; de Haan J, Boonstra PW, van Oeveren W (1993). Activation of fibrinolysis in the pericardial cavity during CPB. *J Thorac Cardiovasc Surg* 1993; 106: 828-33 Print ISSN: 0022-5223 Online ISSN:1524-0274

Thys DM (2009). Cardiac Anesthesia: Thirty years Later-The second Annual Arthur E. Weyman Lecture *Anesth Analg* 2009; 109:1782-90 Print ISSN: 0003-2999; Online ISSN: 1526-7598

Tolwani A, Paganini E, Joannidis M, Zamperetti N, Verbine A, Vidyasagar V, Clark W, Ronco C. (2008). Treatment of patients with cardiac surgery associated-acute kıdney injury. *Int J Artif Organs* 2008; 31: 190-196 Print ISSN:0391-3988 Online ISSN: 1724-6040

Tritapepe L, Landoni G, Guarracino F, Pompei F, Crivellari M, Maselli D, De Luca M, Fochi O, D'Avolio S, Bignami E, Calabrò MG, Zangrillo A (2007). Cardiac protection by volatile anesthetics. A multicenter randomized, controlled study in patients undergoing coronary artery bypass grafting with cardiopulmonary bypass. *Eur J Anesthesi*ol 2007; 24: 323-331 Print ISSN: 0265-0215 Online ISSN: 1365-2346

Tsai SK, Lee C, Kwan WF, Chen BJ (1992) Recovery of cognitive functions after anesthesia with desflurane or isoflurane and nirous oxide. *Br J Anaesth* 1992; 69: 255-8 Online ISSN:1471-6771 Print ISSN:0007-0912

Umscheid CA, Kohl BA, Williams K (2007). Antifibrinolytic use in adult cardiac surgery. *Curr Opin Hematol* 2007; 14: 455-467 ISSN: 1065-6251

Van den Berghe G, Wouters P, Weekers F, Verwaest C, Bruyninckx F, Schetz M, Vlasselaers D, Ferdinande P, Lauwers P, Bouillon R. (2001). Intensive insulin therapy in the critically ill patients. *N Engl J Med Online* 2001; 345: 1359-1367 ISSN 1533-4406 Print ISSN 0028-4793

Vuylsteke A; Djaiani G, Kneeshow J, Bethune DW (1996). Amnestic awareness during cardiac surgery: comparison of three different regimens. *Br J Anaesth* 1996; 76:A81 Online ISSN:1471-6771 Print ISSN:0007-0912

Wahrborg P, Booth JE, Clayton T et al (2004). SoS Neuropsycology substudy investigators. Neuropsycological outcome after percutaneous coronary intervention or coronary artery bypass grafting; results from the sten tor surgery (SoS) Trial. *Circulation* 2004; 110: 3411-3417 ISSN 0009-7322

Waldermar G; Schmidt JF, Andersen AR, Vorsstrup S, Ibsen H, Paulson OB (1989). Angiotensin converting enzyme inhibition and cerebral blood flow autoregulation in normotensive and hypertensive man. *J Hypertens..* 1989; 7: 229-35 Print ISSN: 0263-6352. Online ISSN: 1473-5598

Warltier DC; al-Wathiqui MH, Kampine JP, Schmeling WT (1988). Recovery of contractile function in stunned myocardium in chronically instrumented dogs is enhanced by halothane or isoflurane. *Anesthesiology* 1988; 69: 552-65 Online ISSN:1528-1175 Print ISSN:0003-3022

Warren O, Mandal K, Hadjianastassiou V, Knowlton L, Panesar S, John K, Darzi A, Athanasiou T. (2007). Recombinant activated factor VII in cardiac surgery: A systematic review. *Ann Thorac Surg* 2007; 83: 707-714 Online ISSN: 1552-6259 Print ISSN: 0003-4975

Wong DT, Cheng DC, Kustra R, Tibshirani R, Karski J, Caroll-Munro J, Sandler A (1999). Risk factors of delayed extubation, prolonged lenght of stay in the intensive care unit, and mortality in patients with fast-track cardiac anesthesia: A new Cardiac risk score. Anesthesiology 1999; 91: 936-944 Online ISSN:1528-1175 Print ISSN:0003-3022

2

Anaesthetic Considerations for Congenital Heart Disease Patient

Mohammad Hamid
Aga Khan University
Pakistan

1. Introduction

Incidence of congenital heart disease (CHD) is about 0.8%[1] and most of these CHD children (80%) survive to adulthood in developed countries due to early diagnosis and intervention along with improved surgical and anaesthetic techniques. But the situation is different in most of the third world countries, where 90% of these children receive suboptimal or no care[2]. These patients commonly admitted in the hospital for procedures like cardiac catheterization, radiological procedures[3 4], dental and cardiac surgery.

There is increased risk of mortality and morbidity[5] under anaesthesia as their anaesthetic management in the operating room is challenging in several respect. Few heart defects are so complex that you need to involve paediatric cardiologist and intensivist for complete understanding of anatomy and pathophysiology of heart defect.

Adult population with congenital heart defects has also increased[6 7] over the years and poses more challenges for anaesthesiologist in perioperative period. It is now expected that soon there will be more adult with congenital heart defects than children. Grown up congenital heart (GUCH) is a separate entity, which requires expertise of different disciplines to prevent associated morbidity and mortality[8] during operations (cardiac or non cardiac) particularly in uncorrected defects and in pregnant patients.

When a cardiac defect is recognized in a paediatric patient then the presence of other cardiac and extracardiac lesion is a possibility. The incidence of extra cardiac malformation is as high as 20 - 45% and chromosomal abnormalities in these CHD patients is found to be 5-10%.

Perioperative anaesthetic considerations include preoperative evaluation, management of hypoxaemia, shunt, polycythaemia, pulmonary hypertension and ventricular dysfunction.

2. Classification

Several classifications of CHD have been introduced. Two are given below

2.1 Cyanotic/Acyanotic CHD

2.1.1 Acyanotic

a. Ventricular Septal Defect (VSD)
b. Atrial Septal Defect (ASD)
c. Patent Ductus Arteriosus (PDA)
d. Atrio ventricular Septal Defect (AVSD)

e. Pulmonary Stenosis (PS)
f. Aortic Stenosis (AS)
g. Coarctation of the Aorta

2.1.2 Cyanotic CHD
a. Tetralogy of Fallot
b. Transposition of the Great Arteries (TGA)
c. Total Anomalous Pulmonary Venous Return(TAPVR)
d. Tricuspid Atresia
e. Truncus Arteriosus
f. Uncommon, each <1% of CHD, pulmonary atresia, Ebstein's anomaly.

2.2 Classification on the basis of pulmonary and systemic flow
1. Excessive Pulmonary Blood Flow
   a. VSD, ASD, PDA, PAPVR
2. Inadequate Pulmonary Blood Flow
   a. Tetralogy of Fallot, Pulmonary atresia
3. Inadequate or obstruction to systemic blood flow
   a. Coarctation of Aorta
4. Abnormal Mixing
   a. TGA

3. Preoperative consideration

Three type of paediatric CHD patients are expected to come for evaluation.
1. Patients with uncorrected cardiac defect
2. Patients who had previous palliative surgery
   a. ToF with BT shunt
   b. Atrial septostomy for TGA
3. Patients in whom total correction has been done but they may have residual defects requiring certain procedures[9]

Preoperative evaluation should include detailed information about cardiac lesion, altered physiology and its implications. There are few questions which should be clearly answered during preoperative evaluation of these CHD patients. These includes
a. Complete understanding of the anatomical changes due to cardiac defect or palliative procedure
b. Direction and amount of shunting
c. Presence and severity of pulmonary hypertension
d. To what extent pulmonary flow reduced or increased?
e. Degree of hypoxaemia, Polycythaemia
f. Coagulation abnormalities
g. What associated pathophysiological findings likely will influence the management?
h. Functional status of the patient

Fatigue, headache, visual disturbances, depressed mentation and paraesthesia of toes and fingers are presenting symptoms of polycythaemia. History of cyanosis and congestive heart failure (CHF) are major manifestations of CHD. Fatigue and dyspnoea on feeding and irritability indicate poor functional status. Cyanosis occurs due to decrease pulmonary flow

anatomically or functionally (Mixing lesion). Cyanosis may be permanent or appear intermittently. Cyanosis may not be seen in new born due to presence of faetal haemoglobin which is highly saturated at a given PaO2.
High pulmonary flow leads to pulmonary edema. Failure to thrive and feeding problems are common in patients with history of repeated pulmonary congestion. Patient may presents with tachycardia, tachypnoea, irritability, cardiomegaly and hepatomegaly. The right ventricular function should also be assessed as it is equally important in paediatric CHD patient.
Try to avoid dehydration in cyanotic CHD patients by allowing clear liquids two hours prior to surgery (Table 1). Children also have low glycogen stores which makes them vulnerable to hypoglycemia. If timing of surgery uncertain then start an intravenous line and give glucose containing solution. Midazolam[10 11] is a preferred sedative in the doses of 0.5 to 1mg/kg or even higher doses in few studies given orally half hour before surgery (Table 2). If patient is on prostaglandin (PGE1) infusion then it should be continued.

2hrs	Clear liquids (water, apple juice, pedialyte)
4hrs	Breast milk
6hrs	Formula & Cow milk
6hrs	Solids

Table 1. NPO Orders

Age	**Premedication**
< 6 months	None
6 months to 8 years	Midazolam Oral 0.5- 1.0mg/kg (Max. 12 mg) Intravenously 0.05 - 0.2mg/kg Chloral hydrate 40 - 50mg/kg
> 8 years	Midazolam 7.5 mg PO Morphine 0.1mg/kg IM Ketamine 4mg/kg IM

Table 2. Premedication orders

4. Investigation

Polycythaemia is very common which increases blood viscosity and leads to thrombosis and infarction in cerebral, renal and pulmonary region. Although polycythaemia leads to intravascular volume expansion but at the same time reduces plasma volume. Coagulation abnormalities also occur due to hypofibrinogenaemia and factor deficiencies. Platelet count, PT and PTT should be ordered in all patients coming for surgery. Preoperative phlebotomy can be performed in patients with symptomatic hyperviscosity and haematicrit > 65%.

Electrolyte abnormalities are commonly seen in patients who receive diuretics and parental nutrition. Hypocalcaemia commonly found in patients with Di George syndrome.
ECG may show ventricular strain or hypertrophy pattern. Echocardiography is used for doppler and color flow mapping while catheterization is used for information about pressures in different chambers, magnitude of shunt and coronary anatomy. Examine chest X-Ray for heart position (Dextrocardia) and size, atelectasis, acute respiratory infection, vascular markings and elevated hemidiaphragm. High pulmonary flow will leads to increased pulmonary marking while reduced flow causes oligaemic lung fields.
Neurological assessment and MRI[12] may also be needed in these patients. Delayed brain development is associated with certain CHD. Fetal MRI can help in early assessment of immature brain.

5. Intraoperative considerations

Presence of CHD in paediatric patients poses a great challenge for anaesthetist[13] as morbidity and mortality is quite high. Incidence of cardiac arrest in these paediatric patients under anaesthesia is higher[14] than non CHD patients and mainly due to pharmacological interaction and over dose[5].
Intravenous line must be placed in all patients even for minor procedure. All intravenous tubings should be free of air bubble. Polycythaemic patient must be well hydrated before induction either by IV or orally.
Sevoflurane[15] is preferred over halothane due to better haemodynamic stability in CHD patients. Most of the CHD patients tolerate inhalation induction with sevoflurane while patients with poor cardiac function, may not tolerate inhalation induction. Ionotropes should be continued if patient is on ionotropes.

5.1 Monitoring

Monitoring in paediatric CHD is the same as in adult cardiac surgery but there are few differences and considerations during surgery. Monitoring during surgery ranges from simple ECG to blood glucose, which is controversial due to non availability of evidence that tight blood sugar control improves outcome[16].

5.1.1 Electrocardiogram

Although ECG can be helpful in the detection of ST changes but is mainly used for arrhythmia detection in paediatric patients. Even arrhythmia detection is difficult due to baseline tachycardia. Skin should be prepared for electrode by rubbing with alcohol pad or swab. Three leads system is commonly used while in older children five leads system can also be used.

5.1.2 Blood pressure monitoring

Non invasive monitoring

Non invasive blood pressure should always be monitored even in the presence of arterial line. Cuff should be 20% wider than the diameter of limb where non invasive blood pressure is monitored. Smaller cuff results in erroneously high pressure while larger cuff will give lower pressures.

Invasive pressure monitoring

It not only provides beat to beat continuous blood pressure monitoring but also provides easy access for blood sampling. Pressure monitoring tubing and stopcocks should be free of air to prevent air embolism and damping of system. It is also a major source of fluid overload as system continuously flushes 2-4 ml/hr per invasive line. In addition a quick flush also pushes about 1-2 ml of fluid per second . Dextrose can be used but usually normal saline is the flushing solution as bacterial growth is less likely.

5.1.3 Central venous pressure

Central venous access not only helpful in monitoring but also provides a reliable route for drugs, fluid and blood. Right internal jugular vein (Table 3) is commonly used due to its straight course to right atrium while left side is avoided due to concerns about its persistent connection to left SVC (which may be ligated during surgery). Alternatively femoral and subclavian veins can also be used.

Weight	CVP
< 5kg or less than one year	4F, 5cm
5 - 20 kg	4F, 8cm
>20 kg	5F, 8 or 13cm
Adult	7F

Table 3. Central venous catheter (Internal Jugular Vein) size according to weight

5.1.4 Pulse oximeters

Usually two oximeters are placed , one in the upper limb and other in the lower extremity. Pulse oximeter uses two light emitting diodes and one photodiode for detection of red and infra red lights.

Accuracy of pulse oximeter is affected by

1. Hypotension
2. Hypothermia
3. Electrocautery
4. Artifacts due to
   a. Thick skin
   b. Dark color
   c. Bright outside light
   d. Presence of dyes like indocyanine green and methylene blue
5. Abnormal haemoglobins
   a. Met Hb
   b. Carboxy Hb

Not affected by fetal hemoglobin.

5.1.5 Cerebral oximeter

Transcranial near-infrared spectroscopy (NIRS)[17] is a sensitive measure of regional hypoperfusion. It measures all haemogloblins and useful in non pulsatile cardiopulmonary bypass and circulatory arrest. Cerebral oximeter detects intravascular haemoglobin oxygen saturation of cerebral cortex.

5.1.6 Echocardiography

Intraoperative transesophageal echocardiography (TEE) plays a critical role in improving surgical outcome in CHD surgeries by confirming diagnosis and identifying residual defects. It is also helpful in the placement of devices in catheterization lab. Micromultiplane TEE probe and three dimensional technologies are new advances in echocardiography. Epicardial echocardiography is an alternative option in institutions where smaller TEE probe is not available[18]. Adult TEE probe can be used in patient weighing more than 20Kg.

Arterial blood gases and blood glucose should also be done frequently. Tight blood glucose control is suggested by certain authors as high blood sugar is toxic to mitochondria.

Intraoperative management

Anaesthetic management during surgery depends on presence or absence of shunt, pulmonary hypertension, hypoxaemia, Ventricular dysfunction, pulmonary flow and arrhythmia.

5.2 Shunt

Shunting through these defects depends upon diameter of defect and balance between systemic and vascular resistance. Balance between systemic vascular resistance (SVR) and pulmonary vascular resistance (PVR) is essential in the anaesthetic management of patient with shunts.

Normal pulmonary: Systemic ratio (Qp:Qs ratio) is 1:1 which indicate either no shunting or bidirectional shunt of equal magnitude. Qp:Qs ratio of 2:1 indicate left to right shunt while less than 1:1 ratio (0.8:1) means right to left shunt. The ratio is estimated from oxygen saturation measurements at pulmonary veins, pulmonary artery, systemic arterial and mixed venous blood.

5.2.1 Left to right shunt

1. Atrial septal defect (ASD)
2. Ventricular septal defect (VSD)
3. patent ductus arteriosus (PDA)
4. Atrio ventricular (AV) canal defects
5. Complete anamolous venous return (CAVR)
6. Partial anomalous venous return (PAVR)
7. Artificial Blalock taussig (BT shunt)

L -R shunt reduces greatly with drop in SVR or an increase in PVR. It leads to excess pulmonary blood flow. Patients are usually acynotic but deterioration in gas exchange may result from pulmonary congestion. Avoid 100% oxygen and hyperventilation in patients with L → R shunt.

Patients with PDA are vulnerable to coronary ischaemia[11] due to ongoing pulmonary runoff during the diastolic phase. Therefore diastolic blood pressure (DBP) should be monitored during surgery. Diameter of Modified Blalock Taussig shunt is fixed so its output is proportional to SVR and in case of systemic hypotension, the pulmonary blood flow will be reduced. Blood pressure in the arm will be low due to BT shunt, so use contralateral limb.

5.2.2 Right to left

These intra cardiac shunts lead to prolong inhalation induction. **R → L shunt** (e.g. tetralogy of fallot (TOF) or shunt reversal[12] occur when SVR drops or PVR increases. Hypercyanotic spell under anaesthesia will respond to volume, Increase SVR with alpha agonists such as Phenylephrine.

5.3 Hypoxaemia

Inadequate pulmonary blood flow and/or admixture of deoxygenated with oxygenated blood in systemic circulation are usually responsible for ischaemia. In addition pulmonary congestion with inadequate exchange of gases can also leads to hypoxaemia.

Persistent hypoxaemia leads to following changes

a. Slightly ↑ HR
b. Hyperventilation
c. Polycythaemia
d. Chemoreceptor response to hypoxaemia reduced
e. Cerebral and myocardial oxygenation maintain but Visceral and muscular oxygenation reduced
f. Reduced metabolic activity of many organs
    a. Growth retardation
g. Myocardial ischaemia can occur
h. Myocardial dysfunction
i. Down regulation of β - receptors

The anaesthetic management includes adequate hydration, maintenance of systemic blood pressure, minimizing additional resistance to pulmonary blood flow and avoids sudden increase in oxygen demand (crying, struggling, and inadequate level of anaesthesia).

5.4 Pulmonary hypertension (HTN)

During early stages, the pulmonary HTN is reactive and responds to hypothermia, stress, pain, acidosis, hypercarbia, hypoxia and elevated intrathoracic pressure but later pulmonary HTN becomes fixed. This last stage, where pulmonary vascular resistance exceeds SVR and symptoms appear due to R → L shunt, is the Eisenmenger syndrome[13].

Anaesthetic risk is quite high including right ventricular failure, bronchospasm, pulmonary hypertensive crisis and cardiac arrest. Anaesthetic management focus on preventing further increase in R-L shunt by keeping SVR high and PVR low, maintaining myocardial contractility and prevention of arrhythmia and hypovolemia.

5.5 Ventricular dysfunction

Chronic volume overload (Large shunts, valvular regurgitation), Obstructive conditions and cardiac muscle diseases leads to reduced ventricular function. Blood gas and X-Ray may show metabolic acidosis and pulmonary edema respectively. Patients are usually on digoxin, diuretics and ionotropes.

Anaesthetic considerations includes

1. Preoperative optimization of following before surgery
    a. Ionotopes
    b. Diuretics
    c. Digoxin
    d. Antiarrhythmics or ablation in patients with arrhythmia
2. Preoperative CBC and electrolytes
3. Etomidate and fentanyl provide cardiovascular stability at the time of induction
4. Avoid or limit the use of inhalation anaesthetics due to associated myocardial depression
5. Maintain normal sinus rhythm
6. Maintain preload during anaesthesia.
7. After load reduction in certain situations

5.6 Miscellaneous concerns

5.6.1 Neurological outcome

There is growing concern about their quality of life and neurocognitive function, as the long term survival of these children is now possible. 20 -50% may develop neurological impairment due to chronic hypoxaemia, prolong deep hypothermic circulatory arrest and prolong exposure to anaesthetics. Non pulsatile low flow during cardiopulmonary bypass causing ischaemia/reperfusion injury may also play a part[19].

Brain adapts to chronic hypoxia due to presence of NMDA 2B receptors in early life. Cortical neurons may reduce by 30% due to chronic hypoxia causing reduction in brain volume. But this reduction is compensated when normoxia develops after surgery. Although most of the article have supported the use of high dose narcotics in over all outcome but at present there is no concrete evidence about best anaesthetic agents for congenital heart surgery.

5.6.2 Coagulation disturbances

Coagulation abnormalities are very common in CHD patients particularly in cyanosed and polycythaemic patient.

Coagulation derangement associated with polycythaemia includes:

1. Decreased platelet count and function
2. Primary fibrinolysis
3. Impaired coagulation factors production
4. Contracted serum volume

Use of blood products is common in paediatric cardiac surgery due to coagulopathy during surgery and several strategies have been instituted to minimize this practice. Preoperative exchange transfusion of 20 ml/kg FFP to replace same amount of blood is an effective method to counter coagulopathy. Antifibrinolytics like aprotinin and tranexamic acid[20] have been used for this purpose. Aprotinin is no longer recommended in cardiac surgery due to higher incidence of renal failure, stroke and myocardial infarction while the use of tranexamic acid has increased.

Tranexamic acid as a part of blood saving strategy is given as a bolus of 100mg/kg followed by 10 mg/kg/hr infusion. Whole blood transfusion is quite effective in coagulopathic patients. Factor VII in the dose of 90 microgram/kg is increasingly used in paediatric congenital heart surgeries.

5.6.3 Grown up congenital heart (GUCH)

Pregnancy

Increased in blood volume during pregnancy may further aggravate the situation and patient may develop arrhythmias, pulmonary congestion and heart failure. Consideration during pregnancy ranges from termination of pregnancy to the safe delivery by caesarean section. A multidisciplinary approach involving obstetrician, paediatric cardiac surgeon, paediatric cardiologist, intensivist, anaesthetist and neonatologist is essential in decision making process.

Anaesthetic challenges and considerations include

1. Invasive line monitoring according to the severity of cardiac defect
2. Slow infusion of lowest effective dose of oxytocin as vigorous uterine contraction leads to high pre load
3. Use of inline air filter
4. Reduction in SVR should be avoided
5. Coagulation abnormalities should also be considered
6. Prevention of thromboembolic events

Eisenmenger

Most of the patients with Eisenmenger started with simple correctable cardiac defects but eventually leads to severe pulmonary hypertension (PVR > 800 dynes/cm^{-5}) which does not respond to pulmonary vasodilators. Hypoxaemia, myocardial dysfunction and arrhythmia is a common finding.

Perioperative risk includes

1. Arrhythmia
2. Cardiac arrest
3. Pulmonary hypertensive crisis
4. Bleeding
5. Thrombosis

Anaesthetic management includes

1. Phlebotomy in hyperviscosity syndrome
2. Avoid dehydration in preoperative period

1. Avoid myocardial depressants
2. Keep SVR high
3. Try to reduce PVR
4. Regional anaesthesia can be used but general anaesthesia is preferred
5. Postoperative pain should be adequately managed
6. Will require intensive care after surgery

6. Common CHD

6.1 Ventricular septal defect (VSD)

VSD is the most common congenital heart defect. It may be an isolated cardiac defect or may be associated with other cardiac defects like ASD, PDA or a part of complex defects (tetralogy, AV canal defect). Communication between two ventricles can be of any size and can occur at any part of septum. Most common type of VSD is peri membranous (also called subaortic or infracristal). Other less common defects are subpulmonary (Supra cristal, infundibular or outlet type), Inlet type (canal type) and muscular. Spontaneous closure is possible in muscular and membranous type of defects.

Smaller defects are not associated with large shunting of blood from left ventricle to right ventricle may not diagnose early in life but they are prone to infective endocarditis. Whereas larger defects cause shunting of blood from left to right ventricle this led to higher pulmonary blood flow and consequently pulmonary congestion. Due to early development of symptoms these patients diagnosed earlier. During systole LV ejects blood not only in the aorta but also in the pulmonary artery causing volume overload of pulmonary vessels, atria and left ventricle. These patients will develop high pulmonary vascular resistance (PVR) and if untreated will leads to Eisemenger.

A device like amplatzer can be placed to close few of these defects by interventional cardiologist. This procedure is performed in the cath lab as a daycare procedure but there are certain criteria needs to be fulfilled. There should be an adequate rim around the defects where amplatzer can be placed. Surgically VSD can be approached through ventricle, aorta, pulmonary artery or right atrium.

Anaesthetic considerations

Always consider high pulmonary vascular resistance in these patients and be ready to treat high PVR and right ventricular failure by inhaled NO, dobutamine and milrinone. Desirable haemodynamic goals by anaesthetists are to have slightly higher preload and pulmonary vascular resistance while keeping the SVR on the lower side and at the same time maintaining heart rate and contractility. Up to 10% of patients may develop conduction abnormalities after VSD repair which may be transient or permanent.

Intraoperative transesophageal echocardiography (TEE) will be beneficial in recognizing residual defects, intracardiac air and right ventricular function. Smaller VSD are sometimes becomes apparent after closure of large defect. In uncomplicated VSD closure patient can be extubated in the operating room.

6.2 Atrial septal defect (ASD)

Normally there is no communication between right and left atria due to presence of a septum. This atrial septum composed of septum primum and septum secundum which merges with endocardial cushion, superior and inferior vena cava.

Several types of defects can occur in this septum leading to shunting across. Apart from secundum defect other less common are primum, sinus venosus and coronary sinus type.

Most common defect is **ostium secundum** which usually located in the centre (also called fossa ovalis type) and occurs due to deficient septum primum. It may be single or have several small defects called fenestrated type. Patent foramen ovale commonly seen at the same site in 25 - 30% of normal patients. Usually PFO do not permit left to right shunting but right to left shunting can occurs if right atrial pressure exceeds left atrial pressure (sneezing, valsalva)

Sinus venosus defect is usually associated with partial anomalous pulmonary venous drainage and appears either at the junction of superior vena cava and atrial septum (High up) or at the junction of inferior vena cava and septum (located lower part of septum). Repair some time may cause injury to SA node.

Ostium primum defect is due to failure of fusion between endocardial cushion and lower part of interatrial septum leading to communication between two atria and usually associated with cleft at anterior mitral leaflet.

Coronary sinus type defect is due to absence of wall between left atrium and coronary sinus leading to communication between left and right atrium. It may be associated with persistent left SVC.

Left to right shunting depends on the size of defects and compliance of ventricles as shunting usually occurs during diastole when both mitral and tricuspid valves are open. If the defect is small (less than 5 mm) then it's called restrictive type while larger defects are non restrictive and associated with right atrial dilatation, RV volume overload and increased pulmonary blood flow. Spontaneous closure is possible but most require device closure by cardiologist or surgery.

Anaesthetic considerations

Inhalation induction in infants and very young and intra venous induction in older children is acceptable technique. Intramuscular ketamine can be alternative for induction or intra venous line placement in some children. Pulmonary hypertension is generally not seen in these patients and their management is usually simple with the goals of higher preload and slightly high PVR to reduce pulmonary flow. Presence of ASD is not usually poses higher risk for infective endocarditis.

TEE is helpful to see the residual ASD, mitral valve repair (primum type), four pulmonary veins opening in left atrium (Sinus venosus type). Tracheal extubation in the operating room will help in minimizing the charges.

6.3 Tetralogy of Fallot (ToF)

ToF is the most common cyanotic CHD, accounting for 10% of all CHD. It comprises of four anatomical defects: (i) VSD (ii) RVOT obstruction (iii) RV hypertrophy (iv) Over riding of aorta.

VSD is usually large, non restrictive which led to equalization of RV and LV pressures and shunting through VSD depends primarily on systemic and pulmonary vascular resistance. RVOT obstruction is dynamic due to hypertrophied infundibulum but fixed obstruction can also occur due to v pulmonary valve stenosis.

Due to reduce pulmonary flow, main and branched pulmonary arteries hypoplasia may also be seen. Right ventricular hypertrophy is more marked when VSD is restrictive. ToF may also be associated with certain defects like anomalous origin of LAD crossing the RVOT, pulmonary atresia, absent pulmonary valve and complete AV canal defect.

Palliative surgery

The classic Blalock Taussig shunt was performed in 1944 to relieve the ToF related cyanosis where end to side anastomosis of subclavian artery to pulmonary artery was performed. Today modified BT shunt is the most commonly performed palliative procedure in CHD patients where a synthetic graft is interpositioned between subclavian artery and ipsilateral pulmonary artery.

Complete surgical repair

First total correction was performed by Lillehei in 1954. Surgical correction involves infundibular muscle resection through right ventriculotomy or transpulmonarry approach.

Pulmonary valve is removed or dilated accordingly and a transannular patch is placed. VSD is also closed at the same setting. Main Pulmonary artery and its branches are also inspected for narrowing. Some centres creates small ASD to counteract high right sided pressures. There is trend towards early total correction rather than palliative surgery which is followed by total correction.

Anaesthetic management

Goal of anaesthetic management is to avoid low SVR and ionotropes before bypass. If patient is on prostaglandin E1 then it should be continued in pre bypass period. Avoid catecholamine release in preoperative phase and at the time of induction by providing good premedication and adequate analgesia and anaesthesia.

Induction can be done with ketamine and fentanyl if intravenous line is in place. Inhalation induction can also be performed while maintaining SVR. Remember infundibular stenosis increased by increasing contractility and heart rate, so minimize noxious stimulus avoid catecholamine release. This is achieved by high dose fentanyl at the maintenance phase. Arterial line and central line should be placed after induction and intubation.

Acute desaturation at any time should be considered as tet spell and treated by analgesics and volume. Phenylephrine should also be available to treat low systemic vascular resistance and hypotension. Steroids given at the time of induction can help in reducing release of inflammatory markers during cardio pulmonary bypass.

TEE is helpful in assessing residual VSD and infundibular stenosis and degree of pulmonary regurgitation. In case of tet spell, give 100% O2, Phenyl ephrine, volume, increase depth of anaesthesia, hyperventilate and give bicarbonate. In addition esmolol or proponol can be tried to reduce infundibular spasm.

During postbypass period be ready for arrhythmias and heart block, RV dysfunction and coagulopathy. Ionotrpic support is mandatory in postbypass period along with high filling pressure particularly if right ventriculotomy was performed. Blood products should be available and antifibrinolytics should be started for coagulopathy.

6.4 Patent ductus arteriosus (PDA)

Ductus arteriosus is a normal communication in fetus, which constrict and closes within 10-15 hrs of birth and later closed anatomically by fibrosis in 2 – 3 weeks. Various mechanism have been described for initial functional closure, which includes increased PaO2, absence of placental derived prostaglandins and presence of catecholamines and bradykinins in new born.

Ductus venosus provides a communication between junction of main and left pulmonary artery and lesser curvature of descending aorta after left subclavian artery origin. Higher incidence of patent ductus arteriosus is seen in premature, females, children living at high altitude and associated with maternal rubella.

It provides left to right shunt causing high pulmonary flow and volume load on left atrium and ventricle. Pulmonary congestion and recurrent infection is commonly seen if remain open.

Medical management includes three doses of indomethacin. If medical management fails then either transcatheter or surgical closure becomes necessary. Surgical techniques include ligation via left thoracotmyn sternotomy or recently by video assisted thoracoscopy.

Anaesthetic considerations

Anaesthesia management is planned according to prematurity, degree of pulmonary congestion and PVR and surgical technique. During surgery aorta, left pulmonary artery and left main bronchus can be mistakenly ligated instead of ductus arteriosus. Remember to place a pulse oximeter at lower extremity to diagnose ligation of aorta. In addition, DBP will rise as soon as PDA is ligated, which will confirm the identification.
Invasive monitoring is not essential in uncomplicated PDA but arterial line can be placed in patients with comorbids to check beat to beat pressure and diagnosis and correction of acidosis. Limit Left to right shunt by keeping FiO_2 low and $PaCO_2$ between 40–50 mmHg. Blood should be available in the room as bleeding is a possibility.

6.5 Common atrioventricular canal (CAVC)

It is also called endocardial cushion defect and results from failure of endocardial cushions to fuse with lower part of atrial and upper portion of ventricular septum. In addition, atrioventricular valves will also be abnormal. There are three different types of CAVC exist.

1. Partial atrioventricular canal or Ostium primum defect
   a. Usually interatrial communication and cleft mitral valve
   b. Two separate AV valves
2. Transitional atrioventricular canal defect
   a. Ostium primum plus
   b. Partially separated AV valves
   c. Small to moderate VSD partially closed by chordate attachment
3. Complete atrioventricular canal defect
   a. Large non restrictive ostium primum
   b. Large VSD
   c. Large common single atrioventricular valve

Left to right shunting and regurgitation leads to volume loading of both atria and both ventricles. Patient will develops pulmonary congestion and pulmonary hypertension. Surgery usually performed at the age of 2-5 years and in some cases earlier.

Anaesthetic management

Management depends on severity of pulmonary hypertension and degree of left to right shunting. FiO2 and ventilation is manipulated along with use of NO and analgesics to reduce pulmonary hypertension. Ionotropic support will be required after bypass. TEE will be useful in detecting residual defects and ventricular function. LA line along with other invasive lines will help in deciding about escalation in ionotropes.

6.6 Anomalous pulmonary venous connection

Two types of abnormal communication are seen. Both of these defects may be associated with other cardiac lesions like ASD, VSD and PDA.

1. Partial anomalous pulmonary venous connection
   a. At least one pulmonary vein is connected to right atrium either directly or indirectly. Most common is right upper pulmonary vein opening in the superior vena cava. These patients may remain asymptomatic for long time.

2. Total anomalous pulmonary venous return (TAPVR)
    a. All four pulmonary veins opens in the right atrium.
    b. Four types of TAPVR exist
        i. Supra cardiac
            - Pulmonary veins converge and drains into a vertical vein which then drains into right atrium via innominate V or SVC
        ii. Cardiac
            - Common pulmonary confluence drains into coronary sinus
        iii. Infra cardiac or infra diaphragmatic
            - A common confluence of pulmonary vein passes through diaphragm and drains in the portal system which then drains into inferior vena cava.
        iv. Mixed
            - Pulmonary veins drains at two or more levels.

Pathophysiology of TAPVR depends on obstructed or non obstructed pulmonary venous return. Obstruction will leads to pulmonary venous hypertension and higher back pressures.

Anaesthetic considerations

PAPVR is associated with higher pulmonary blood flow, so main aim would be to reduce pulmonary blood flow. Patients with obstructed TAPVR are sicker and will need higher PaO2, ionotropic support and repeated blood gases to control acidosis. Post bypass period require high PaO2, hyperventilation, ionotropic support, good sedation, paralysis and NO. Intraoperative TEE is usually not done to avoid further obstruction of pulmonary veins but TTE and epicardial echo can be performed to look at venous return in the left atrium.

6.7 Transposition of the great vessels

Transposition is a common CHD which is associated with high mortality without intervention. Atrial septostomy is usually performed in the catheterization laboratory to stabilize the patient before surgery. PgE1 should be continued before bypass to keep the duct opens. Coronary artery[21] should be preoperatively assessed as abnormal location of coronaries creates surgical difficulties.

Anaesthetic considerations

Anaesthetic goal is to avoid reduction in cardiac output and systemic vascular resistance while keeping the PVR lower relative to SVR. Increased pulmonary blood flow due to reduced PVR will leads to increased mixing of blood and better saturation. Pulmonary resistance can be reduced by following measures:

1. Inhaled nitric oxide (NO)
2. Nebulized PGI2
3. Sildenafil (Oral and preferably intravenous)
4. Ventilatory interventions
    a. Increased FiO2
    b. Reduced carbon dioxide

c. Alkalotic PH

5. At the same time avoid hypoxia, hypercarbia, acidosis, hypothermia, high and low tidal volume, high PEEP and hypoglycaemia in neonates.

7. Postoperative pain management

High dose opioids are given during paediatric congenital heart surgery and analgesic effect continues in postoperative period. Good intraoperative and postoperative analgesia is associated with improved surgical outcome[22]. Morphine in the doses of 25 microgram/kg/hr will provide adequate analgesia and moderate sedation during postoperative period while additional sedatives are needed in intubated patients. Larger doses are needed in infants and young children basically due to high clearance.

Fentanyl at the doses of 1-5 microgram/kg/hr can be given instead to provide continuous analgesia but associated with less sedation then morphine. Non opioid analgesics like acetaminophen and ketamine can also be used as an adjunct to opioid analgesia. Ketamine is given intravenously as a bolus or in the form of continuous infusion at the rate of 10 - 45 microgram/kg/min.

8. Anaesthesia for catheterization laboratory procedures

Diagnostic and interventional cardiology plays a major in the management of congenital heart patients. General anaesthesia for these procedures is associated with low risk of morbidity and mortality[23]. Some of the challenges faced by anaesthesiologist in cath lab include

1. Usually located far away from operating rooms
2. Not equipped with recovery room
3. Transfer of critically ill patient from intensive care to cath lab or vice versa can create several problems
4. Rooms are usually undersized
5. Not properly illuminated
6. Access to patients airway is difficult
7. Monitoring interference with cath lab equipment
8. Contrast material use and its complications like contrast induced nephrotoxicity and vasovagal reaction
9. Radiation exposure
    a. Always use shielding devices like gown, glasses and thyroid collar
    b. Keep a distance from radiation source
    c. Minimize exposure time
    d. Different resident and consultant should rotate rather than assigning one person for cath procedures

Catheterization procedures should only be performed in centers where facilities for paediatric heart surgery are available. Catheterization procedures can be performed under local, monitored anaesthesia care (MAC) and general anaesthesia. There are several difficulties which make these procedures lengthy and complicated. Difficulties during procedure vary from intravenous access by anaesthesiologist to arterial and venous access by cardiologist. Necessary equipment for intubation and drugs for resuscitation should be available as cardiac arrest in these patients is not uncommon[24] when sedation is given for the procedure.

Although cardiologists do give sedation for certain procedures but another person with ability to resuscitate the patient should be available in cath lab. Laryngeal mask airway (LMA) is well tolerated by most of the patients but those patients who can develop airway obstruction (Down's syndrome) during procedure should be intubated before the start of procedure. Intubation should also be done on those patients who need TEE. Anaesthesiologist has to be very careful during TEE manipulation. High doses of analgesia are not required and only local anaesthesia infiltration at access site is sufficient.

9. Complications

Expected complications during the procedure include

1. Arrhythmias
   a. Mechanical reasons, electrolyte disturbance and hypercarbia
2. Brachial plexus neuropathy due to stretching of nerve plexus during positioning
3. Hypothermia
4. Vascular damage at access site
5. Bleeding
6. Congestive heart failure
7. Tamponade

Use of ionotropes and vasopressors should be intentionally reduced, when anaesthesia is given for electrophysiological studies to minimize arrhythmias.

10. References

[1] Mohindra R, Beebe DS, Belani KG. Anaesthetic management of patients with congenital heart disease presenting for non-cardiac surgery. *Ann Card Anaesth* 2002;5(1):15-24.

[2] Doherty C, Holtby H. Pediatric cardiac anesthesia in the developing world. *Paediatr Anaesth*;21(5):609-14.

[3] Poortmans G. Anaesthesia for children with congenital heart disease undergoing diagnostic and interventional procedures. *Curr Opin Anaesthesiol* 2004;17(4):335-8.

[4] Frascaroli G, Fuca A, Buda S, Gargiulo G, Pace C. [Anesthesia for non-cardiac surgery in children with congenital heart diseases]. *Minerva Anestesiol* 2003;69(5):460-7.

[5] Odegard KC, DiNardo JA, Kussman BD, Shukla A, Harrington J, Casta A, et al. The frequency of anesthesia-related cardiac arrests in patients with congenital heart disease undergoing cardiac surgery. *Anesth Analg* 2007;105(2):335-43.

[6] Seal R. Adult congenital heart disease. *Paediatr Anaesth*;21(5):615-22.

[7] Cannesson M, Piriou V, Neidecker J, Lehot JJ. [Anaesthesia for non cardiac surgery in patients with grown-up congenital heart disease]. *Ann Fr Anesth Reanim* 2007;26(11):931-42.

[8] Hamid M, Khan MA, Akhtar MI, Hameedullah, Saleemullah, Samad K, et al. Grown up congenital heart disease patient presenting for non cardiac surgery: anaesthetic implications. *J Pak Med Assoc*;60(11):955-9.

[9] Larsen SH, Emmertsen K, Johnsen SP, Pedersen J, Hjortholm K, Hjortdal VE. Survival and Morbidity Following Congenital Heart Surgery in a Population-based Cohort of Children-up to 12 Years of Follow-up. *Congenit Heart Dis.*

[10] Cox RG, Nemish U, Ewen A, Crowe MJ. Evidence-based clinical update: does premedication with oral midazolam lead to improved behavioural outcomes in children? *Can J Anaesth* 2006;53(12):1213-9.

[11] Masue T, Shimonaka H, Fukao I, Kasuya S, Kasuya Y, Dohi S. Oral high-dose midazolam premedication for infants and children undergoing cardiovascular surgery. *Paediatr Anaesth* 2003;13(8):662-7.

[12] Sigal-Cinqualbre A, Lambert V, Ronhean A, Paul JF. [Role of MSCT and MRI in the diagnosis of congenital heart disease.]. *Arch Pediatr.*

[13] [Anaesthesia for noncardiac surgery in children with congenital heart disease]. *Srp Arh Celok Lek*;139(1-2):107-15.

[14] Thiagarajan RR, Laussen PC. Mortality as an outcome measure following cardiac surgery for congenital heart disease in the current era. *Paediatr Anaesth*;21(5):604-8.

[15] Russell IA, Miller Hance WC, Gregory G, Balea MC, Cassorla L, DeSilva A, et al. The safety and efficacy of sevoflurane anesthesia in infants and children with congenital heart disease. *Anesth Analg* 2001;92(5):1152-8.

[16] Steven J, Nicolson S. Perioperative management of blood glucose during open heart surgery in infants and children. *Paediatr Anaesth*;21(5):530-7.

[17] Amigoni A, Mozzo E, Brugnaro L, Tiberio I, Pittarello D, Stellin G, et al. Four-side near-infrared spectroscopy measured in a paediatric population during surgery for congenital heart disease. *Interact Cardiovasc Thorac Surg*;12(5):707-12.

[18] Kamra K, Russell I, Miller-Hance WC. Role of transesophageal echocardiography in the management of pediatric patients with congenital heart disease. *Paediatr Anaesth*;21(5):479-93.

[19] Wise-Faberowski L, Loepke A. Anesthesia during surgical repair for congenital heart disease and the developing brain: neurotoxic or neuroprotective? *Paediatr Anaesth*;21(5):554-9.

[20] Schindler E, Photiadis J, Sinzobahamvya N, Dores A, Asfour B, Hraska V. Tranexamic acid: an alternative to aprotinin as antifibrinolytic therapy in pediatric congenital heart surgery. *Eur J Cardiothorac Surg*;39(4):495-9.

[21] Tangcharoen T, Bell A, Hegde S, Hussain T, Beerbaum P, Schaeffter T, et al. Detection of coronary artery anomalies in infants and young children with congenital heart disease by using MR imaging. *Radiology*;259(1):240-7.

[22] Wolf AR, Jackman L. Analgesia and sedation after pediatric cardiac surgery. *Paediatr Anaesth*;21(5):567-76.

[23] Swiatnicka-Lucinska M, Markiewicz M, Moszura T, Krajewski W. [Complications during anaesthesia for diagnostic and interventional cardiac procedures in children with congenital heart defects]. *Anestezjol Intens Ter* 2009;41(3):130-4.

[24] Ramamoorthy C, Haberkern CM, Bhananker SM, Domino KB, Posner KL, Campos JS, et al. Anesthesia-related cardiac arrest in children with heart disease: data from the Pediatric Perioperative Cardiac Arrest (POCA) registry. *Anesth Analg*;110(5):1376-82.

3

Data Integration and Management in Cardiac Surgery

Alessandro Taddei[1,2], Maurizio Mangione[1], Paolo Marcheschi[1] and Stefano Dalmiani[1]
[1]*Medical Informatics, Gabriele Monasterio CNR / Tuscany Region Foundation,*
[2]*CNR Institute of Clinical Physiology, G. Pasquinucci Heart Hospital, Massa Italy*

1. Introduction

Today information and communication technology is widely applied in health care. A variety of Information Systems for management of both administrative, government and clinical tasks have been developed and largely implemented in hospitals. Cardiac surgery setting is peculiar in terms of complexity of health-care information management, involving in addition to general tasks related to hospital patient care (ADT, DRG billing, cost evaluation, multimodality diagnostic examinations, laboratory tests, ward and nursing care, anesthesia and surgical interventions, follow-up) specific procedures for cardiac function evaluation and care (cath-lab, radiology), heart surgery (from minimal invasive to open heart operations with assisted circulation), intensive care unit monitoring.

Given the huge amount of different heterogeneous sources of patient data, both administrative and clinical, integration is crucial to allow comprehensive medical decision making, effective care planning and proper resource control. Actually few systems achieve this objective even if interoperability in health care has been promoted by many international initiatives (HL7, ANSI, CEN, DICOM).

Aim of this paper is to report our experience in developing an integration system to manage health care in its technological, administrative and clinical aspects, in respect of high quality care and cost-effectiveness evaluation.

Almost 15 years ago the Hospital Information System (HIS) was first developed at National Research Council (CNR), Institute of Clinical Physiology (IFC), in Pisa by the SPERIGEST project (supported by Italian National Health Ministry, 1995-98) (Macerata, 1995) for the integration of resources in Cardiology. Later, extension of HIS at G.Pasquinucci Heart Hospital (GPH), IFC-CNR's section in Massa, 60 kilometers from Pisa, specialized in Cardiology and Cardiac Surgery (both adult and pediatric), required both adaptation and development. In 2007 IFC-CNR health-care activities converged into the "G.Monasterio Foundation" (FGM) by the joint effort of CNR, Tuscany Region and Universities.

A networked computer-based information systems was implemented, based on three levels of data archiving (administration, clinical system and functional units, i.e. diagnostic laboratories, care units, Operating Rooms) and on two modalities for data exchange

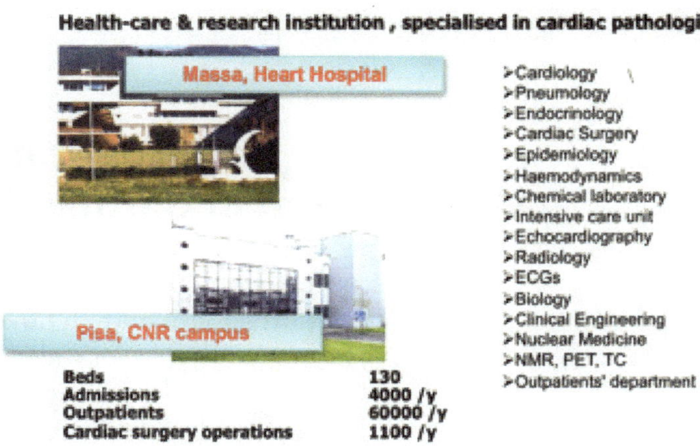

Fig. 1. Gabriele Monasterio CNR / Tuscany Region Foundation, Pisa and Massa, Italy

(middleware data integration into the central clinical database ARCA and Web distribution of health care information over the HIS network). PACS was set up using Open Source DICOM utilities. The computer-network infrastructure, interconnecting GPH with the head institution in Pisa, allows achieving full access to patient information from any workstation. Secure Web technology was applied for distribution of health care information within hospital Intranet and also outside by Extranet.

The project of the information system was aimed at collecting, archiving and integrating all data related to patient care, from the visit in ambulatory to hospital admission, diagnostic procedures, cardiac surgery intervention and finally discharge and follow-up. The different

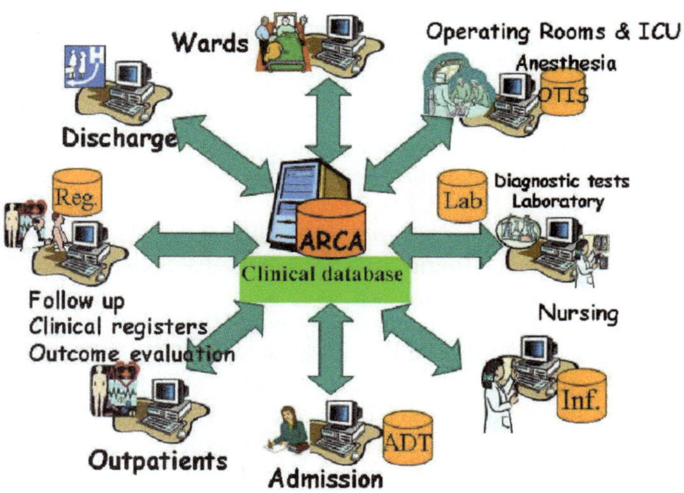

Fig. 2. The clinical information system: patient data flows

sources of patient information were integrated by middleware into the central hospital database (ARCA) which represents the clinical repository. Network connection between GPH and IFC is currently fast enough (8 Mb/s and recently up to 200 Mb/s) to guarantee effective access to patient data, archived in the ARCA repository located in Pisa (SQL IBM DB2/2, recently migrated into Oracle DB).

2. Electronic medical record

Transition from conventional paper-based towards electronic medical record (EMR) required, first, to set up regular and comprehensive patient information flow from health care units into ARCA repository (Taddei et al., 2003). Each diagnostic or care unit (ECG, echocardiography, cath lab, chemical lab, nursing system) as well as the Operating Room Theatre and the Intensive Care Unit were provided with computer-based systems for recording patient data and transferring reports into EMR. Structured data entry was generally implemented in addition to free text. Standard ICD9-CM codes of diagnoses and

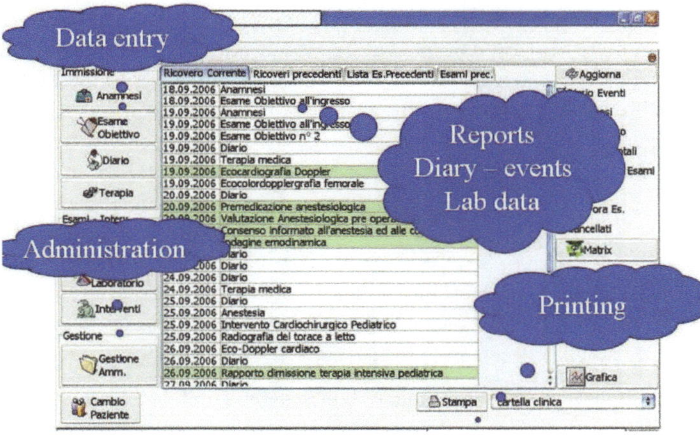

Fig. 3. The main GUI of the Electronic Medical Record

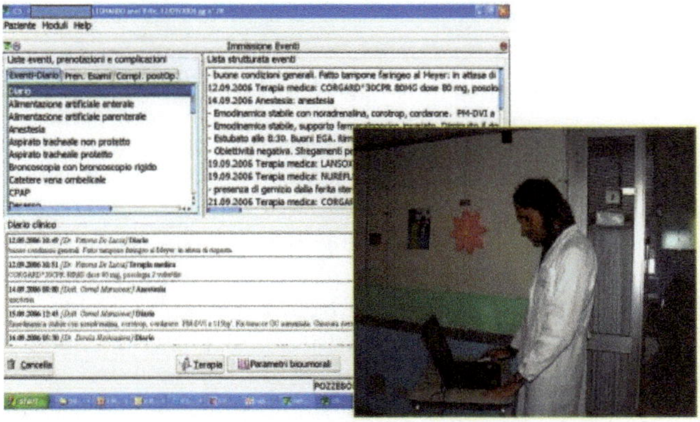

Fig. 4. Accessing the medical record in the ward by Wi-Fi connected laptop

procedures were applied for filling in DRG forms. EMR user interface was set up extending the model already used in Cardiology departments of IFC-CNR in Pisa (Carpeggiani et al.,

2000). Use of Java language allowed to deploy EMR on any platforms (MS-Windows, Mac, Linux). Safe wireless networks were installed in the wards of both adult and pediatric cardiac departments to allow use of mobile EMR workstations at patient bed.

3. Operating room theatre

Development of HIS at GPH started with the set up of the Anesthesia Information Management system (Taddei et al., 2000) for documentation of anesthesia procedure during cardiac surgery operations. Commercial software (OTIS by Dedalus Inc.) for anesthesia data entry with on-line acquisition from OR equipment was adapted and integrated with HIS. Three phases were distinguished: preoperative patient identification and characterization, importing data from ARCA repository; intra-operative data entry (drugs, events, notes) and automatic data capture from OR equipment; post-operative ICU ordering, anesthesia record printing and data exporting to ARCA repository. Material data entry system was developed for resource management during operations. For each anesthesia record a surgery record was created automatically (by trigger on intervention start) in order to facilitate reporting by operators and to achieve OR register.

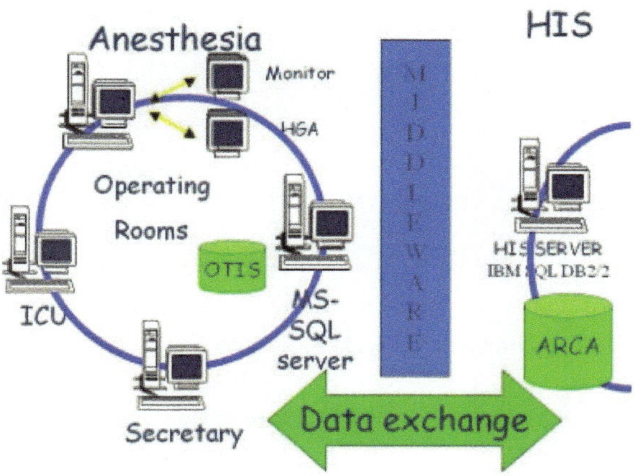

Fig. 5. Anesthesia Information System integrated with Hospital Information System

Recently a new Anesthesia Information Management System has been developed at the Heart Hospital in Massa (Cossu et al., 2011). It was specialized for recording anesthesia-related perioperative patient data during cardiac surgery on either adult or pediatric patients. The system was aimed at integrating patient data (clinical, instrumental and administrative) partly filled in by operator (anesthetist or anesthesia technician) through the Graphical User Interface, partly SQL-retrieved from Hospital Information System (Oracle), repository of patient electronic medical records, and partly gathered, by HL7, from Operating Room instrumentation (monitors, anesthetic machine and blood gas analyzer). Software was created in Java, achieving reliability and cross-platform capability. First, it was crucial to define requirements by interaction with anesthetists and later by cycles of test, revising and correction. GUI, designed to better ergonomics, was divided into modules, each for a corresponding task or phase of anesthesia. Specific forms are provided for documentation of induction phase, for recording staff, drug administrations (bolus or drip),

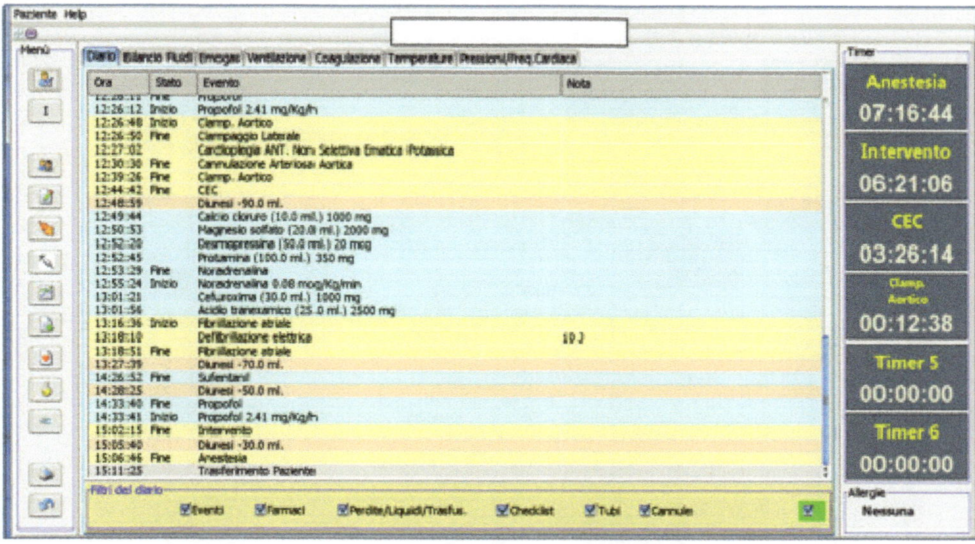

Fig. 6a. The main GUI of the new Anesthesia Information System: the diary (middle), the event counters (right), the tags for access to data views (top), the diary filters (bottom)

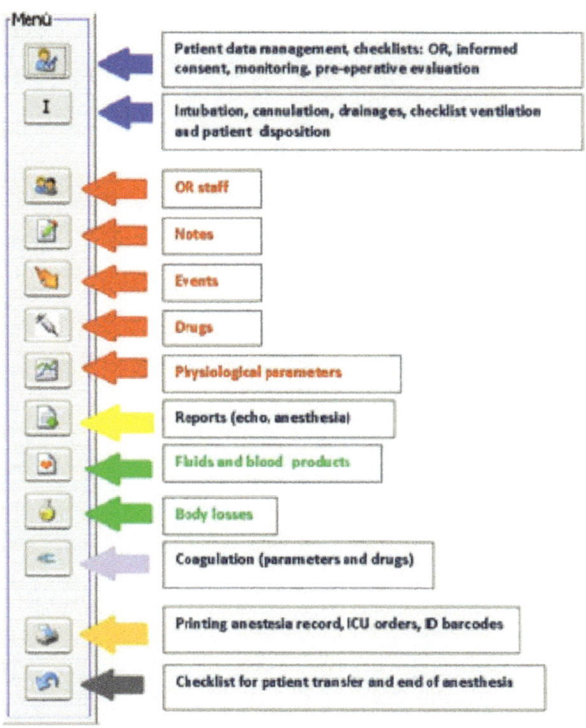

Fig. 6b. Data entry and printing

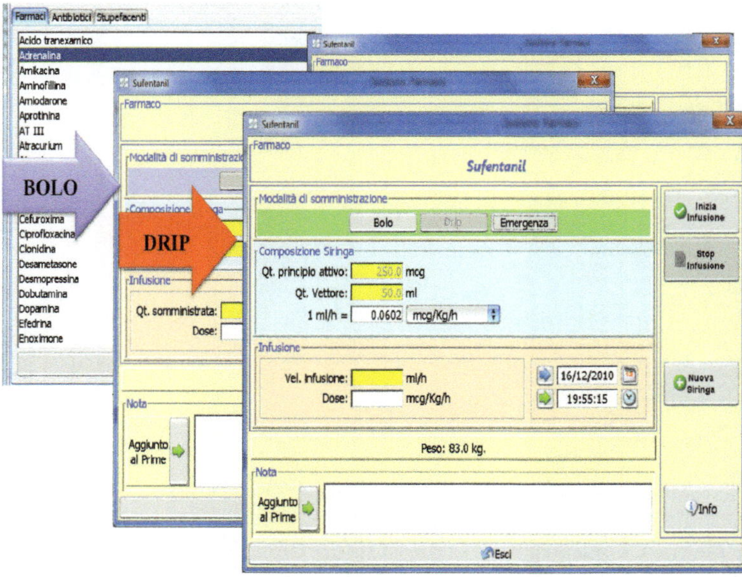

Fig. 7. Recording bolo/drip drug administrations and computing dosages and quantities

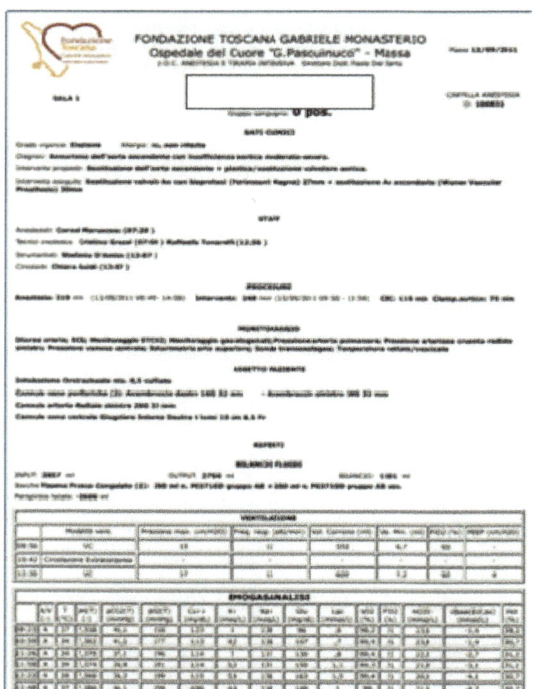

Fig. 8. Printout of anesthesia record

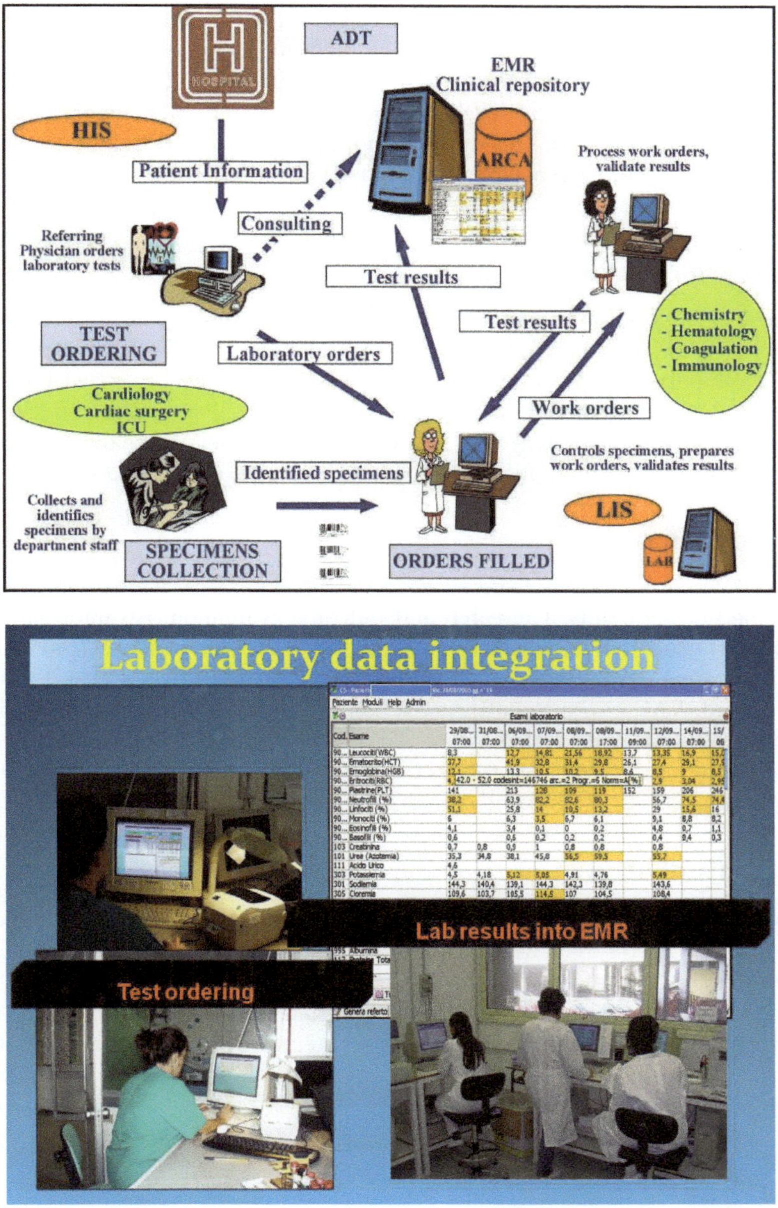

Fig. 9. From test ordering in the wards to laboratory processing and EMR reporting

fluid or blood administrations or losses, and any event of interest, for displaying physiological parameters, for echocardiography reporting. List of anesthesia-related information, fluid balance, lists or trends of physiologic, blood, ventilation, coagulation or monitoring parameters are represented. Counters for timing of main phases (e.g. anesthesia, surgery, ECC) are provided. Operation reports for surgeon's convenience are automatically created in the HIS medical record at start of surgery. HTML reports are created, retrieving data from anesthesia database (Oracle), and printed out: "the anesthesia report", i.e. the medical and legal document, and the "ICU report" addressed to personnel taking care of operated patient. AIMS was introduced in ORs since March 2011, using medical-grade computers close to patient bed. This system, adopting advanced IT solutions (Java, HL7, database relational), could be potentially deployed to other institutions, not limiting to cardiac interventions.

4. Laboratory information system

The LIS was integrated with the HIS to automate the testing process from clinical departments to laboratory and back into EMR (Taddei et al., 2005). Laboratory workflow consists of three parts: (a) test ordering by clinical staff, printing bar-coded ID labels and transmitting orders by network to laboratory; (b) processing test requests and controlling identified specimens by laboratory staff, providing work orders to analytical instruments and validation of results authorizing delivery into the hospital clinical repository.

5. Clinical registers

International reference data sets were adopted to characterize cardiac patients developing registers, aimed at both clinical research and outcome evaluation. An information model was created for structured data management to build clinical registers (Dalmiani et al., 2002). Registers were partially filled in automatically by data retrieved from EMR or from anesthesia record. EACTS congenital heart surgery dataset was adopted as reference for pediatric patients (EACTS database), while National Society of Cardiac Surgery dataset for adults undergoing cardiac surgery (SICCH database). Standard risk scores were derived from datasets (Euroscore for adult and Aristotle for pediatric cardiac surgery).

6. Web data distribution

Distribution of health care information over HIS network was achieved by the use of Web technology. HTTPS Web server was installed for secure access to clinical data recorded in ARCA repository. Web clinical site was developed for allowing authorized users, through password control, to browse into patient clinical data from any workstation over HIS network or even from Internet by VPN connection. First, CGI applications in C language

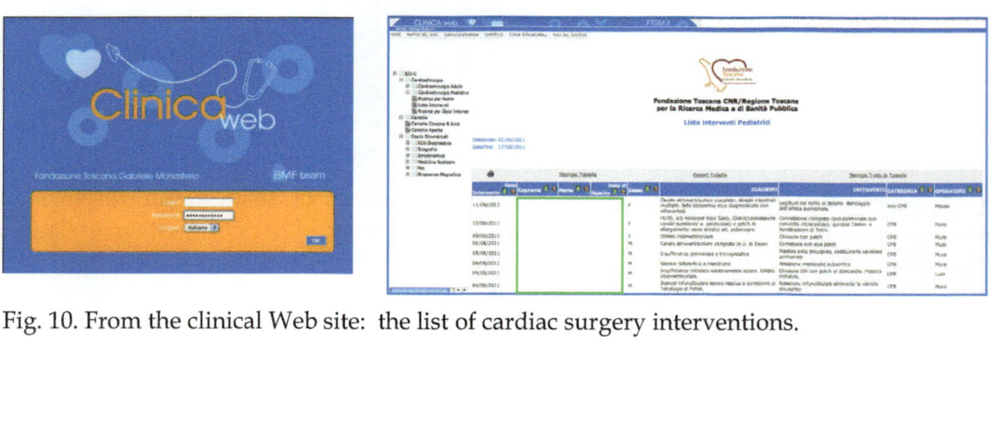

Fig. 10. From the clinical Web site: the list of cardiac surgery interventions.

and in NetData script (IBM) were realized and later Java servlets and PHP4 applications were developed. Tabular or graphic views were implemented for reporting medical records of in- and outpatients, discharge letters, lists of patients and diagnostic reports, cardiac surgery and anesthesia data. Data, downloaded from the web site, were further processed by statistical packages. Later a new web information systems (BMF) allowing deep user access control was developed; all administrative, clinical and government web applications were migrated and adapted (Mangione, 2006).

7. RIS-PACS

Using Open-Source utilities (DCM4CHE), the PACS for different DICOM modalities (CR, CT, XA, US) was set up, while viewer/processing workstations (OSIRIX) were installed for both reporting and consultation (OSIRIX). According to conformance statement of DICOM server (DCM4CHE) and modality equipment Work-List service was implemented was applied to get patient lists from HIS, thus allowing to identify examinations. Radiology workflow include the following steps: examination reservations (1) (in-or outpatients); execution of examinations, identified by worklist and recorded on DICOM server (2a,b); examination reporting on review workstation (3b) or on conventional films (3a); report data entry and printing by EMR (Taddei et al., 2008). Data security was maintained by RAID architecture and using CD/DVD automated DICOM backup systems.

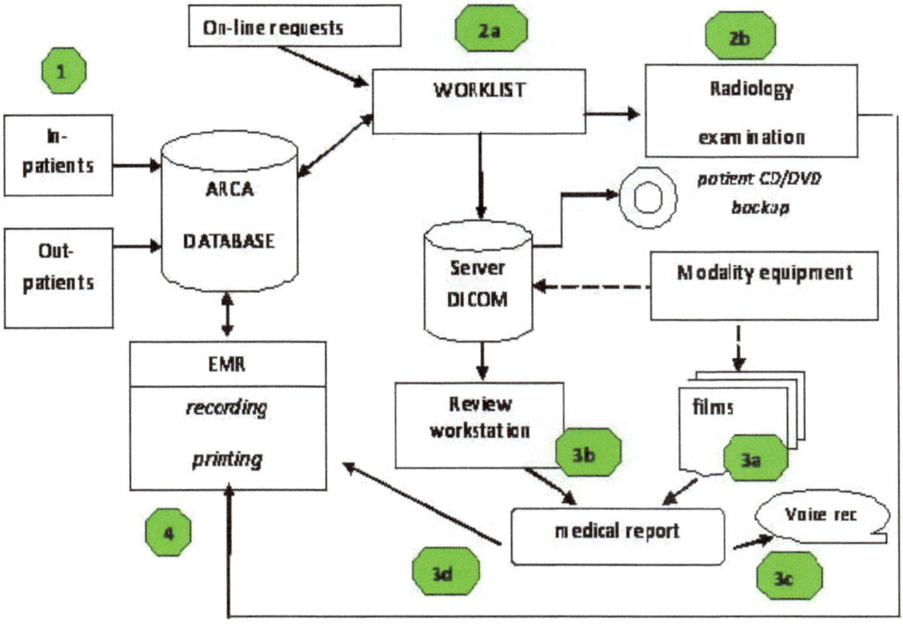

Fig. 11. The RIS structure

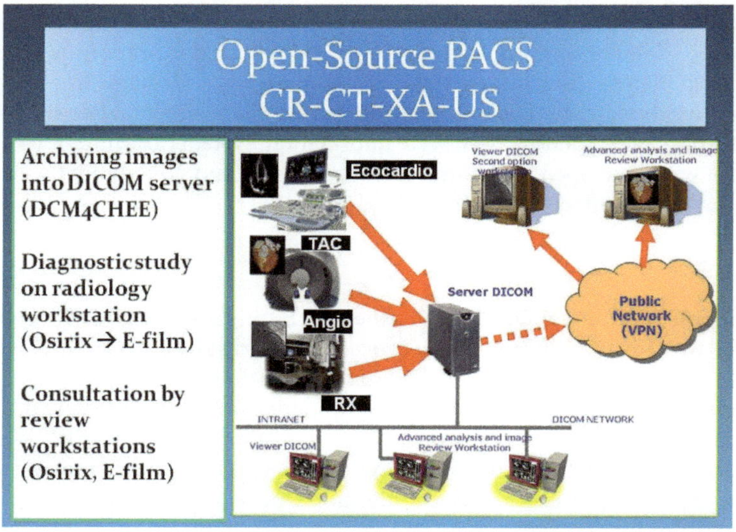

Fig. 12. The PACS

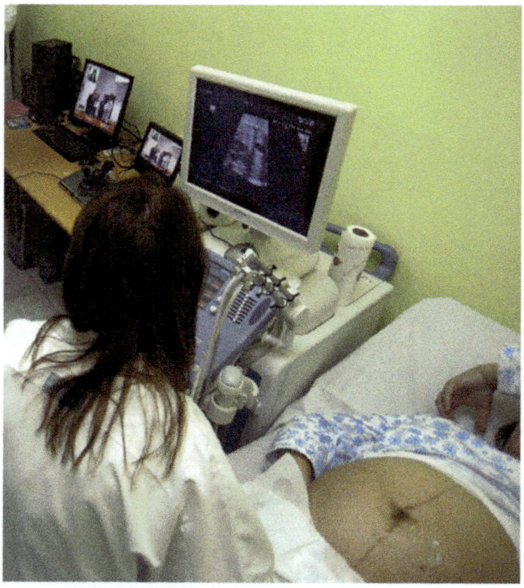

Fig. 13. Fetal tele-echocardiography

8. Telemedicine

Recently telemedicine applications were implemented by on-line secure transmission over Internet of echocardiography and angiography images over public network (project for tele-diagnosis between Balkan countries and GPH - Massa) (Taddei, 2011; Gori et al., 2010). Real-time capability is crucial for allowing specialists to drive remotely proper echo scanning of cardiac structures in patient or foetus with suspected congenital heart disease.

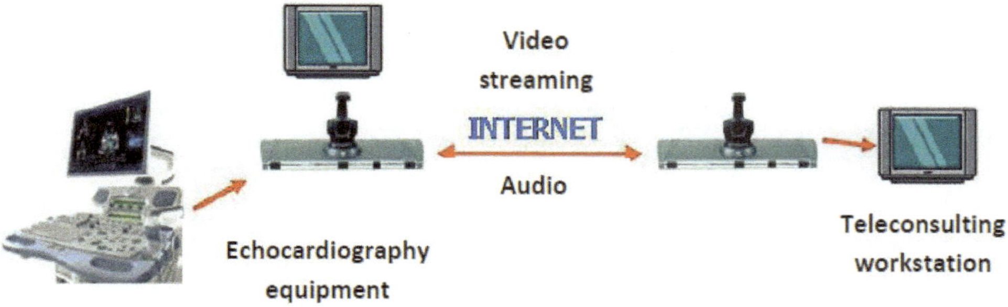

Fig. 14. Use of videoconferencing equipment in tele-echocardiography

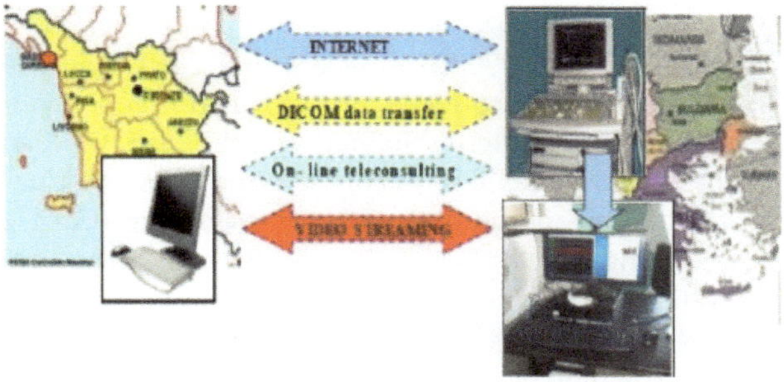

Fig. 15. Tele-consulting for collaborative diagnosis and care planning: diagnostic images are transferred via Internet (on-line or off-line) from remote clinical centers to the reference one.

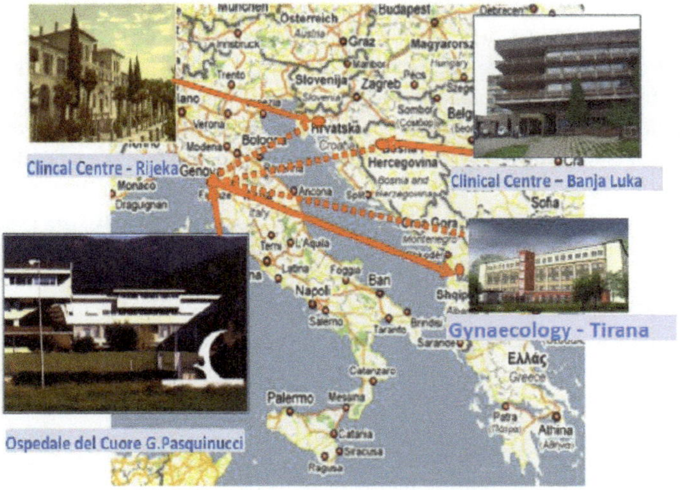

Fig. 16. Tele-consulting network between Massa Hospital and Balkan Centers

Tele-echocardiography was initially implemented in pediatric centers of Banja Luka and Rijeka and Gynecology University Hospital in Tirana, using videoconferencing equipment for transmitting on-line over Internet sequences of diagnostic images. Limitations in terms of functionality, versatility, scalability and cost/effectiveness suggested exploitation of Open-Source technology to set up low-cost devices implementing both live and store-and-forward teleconsulting as well as videoconference and image storage/management.
These devices are generally prone to promote collaborative health-care in various medical fields even in remote Countries not able to acquire expensive medical technology.

9. Conclusion

While information systems for reporting diagnostic, clinical and cardiac surgery activities have been in use at GPH for more than ten years, since 2005, EMR is daily used on all the patients admitted in the clinical departments (Cardiology, Cardiac Surgery and ICU). In order to assure confidentiality, EMR access is allowed only to authorized health care personnel using a personal password to login.
So far at GPH in Massa more than 30000 inpatient and 240000 outpatient records were processed and archived, including up to 12000 cardiac surgery reports (adult and pediatric).
The HIS, developed by the efforts of interdisciplinary teams of IFC-CNR and GPH during the last fifteen years, despite initial difficulties, mainly due to adoption of new technology, was finally effective for both clinical and administrative management (Carpeggiani et al., 2008). Data integration and archiving allowed hospital personnel (physicians, nurses, secretary and administration officers, director) to access clinical records easily and reliably with benefits to overall health-care process. Particularly EMR in the ward promoted staff inter-communication and comprehensive documentation of patient care during hospitalization. Actually a series of technical measures, continuously updated, were needed for assuring data security, confidentiality and integrity, given the continuous exposure to intrusion risks on networks. Technical services were organized to provide 24-hour assistance and support.
Currently medical records need to be printed out after patient discharge and signed by the responsible of department, just achieving a legal value. Application (under development) of both electronic signature and official clinical data storage systems, according to regulatory laws, will allow to authenticate electronic documents achieving a real paperless medical record. Policies for data access, backup and storage will be revised and updated.
Adoption of standard dataset for the characterization of cardiac patients was crucial to achieve comprehensive registers allowing to benchmark surgeons' practice by making prospective prediction of patient outcome according to multicenter risk stratification models. Uploading pediatric cardiac surgery records on international EACTS database it was possible to qualify the GPH centre as one of the best ones in terms of outcome during the last years.
Actually revision of both database architectures (Oracle DBMS) and clinical applications according to health-care data exchange standards (HL7 v3, IHE) (HL7 standard) is currently under development aimed at improving performance of information systems, safeguarding their security and also to assure multicenter interoperability.

10. Acknowledgment

We thank the information technology teams of both Heart Hospital in Massa (Andrea Gori, Emiliano Rocca, Giacomo Piccini and Tiziano Carducci) and of Hospital section in Pisa

(Alessio Ciregia, Mario Cossu, Mauro Raciti, Cristina Salvatori, Andrea Trabucco, Fabrizio Conforti, Giuseppe Di Guglielmo, Gavino Marras) for help, suggestions and advice in setting up applications. Moreover our appreciation for collaborative efforts and suggestions to the clinical staff involved in cardiology, cardiac surgery, anesthesia and radiology (particularly Bruno Murzi, Nadia Assanta, Sergio Berti, Paolo Del Sarto, Mattia Glauber, Dante Chiappino, Pierantonio Furfori and Umberto Paradossi).

11. References

Carpeggiani, C.; Dalmiani, S.; Taddei, A.; Macerata, A.; Franchi, D.; Michelassi, C.; Chelozzi, L.; Emdin, M.; Benassi, A. & L'Abbate, A. (2000). Use of an electronic medical record in a department of Cardiology. In: *Computers in Cardiology*, vol.27, pp. 291-294, IEEE.

Carpeggiani, C.; Macerata, A.; Taddei, A,; Benassi, A. & Donato, L. (2008). Sviluppo, applicazione e valutazione di un sistema integrato gestionale e clinico nel campo delle malattie cardiovascolari: dieci anni di esperienza. *G Ital Cardiol*, vol. 9, pp. 558-565.

Cossu, M.; Furfori, P.; Taddei, A.; Mangione, M. & Del Sarto, P. (2011). Anesthesia Information Management System in Cardiac Surgery. In: *Proceedings of Computing in Cardiology*, Hangzhou, China, September, 2011.

Dalmiani, S.; Taddei, A.; Glauber, M. & Emdin, M. (2002). An informative system for structured data management to build a cardiological multidimensional database. In: *Computers in Cardiology*, vol.29, pp. 369-372, IEEE.

DCM4CHE. Available from: http://www.dcm4che.org/

EACTS database. Available from: http://www.eactscongenitaldb.org/

Gori, A.; Taddei, A.; Mota, D.; Rocca, E.; Carducci, T.; Piccini, G.; Ciregia, A.; Marcheschi, P.; Assanta, N.; Murzi, B. & Ricci, G. (2010). Open Source teleconsulting system for international cooperative medical decision making in congenital heart diseases. In: *Computing in Cardiology*, vol.37, pp. 481-484, IEEE.

HL7 standard. Available from: http://www.hl7.org/

Macerata, A.; Landucci, L. & al. (1995). Networking for health care administration and delivery: the information system at the CNR Institute of Clinical Physiology. *Proceedings of Health Telematics '95*, pp. 113-118, Pisa, Italy.

Mangione, M. BMF - Bio Medical Framework (2006). Technical Report, National Research Council, Institute of Clinical Physiology, Pisa, Italy.

OSIRIX. Available from: http://www.osirix-viewer.com/

SICCH Database. Available from: http://www.sicch.org/ sections/Database_Nazionale/index.html

Taddei, A.; Dalmiani, S.; Piccini, G.; Vellani, A.; Carducci, T.; Buffa, M.; Scebba , L.; Glauber, M.; Murzi, B.; Biagini, A. & Macerata, A. (2003). Data integration in cardiac surgery and resource management. In: *Computers in Cardiology*, vol.30, pp. 279-282, IEEE

Taddei, A.; Fiaschi, A.; Kraft, G.; Fania, A.; Furfori, P.; Del Sarto, P. & Santoli, F. (2000). Integrated system for anesthesia records in cardiac surgery. In: *Computers in Cardiology*, vol.27, pp. 789-792, IEEE.

Taddei, A.; Pisani, P.; Vellani, A.; Dalmiani, S.; Piccini, G.; Carducci, T.; Kraft, G.; Rocca, E.; Storti, S.; Andrenelli, A.; Parri. M.S.; Cardillo, M.; Lauciello, P.; Gwynne, S. & Macerata, A. (2005). Laboratory Data Integration into Medical Record. In: *Computers in Cardiology*, vol.32, pp. 909-912, IEEE .

Taddei, A.; Dalmiani, S.; Vellani, A.; Rocca, E.; Piccini, G.; Carducci, T.; Gori, A.; Borghini, R.; Marcheschi, A.; Mazzarisi, A.; Salvatori, C. & Macerata, A. (2008). Data Integration in Cardiac Surgery Health Care Institution: Experience at G. Pasquinucci Heart Hospital. In: *Computers in Cardiology*, Vol.35, pp. 287−290, ISSN 0276−6574.

Taddei, A. (2011). How we set up telemedicine for diagnosis and care of heart defects in the foetus and newborn. In: E-journal of the ESC Council for Cardiology Practice, Vol.9, N°33. Available from:
http://www.escardio.org/communities/councils/ccp/e-journal/volume9/Pages/telemedicine-open-source-technology-congenital-heart-disease-foetus-newborn-Alessandro-Taddei.aspx

4

Perioperative Organ Protection in Cardiac Surgery

Maria Carmona[1], Matheus Vane[1] and Luiz Malbouisson[2]
[1]*Discipline of Anesthesiology, University of São Paulo Medical School, São Paulo*
[2]*Postoperative ICU, Institute of General Hospital, University of São Paulo Medical School, São Paulo*
Brazil

1. Introduction

Perioperative organ protection refers to the set of strategies to lessen the intensity of the surgical and anesthetic stress. A better understanding of mechanisms involved in tissue hypoperfusion, ischemia-reperfusion phenomena, and the protection triggered by certain anesthetic techniques, drugs and adjuvants have been very useful in perioperative organ protection, especially in patients with comorbidities and / or undergoing high risk surgical procedures.

2. Myocardial protection

Among the methods used during cardiac anesthesia, the use of anesthetic drugs and techniques that increase tolerance to ischemia and contribute to protect myocardial function have been gaining importance in clinical practice and may influence the postoperative course. Myocardial ischemia triggers a cascade of cellular events that start mildly and become increasingly deleterious as the ischemic time passes. Although reperfusion is the end of the ischemic process and is essential for the restoration of normal cell function and survival, it may paradoxically amplify the damage secondary to ischemia and compromise postoperative outcome.

Effects of Anesthetics drugs: For more than three decades, there is growing evidence that inhaled volatile anesthetics can protect the myocardium from ischemic reversible and irreversible injuries (1). The mechanisms by which these drugs promote cardioprotection are not fully known and it is suggested that the mechanism induced by inhaled anesthetics seems to mimic the ischemic preconditioning. Halogenated anesthetics reduce blood pressure, cause depression in myocardial contractility, coronary vasodilation, slow the conduction of electrical stimuli and attenuate the activity of the sympathetic nervous system, which contributes to decrease the myocardial oxygen consumption. However, mechanisms other than the adequacy of oxygen supply and consumption appear to be related to the cardioprotection conferred by inhaled anesthetics, such as the preservation of high energy phosphates(2). The modulation of calcium influx to the cardiomyocyte(3) and the inhibition of the sodium - calcium pump, with increased expression of calcium channels induced by ischemia-reperfusion injury, are also related with the inhaled anesthetics (4).

Some authors have suggested that concentrations around one minimum alveolar concentration (MAC) of various halogenated anesthetics produce similar effects on the intensity of myocardial protection(5). The inhaled anesthetics have shown consistent effects on myocardial protection in animal models of ischemia-reperfusion, and clinical studies have been conducted to verify these benefits in clinical practice.

Myocardial protection during anesthesia aims to decrease the myocardial oxygen consumption, adapting it to the momentary tissue supply and / or cardiac cells become more resistant to ischemia, attenuating the magnitude of the injury induced by ischemia-reperfusion and its deleterious immediate and late consequences, such as myocardial infarction (MI), arrhythmias, ventricular dysfunction, cardiogenic shock and increased perioperative mortality.

The extent and severity of tissue injury after coronary occlusion is not determined at the onset of ischemia and may be modified by methods of myocardial protection. A great number of experimental studies have investigated the mechanisms of ischemia and modalities of myocardial protection, although only a few therapeutic interventions have been shown to be clinically effective. Despite advances in understanding the determinants of coronary blood flow, the relationship between supply and consumption of oxygen, and the cellular mechanisms triggered by ischemia, the incidence of perioperative MI is still high(6, 7).

During ischemia, oxygen supply is below regional metabolic needs, resulting in depletion of cellular reserves of ATP. In this situation, there is a reduction in the efficiency of the ATP-dependent sodium (Na+) potassium (K+) pump, increasing the levels of intracellular Na+. Hydrogen ion (H+) accumulates intracellularly as a result of decreased excretion of metabolic wastes, inhibition of $NADH_2$ mitochondrial oxidation and ATP break down. The accumulation of intracellular H+ promotes an increase in exchange of H+ by Na+ in an attempt to keep cell pH in its normal range, increasing the intracellular levels of Na+ even higher, causing increased levels of intracellular calcium (Ca2+) due to the exchange of Na+ by Ca2+(8, 9). High levels of intracellular Ca2+ promote activation of protein kinases with degradation of proteins and phospholipids culminating in a decrease of the maximum force generated by calcium-dependent myofilaments. After the onset of ischemia, the production of free radicals derived from neutrophils and mitochondria also contributes to the degradation of proteins and phospholipids, which are the main constituents of the cells structure and enzymes(10-12).

The injury installed after the onset of ischemia appears to be amplified when coronary vessels are damaged and the endothelial cells are swollen, reducing the efficiency of gas exchange. The vascular smooth muscle cells and endothelial cells with abnormal function loose the ability to promote vasodilation and to pair the regional blood flow to the momentary needs. Neutrophils play a central role in the spread of cell injury. These cells are attracted by dysfunctional endothelial cells and migrate into the extravascular space, releasing free radicals, cytokines and pro-inflammatory substances, worsening the endothelial, smooth muscle and cardiomyocyte injuries (13). The aggregation of neutrophils and platelets causing microvascular obstruction contributes to the decoupling of the supply / demand relationship (11, 14). The time required for synthesis of damaged proteins would explain the period required for recovery of myocardial function after ischemia-reperfusion injury (15, 16). In combination with high levels of intracellular calcium, there is a major increase in the production of oxygen free radicals due to reperfusion with oxygenated blood. Free radicals such as superoxide (O2-), hydroxyl (OH-) and hydrogen peroxide (H2O2) are extremely reactive and are able to damage all cellular components indistinctly, increasing the damage induced by ischemia. The clinical consequences can range from reversible myocardial dysfunction that persists after reperfusion, known as myocardial stunning, up to MI (10, 12). The development of micro-perioperative ischemic areas is recognized as a problem that can lead to low cardiac output syndrome and death in surgical patients. The perioperative myocardial infarction can occur due to increased consumption of oxygen from the induction of anesthesia until postoperative recovery.

The ischemic preconditioning is an endogenous adaptive and protective response against prolonged myocardial ischemia(17). Despite being initially promising to reduce the incidence and extent of MI, this method of myocardial protection may also decrease the incidence of reversible myocardial dysfunction and post-ischemic dysfunction of the coronary circulation(18). Several membrane receptors seems to be involved in the phenomenon of ischemic preconditioning including α-1, β, opioid and adenosine receptors(19).

In cardiac surgery, the observed systemic inflammatory response is the result of direct surgical trauma, ischemia-reperfusion injury and extracorporeal circulation(20) and cardiac injury can be triggered by ischemia, reperfusion, and also by local effects of mediators of the inflammatory response. Additionally, the heart itself may release locally inflammatory mediators and oxygen free radicals that can contribute to the worsening of the cardiac function. Myocardial protection strategies during cardiac surgery aimed at limitation of the reperfusion injury and systemic inflammatory response are essential to reduce mortality, although many anesthetics may have cardioprotective actions, the diversity of proposed mechanisms for protection (e.g. attenuation of calcium influx, anti-inflammatory and anti-oxidants effects, pre and post conditioning). A randomized study comparing the effects of total intravenous anesthesia (TIVA) and balanced anesthesia with desflurane or sevoflurane on the release of troponin T in the post operative period with 414 patients undergoing coronary artery bypass grafting with cardiopulmonary bypass observed that although the maximum postoperative troponin T did not differ between groups, the mortality rate after one year was 12.3% in the TIVA group, 3.3% in the sevoflurane group and 6.7% in the desflurane group(21).

Clinical studies have suggested the cardioprotective effects of volatile anesthetics and the effects of these agents on the early and late morbidity and mortality requires further investigation. The administration of inhaled anesthetics in post-ischemic period can also be cardioprotective by attenuating the reperfusion damage. This mechanism may be useful in situations where the patients has already suffered or is suffering an ischemic event(22, 23).

The contribution of endogenous opioids for organic adaptation to hypoxia and protection against ischemia-reperfusion injuries by opioid receptor agonists has been demonstrated experimentally in several animal models (24) (25). Morphine administered before occlusion of left anterior descending artery caused a decrease in the infarction zone from 54% to 12% of the area at risk in rats(26). This reduction in the infarct area induced by morphine was also observed in isolated heart models, in *in situ* hearts and in cardiomyocytes(27). It was also observed an improvement in ventricular contractility after ischemic episodes with morphine and fentanyl (28). Besides participating in the triggering of the cascade of ischemic preconditioning, opioids also seem to mediate the memory phase in some animal species and the opioid-induced cardioprotection appears to be modulated by the activation of cardiac receptors, independent of the action of these drugs on the central nervous system [40-41].

It has been proposed that opioid-induced cardioprotection is processed by the activation of ATP-dependent potassium channels, possibly in the mitochondrial membrane(29). However, the intracellular pathway that makes the transduction triggered by the sigma receptor stimulation to the end effectors is still unclear. Other intracellular pathways of cardioprotection induced by opioids appear to be related to the activation of inhibitory G protein and protein kinase C1 (30).

On the other hand, some studies suggest that propofol can attenuate the mechanical dysfunction after myocardial ischemia, improving functional and metabolic recovery(31). Propofol can decrease the concentration of free radicals and its deleterious effects(32) and it is also able to reduce the intracellular influx of calcium and attenuate neutrophil activity, interfering with critical phases of myocardial reperfusion(33). Although some degree of myocardial protection appears to be conferred by propofol when administered during the reperfusion phase in experimental models of isolated rat heart, the protective effect of propofol appears to be momentary and it is not considered an agent capable of inducing preconditioning or myocardial protection. Sevoflurane, but not propofol, seems to be able to preserve post-operative myocardial function with evidence of reduced myocardial cell injury after coronary artery bypass graft (CABG) (34). On the other hand, the continuous infusion of propofol at the dose of 120 mcg/kg/min, initiated 10 minutes before cardiopulmonary bypass (CPB), resulted in lower levels of troponin I and elevated the cardiac index when compared to isoflurane and lower doses of propofol(35).

Despite the well-established role of ketamine as an anesthetic agent in congenital heart surgery and in patients with circulatory shock, this drug seems to block ischemic preconditioning and enhance myocardial injury. Ketamine reduces the production of 1, 4, 5-triphosphate inositol and inhibits ATP-dependent potassium channels in the sarcoplasmic membrane(36). Barbiturates have also been classified as medications that can inhibit myocardial protection induced by ischemic preconditioning (37).

Adjuvant drugs for myocardial protection: Several medications have been investigated preoperatively, intraoperatively or directly administered in the cardioplegic solution before the start of CPB. Beta-adrenergic antagonists can reduce myocardial oxygen consumption, reduce the sympathetic tone, and stabilize cell membranes. If there is no contraindications for its use, the administration of beta-adrenergic antagonists in the early hours after acute MI, modulating the intense adrenergic stimulation(38), can be beneficial in reducing mortality and complications(39).

Regarding the $\alpha 2$ receptor agonists, clonidine seems to be less effective than high thoracic epidural anesthesia in reducing perioperative stress and troponin release in patients undergoing CABG (40). Additionally, experimental and small clinical trials showed encouraging results for the improvement of myocardial performance in patients undergoing cardiac surgery with the infusion of a solution containing glucose, insulin and potassium (GIK) (41). The mechanism by which GIK solution promotes cardioprotection seems to be related to the restoration of the activity of the ATP-dependent potassium channels by insulin, since glucose decreases the activity of this channel and insulin infusion can decrease apoptosis induced by ischemia and reperfusion(42). However, despite the beneficial effects observed experimentally and in small studies, the benefit of GIK in high-risk patients undergoing CABG has not been demonstrated.(43).

Thoracic Epidural Anesthesia: Thoracic epidural anesthesia with local anesthetics has been used as a technique capable of promoting perioperative analgesia and reduction of myocardial oxygen consumption by blocking the roots of the thoracic sympathetic fibers from T1 to T5, which provide sympathetic innervation to the heart. The cardioprotection conferred by thoracic epidural anesthesia is related to an improvement in the myocardial oxygen supply induced by the sympathetic blockade, which causes reduction of myocardial oxygen consumption secondary to bradycardia, reduction of the cardiac output, a decrease in systemic vascular resistance and an improvement in the regional perfusion by a post stenotic vasodilation of the segments of arteries partially obstructed. Some studies have shown that thoracic epidural anesthesia can attenuate the endocrine-metabolic response secondary to surgery, with reduction of release and in serum levels of catecholamines, which contributes to a decrease in oxygen consumption(44).This improvement in myocardial oxygen balance is demonstrated clinically by improvement in angina in patients with coronary artery disease (45).

The efficiency of thoracic epidural analgesia allows lower doses of systemic opioids, thereby reducing the time of tracheal intubation and pulmonary morbidity in postoperative cardiac surgery(46). However, despite the beneficial effects of thoracic epidural anesthesia on myocardial oxygen balance, no direct mechanism to increase myocardial tolerance to ischemia and reperfusion has been described, and the additional risk of the procedure in patients under effects of heparin should be considered. In a meta-analysis of 15 studies and 1178 patients the use of thoracic epidural anesthesia in CABG was not effective in reducing mortality (0.7% versus 0.3% general anesthesia) nor the incidence of myocardial infarction (2.3% versus 3.4% general anesthesia). On the other hand, a significant decrease in the incidence of arrhythmia (OR 0.52), pulmonary complications (OR 0.41) and duration of tracheal intubation was evidenced. Analgesia with spinal opioids showed no effect on mortality, incidence of myocardial infarction, arrhythmias, mortality and duration of intubation when compared with general anesthesia(47). In patients undergoing off-pump coronary artery bypass surgery, the addition of thoracic epidural to general anesthesia can reduce the incidence of postoperative arrhythmias and improves pain control and overall quality of recovery, allowing earlier extubation and hospital discharge(48).

Myocardial protection during cardiopulmonary bypass: The technique of myocardial protection used for most CABG is the infusion of hypothermic cardioplegic solution, with blood or crystalloids. Early reports cardioplegia date from the 50's, describing electrochemical cardiac arrest in diastole induced by potassium citrate solutions, allowing the cardiac surgery to be performed on a stopped and flaccid heart(49). However, this solution was associated with high incidence of myocardial necrosis. Cardioplegic solutions rich in potassium have been abandoned in the mid 70's when it was found that myocardial necrosis was related to its high concentration and hypertonicity. Until the 80's, the use of hypothermic crystalloid cardioplegic solution was the main technique for myocardial protection during cardiac surgery. From the 80's, studies have shown that cardioplegic solutions with potassium and blood promoted more efficient myocardial protection than the crystalloid solution. This was observed by a decrease in the release of CK-MB and in the incidence of perioperative infarction(50). Since then, cardioplegic solutions with blood and potassium have been the cornerstone of myocardial protection with a defined role in intraoperative heart protection. The technique for the infusion of cardioplegic solutions most commonly used is antegrade and intermittent infusion in the aorta, proximal to the heart, after aortic clamping, or directly into the coronary artery ostia, especially when there is associated aortic valve disease. Recently, it has been proposed the infusion of retrograde cardioplegic solutions in the coronary sinus. This technique assumes the possibility of maintaining uninterrupted infusion and distribution of the solution to regions irrigated by stenotic coronary vessels, improving the sub-endocardial protection(51). The optimal temperature for cardioplegia is controversial. Solutions at temperatures below 15°C seem to be more effective in reducing myocardial oxygen consumption, lactate production and markers of cellular hypoxia than solutions at room temperature. However, solutions with temperature around 27 ° C seem to have better recovery of left ventricular function in the immediate postoperative period and lower incidence of arrhythmias, need for defibrillation and bleeding volumes (52). Another controversial issue is the time interval between infusions of cardioplegia, being 20 to 25 minutes the mean used by surgeons. Also, there are no consensuses neither on the optimal dose of cardioplegic solution to be infused nor about the addition of substrates such as l-arginine, anti-arrhythmics or beta-adrenergic antagonists.

Therapeutic hypothermia has been another strategy to reduce myocardial injury secondary to ischemia during CPB. The mechanism by which hypothermia exerts its protective role in the myocardium is not completely understood. The classic explanation is a decrease in oxygen consumption induced by a reduction in the cellular metabolic activity and enzymatic reactions, which could limit the areas of myocardial ischemia in regions at risk. In humans cooled to 32 °C, the total body oxygen consumption is decreased by 45%, unrelated to changes in arterial oxygen saturation(53). The increase in the oxygen affinity to hemoglobin is compensated by increasing its blood solubility. As the temperature decreases, myocardial oxygen consumption decreases, being less than 1% at 12 ° C(54). This cardioprotective effect is independent of hypothermia-induced bradycardia because it persists after heart rate normalization using a pacemaker(55). The decreased metabolic activity, however, does not seem to be the sole mechanism related to cardioprotection induced by hypothermia. There are evidences of reduction in lipid peroxidation, in free radical production, and lower values of extracellular 2, 3-dihydrobenzoic acid, an indicator of free radical production. Hypothermia helps in the preservation of cell's ATP reserves during ischemia. Animal models of acute MI shows that the cardioprotective effects of hypothermia include: smaller infarct size, preservation of microvascular flow and maintenance of cardiac output. The intensity and duration of hypothermia are determined according to the surgical procedure to be performed. Despite the beneficial effects of hypothermia on organ protection, increasing the duration of hypothermia seems to have paradoxical effects, worsening ischemia-reperfusion myocardial injury. Deep hypothermia for prolonged periods may exacerbate intracellular calcium overload and induce the formation of peroxides and reactive oxygen species(56). Other undesirable side effects of hypothermia are electrolyte disturbances, which is related to coagulopathy and immunosuppression(57), increase in systemic vascular resistance, changes in metabolism and clearance of drugs.

3. Neurologic protection

Neurological injuries after cardiac surgery involve a number of disorders that includes stroke, encephalopathy, and cognitive dysfunction(58). In a large multicenter prospective investigation, it was found that around 6.1% of patients had some type of postoperative neurological complication (59), half of them with type I neurological outcomes, involving death as a result of cerebral injury, nonfatal strokes, transient ischemic attack and stupor. The other half had type II neurological outcome with intellectual function deterioration or seizures(59). In another large study, when no stroke or encephalopathy was present, the hospital mortality was 1.4%, but patients with sustained cerebrovascular accident presented a mortality of 22%, whereas those with encephalopathy had a hospital mortality of 7.5%(60).

The risk factors that are associated with neurological disorders after CPB include history of cardiac failure, diabetes, the presence of extracoronary vascular disease, difficult weaning from bypass; intraoperative mean arterial pressure levels of less than 40 mmHg, and a large drop in hemoglobin levels during surgery (61).

Along with other mechanisms, embolism has been related to neurological disorders in postoperative period and, according to size, embolus can be divided into macro (greater than 200 micrometers) or microemboli (less than 200 micrometers)(62). The clinical manifestations depends on the size of emboli and, consequently, on vessel diameter that it occludes(62). Macroembolus might result in hemiplegia, while a solitary microembolus is unlikely to have an important clinical effect, excluding very susceptible tissues (i.e. retina)(62). The microembolus may have greater clinical manifestations when they are numerous, showing a diffuse lesion in the central nervous system(62). The types of emboli are constituted of gas bubbles (air or anesthetics, in particular nitrous oxide), biologic aggregates (thrombus, platelet aggregates, and fat), inorganic debris (fragments of polyvinyl chloride tubing, and atheroembolism) (62, 63). Another mechanism implied in postoperative neurological disorder is the excitotoxicity, which involves the damage of neurons induced by excessive stimulation with neurotransmitters, in special glutamate, causing acute neuron necrosis during and immediately after the exposure and delayed-onset apoptosis(64).

Neuroprotective strategies include the prevention of: hyperthermia (>37°C) during the rewarming phase; of rapid rewarming after hypothermic CPB; of hyperglycemia; and of introduction of emboli and fat globules by cardiotomy suction(60). Regarding the aorta, the minimization of its manipulation and epiaortic scanning to detect unrecognized aortic atheroma helps to reduce atheroembolism(60). Also, arterial line filters should be used(60). No class I recommendations to minimize neuronal excitotoxicity have been proposed yet. These strategies focus on micro and macroemboli reduction and prevention of hypoperfusion and ischemia(60).

The potential neuroprotective action of volatile anesthetics is related to an increase in cerebral blood flow in ischemic regions, the suppression of seizures, reduced brain metabolism, inhibition of lactic acidosis and the release of excitatory neurotransmitters, preventing the pathological influx of Ca^{2+} and Na^{+}, inhibition of lipid peroxidation, reducing the formation of free radicals and stimulation of anti-apoptotic processes. This diversity of cited neuroprotective mechanisms resulted from studies that used different anesthetic conditions and different models of cerebral ischemia and incorporated different controls of physiological variables including brain temperature and plasma glucose. Experimental studies of hemispheric ischemia, global or incomplete demonstrated that volatile anesthetics can reduce the size of cerebral infarction and improves neurological recovery when administered before the ischemic test(65-69). This neuroprotective effect appears to be partly related to the maximal suppression of cerebral metabolism of volatile anesthetics at concentrations above 2 CAM, concentration which corrects the imbalance between supply and oxygen consumption(67). The volatile agents also decrease the frequency and increase the time onset of ischemic depolarization(70) and partially inhibit the release of lactate dehydrogenase resulting from the activity of NMDA (N-methyl-D-aspartate) and AMPA (alpha-amino-D-hydroxy-5-methyl-4-isoxazol-propionate) receptors(71).

These experimental data are consistent with clinical observations, where patients anesthetized with sevoflurane were more tolerant to reductions in cerebral blood flow during carotid endarterectomy (72). Similarly, the incidence, extent, and duration of the episodes of cerebral oxygen deprivation seem to be lower in neurosurgical patients anesthetized with volatile anesthetics.

Some intravenous anesthetics have been implicated to have neuroprotective properties. The effects of barbiturates on neuroprotection were at first attributed to the reduction in the cerebral metabolism, but recent studies have shown that this does not appear to be the sole mechanism involved(73). Although barbiturates are well-known to have neuroprotective properties, a review done with randomized or quasi randomized trials by Cochrane from December 1996 to April 1999 showed no evidences that barbiturates in severe head injury could improve outcomes(74). This review also concluded that barbiturates would cause a decrease in blood pressure that would offset the reduction in the intracranial pressure effect, and this could deteriorate the cerebral perfusion pressure(74).

Propofol has been shown to have in vitro(75) and in vivo(76) neuroprotection properties, but this profile is still controversial(77, 78). For ketamine, the widely known concept that it causes an increase in the intracranial pressure is currently under review. In mechanically ventilated head-trauma patients sedated with propofol, doses up to 5mg/kg of ketamine did not alter cerebral hemodynamics nor increased the intracranial pressure(79). As with propofol, ketamine's neuroprotective properties are still controversial.

Controlled hypothermia has also neuroprotective properties, especially after CPR. Patients under controlled hypothermia presented with better neurologic outcomes and lower mortality rates after cardiac arrest than under mild to moderate hypothermia(80-82). Close monitoring should be made in patients during controlled hypothermia due to risks of coagulopathy and bleeding, mainly after percutaneous coronary interventions, arrhythmias and electrolytes disturbances(82, 83). The association of neuroprotective intravenous anesthetics and hypothermia can have an even higher neurologic protection.

Considering the spinal cord, it is known that paraplegia is one of the most devastating complications of aortic surgery and an understanding of spinal cord perfusion has become important in the attempt to minimize the frequency of spinal cord injury(84). Monitorization of somatosensory-evoked potential, motor-evoked potential, strategies of spinal fluid drainage, distal perfusion, and specific surgical techniques in addition to the protection of hypothermia and anesthetic drugs can contribute to optimize the outcome.

4. Pulmonary protection

The changes in lung function have been reported since the first heart surgery with extracorporeal circulation(85), with a low incidence of respiratory distress syndrome and a high incidence of atelectasis . During cardiac surgery with cardiopulmonary bypass, lungs are exposed to insults of mechanical ventilation(86), ischemia-reperfusion injury, hypothermia(87), blood transfusions(88, 89) and contact of blood with non endothelized circuit and membrane oxygenator. All of these situations triggers inflammatory reaction and cause lung injury. The resultant alterations in respiratory function observed on postoperative period can prolong mechanical ventilation. Despite major advances in surgical, anesthetic techniques, and equipment for cardiopulmonary bypass, pulmonary complications, which are expressed mainly in the postoperative period, remains a great challenge and are important causes of morbidity and mortality (90, 91).

Although off-pump surgeries can reduce pulmonary changes, it doesn't avoid completely postoperative respiratory changes. Many strategies can be used to minimize or prevent lung injury related to cardiopulmonary bypass, such as (87) reduction the length of cardiopulmonary bypass, the use of miniaturized CPB circuits, heparin-coated circuits and filters can be helpful. The adequate myocardial protection, as well abbreviation of pulmonary ischemia-reperfusion, is important in the prevention of postoperative lung dysfunction. Routine use of antifibrinolytic and corticosteroids have controversial effects in the postoperative respiratory outcome.

5. Renal protection

The sensibility of kidneys to ischemic insults can culminate in acute kidney injury (AKI), more common in large surgeries and where extensive bleeding is present, especially if associated with hemodynamic instability, and is an independent risk factor for hospital mortality(92). Although acute renal failure requiring renal replacement therapy after cardiac surgery is rare, it has a devastating impact on outcome(93).

The incidence of postoperative AKI involves multifactorial mechanism, including hemodynamic, inflammatory and nephrotoxic factors(94). The risk factors for post-operative renal injury include increased intra-abdominal pressure, hyperglycemia, inadequate maintenance of the intravascular volume, the use of nephrotoxic drugs (i.e. radiologic contrast), duration of the CPB, and postoperative drugs(95). Also, the inflammatory response associated with the surgery, the formation oxygen-reactive species, and immune response can promote renal injury(96).

Some strategies have been suggested to prevent AKI in perioperative setting. Hypovolemia is attributed as an important risk factor for AKI and fluid therapy is implicated in diminishing the incidence of renal dysfunction, although no controlled randomized trial has directly addressed this issue(96). Currently, restrictive fluid replacement, based on goals rather than pre-defined values appear to reduce morbidity following colorectal surgery. One strategy based therapy is associated with the use of esophageal Doppler, using corrected flow time in the descending aorta and stroke volume response to a fluid challenge(97, 98). Intraoperative intravascular volume loading to optimize stroke volume is associated with a more rapid postoperative recovery and a reduced hospital stay(98). The recommendation for fluid resuscitation is to avoid 10% hydroxyl-ethyl starch 250/0.5, strategies for patients with risk of contrast nephropathy (listed below), prophylactic volume expansion with crystalloids to prevent AKI, especially with known nephrotoxic drugs(99). Also, based on the same Joannidis et al. recommendations, loop diuretics should not be used to prevent AKI(99).

Iodinated contrast has also been associated with AKI. Currently, N-Acetylcysteine and isotonic intravenous bicarbonate have been investigated, but the data supporting these interventions are controversial mainly due to methodological limitations(100). Atrial natriuretic peptide, statins and prostaglandin analogs are under study and there are some evidence of their benefit, but no large, adequately power study is present(100). Currently no grade IA recommendation exists regarding renal protection to iodinated contrasts. Prophylactic volume expansion without hydroxy-ethyl starch and sodium bicarbonate for emergency procedures appears to be beneficial in patients at risk of contrast nephropathy(99).

Pharmacological interventions, such as the use of fenoldopam, are currently under study, but large trials with adequate power are still needed in order to recommend the routine for prevention of renal failure. Atrial natriuretic peptide (ANP) is another drug implicated in renal protection, and low doses of ANP can provide better outcomes when used in low doses in the prevention of AKI and in the postsurgery management(96, 101). Inhalational and intravenous anesthetics can also have effects on renal protection(102). When comparing propofol and sevoflurane, propofol was associated with renal protection during an episode of ischemia and reperfusion in a swine model with lower levels of plasma creatinine(103). Also, lower neutrophil infiltrates, plasmatic cytokines, free radical production, lipid peroxidation and inducible nitric oxide synthase activity were found when propofol was used, suggesting a possible renal protection(103).

In conclusion, only a few recommendations exist regarding renal protection. Most of them are common sense based, maintaining adequate blood pressure, fluid therapy and avoiding the use of nephrotoxic drugs(99, 102).

6. Liver protection

Hepatic injury in cardiac surgery is not frequent but is associated with significant morbidity and mortality. High index of suspicion postoperatively will lead to earlier treatment directed at eliminating or minimizing ongoing hepatic injury while preventing additional metabolic stress from ischemia, hemorrhage, or sepsis(93). Protection may be conferred by modulating the perfusion protocol during bypass and pharmacological interventions which modify the inflammatory response to surgery(104).

The principle underlying the protective ischemic preconditioning is a limitation to the exposure of the liver to ischemia, thus allowing the activation of natural defense mechanisms against subsequent injury(105). Several mechanisms of injury determined by a period of ischemia followed by reperfusion are known. These mechanisms, involving cytokines and oxygen free radicals, determine both local and systemic injury(106) and the nitric oxide plays a crucial role in protection. This effect can last for a few days(107). The possibility of remote (inter organ) preconditioning is a recent observation in which brief ischemia of one organ has been shown to confer protection on distant organs, such as liver, without direct stress to the organ(108), but effective clinical use of this resource needs additional studies.

Despite many advances in preoperative evaluation, technological, pharmacological, surgical, and anesthetic techniques, cardiac surgery continues to cause major organ derangement. There are many unanswered questions regarding perioperative organ protection and many promising therapies may continue to improve postoperative outcome. Considering the evolution of anesthetic and surgical techniques, patients are currently submitted to surgery with severe diseases and extreme ages. Anesthesiologists are often faced with patients who have heart disease or hemodynamic instability. The combination of anesthetic and postoperative sedation with appropriate cardioprotective anesthetics agents may contribute to the prevention of organ dysfunction and contribute to the reduction of perioperative morbidity and mortality.

7. References

[1] Bland JH, Lowenstein E. Halothane-induced decrease in experimental myocardial ischemia in the non-failing canine heart. Anesthesiology. 1976;45(3):287-93.

[2] Freedman BM, Hamm DP, Everson CT, Wechsler AS, Christian CM, 2nd. Enflurane enhances postischemic functional recovery in the isolated rat heart. Anesthesiology. 1985;62(1):29-33.

[3] Bosnjak ZJ. Effects of volatile anesthetics on the intracellular calcium transient and calcium current in cardiac muscle cells. Adv Exp Med Biol. 1991;301:97-107.

[4] Kersten JR, Lowe D, Hettrick DA, Pagel PS, Gross GJ, Warltier DC. Glyburide, a KATP channel antagonist, attenuates the cardioprotective effects of isoflurane in stunned myocardium. Anesth Analg. 1996;83(1):27-33.

[5] Kato R, Foex P. Myocardial protection by anesthetic agents against ischemia-reperfusion injury: an update for anesthesiologists. Can J Anaesth. 2002;49(8):777-91.

[6] Mangano DT, Browner WS, Hollenberg M, Li J, Tateo IM. Long-term cardiac prognosis following noncardiac surgery. The Study of Perioperative Ischemia Research Group. Jama. 1992;268(2):233-9.

[7] Zaugg M. Perioperative organ protection. Preface. Best Pract Res Clin Anaesthesiol. 2008;22(1):vii-viii.

[8] Opie LH. Oxygen lack: ischemia and angina. In: Opie LH, editor. The Heart Physiology, from cell to ciculation. 3 ed. Philadelphia: Lippincott-Raven; 1998. p. 515-41.

[9] Opie LH. Myocardial reperfusion: new ischemic syndromes. In: Opie LH, editor. The Heart Physiology, from cell to ciculation. 3 ed. Philadelphia: Lippincott-Raven; 1998. p. 563-88.

[10] Opie LH. Myocardial stunning--we do not know the mechanism nor is there "overwhelming evidence" for a major role of free radicals. Basic Res Cardiol. 1998;93(3):152-5.

[11] Maxwell SR, Lip GY. Free radicals and antioxidants in cardiovascular disease. Br J Clin Pharmacol. 1997;44(4):307-17.

[12] Bolli R, Marban E. Molecular and cellular mechanisms of myocardial stunning. Physiol Rev. 1999;79(2):609-34.

[13] Jordan JE, Zhao ZQ, Vinten-Johansen J. The role of neutrophils in myocardial ischemia-reperfusion injury. Cardiovasc Res. 1999;43(4):860-78.

[14] Maxwell SR, Lip GY. Reperfusion injury: a review of the pathophysiology, clinical manifestations and therapeutic options. Int J Cardiol. 1997;58(2):95-117.

[15] Friedrich P. The intriguing Ca2+ requirement of calpain activation. Biochem Biophys Res Commun. 2004;323(4):1131-3.

[16] Perrin C, Ecarnot-Laubriet A, Vergely C, Rochette L. Calpain and caspase-3 inhibitors reduce infarct size and post-ischemic apoptosis in rat heart without modifying contractile recovery. Cell Mol Biol (Noisy-le-grand). 2003;49 Online Pub:OL497-505.

[17] Murry CE, Jennings RB, Reimer KA. Preconditioning with ischemia: a delay of lethal cell injury in ischemic myocardium. Circulation. 1986;74(5):1124-36.

[18] Rubino A, Yellon DM. Ischaemic preconditioning of the vasculature: an overlooked phenomenon for protecting the heart? Trends Pharmacol Sci. 2000;21(6):225-30.

[19] Schultz JJ, Hsu AK, Gross GJ. Ischemic preconditioning is mediated by a peripheral opioid receptor mechanism in the intact rat heart. J Mol Cell Cardiol. 1997;29(5):1355-62.

[20] Suleiman MS, Zacharowski K, Angelini GD. Inflammatory response and cardioprotection during open-heart surgery: the importance of anaesthetics. Br J Pharmacol. 2008;153(1):21-33.

[21] De Hert S, Vlasselaers D, Barbe R, Ory JP, Dekegel D, Donnadonni R, et al. A comparison of volatile and non volatile agents for cardioprotection during on-pump coronary surgery. Anaesthesia. 2009;64(9):953-60.

[22] Feng J, Fischer G, Lucchinetti E, Zhu M, Bestmann L, Jegger D, et al. Infarct-remodeled myocardium is receptive to protection by isoflurane postconditioning: role of protein kinase B/Akt signaling. Anesthesiology. 2006;104(5):1004-14. Epub 2006/04/29.

[23] Feng J, Lucchinetti E, Ahuja P, Pasch T, Perriard JC, Zaugg M. Isoflurane postconditioning prevents opening of the mitochondrial permeability transition pore through inhibition of glycogen synthase kinase 3beta. Anesthesiology. 2005;103(5):987-95. Epub 2005/10/27.

[24] Mayfield KP, D'Alecy LG. Role of endogenous opioid peptides in the acute adaptation to hypoxia. Brain Res. 1992;582(2):226-31.

[25] Chien S, Oeltgen PR, Diana JN, Salley RK, Su TP. Extension of tissue survival time in multiorgan block preparation with a delta opioid DADLE ([D-Ala2, D-Leu5]-enkephalin). J Thorac Cardiovasc Surg. 1994;107(3):964-7.

[26] Schultz JE, Hsu AK, Gross GJ. Morphine mimics the cardioprotective effect of ischemic preconditioning via a glibenclamide-sensitive mechanism in the rat heart. Circ Res. 1996;78(6):1100-4.

[27] Miki T, Cohen MV, Downey JM. Opioid receptor contributes to ischemic preconditioning through protein kinase C activation in rabbits. Mol Cell Biochem. 1998;186(1-2):3-12.

[28] Kato R, Ross S, Foex P. Fentanyl protects the heart against ischaemic injury via opioid receptors, adenosine A1 receptors and KATP channel linked mechanisms in rats. Br J Anaesth. 2000;84(2):204-14.

[29] Huh J, Gross GJ, Nagase H, Liang BT. Protection of cardiac myocytes via delta(1)-opioid receptors, protein kinase C, and mitochondrial K(ATP) channels. Am J Physiol Heart Circ Physiol. 2001;280(1):H377-83.

[30] Kato R, Foex P. Fentanyl reduces infarction but not stunning via delta-opioid receptors and protein kinase C in rats. Br J Anaesth. 2000;84(5):608-14.

[31] Kokita N, Hara A, Abiko Y, Arakawa J, Hashizume H, Namiki A. Propofol improves functional and metabolic recovery in ischemic reperfused isolated rat hearts. Anesth Analg. 1998;86(2):252-8.
[32] Murphy PG, Myers DS, Davies MJ, Webster NR, Jones JG. The antioxidant potential of propofol (2,6-diisopropylphenol). Br J Anaesth. 1992;68(6):613-8.
[33] Nakae Y, Fujita S, Namiki A. Propofol inhibits Ca(2+) transients but not contraction in intact beating guinea pig hearts. Anesth Analg. 2000;90(6):1286-92.
[34] De Hert SG, ten Broecke PW, Mertens E, Van Sommeren EW, De Blier IG, Stockman BA, et al. Sevoflurane but not propofol preserves myocardial function in coronary surgery patients. Anesthesiology. 2002;97(1):42-9.
[35] Xia Z, Huang Z, Ansley DM. Large-dose propofol during cardiopulmonary bypass decreases biochemical markers of myocardial injury in coronary surgery patients: a comparison with isoflurane. Anesth Analg. 2006;103(3):527-32. Epub 2006/08/26.
[36] Ko SH, Lee SK, Han YJ, Choe H, Kwak YG, Chae SW, et al. Blockade of myocardial ATP-sensitive potassium channels by ketamine. Anesthesiology. 1997;87(1):68-74.
[37] Tsutsumi Y, Oshita S, Kitahata H, Kuroda Y, Kawano T, Nakaya Y. Blockade of adenosine triphosphate-sensitive potassium channels by thiamylal in rat ventricular myocytes. Anesthesiology. 2000;92(4):1154-9.
[38] Hoar PF, Stone JG, Faltas AN, Bendixen HH, Head RJ, Berkowitz BA. Hemodynamic and adrenergic responses to anesthesia and operation for myocardial revascularization. J Thorac Cardiovasc Surg. 1980;80(2):242-8.
[39] Piriou V, Aouifi A, Lehot JJ. [Perioperative beta-blockers. Part two: therapeutic indications]. Can J Anaesth. 2000;47(7):664-72.
[40] Loick HM, Schmidt C, Van Aken H, Junker R, Erren M, Berendes E, et al. High thoracic epidural anesthesia, but not clonidine, attenuates the perioperative stress response via sympatholysis and reduces the release of troponin T in patients undergoing coronary artery bypass grafting. Anesth Analg. 1999;88(4):701-9.
[41] LaDisa JF, Jr., Krolikowski JG, Pagel PS, Warltier DC, Kersten JR. Cardioprotection by glucose-insulin-potassium: dependence on KATP channel opening and blood glucose concentration before ischemia. Am J Physiol Heart Circ Physiol. 2004;287(2):H601-7.
[42] Zhang HF, Fan Q, Qian XX, Lopez BL, Christopher TA, Ma XL, et al. Role of insulin in the anti-apoptotic effect of glucose-insulin-potassium in rabbits with acute myocardial ischemia and reperfusion. Apoptosis. 2004;9(6):777-83.
[43] Lell WA, Nielsen VG, McGiffin DC, Schmidt FE, Jr., Kirklin JK, Stanley AW, Jr. Glucose-insulin-potassium infusion for myocardial protection during off-pump coronary artery surgery. Ann Thorac Surg. 2002;73(4):1246-51; discussion 51-2.
[44] Kirno K, Friberg P, Grzegorczyk A, Milocco I, Ricksten SE, Lundin S. Thoracic epidural anesthesia during coronary artery bypass surgery: effects on cardiac sympathetic activity, myocardial blood flow and metabolism, and central hemodynamics. Anesth Analg. 1994;79(6):1075-81.
[45] Gramling-Babb PM, Zile MR, Reeves ST. Preliminary report on high thoracic epidural analgesia: relationship between its therapeutic effects and myocardial blood flow as assessed by stress thallium distribution. J Cardiothorac Vasc Anesth. 2000;14(6):657-61.

[46] Scott NB, Turfrey DJ, Ray DA, Nzewi O, Sutcliffe NP, Lal AB, et al. A prospective randomized study of the potential benefits of thoracic epidural anesthesia and analgesia in patients undergoing coronary artery bypass grafting. Anesth Analg. 2001;93(3):528-35.
[47] Liu SS, Block BM, Wu CL. Effects of perioperative central neuraxial analgesia on outcome after coronary artery bypass surgery: a meta-analysis. Anesthesiology. 2004;101(1):153-61.
[48] Caputo M, Alwair H, Rogers CA, Pike K, Cohen A, Monk C, et al. Thoracic epidural anesthesia improves early outcomes in patients undergoing off-pump coronary artery bypass surgery: a prospective, randomized, controlled trial. Anesthesiology. 2011;114(2):380-90. Epub 2011/01/20.
[49] Karthik S, Grayson AD, Oo AY, Fabri BM. A survey of current myocardial protection practices during coronary artery bypass grafting. Ann R Coll Surg Engl. 2004;86(6):413-5.
[50] Fremes SE, Christakis GT, Weisel RD, Mickle DA, Madonik MM, Ivanov J, et al. A clinical trial of blood and crystalloid cardioplegia. J Thorac Cardiovasc Surg. 1984;88(5 Pt 1):726-41.
[51] Nicolini F, Beghi C, Muscari C, Agostinelli A, Maria Budillon A, Spaggiari I, et al. Myocardial protection in adult cardiac surgery: current options and future challenges. Eur J Cardiothorac Surg. 2003;24(6):986-93.
[52] Hayashida N, Weisel RD, Shirai T, Ikonomidis JS, Ivanov J, Carson SM, et al. Tepid antegrade and retrograde cardioplegia. Ann Thorac Surg. 1995;59(3):723-9.
[53] Bigelow WG, Lindsay WK, Greenwood WF. Hypothermia; its possible role in cardiac surgery: an investigation of factors governing survival in dogs at low body temperatures. Ann Surg. 1950;132(5):849-66.
[54] Niazi SA, Lewis FJ. Effects of carbon dioxide on ventricular fibrillation and heart block during hypothermia in rats and dogs. S Forum. 1955;5:106-9.
[55] Hale SL, Kloner RA. Myocardial temperature in acute myocardial infarction: protection with mild regional hypothermia. Am J Physiol. 1997;273(1 Pt 2):H220-7.
[56] Kumar K, Wu X, Evans AT, Marcoux F. The effect of hypothermia on induction of heat shock protein (HSP)-72 in ischemic brain. Metab Brain Dis. 1995;10(4):283-91.
[57] Valeri CR, MacGregor H, Cassidy G, Tinney R, Pompei F. Effects of temperature on bleeding time and clotting time in normal male and female volunteers. Crit Care Med. 1995;23(4):698-704.
[58] Hogue CW, Jr., Palin CA, Arrowsmith JE. Cardiopulmonary bypass management and neurologic outcomes: an evidence-based appraisal of current practices. Anesth Analg. 2006;103(1):21-37. Epub 2006/06/23.
[59] Roach GW, Kanchuger M, Mangano CM, Newman M, Nussmeier N, Wolman R, et al. Adverse cerebral outcomes after coronary bypass surgery. Multicenter Study of Perioperative Ischemia Research Group and the Ischemia Research and Education Foundation Investigators. N Engl J Med. 1996;335(25):1857-63. Epub 1996/12/19.
[60] Baumgartner WA. Neuroprotection in cardiac surgery. Ann Thorac Surg. 2005;79(6):S2254-6. Epub 2005/05/28.

[61] Shaw PJ, Bates D, Cartlidge NE, French JM, Heaviside D, Julian DG, et al. An analysis of factors predisposing to neurological injury in patients undergoing coronary bypass operations. Q J Med. 1989;72(267):633-46. Epub 1989/07/01.
[62] Blauth CI. Macroemboli and microemboli during cardiopulmonary bypass. Ann Thorac Surg. 1995;59(5):1300-3. Epub 1995/05/01.
[63] Blauth CI, Cosgrove DM, Webb BW, Ratliff NB, Boylan M, Piedmonte MR, et al. Atheroembolism from the ascending aorta. An emerging problem in cardiac surgery. J Thorac Cardiovasc Surg. 1992;103(6):1104-11; discussion 11-2. Epub 1992/06/01.
[64] Ankarcrona M, Dypbukt JM, Bonfoco E, Zhivotovsky B, Orrenius S, Lipton SA, et al. Glutamate-induced neuronal death: a succession of necrosis or apoptosis depending on mitochondrial function. Neuron. 1995;15(4):961-73. Epub 1995/10/01.
[65] Engelhard K, Werner C, Reeker W, Lu H, Mollenberg O, Mielke L, et al. Desflurane and isoflurane improve neurological outcome after incomplete cerebral ischaemia in rats. Br J Anaesth. 1999;83(3):415-21.
[66] Miura Y, Grocott HP, Bart RD, Pearlstein RD, Dexter F, Warner DS. Differential effects of anesthetic agents on outcome from near-complete but not incomplete global ischemia in the rat. Anesthesiology. 1998;89(2):391-400.
[67] Nellgard B, Mackensen GB, Pineda J, Wellons JC, 3rd, Pearlstein RD, Warner DS. Anesthetic effects on cerebral metabolic rate predict histologic outcome from near-complete forebrain ischemia in the rat. Anesthesiology. 2000;93(2):431-6.
[68] Soonthon-Brant V, Patel PM, Drummond JC, Cole DJ, Kelly PJ, Watson M. Fentanyl does not increase brain injury after focal cerebral ischemia in rats. Anesth Analg. 1999;88(1):49-55.
[69] Werner C, Mollenberg O, Kochs E, Schulte JaE. Sevoflurane improves neurological outcome after incomplete cerebral ischaemia in rats. Br J Anaesth. 1995;75(6):756-60.
[70] Patel PM, Drummond JC, Cole DJ, Kelly PJ, Watson M. Isoflurane and pentobarbital reduce the frequency of transient ischemic depolarizations during focal ischemia in rats. Anesth Analg. 1998;86(4):773-80.
[71] Kimbro JR, Kelly PJ, Drummond JC, Cole DJ, Patel PM. Isoflurane and pentobarbital reduce AMPA toxicity in vivo in the rat cerebral cortex. Anesthesiology. 2000;92(3):806-12.
[72] Grady RE, Weglinski MR, Sharbrough FW, Perkins WJ. Correlation of regional cerebral blood flow with ischemic electroencephalographic changes during sevoflurane-nitrous oxide anesthesia for carotid endarterectomy. Anesthesiology. 1998;88(4):892-7.
[73] Kawaguchi M, Furuya H, Patel PM. Neuroprotective effects of anesthetic agents. J Anesth. 2005;19(2):150-6. Epub 2005/05/06.
[74] Roberts I. Barbiturates for acute traumatic brain injury. Cochrane Database Syst Rev. 2000(2):CD000033. Epub 2000/05/05.
[75] Rossaint J, Rossaint R, Weis J, Fries M, Rex S, Coburn M. Propofol: neuroprotection in an in vitro model of traumatic brain injury. Crit Care. 2009;13(2):R61. Epub 2009/04/29.

[76] Engelhard K, Werner C, Eberspacher E, Pape M, Stegemann U, Kellermann K, et al. Influence of propofol on neuronal damage and apoptotic factors after incomplete cerebral ischemia and reperfusion in rats: a long-term observation. Anesthesiology. 2004;101(4):912-7. Epub 2004/09/28.
[77] Tsai YC, Huang SJ, Lai YY, Chang CL, Cheng JT. Propofol does not reduce infarct volume in rats undergoing permanent middle cerebral artery occlusion. Acta Anaesthesiol Sin. 1994;32(2):99-104. Epub 1994/06/01.
[78] Zhu H, Cottrell JE, Kass IS. The effect of thiopental and propofol on NMDA- and AMPA-mediated glutamate excitotoxicity. Anesthesiology. 1997;87(4):944-51. Epub 1997/11/14.
[79] Albanese J, Arnaud S, Rey M, Thomachot L, Alliez B, Martin C. Ketamine decreases intracranial pressure and electroencephalographic activity in traumatic brain injury patients during propofol sedation. Anesthesiology. 1997;87(6):1328-34. Epub 1998/01/07.
[80] Mild therapeutic hypothermia to improve the neurologic outcome after cardiac arrest. N Engl J Med. 2002;346(8):549-56. Epub 2002/02/22.
[81] Bernard SA, Gray TW, Buist MD, Jones BM, Silvester W, Gutteridge G, et al. Treatment of comatose survivors of out-of-hospital cardiac arrest with induced hypothermia. N Engl J Med. 2002;346(8):557-63. Epub 2002/02/22.
[82] Peberdy MA, Callaway CW, Neumar RW, Geocadin RG, Zimmerman JL, Donnino M, et al. Part 9: post-cardiac arrest care: 2010 American Heart Association Guidelines for Cardiopulmonary Resuscitation and Emergency Cardiovascular Care. Circulation. 2010;122(18 Suppl 3):S768-86. Epub 2010/10/22.
[83] Nielsen N, Hovdenes J, Nilsson F, Rubertsson S, Stammet P, Sunde K, et al. Outcome, timing and adverse events in therapeutic hypothermia after out-of-hospital cardiac arrest. Acta Anaesthesiol Scand. 2009;53(7):926-34. Epub 2009/06/25.
[84] Griepp RB, Griepp EB. Spinal cord perfusion and protection during descending thoracic and thoracoabdominal aortic surgery: the collateral network concept. The Annals of thoracic surgery. 2007;83(2):S865-9; discussion S90-2.
[85] Nahas RA, Melrose DG, Sykes MK, Robinson B. Post-Perfusion Lung Syndrome: Role of Circulatory Exclusion. Lancet. 1965;2(7406):251-4.
[86] Zupancich E, Paparella D, Turani F, Munch C, Rossi A, Massaccesi S, et al. Mechanical ventilation affects inflammatory mediators in patients undergoing cardiopulmonary bypass for cardiac surgery: a randomized clinical trial. The Journal of thoracic and cardiovascular surgery. 2005;130(2):378-83.
[87] Apostolakis EE, Koletsis EN, Baikoussis NG, Siminelakis SN, Papadopoulos GS. Strategies to prevent intraoperative lung injury during cardiopulmonary bypass. Journal of cardiothoracic surgery.5:1.
[88] Koch C, Li L, Figueroa P, Mihaljevic T, Svensson L, Blackstone EH. Transfusion and pulmonary morbidity after cardiac surgery. The Annals of thoracic surgery. 2009;88(5):1410-8.
[89] Triulzi DJ. Transfusion-related acute lung injury: current concepts for the clinician. Anesthesia and analgesia. 2009;108(3):770-6.

[90] Hammermeister KE, Burchfiel C, Johnson R, Grover FL. Identification of patients at greatest risk for developing major complications at cardiac surgery. Circulation. 1990;82(5 Suppl):IV380-9.

[91] Mangano DT. Myocardial ischemia following surgery: preliminary findings. Study of Perioperative Ischemia (SPI) Research Group. J Card Surg. 1990;5(3 Suppl):288-93.

[92] Abelha FJ, Botelho M, Fernandes V, Barros H. Determinants of postoperative acute kidney injury. Crit Care. 2009;13(3):R79. Epub 2009/05/26.

[93] Diaz GC, Moitra V, Sladen RN. Hepatic and renal protection during cardiac surgery. Anesthesiology clinics. 2008;26(3):565-90.

[94] Rosner MH, Portilla D, Okusa MD. Cardiac surgery as a cause of acute kidney injury: pathogenesis and potential therapies. Journal of intensive care medicine. 2008;23(1):3-18.

[95] Reddy VG. Prevention of postoperative acute renal failure. J Postgrad Med. 2002;48(1):64-70. Epub 2002/06/26.

[96] Brienza N, Giglio MT, Marucci M. Preventing acute kidney injury after noncardiac surgery. Curr Opin Crit Care. 2010;16(4):353-8. Epub 2010/07/06.

[97] Chytra I, Pradl R, Bosman R, Pelnar P, Kasal E, Zidkova A. Esophageal Doppler-guided fluid management decreases blood lactate levels in multiple-trauma patients: a randomized controlled trial. Crit Care. 2007;11(1):R24. Epub 2007/02/23.

[98] Sinclair S, James S, Singer M. Intraoperative intravascular volume optimisation and length of hospital stay after repair of proximal femoral fracture: randomised controlled trial. BMJ. 1997;315(7113):909-12. Epub 1997/11/15.

[99] Joannidis M, Druml W, Forni LG, Groeneveld AB, Honore P, Oudemans-van Straaten HM, et al. Prevention of acute kidney injury and protection of renal function in the intensive care unit. Expert opinion of the Working Group for Nephrology, ESICM. Intensive Care Med. 2010;36(3):392-411. Epub 2009/11/19.

[100] Weisbord SD, Palevsky PM. Strategies for the prevention of contrast-induced acute kidney injury. Curr Opin Nephrol Hypertens. 2010;19(6):539-49. Epub 2010/07/14.

[101] Nigwekar SU, Navaneethan SD, Parikh CR, Hix JK. Atrial natriuretic peptide for preventing and treating acute kidney injury. Cochrane Database Syst Rev. 2009(4):CD006028. Epub 2009/10/13.

[102] Stafford-Smith M. Evidence-based renal protection in cardiac surgery. Seminars in cardiothoracic and vascular anesthesia. 2005;9(1):65-76.

[103] Rodriguez-Lopez JM, Sanchez-Conde P, Lozano FS, Nicolas JL, Garcia-Criado FJ, Cascajo C, et al. Laboratory investigation: effects of propofol on the systemic inflammatory response during aortic surgery. Can J Anaesth. 2006;53(7):701-10. Epub 2006/06/29.

[104] Ohri SK, Velissaris T. Gastrointestinal dysfunction following cardiac surgery. Perfusion. 2006;21(4):215-23.

[105] Peralta C, Bulbena O, Xaus C, Prats N, Cutrin JC, Poli G, et al. Ischemic preconditioning: a defense mechanism against the reactive oxygen species generated after hepatic ischemia reperfusion. Transplantation. 2002;73(8):1203-11.

[106] Koti RS, Seifalian AM, Davidson BR. Protection of the liver by ischemic preconditioning: a review of mechanisms and clinical applications. Dig Surg. 2003;20(5):383-96.

[107] Banga NR, Homer-Vanniasinkam S, Graham A, Al-Mukhtar A, White SA, Prasad KR. Ischaemic preconditioning in transplantation and major resection of the liver. Br J Surg. 2005;92(5):528-38.

[108] Tapuria N, Kumar Y, Habib MM, Abu Amara M, Seifalian AM, Davidson BR. Remote ischemic preconditioning: a novel protective method from ischemia reperfusion injury--a review. The Journal of surgical research. 2008;150(2):304-30.

5

Perioperative Management of Pulmonary Hypertension

Theofani Antoniou[1] and Kassiani Theodoraki[2]
[1]*Onassis Cardiac Surgery Center, Athens*
[2]*Areteion University Hospital,*
University of Athens School of Medicine, Athens
Greece

1. Introduction

Pulmonary hypertension (PH) was first described over 100 years ago, but a thorough understanding of its pathogenesis and a successful approach to curing the disease still remain under investigation.

Advanced research in the field of PH has enhanced our understanding of this entity and has led to new therapies. PH is rare but can affect people of all ages and is associated with several seemingly unconnected diseases.

2. Definition

PH refers to increased pressure in the arterial site of the pulmonary circulation and is defined as persistent elevation of mean pulmonary arterial pressure (MPAP) above 25 mmHg.

The current hemodynamic definition of PH is described in **Table 1**. The first clinical classification of PH was proposed at the first international conference on primary pulmonary hypertension endorsed by the World Health Organization (Hatano & Strassert, 1975). The previous version of the European Society of Cardiology (ESC) PH guidelines adopted the Evian-Venice classification proposed at the second and third World meeting on PH in 1998 and 2003 respectively (Galiè et al., 2004). According to these classifications, clinical conditions associated with PH are divided in five groups according to pathological, pathophysiological and therapeutic characteristics. During the fourth World symposium on PH held in Dana Point, California, the consensus agreement of experts worldwide was to maintain the general philosophy and organization endorsed by the Evian-Venice classifications while at the same time amending some specific points so as to improve clarity and to take into account new information (Galiè et al., 2009). Accordingly, PH can be classified into six clinical groups with specific characteristics (**Table 2**).

Anesthesiologists encounter patients with PH in a variety of situations in the operating room (Tidswell & Higgins, 2007). The most common underlying pathology of cardiac surgery patients which leads to PH is due to left-sided valvular heart disease, left-sided ventricular heart disease and shear stress from increased pulmonary blood flow due to intracardiac shunts.

Definition	Characteristics	Clinical group(s)
PH	MPAP ≥25 mmHg	All
Pre-capillary PH	MPAP ≥25 mmHg PCWP ≤15 mmHg CO normal or reduced	1. Pulmonary arterial hypertension 3. PH due to lung diseases 4. Chronic thromboembolic pulmonary hypertension 5. PH with unclear and-or multifactorial mechanisms
Post-capillary PH	MPAP ≥25 mmHg PCWP >15 mmHg CO normal or reduced	2. PH due to left heart disease
Passive	TPG ≤12 mmHg	
Reactive (out of proportion)	TPG >12 mmHg	

Table 1. Hemodynamic definition of pulmonary arterial hypertension.
CO, cardiac output; MPAP, mean pulmonary arterial pressure; PH, pulmonary hypertension; PCWP, pulmonary capillary wedge pressure; TPG, transpulmonary pressure gradient (MPAP-PCWP)

Data from the multinational database EuroSCORE have demonstrated that PH is an independent risk factor for increased morbidity and mortality in patients undergoing heart surgery (Roques et al., 1999).

3. Pathophysiology

Highlighting the pathophysiology of PH can help us properly manage acute PH in the specific context of cardiac surgery.

The cause of PH in the case of mitral or aortic valve disease, especially when PH is a complication of stenotic valve disease, is quite complex. Increased left arterial pressures result in chronic obstruction to venous drainage in the pulmonary vasculature, causing remodeling of the pulmonary vascular bed and ultimately PH.

The molecular pathophysiological mechanism of PH has been recently reviewed. The PH 'phenotype' is characterized by endothelial dysfunction, a decrease ratio of apoptosis / proliferation in the pulmonary artery muscle cells and a thickened disordered adventitia in which there is excessive activation of adventitial metalloproteases (McLaughlin et al., 2009).

The fundamental functions of the endothelium include: regulating the vascular tone, coordinating vascular cell growth, controlling inflammatory and immunological processes as well as maintaining the balance between thrombotic and fibrotic activities. Each of these functions is controlled by a finely tuned network of activating and inhibiting compounds.

In the case of PH, the endothelium is characterized by increased production of vasoconstrictor / mitogenic mediators, such as endothelin and thromboxane, and deficient

1. Pulmonary arterial hypertension (PAH)
- 1.1 Idiopathic
- 1.2 Heritable
  - 1.2.1 BMPR2
  - 1.2.2 ALK1, endoglin (with or without hereditary hemorrhagic telangiectasia)
  - 1.2.3 Unknown
- 1.3 Drugs and toxins induced
- 1.4 Associated with
  - 1.4.1 Connective tissue diseases
  - 1.4.2 HIV infection
  - 1.4.3 Portal hypertension
  - 1.4.4 Congenital heart disease
  - 1.4.5 Schistosomiasis
  - 1.4.6 Chronic hemolytic anemia
- 1.5 Persistent pulmonary hypertension of the newborn

1a. Pulmonary venoocclusive disease and-or pulmonary capillary hemangiomatosis

2. Pulmonary hypertension due to left heart disease
- 2.1 Systolic dysfunction
- 2.2 Diastolic dysfunction
- 2.3 Valvular disease

3. Pulmonary hypertension due to lung diseases and/or hypoxia
- 3.1 Chronic obstructive pulmonary disease
- 3.2 Interstitial lung disease
- 3.3 Other pulmonary diseases with mixed restrictive and obstructive pattern
- 3.4 Sleep-disordered breathing
- 3.5 Alveolar hypoventilation disorders
- 3.6 Chronic exposure to high altitude
- 3.7 Developmental abnormalities

4. Chronic thromboembolic pulmonary hypertension

5. Pulmonary hypertension with unclear and-or multifactorial mechanisms
- 5.1 Hematological disorders: myeloproliferative disorders, splenectomy
- 5.2 Systemic disorders: sarcoidosis, pulmonary Langerhans cell histiocytosis, lymphangioleiomyomatosis, neurofibromatosis, vasculitis
- 5.3 Metabolic disorders: glycogen storage disease, Gaucher disease, thyroid disorders
- 5.4 Others: Tumoural obstruction, fibrosing mediastinitis, chronic renal failure on dialysis

Table 2. Updated clinical classification of pulmonary hypertension (Dana Point, 2008). *ALK-1, activin receptor-like kinase 1 gene; BMPR2, bone morphogenetic protein receptor, type 2; HIV, human immunodeficiency virus*

production of vasodilators, such as prostacyclin (Christman et al., 1992; Giaid et al., 1993; Stewart et al., 1991). Elevated levels of fibrinopeptide A and plasminogen activator inhibitor-1 and reduced levels of tissue plasminogen activator contribute to a procoagulant state. Endothelial injury may also expose the underlying smooth muscle cells to circulating mitogens and growth factors that stimulate cell proliferation.

The so-called endothelium-dependent mechanism is that receptors located on the surface of the endothelial cells react to various stimulators or mediators and subsequently change signals. Via a cascade of reactions, the presence of shearing forces or mediators such as bradykinine and acetylcholine leads to the formation of so-called second messenger substances such as cyclic adenosine monophosphate (cAMP) or guanosine monophosphate (cGMP). These substances exert vasodilator effects and are responsible for smooth muscle relaxation.

Nitric oxide (NO) is a vasodilator and inhibitor of platelet activation and vascular smooth muscle proliferation. The effects of NO are mediated by cGMP, which is rapidly inactivated by phosphodiesterase.

Vascular dilatation occurs via the NO-triggered proliferation of endothelial-dependent hyperpolarizing factors which, through the activation of tension dependent potassium channels leads to relaxation of the smooth muscle cell. NO leads to an increase in the production of prostacyclin. Other potassium channels (ATP-dependent, Ca++ - dependent) are also involved in the regulation of the myosin-actin-calcium interaction.

On the contrary, hypoxia or specific mediators (e.g. thrombin, metabolites of arachidonic acid, angiotensin II and endothelin) lead to vasoconstriction. They also function through signal transduction via various receptors on the endothelial cells themselves or on the smooth muscle cells.

Prostacyclin and thromboxane A_2 are major arachidonic acid metabolites. Prostacyclin is a potent vasodilator, inhibits platelet activation and has antiproliferation properties, whereas thromboxane A_2 promotes proliferation and platelet activation In PH, the balance between the two molecules is shifted towards thromboxane A_2.

Endothelin-1 (ET-1) is a potent vasoconstrictor produced by endothelial cells, which exerts potent vasoactive properties by binding to specific receptors (ET_A and ET_B) on vascular endothelial and smooth muscle cells. Following the bonding of ET-1 to the ET_A receptor, phospholipase C is activated which consecutively leads to the accumulation of inositol-triphosphates and intracellular calcium. Through this mechanism, vasoconstriction as well as cell proliferation take place in various tissues. Activation of the ET_B receptor upon the endothelial cells not only leads to the release of NO and prostacyclin and consequence vasodilatation, but also inhibits expression of the endothelin converting enzyme upon endothelial cell and apoptosis. Pulmonary clearance of circulating ET-1 as well as its reentrance into the endothelial cells is also regulated via these receptors.

Serotonin (5-hydroxytryptamine, 5-HT) (Jain et al., 2007) is a pulmonary vasoconstrictor and promotes pulmonary artery smooth muscle cells hypertrophy and hyperplasia. There is a transporter for 5-HT that controls serotonin uptake and clearance, which is located on the surface of platelets, neurons, and pulmonary endothelial cells. The presence of elevated levels of 5-HT in the blood of patients with PH suggests that this substance also plays a role in the pathogenesis of PH.

In summary, PH can simply be explained as a functional disturbance of the endothelium, caused by an imbalance between the dilative and contractive mechanisms within the vascular resistance of the pulmonary vascular bed. These functional changes occur together with morphological alterations within the pulmonary vasculature.

Thus, NO, endothelin and prostacyclin also have a direct influence upon the thrombocytes, the endothelial-leukocyte interaction as well as vascular cell proliferation. This imbalance leads to thrombotic tendency, vasoconstriction and proliferation.

3.1 Pathophysiology of post bypass exacerbation of PH

Post bypass pulmonary vasoconstriction has been demonstrated in a variety of experimental models as well as in the clinical setting and there is increased evidence that the severity of the vasoconstriction correlates with the extent of cardiopulmonary bypass (CPB)-induced endothelial injury (Riedel, 1999).

Endothelial injury and dysfunction is promoted by acidosis, hypoxia, shear stress from increased pulmonary blood flow (left-to-right intracardiac shunts), and fibrin from thromboembolism. Leukocyte activation, oxygen free radicals such as superoxide, hydroxyl radicals and peroxynitrate, tumor necrosis factor α, interleukin-1, elastases and inflammatory mediators are involved in this process.

The most important mechanism underlying this endothelial dysfunction in the setting of cardiac surgery could be ischemia/reperfusion injury, with associated inflammatory cell and complement activation. Ischemia/reperfusion injury due to inadequate flow in the bronchial circulation plays a pivotal role in the exacerbation of post-CPB PH (Matuschak, 1999).

In summary, intraoperative pulmonary vasoconstriction is a result of complex interactions between various perioperative factors: *preoperative status* of the pulmonary vascular bed (valvular pathology, shear stress), *intraoperative vasospastic stimuli* (hypoxia, hypercarbia, acidosis, ischemia/reperfusion injury, inflammatory mediators, free radical formation, pulmonary leukosequestration, excess thromboxane or endothelin production and microemboli) and *postoperative factors* (atelectasis, adrenergic tone, hypoxic pulmonary vasoconstriction). Preexisting pulmonary hypertension, increased pulmonary blood flow states, in combination with intraoperative hypoxia, acidosis, hypothermia, and microembolism may exacerbate CPB-induced pulmonary hypertension.

The final result of this pathophysiology is the imbalance between vasoconstrictor and vasodilator factors at the pulmonary vascular bed, that is reduction in prostacyclin (PGI_2) and NO levels and an increase in thromboxane A_2, catecholamines, adhesion molecules and endothelin levels.

This can culminate to a life- threatening situation and disconnecting the patient from the extracorporeal circulation may prove particularly laborious, because of right ventricular failure.

Moreover, after discontinuation from bypass there is need for heparin reversal and this is accomplished by the administration of protamine. Protamine administration is commonly associated with hypotension due to systemic vasodilatation. This is suggested to be mediated by the release of NO (Raikar, 1996). A rare reaction brought about by protamine administration, which may be mediated by the release of complement pathway anaphylatoxins (C3a and C5b) and / or cyclooxygenase products (e.g. thromboxane A_2), may lead to catastrophic pulmonary hypertension and subsequent right ventricular failure.

4. Clinical impact of post bypass exacerbation of PH

Independent of the exact cause, the exacerbation of preexisting PH can lead to a further increase in the right ventricular afterload and distension of an already dysfunctional right ventricle, resulting in increased right ventricular free wall tension and myocardial oxygen consumption.

Normally, the pulmonary circulation is a low pressure, high flow vascular bed accommodating the entire cardiac output with each heartbeat. Elevated pulmonary vascular resistance (PVR) may significantly contribute to right ventricular dysfunction, which may compromise the preload of the left ventricle inducing systemic hypotension. In patients with pathologically increased PVR, the right ventricle and left ventricle are interdependent and have similar vitally important functions. Right ventricular dilatation causes shifting of the intraventricular septum towards the left ventricle, leading to a smaller underfilled left ventricular cavity. The normal thin walls and crescent shape of the right ventricle result in a highly compliant right ventricular chamber, which is able to accommodate large increases in volume. However, the right ventricular adaptive mechanisms are not well suited to acute, large increases in pressure, (Fischer et al., 2003), as this may happen after CPB.

Furthermore systemic hypotension decreases right ventricular coronary perfusion pressure and oxygen delivery. Therefore, a vicious circle starts that can lead to exacerbation of right ventricular dysfunction.

5. Diagnosis of PH

The existence of sophisticated monitoring in this particular group of patients is deemed necessary because early diagnosis and prompt institution of therapy for acute PH is required in order to prevent right ventricular failure.

Diagnosis is aided by awareness of existing preoperative risk factors, such as valvular pathology or intracardiac shunts that are associated with PH. The development of acute PH will result in clinical signs of relatively rapid onset relating to the development of tricuspid regurgitation: prominent central venous atrioventricular pulsatile pressure waveforms, right-sided heart failure and a holosystolic murmur at the lower border of the sternum that increases in intensity during inspiration.

Pulmonary artery pressure catheterization and transesophageal echocardiography (TOE) constitute a valid monitoring tool for early detection of acute PH.

Pulmonary artery pressure catheterization will demonstrate elevated right atrial pressure, right ventricular end-diastolic pressure and pulmonary artery pressure with normal or low pulmonary wedge pressures. In the case of right ventricular dysfunction without pulmonary vasoconstriction, the pulmonary artery pressure may also be normal. Hemodynamic parameters calculated and derived by thermodilution will reflect elevated PVR and a reduction in right ventricular stroke work index and right ventricular stroke work index / central venous pressure relationship and a reduction in cardiac output or right ventricular ejection fraction.

TOE is an invaluable tool in the diagnosis of PH and right ventricular dysfunction, demonstrating both right ventricular volume and pressure overload. The two- dimension mode provides a subjective view of the increased ratio of right ventricle-to- left ventricle chamber size, paradoxical septal bulging, and deterioration in right ventricular function as seen on five-chamber and 4-chamber long axis views (Figure 1).

Color flow mapping will often reveal pulmonary and tricuspid regurgitation. The use of continuous wave Doppler across the regurgitant tricuspid valve allows quantification of the

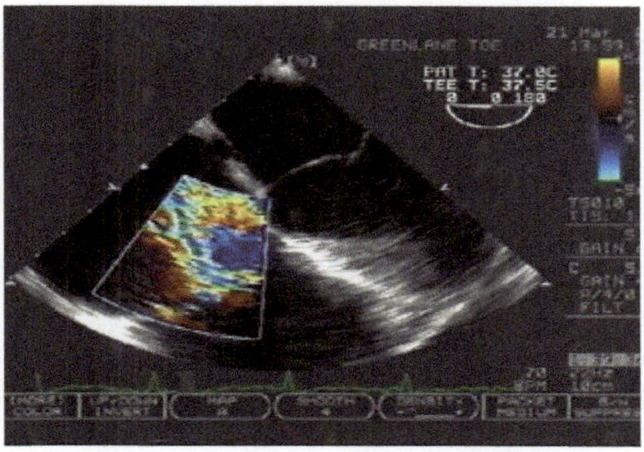

Fig. 1. Severe tricuspid regurgitation and enlargement of the right ventricle caused by severe pulmonary hypertension

pressure gradient across the valve and thereby an estimation of the pulmonary artery pressure.

Also TOE has been proved to be a useful tool in the continuous assessment of the results of the applied therapeutic strategy.

6. Treatment of PH

Therapeutic strategies should be aimed at the prevention of acute perioperative PH or at the prevention of further increases in the already existing PH. The cornerstone of treatment lies in prevention of right ventricular failure brought about by the abrupt increase of right ventricular afterload, since impaired RV function is associated with poor outcome in the surgical and non-surgical setting.

It is important to underline that the treatment of perioperative PH in cardiac surgery patients should start as promptly as possible. If clinicians do not react early, a vicious circle may start and the discontinuation from CPB may prove extremely difficult. Right ventricular failure and low cardiac output can occur several hours after weaning from CPB, so a high level of vigilance is required during the entire postoperative period.

The incidence of postoperative acute refractory right ventricular failure is only about 0.1% after cardiotomy, but this can rise to around 2-3% after heart transplantation and even to 20-30% when a left ventricular assist device has been implanted (Kaul & Fields, 2000).

The appropriate treatment in order to prevent right ventricular failure is based on the following principles (Winterhalter et al., 2010):

- Avoidance of factors that are well known to exacerbate PH, such as hypoxemia, hypercarbia, acidosis, hypervolemia, hypothermia, and light anesthesia.
- Optimization of right ventricular preload: If the right atrial pressure is low, volume infusion is indicated. If it is high, diuretics and nitroglycerin are preferable.
- Improvement of right ventricular contractility: The administration of inotropes, such as epinephrine, dobutamine or the phosphodiesterase-3-inhibitor milrinone may be useful to raise right ventricular contractility.
- Minimization of right ventricular afterload: This can be accomplished by different strategies. The use of intravenously or inhalable vasodilators such as milrinone, nitroprusside, NO or the stable prostacyclin analogue iloprost can be administered.

Readministration of heparin and postoperative reinstitution of CPB may be necessary in refractory cases.

6.1 Intravenous vasodilators

The main goal of pulmonary vasodilatation is to lower right ventricular impedance, so as to decrease afterload and thus improve ventricular performance.

Traditional methods of treatment for perioperative PH included nitrates, prostaglandins, phospodiesterase -3 inhibitors and calcium channel blockers. The aforementioned therapeutic modalities represent three distinct pharmacological pathways.

Nitrates (sodium nitroprusside-SNP, nitroglycerin-NTG) are NO donors, releasing NO spontaneously, which is normally located in biological tissues. Both agents decrease PVR, but because of their nonselectivity, they often decrease systemic blood pressure to a degree that impairs right ventricular perfusion and can cause ischemia.

Normally, the right ventricle is perfused during the entire cardiac cycle. In the presence of PH, the hypertrophic right ventricle generates elevated intracavital and intramural pressures, limiting the period of perfusion predominantly to diastole, thereby increasing the risk of right ventricular ischemia and failure in the presence of systemic hypotension. Therefore, nitrates can compromise right ventricular perfusion through their hypotensive action in the arterial part of the circulation. Furthermore, these drugs increase venous admixture by dilatation of pulmonary vessels supplying poorly ventilated alveoli and therefore abolishing the protective effect of hypoxic pulmonary vasoconstriction.

Prostacyclins (prostacyclin PGI_2, prostaglandin-E_1 PGE_1) have been reported to have beneficial effects on pulmonary artery pressure and right ventricular function perioperatively. They act by stimulating adenylate cyclase to generate cAMP, but they also act non-selectively when administered intravenously and systemic hypotension limits their clinical effectiveness.

Phosphodiesterase-3 inhibitors (whose milrinone is the major representative) cause vasodilatation via inhibition of enzyme phosphodiesterase-3, increasing cAMP, which causes vasodilatation.

Calcium channel blockers also induce systemic vasodilatation but without sparing the systemic circulation.

Due the lack of selectivity to the pulmonary circulation of the aforementioned agents and the risk of a massive drop in the systemic blood pressure and right ventricular perfusion pressure, their administration should be avoided (Kieler-Jensen et al., 1993).

On the other hand, the importance of inhalable vasodilators has risen continuously over recent years. The advantage of these inhalable substances is their pulmonary selectivity and the subsequent reduction of systemic side effects, such as systemic hypotension. Also, the probability of ventilation-perfusion mismatch is low, as by inhalation primarily blood vessels close to the ventilated alveoli are dilated. The risks of shunt development and severe hypoxia are thus eliminated (Walmrath et al., 1997).

6.2 Inhalable vasodilators

The administration of inhalable pulmonary vasodilators, such as inhaled nitric oxide (NO), prostaglandins, NO donors (SNP-NTG) and milrinone is preferable over intravenous agents because of their pulmonary selectivity which is exerted without a concurrent increase in shunt fraction.

Inhaled NO: NO stimulates soluble guanylate cyclase (sGC) and increases cGMP. The latter activates cGMP- dependent protein kinases that are abundant in the cerebellum, smooth and cardiac myocytes, platelets, and leukocytes (Lucas et al., 2000). In turn, these kinases mediate a cGMP-induced decrease in intracellular calcium concentration in vascular smooth muscle and vasodilatation (Hanafy et al., 2001).

Inhaled NO is a selective pulmonary vasodilator without clinically significant effect on blood pressure and cardiac output. Its selective action results from the fixation of NO to the heme moiety of the hemoglobin molecule after passing through the pulmonary vessel wall. NO is then oxidized to nitrogen dioxide (NO_2) and nitrogen trioxide (NO_3). Hemoglobin is transformed to methemoglobin, which is secondarily reduced to hemoglobin by methemoglobin reductase. Although NO has no systemic hemodynamic effects, it does have extrapulmonary activity (Wang et al., 2003). That is, it interferes with platelet and leukocyte functions, fibrinolysis, and reperfusion injury by inhibiting expression of adhesion molecules at leukocyte surfaces and by activation of sCG, which lead to a rapid increase in platelet cGMP and inhibition of platelet aggregation. NO-induced favorable effect on cardiac function is based on reduction of right ventricular afterload. Even in patients with severe right ventricular dysfunction, NO improves cardiac output and right ventricular ejection fraction (Bhorade et al., 1999).Most of the studies used doses of 20 parts per million (ppm) (range 10-40 ppm). It is reasonable to start NO at the lowest possible dose and titrate upwards as required in patients with pulmonary hypertension.

Toxicity from NO results from the formation of methemoglobin, NO_2 and peroxynitrite. Life-threatening increases in PVR have been noted with acute withdrawal of NO. To prevent rebound pulmonary hypertension, NO should be tapered off progressively without any attempt to discontinue it completely if FiO2 is higher than 50%. However, these disadvantages of NO therapy have called for research on inhaled alternatives to NO.

Prostaglandins

- Inhaled **prostacyclin** (PGI_2)

Prostacyclin is a member of the prostaglandin family derived from arachidonic acid.

Inhaled **prostacyclin** seems to be the more favorable agent because of its lack of toxicity, ease of application, and reduced cost. Similar to NO, it is produced by the vascular endothelium and is involved in the regulation of vascular tone and in localized thrombotic and inflammatory processes. PGI_2 stimulates the endothelial release of NO, while NO, in turn, increases the synthesis of endogenous PGI_2. In vivo, PGI_2 is spontaneously hydrolyzed to its inactive metabolite 6-keto-prostaglandin-F_{1a} with a half life of 3-6 min.

Inhaled PGI_2 produces comparable effects to NO. The two agents have been compared in both animal and clinical studies, which have showed that inhaled PGI_2 produces greater decreases in PVR while NO induces greater improvements in oxygenation (Lowson, 2002). Moreover, Fattouch et al (Fattouch et al., 2005) have shown similar effectiveness for NO and inhaled prostacyclin in the treatment of pulmonary hypertension after mitral valve replacement in a randomized, double-blinded clinical trial. PGI_2 and its metabolites are remarkably non-toxic compared with NO. A prominent side-effect of inhaled PGI_2 is inhibition of platelet aggregation. Impaired in vitro platelet aggregation was noted after 2h of inhaled PGI_2 in patients undergoing cardiac surgery, but was not associated with an increase in chest tubes drainage or transfusion requirements even when therapy was continued for 6 h (Lowson, 2002). Systemic hypotension is another potential side effect of inhaled PGI_2, suggesting that there is a minimal absorption of inhaled PGI_2 from the lungs into the systemic circulation. Moreover, abrupt withdrawal of inhaled PGI_2 may cause rebound increases in PH. (Lowson, 2002)

Variable dose delivery, alteration of ventilation volumes, pressures, FiO2, and solvent evaporation with drug-concentrating effect are other obvious disadvantages. Plasma half-life of prostacyclin is 3 to 6 minutes.

- **Iloprost**

Iloprost is a more stable carbacyclin derivative of prostacyclin and can be administered intermittently, as the hemodynamic effects of a single dose are sustained for approximately 60-120 min, although the plasma half-life time of intravenously administered iloprost is known to be between 20-30 min (Theodoraki et al., 2002). This form of treatment appears to be promising combining the advantages of NO and the lack of problems of intravenous administration. Iloprost causes a significant reduction in MPAP and PVR and a significant increase in cardiac output after its administration since there is a substantial reduction in right ventricular afterload. It cannot be ruled out that a decrease in systemic vascular resistance (SVR) may occur during its administration but not to a degree that can affect arterial blood pressure dramatically.

Aerosolized iloprost has been described as a more potent pulmonary vasodilator than NO in patients with PH (Winterhalter et al., 2008). Its longer half-life firstly confers effective protection against the rebound phenomenon and, secondly, may facilitate the pharmacological effective transfer of the inhaler material from the pulmonary into the systemic arterial circulation.

Iloprost remains stable at room temperature and does not undergo any molecular changes on exposure to light, in comparison to PGI_2 (Fattouch et al., 2003). Also, inhaler iloprost can be rapidly and simply administered intraoperatively, irrespective of ventilator type. Unlike the situation with NO, inhaled iloprost treatment can also be continued with an ultrasonic nebulizer during weaning from the ventilator and after extubation.

Episodes of PH during heart transplantation procedures can be successfully treated with the administration of iloprost without unwanted side effects or significant systemic impact (Theodoraki et al., 2006).

Right heart failure after left ventricular assist device (LVAD) implantation is an acute life-threatening event. In patients with intraoperative severe acute right heart failure after implantation of a LVAD, successful weaning from CPB was possible after inhaled iloprost was added (Winterhalter et al., 2006).

In addition to its beneficial hemodynamic profile, aerosolized iloprost also exerted beneficial effects on arterial oxygenation, which probably reflected the more potent effects of iloprost on the pulmonary vascular bed and the more pronounced increase of mixed-venous oxygen saturation (Hoeper et al., 2000).

- **NO donors**

Inhaled NTG decreases PH without producing systemic vasodilatation (Yurtseven et al., 2003). Further studies are warranted to define their potential utility because nebulization of these drugs does not require an expensive apparatus like the one required for NO nebulization.

- **Phosphodiesterase - 3 inhibitors**

Milrinone inhibits the breakdown of cAMP, thereby promoting pulmonary vasodilatation. There are few recent studies which demonstrated the beneficial effects of inhaled milrinone on PH during weaning of patients from CPB.

Inhaled milrinone prevents pulmonary endothelial dysfunction after CPB, and its hemodynamic and oxygenation profiles are safer than those of intravenous milrinone (Lamarche et al., 2005).

6.2 Combination therapy

NO and PGI_2 / iloprost cause vasodilatation via two different intracellular signal pathways by relaxing smooth muscle cells. After diffusion into the smooth muscle cells, NO causes vascular smooth muscle cell relaxation by stimulating guanylate cyclase, leading to an increase in 3,5-cGMP and a reduction in intracellular calcium concentration. By contrast, PGI_2 / iloprost result in an increase in intracellular cyclic 3,5 cAMP concentrations, causing calcium-activated potassium channels to open through activation of adenyl-cyclase. However these drugs can be administered as combination therapy.

6.3 Other drugs

Adenosine activates adenylate cyclase and stimulates the generation of cAMP. Adenosine is rapidly inactivated with a plasma half-life of less than 10 seconds. In a study performed on ten patients who received an infusion of low-dose adenosine (50 mg/Kg/min) after weaning from CPB a significant reduction in MPAP and PVR and an increase in CO were demonstrated without adverse side effects without any adverse side effects (Fullenrton et al., 1996).

Phosphodiesterase-5-inhibitors such as zaniprast, dipyridamole, and sildenafil have been studied in the field of PH. There have been reports of variable beneficial effects of these agents on PH after cardiac surgery in combination with NO (Ichinose et al., 2001).

Bosentan is an endothelin antagonist which does not act acutely but has shown promising results as a sole agent and as combination chronic therapy for PH (Channick et al., 2004).

7. Special aspects of PH

7.1 PH in children

PH in children is associated with significant perioperative risk for major complications, including pulmonary hypertensive crisis and cardiac arrest (Friesen & Williams, 2008).

The goals of balanced and cautious anesthetic management are to provide adequate anesthesia and analgesia for the surgical procedure while minimizing increases in PVR and depression of myocardial function.

The development of the aforementioned specific pulmonary vasodilators has led to significant advances in the medical therapy of PH that can be incorporated in the anesthetic management of the pediatric population.

The incidence of complications in children with PH undergoing cardiac catheterization was found to be independent of the method of airway management. Tracheal intubation has been reported to precipitate pulmonary hypertensive crisis and death in critically ill pediatric patients with severe PH, so many anesthesiologists avoid intubation. Similarly, deep extubation can decrease exposure to noxious airway stimulation following selected procedures.

However, similarly to adult patients, PVR can be affected by many other aspects of anesthesia technique such as the inspired oxygen concentration, acid-base management, ventilation mode, drugs, blood products, CPB, pain management and stress response.

Given the multiple factors involved, it is not surprising that no single anesthetic agent has been shown to be ideal for that particular patient population and therefore, balanced anesthesia is preferred.

7.2 Anesthetic drugs

Numerous studies (Fischer et al., 2003; Blaise et al., 2003) investigate the effect of anesthetic drugs on pulmonary vascular tone. In general, it appears that the effect of anesthetic agents on the pulmonary circulation is different from their effect on the systemic circulation, often resulting in an increase in PVR.

Propofol decreases PAP, PVR as well as mean arterial pressure (MAP) after CPB. Propofol infusion to children undergoing cardiac catheterization decreased SVR significantly and cardiac contractility mildly. In addition, patients with cardiac shunts and fixed elevated PVR (Eisenmenger syndrome) may experience oxygen desaturation because the decrease in SVR will augment right-to-left shunt.

Etomidate is known for its lack of systemic hemodynamic effects on patients with heart disease, but its pulmonary vascular effects have not been investigated adequately.

Thiopental has been reported to increase PVR in adults, but in children a decrease of PVR by thiopental has been reported. However, thiopental is a less desirable choice for patient with PH, because it can cause significant myocardial depression and systemic hypotension.

An increase in PVR has been observed with *Ketamine* during spontaneous ventilation, but decreases in PVR have been reported during controlled ventilation. This effect makes ketamine the drug of choice for the anesthetic management of patients with PH, particularly of children with congenital heart diseases.

Benzodiazepines are associated with minimal hemodynamic effects and are considered useful for preanesthetic premedication.

Fentanyl and sufentanil have minimal pulmonary and systemic effects and attenuate pulmonary and vascular response to noxious stimuli in adults as well as in children.

Volatile anesthetics have variable effects on pulmonary vascular tone. Isoflurane and halothane potentiate the vasodilator response to β_1 adrenoceptor activation. Isoflurane, halothane, enflurane and desflurane (but not sevoflurane) inhibit endothelium-dependent relaxation by inhibiting the activity of the adenosine triphosphate-sensitive potassium channels, which mediate the vasodilator effect of many endogenous mediators such as adenosine, PGI_2 and nitric oxide. In general, isoflurane and sevoflurane are associated with clinical pulmonary vasodilatation and are accepted components of a balanced anesthetic technique in patients with PH.

However, volatile anesthetic agents can lead to dose-dependent depression of cardiac contractility and reduction of SVR, which may be problematic. Moreover, volatile anesthetics, when administered in high minimal alveolar concentrations, attenuate hypoxic pulmonary vasoconstriction, thereby exacerbating ventilation-perfusion mismatching.

Nitrous oxide increases the pulmonary vascular tone in adult patients undergoing valve surgery preoperatively and postoperatively. In children, it has shown to have little effect on pulmonary hemodynamics.

8. Conclusion

In the present chapter, we described the pathogenesis and pathophysiology of PH as well as its perioperative management with specific emphasis in the period following cardiac surgery. Aspects of perioperative manipulation aiming at optimizing right ventricular function and the application of novel therapeutic modalities were critically presented and evaluated.

9. References

Blaise, G.; Langleben, D. & Hubert, B. (2003). Pulmonary arterial hypertension: pathophysiology and anesthetic approach. *Anesthesiology*, Vol.99, No.6, pp.1415-1432.

Bhorade, S.; Christenson, J.; O'Connor, M.; Lavoie, A.; Pohlman, A. & Hall, JB. (1999). Response to inhaled nitric oxide in patients with acute right heart syndrome. *Am J Respir Crit Care Med*, Vol.159, No.2, pp.571-579

Channick, RN.; Sitbon, O.; Barst, RJ.; Manes, A. & Rubin, LJ. (2004). Endothelin receptor antagonists in pulmonary arterial hypertension. *J Am Coll Cardiol*, Vol.43, 12 Suppl S, 62S-67S

Christman, BW.; McPherson, CD.; Newman, JH. King, GA.; Bernard, GR.; Groves, BM. & Loyd, JE. (1992). An imbalance between the excretion of thromboxane and prostacyclin metabolites in pulmonary hypertension. *N Engl J Med*, Vol.327, No.2, pp. 70–75

Fattouch, K.; Sbraga, F.; Bianco, G.; Speziale, G.; Gucciardo, M.; Sampognaro, R. & Ruvolo, G. (2005). Inhaler prostacyclin, nitric oxide, and nitroprusside in pulmonary hypertension after mitral valve replacement. *J Card Surg*, Vol.20, No.2, pp.171-176

Fischer, LG.; Van Aken, H. & Burkle, H. (2003). Management of pulmonary hypertension: physiology and pharmacological considerations for anesthesiologists. *Anesth Analg*, Vol. 96, No 6, pp.1603-1616

Friesen, R. & Williams, G. (2008). Anesthetic management of children with pulmonary arterial hypertension. *Pediatric Anesthesia*, Vol.18, No.3, pp.208-216

Fullenrton, DA.; Jones, SD.; Grover, FL. & McIntyre, RC Jr. (1996). Adenosine effectively controls pulmonary hypertension after cardiac operations. *Ann Thorac Surg*, Vol.61, No.4, pp.1118-1123

Galiè, N.; Hoeper, MM.; Humbert, M.; Torbicki, A.; Vachiery, JL.; Barbera, JA.; Beghetti, M.; Corris, P.; Gaine, S.; Gibbs, JS.; Gomez-Sanchez, MA.; Jondeau,G.; Klepetko, W.; Opitz, C.; Peacock, A.; Rubin, L.; Zellweger, M.; & Simonneau, G. (2009). Guidelines for the diagnosis and treatment of pulmonary hypertension: the Task Force for the Diagnosis and Treatment of Pulmonary Hypertension of the European Society of Cardiology (ESC) and the European Respiratory Society (ERS), endorsed by the International Society of Heart and Lung Transplantation (ISHLT). *Eur Heart J*, Vol.30, No.20, pp.2493-2537

Galiè, N.; Torbicki, A.; Barst, R.; Dartevelle, P.; Haworth, S.; Higenbottam, T.; Olschewski, H.; Peacock, A.; Pietra, G.; Rubin, LJ.; Simonneau, G.; Priori, SG.; Garcia, MA.; Blanc, J.; Budaj, A.; Cowie, M.; Dean, V.; Deckers, J.; Burgos, EF.; Lekakis, J.; Lindahl, B.; Mazzotta, G.; McGregor, K.; Morais, J.; Oto, A.; Smiseth, OA.; Barbera, JA.; Gibbs, S.; Hoeper, M.; Humbert, M.; Naeije, R. & Pepke-Zaba, J. (2004). Guidelines on diagnosis and treatment of pulmonary arterial hypertension. The task force on diagnosis and treatment of pulmonary arterial hypertension of the European Society of Cardiology. *Eur Heart J*, Vol.25, No.24, pp.2243-2278

Giaid, A.; Yanagisawa, M.; Langleben, D.; Michel RP.; Levy, R.; Shennib, H.; Kimura, S.; Masaki, T.; Duguid, WP.; & Stewart, DJ. (1993). Expression of endothelin-1 in the lungs of patients with pulmonary hypertension. *N Engl J Med*, Vol.328, No.254, pp.1732–1739

Hanafy, KA.; Krumenacker, JS. & Murad, F. (2001). NO, nitrotyrosine, and cyclic GMP in signal transduction. *Med Sci Monit* Vol.7, No.4, pp.801-819

Hatano, S. & Strassert, T. World Health Organization 1975. Primary pulmonary hypertension. Geneva: WHO; 1975.

Hoeper, MM.; Olschewski, H.; Ghofrani, HA.; Wilkens, H.; Borst, MM.; Niedermeyer, J.; Fabel, H. & Seeger, W. (2000). A comparison of acute hemodynamic effects of inhaled nitric oxide and aerosolized iloprost in primary pulmonary hypertension. *J Am Coll Cardiol*, Vol.35, No.1, pp.176-182

Ichinose, F.; Erana-Garcia, J.; Hromi, J.; Raveh, Y.; Jones, R.; Krim, L.; Clark, MW.; Winkler, JD.; Bloch, KD. & Zapol, WM. (2001). Nebulized sildenafil is a selective pulmonary vasodilator in lambs with acute pulmonary hypertension. *Crit Care Med*, Vol.29, No.5, pp.1000-1005

Jain S, Ventoura H, deBoisblanc B. (2007). Pathophysiology of pulmonary arterial hypertension. *Semin Cardiothorac Vasc Anesth*, Vol.11, No.2, pp.104-109

Kaul, TK & Fields, BL. (2000). Postoperative acute refractory right ventricular failure: incidence, pathogenesis, management and prognosis. *Cardiovasc Surg*, Vol. 8, No.1, pp.1-9

Kieler-Jensen, N.; Milocco, I.; & Ricksten, SE. (1993). Pulmonary vasodilation after heart transplantation. A comparison among prostacyclin, sodium nitroprosside and nitroglycerin on right ventricular function and pulmonary selectivity. *J Heart Lung Transplant*, Vol.12, No.2, pp.179-184

Lamarche, Y.; Malo, O.; Thorin, E.; Denault, A.; Carrier, A.; Roy, J. & Perrault, LP. (2005). Inhaled but not intravenous milrinone prevents pulmonary endothelial dysfunction after cardiopulmonary bypass. *J Thorac Cardiovasc Surg*, Vol.130, No.1, pp.83-92

Lowson, SM. Inhaler alternatives to nitric oxide. (2002). *Anesthesiology*, Vol.96, No.6, pp.1504-1513

Lucas, KA.; Pitari, GM.; Kazerounian, S.; Ruiz-Stewart, I.; Park, J.; Schulz, S.; Chepenik, KP. & Waldman, SA. (2000). Guanylyl cyclases and signaling by cyclic GMP. *Pharmacol Rev*, Vol.52, No.3, pp.375-414

Matuschak, GM. (1997). Pulmonary dysfunction after surgery involving cardiopulmonary bypass: do we understand the mechanisms? *Crit Care Med*, Vol.25, No.11, pp.1778-1780

McLaughlin W.; Archer SL.; Badrsch, DB.; Barst, RJ.; Farber, HW.; Lindner, JR.; Mathier, MA.; McGoon, MD.; Park, MH.; Rosenson, RS.; Rubin, LJ.; Tapson, VF.; Varga, J.; Harrington, RA.; Anderson, JL.; Bates, ER.; Bridges, CR.; Eisenberg, MJ.; Ferrari, VA.; Grines, CL.; Hlatky, MA.; Jacobs, AK.; Kaul, S.; Lichtenberg, RC.; Lindner, JR.; Moliterno, DJ.; Mukherjee, D.; Pohost, GM.; Rosenson, RS.; Schofield, RS.; Shubrooks, SJ.; Stein, JH.; Tracy CM.; Weitz, HH. & Wesley DJ. (2009). ACCF/AHA

2009 Expert Consensus Document on pulmonary hypertension: a report of the American College of Cardiology foundation task force on expert consensus documents and the American Heart Association: developed in collaboration with the American College of Chest Physicians, American Thoracic Society, Inc., and the Pulmonary Hypertension Association. *Circulation*, Vol.119, No.16, pp.2250-2294

Raikar, GV.; Hisamochi, K.; Raikar, BL. & Schaff, HV. (1996). Nitric oxide inhibition attenuates systemic hypotension produced by protamine. *J Cardiovasc Surg*, Vol.111, No 6, pp.1240-1246

Riedel B. (1999). The pathophysiology and management of perioperative pulmonary hypertension with specific emphasis on the period following cardiac surgery. *Int Anesthesiol Clin*, Vol.37, No.2, pp.55-79

Roques, F.; Nashef, SA.; Michel, P.; Gauducheau, E.; de Vincentiis, C.; Baudet, E.; Cortina, J.; David, M.; Faichney, A.; Gabrielle, F.; Gams, E.; Harjula, A.; Jones, MT.; Pintor, PP.; Salamon, R. & Thulin, L. (1999). Risk factors and outcome in European cardiac surgery: analysis of the EuroSCORE multinational database of 19,030 patients. *Eur J Cardiothorac Surg*, Vol.15, No.6, pp.816-822

Stewart, DJ.; Levy, RD.; Cernacek, P. & Langleben, D. (1991). Increased plasma endothelin-1 in pulmonary hypertension: marker or mediator of disease? *Ann Intern Med*, Vol.114, No.6, pp.464–469

Theodoraki, K.; Rellia, P.; Thanopoulos, A.; Tsourelis, L.; Zarkalis, D.; Sfyrakis, P. &Antoniou, T. (2002). Inhaled iloprost controls pulmonary hypertension after cardiopulmonary bypass. *Can J Anaesth*, Vol.49, No.9, pp.963- 967

Theodoraki, K.; Tsiapras, D.; Tsourelis, L.; Zarkalis, D.; Sfirakis, P.; Kapetanakis, E.; Alivizatos, P. & Antoniou, T. (2006). Inhaled iloprost in eight heart transplant recipients presenting with post-bypass acute right ventricular dysfunction. *Acta Anaesthesiol Scand*, Vol.50, No.10, pp.1213-1217

Tidswell, M. & Higgins, TL. (2007). The anesthesiologist and pulmonary arterial hypertension. *Semin Cardiothorac Vasc Anesth*, Vol.11, No.2, pp.93-95

Walmrath, D.; Olschewski, H.; Grimminger, F. & Seeger, W. (1997). NO and alternative inhalational therapy approaches in pulmonary hypertension. *Internist*, Vol.38, No.5, pp. 453-460

Wang, T.; Kebir, D. & Blaise, G. (2003). Inhaled nitric oxide in 2003: a review of its mechanisms of action. *Can J Anesth*, Vol.50, No.8, pp.839-846

Winterhalter, M.; Antoniou, T. & Loukanov, T. (2010). Management of adult patients with perioperative pulmonary hypertension: technical aspects and therapeutic options. *Cardiology*, Vol.116, No.1, pp.3-9

Winterhalter, M.; Fischer, S.; Tessmann, R.; Goerler A.; Piepenbrock, S.; Haverich, A. & Strueber, M. (2006). Using inhaled iloprost to wean from cardiopulmonary bypass after implanting a left ventricular assist device. *Anesth Analg*, Vol.103, No.2, pp.515-516

Winterhalter, M.; Simon, A.; Fischer, S.; Rahe-Meyer, N.; Chamtzidou, N.; Hecker, H.; Zuk, J.; Piepenbrock, S. & Struber, M. (2008). Comparison of inhaled iloprost and nitric oxide in patient with pulmonary hypertension during weaning from cardiopulmonary bypass in cardiac surgery: A prospective randomized trial. *J Cardioth Vasc Anesth*, Vol.22, No.3, pp.406-413

Yurtseven, N.; Karaca, P.; Kaplan, M.; Ozkul, V.; Tuygun, AK.; Canik, S. & Kopman, E. (2003). Effect of nitroglycerin inhalation on patients with pulmonary hypertension undergoing mitral valve replacement surgery. *Anesthesiology*, Vol.99, No.4, pp.855-858

6

Monitoring Outcomes in Highly Specialised Cardiac Surgery

Thomas Kenny and Martin Ashton-Key
National Specialised Commissioning Team
England

1. Introduction

In the UK there are a small number of highly specialised areas of cardiac surgery that are centrally planned, funded and monitored these include Heart Transplantation in children and adults, Extra Corporeal Membrane Oxygenation (ECMO) in children and adults, Pulmonary Endarterectomy, and Ventricular Assist Devices (VAD) as a bridge to cardiac transplantation in children and adults.

In England, the National Specialised Commissioning Team (NSCT) is responsible for planning, funding and monitoring these highly specialised services within the English National Health Service (NHS) (Kenny et al., 2008). In total the NSCT commissions approximately 70 services, each of these service involves is commissioned centrally due to one or more of the following reasons:-

- Rare disease or condition, requiring significant expertise to manage
- Expensive drugs or technology
- Organisationally complex arrangements are needed for optimal management
- Technically demanding techniques or procedures

This chapter will discuss our approach, experience and the impact closely monitoring clinical outcomes has in this area of highly specialised surgery. While much that is written on monitoring outcomes focuses solely on formal data collection, analysis and interpretation we believe this is only a small, although important, part of the process of monitoring clinical outcomes when your aim is improvement of clinical services. Not only does formal data alone not give clear answers, but also they require detailed understanding of the service and interpretation. This is particularly true when the data refer to small volumes of clinical activity.

The small numbers of cases within these highly specialised areas are an issue for both the development of expert performance and for monitoring that performance. There is a significant sensitivity of any aggregate outcomes to the case-mix of the cases operated on and understanding how to interpret the results in a fair, measured, proportionate and transparent manner is essential.

If formal data alone are used for 'performance management' then even if the aim of the appraisal is performance improvement there are two more likely effects. The first is distortion of data and the second is distortion of the service, these occur because they appear to produce the same results, but it is much harder to produce real improvements in any system. Therefore, we strive to ensure that these data are never examined in isolation so that inadvertent or deliberate distortion of either the service or the data are identified and prevented.

1.1 Our philosophy and approach

The basis of our approach is close personal working relationships, collaboration and mutual trust between those providing the service and those monitoring it. Each of these is equally important.

Close personal working relationships because although each of these service has detailed service specifications, exacting standards and a full and complex contract, we have found that when you have to resort to the use of these formal documents then you are unlikely to get the quality of service and the ongoing improvement that these highly complex service need.

Collaboration because there are synergies that arise from the joining of multiple perspectives. In the case of these highly specialised service when the perspectives of the provider, the purchaser and the patient are brought together to develop a service, solve a problem or resolve an issue the solutions are often far stronger and more long-sighted than the solution if only one perspective were considered.

Mutual trust because there are so many opportunities for the development of perverse incentives, short-term gain with long-term losses and gaming of any performance indicators that it is, in our opinion, very challenging to contract with people and organisations where such trust is undermined or becomes compromised.

Into each of these relationships, we believe we bring sensitivity and a thorough understanding of each service that allows us to use appropriately the 'dark art' of interpreting outcomes bases on small numbers.

We also insist on the development of clinical and managerial systems that wrap around these services and provide prompt, timely and appropriate feedback so that expert performance can develop (Klein, 1998). Encourage reflection so that each opportunity for learning from these scarce experiences if optimised for both individual learning and vicariously by the wider team and service. In addition, focus on performance improvement because however far a service has come however good it is, we find that either services improve or they deteriorate. Keeping a service's performance static requires as much if not more effort than improving it and our preference is, by far, for services that improve.

1.2 How the national specialised commissioning team uses the outcome data

Every service commissioned by the National Specialised Commissioning Team is allocated to a Triumvirate of a commissioning manager, a finance manager and a medical advisor. This Triumvirate oversees all elements of the commissioning process on an ongoing basis and through a number of simultaneously delivered processes.

The first process that underpins each service we commission is the development of clinical and service standards. These standards are developed collaboratively, with both our team and the service contributing fully to their development. In spite of this collaborative development, or maybe because of it, the standards are invariably high and most commonly represent, wherever possible, best practice, based on evidence rather than a lowest common denominator consensus.

The second process is formal twice-yearly face-to-face review meetings between each service provider and the Triumvirate. These twice-yearly review meetings cover all elements of the service and include a formal review of clinical audits, feedback on service in the form of complaints, compliments, patients surveys, satisfaction questionnaires and the key clinical outcomes agreed for the service. The focus of the reviews is on how the service is developing and changing because of the information it is receiving from each of the preceding data sources.

The third process is an annual clinical audit day where all the providers of a service meet to go through the clinical outcomes of the service. These outcomes are based on 100% consecutive case-series of outcome reporting i.e. outcomes from every single patient cared for by a service in a given year.

The fourth process specific to the highly specialised cardiac services and the other transplant services takes the form of monthly monitoring of outcomes using the O-E (observed - expected) monitoring and tabular CUSUM (cumulative sum control chart). This monitoring allows each of the service providers and the National Specialised Commissioning Team to track any changes in outcomes in real-time, which allows early identification of any change from that which might be expected and allows the timely questioning of why such variation may have occurred. Details of such investigations are presented in the published UK Cardiothoracic Transplant Audit annual reports, leading to shared learning and shared service development and improvement based on centre level clinical outcome data and timely reporting and analysis.

Throughout each of these processes, our emphasis is on the use of data, from all sources, to provide feedback on the performance of the service and guide them to where the time would be most valuably spent improving.

We apply all of the above principles to all of the services we commission whether they are secure mental health services, diagnostic services, surgical services or those for cardiac transplantation (see www.specialisedservices.nhs.uk for the full list of services commissioned by the National Specialised Commissioning Team). To demonstrate this application we will use heart and lung transplantation as a case study, which includes a detailed reflection on an external review carried out at one of the heart and lung centres that involved a detailed statistical analysis of mortality data that informed the review findings.

We then conclude with summaries of the other nationally commissioned cardiac services and the use of outcome data within them.

2. Heart and lung transplantation

This section includes elements reproduced in full, or paraphrased, with permission from *The Royal College of Surgeons of England Clinical Effectiveness Unit and NHS Blood and Transplant UK Cardiothoracic Audit End of Year Report from the Audit Steering Group to the National Commissioning Group (Rogers et al., 2010)*. (These have been reproduced to ensure technical consistency and accuracy in relation to how transplant related data are collected, analysed and presented.

Heart and lung transplantation has been nationally commissioned in England since 2002. Currently cardiothoracic transplantation is provided by the following hospital Trusts:

- The Newcastle upon Tyne Hospitals NHS Foundation Trust (adults and children)
- University Hospitals Birmingham NHS Foundation Trust (adults only)
- University Hospital of South Manchester NHS Foundation Trust (adults only)
- Papworth Hospital NHS Foundation Trust (adults only)
- Royal Brompton and Harefield NHS Trust (adults only)
- Great Ormond Street Hospital for Children NHS Trust (children only)

Systems for monitoring early and late mortality for heart and lung transplants are linked to data routinely collected by NHS Blood and Transplant (NHSBT), a Special Health Authority within the NHS with responsibility for "*optimising the supply of blood, organs, and tissues and raising the quality, effectiveness and efficiency of blood and transplant services*". (NHS Blood and Transplant, 2011). Data have been recorded on all patients in the UK receiving a first heart, lung or heart and lung transplant since 01 July 1995. Reports using these data have been published annually for all patients receiving a cardiothoracic transplant from 01 July 1995 to present day.

Patient level information is submitted to NHSBT at key steps along the transplant pathway: (i) when the patient is registered on the national transplant waiting list; (ii) at the time of the transplantation; (iii) three months after having the transplant; (iv) and annually thereafter until death. These data are transferred on a monthly basis to the UK Cardiothoracic Transplant Audit team based at the Clinical Effectiveness Unit (CEU) of the Royal College of Surgeons of England (RCS). The data submitted are subjected to on-going process of validation including the use of computer-based validation and case notes reviews, and as a result are robust and reliable.

The database held by NHSBT / Royal College of Surgeons Clinical Effectiveness Unit forms the basis of the UK Cardiothoracic Transplant Audit. The UK Cardiothoracic Transplant Audit is a multi-centre prospective cohort study. The audit has donor, recipient and outcome data on all cardiothoracic transplants undertaken in the UK since July 1995 and allows for prospective and retrospective audit of the outcomes from cardiothoracic transplantation. Because the data are collected in a timely manner as outlined above the data collected also allows real-time monitoring of outcomes for each transplant centre that can be used for monitoring performance.

The audit is undertaken by a project team, overseen by a steering group, comprising the directors of all cardiopulmonary transplant centres in the UK, the director of the Royal College of Surgeons Clinical Effectiveness Unit, and representatives from NHSBT and the National Specialised Commissioning Team. The Steering Group approves all output from the audit prior to publication.

The UK Cardiothoracic Transplant Audit publishes on an annual basis the 30-day, 90-day, 1-year, 3-year, 5-year and 10-year mortality after first intrathoracic transplantation at all cardiopulmonary transplant centres in the United Kingdom. Centre-specific 30-day and 90-day mortality is reported for the more recent cohorts with 1-year and 3-year mortality being presented for the most appropriate recent cohort as well as for the period as a whole. Five and 10-year mortality rates are reported for the entire period as a whole. The Audits are available on the Royal College of Surgeons of England website (www.rcseng.ac.uk/surgical_research_units/ceu/docs.html) (see Rogers et al., 2010).

Results for adult (age ≥ 16 years at transplant) heart and lung transplants and paediatric heart and lung transplants are reported separately. The results for 30-day, 90-day and 1-year mortality after adult heart transplantation and 30-day and 90-day mortality after adult lung transplantation are presented both with and without adjustment for case-mix. The risk models used for case-mix adjustment have all been developed specifically for this audit.

The risk-adjusted estimates of early mortality after adult heart transplant for the most recent cohort of patients available (April 2007 – March 2010 [December 2009 for 90-day mortality]) are shown as funnel plots in Figures 1 and 2.

Figures 1 and 2 highlight that both the 30-day and 90-day mortality for each centre in the UK is within the range expected with no centre experiencing a mortality that was lower or higher than expected.

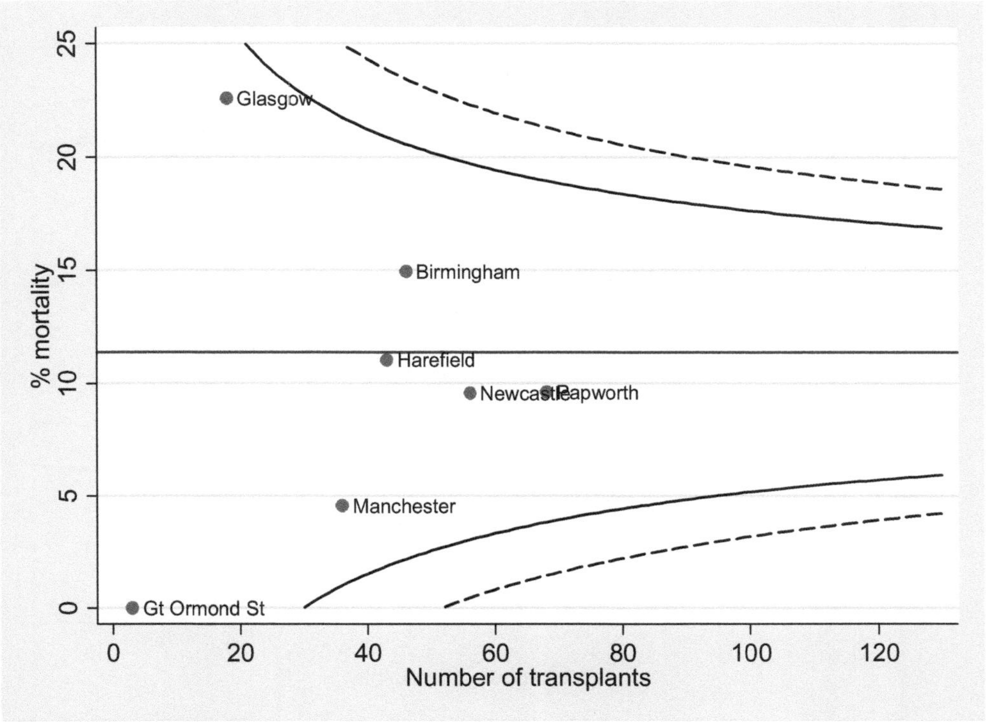

Note: Solid and dashed lines define the 95% and 99% confidence intervals

Fig. 1. Risk-adjusted estimates of early (30-day) mortality after adult heart transplantation, April 2007 - March 2010 (reproduced from the RCS / NHSBT UK Cardiothoracic Transplant Audit, August 2010, (Rogers et al., 2010)).

Data collected since January 2004 are used to continuously monitor 30-day and 90-day mortality, and presented both as a cumulative observed-expected (O-E) mortality and tabular CUSUM in the Annual Audit. For the adult transplant programmes the cumulative observed-expected mortality is presented both with and without risk adjustment. Paediatric recipient outcomes are only presented without risk adjustment.

In addition to the CUSUM monitoring presented in the annual report of the audit, real-time CUSUM monitoring has also been performed on a monthly basis since October 2006. This is especially important because it allows real-time monitoring of mortality outcomes and allows timely identification of any unexpected changes in mortality rates.

The O-E mortality chart plots the cumulative difference between the observed and expected patient mortality. For the continuous monitoring programme expected mortality rates are based on the national average mortality rate for transplants performed between 2000 and 2003, with more recent transplants given more weight. If the trend in the O-E chart goes downwards then this would indicate that the mortality rate observed is lower than might be expected, whilst an upward trend would suggest an observed mortality rate that is higher than expected.

An example of an O-E cumulative mortality chart for the five English centres is given in Figure 3.

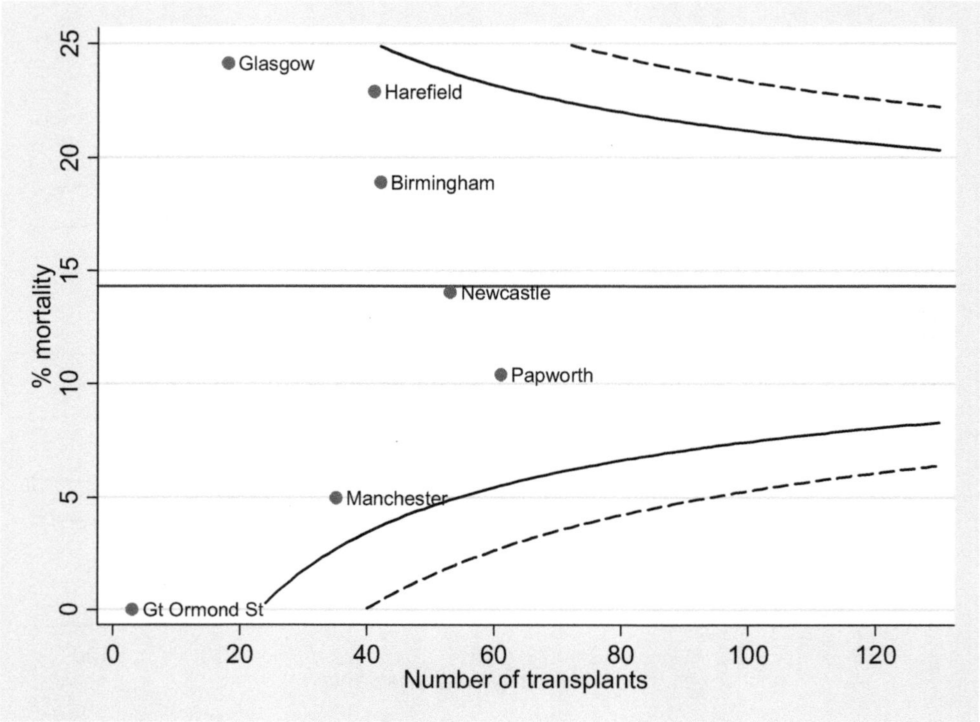

Note: Solid and dashed lines define the 95% and 99% confidence intervals

Fig. 2. Risk-adjusted estimates of early 90-day mortality after adult heart transplantation, April 2007 – December 2009 (reproduced from the RCS / NHSBT UK Cardiothoracic Transplant Audit, August 2010, (Rogers et al., 2010)).

The tabular CUSUM chart is used to signal when a significant increase in mortality rate has been observed. The chart limit is set to signal when there is sufficient evidence to indicate that the mortality rate has doubled. A signal may indicate divergence from the national average. If an individual centre's CUSUM chart signals then following any appropriate investigation to understand what might have caused the signal, the CUSUM chart is reset to enable closer monitoring of the centre's performance in the following months.

Examples of tabular CUSUMs included in the most recent Royal College of Surgeons and NHSBT UK Cardiothoracic Transplant Audit, August 2010, (Rogers et al., 2010) for the 5 English adult cardiothoracic transplant centres are given in Figure 3 (30-day mortality) and Figure 4 (90-day mortality).

The CUSUM charts illustrate that recent 30 and 90-day mortality rates following adult heart transplantation have been as expected at Centre 1, Centre 4 and Centre 5.

However, they also show that Centre 2 experienced more deaths than might be expected in 2007 and Centre 3 experienced more deaths than might be expected in 2008. In all cases, the CUSUM charts signalled and the centres underwent an external review of their service. Since the signals, the 30-day mortality rates have returned to the expected level at each centre. After the signal in 2008, Centre 3 continued to experience more deaths within 90 days

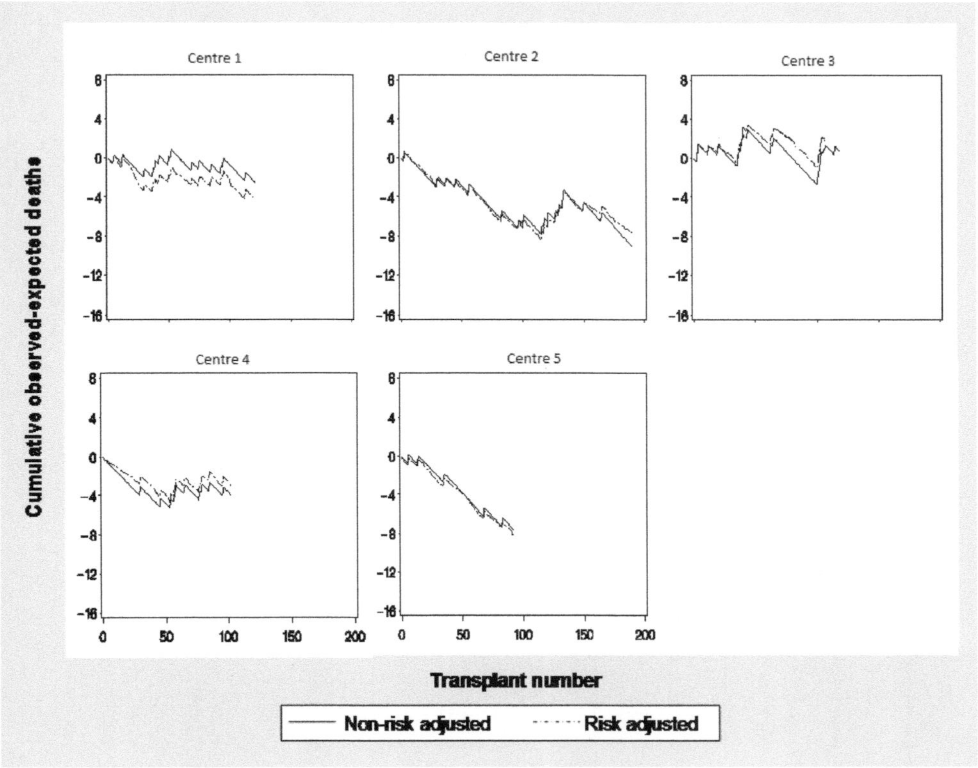

Fig. 3. Cumulative (observed - expected) 30-day mortality after adult heart transplantation, January 2004 to March 2010(reproduced from the RCS and NHSBT UK Cardiothoracic Transplant Audit, August 2010, (Rogers et al., 2010)).

than expected and the 90-day CUSUM chart signalled again. This is because centres are monitored more closely after a signal and the charts are more sensitive.

2.1 Outcome monitoring to ensure maintenance of high quality clinical services

Real-time monitoring of mortality outcomes after heart and lung transplants have led to several reviews of services to understand why variation from expected might have occurred, and to put in place appropriate action plans when necessary. The conclusions of such reviews are published on the National Specialised Commissioning Team's website and are available at www.specialisedservices.nhs.uk.

Included below are some extracts taken from an external review undertaken at Harefield Hospital in 2008, the full report of which is in the public domain and available on the National Specialised Commissioning Team's website (NSCT, 2008). It outlines the background to the review and summarises the additional statistical analyses undertaken on the mortality data available for the service. The extracts below do not include the elements of the actual external review process, the details of which are available in the full report.

These highlight how rapid further analysis of available data can be undertaken to help understand why variability in outcomes might have occurred and demonstrate how this

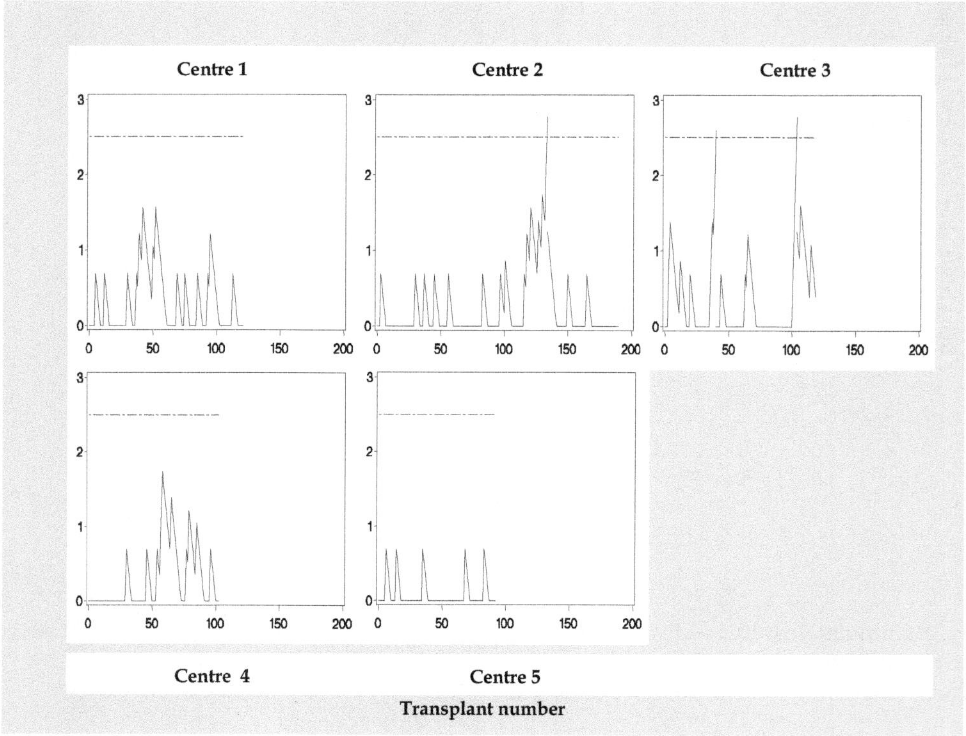

Fig. 4. Tabular CUSUM for 30-day mortality after adult heart transplant unadjusted for patient risk, January 2004 to March 2010 (reproduced from the RCS / NHSBT UK Cardiothoracic Transplant Audit, August 2010, (Rogers et al., 2010)).

understanding can then be used by clinicians and commissioners to support any necessary service changes.

One of the strengths of National Specialised Commissioning is the relationship and understanding that is built up between the commissioning team (medical advisor, commissioning manager and finance manager) with the clinical teams providing the service. This is exemplified in this example by the fact that the clinical team alerted the National Specialised Commissioning Team to a potential issue ahead of any alert signalling at NHSBT, demonstrating good clinical practice.

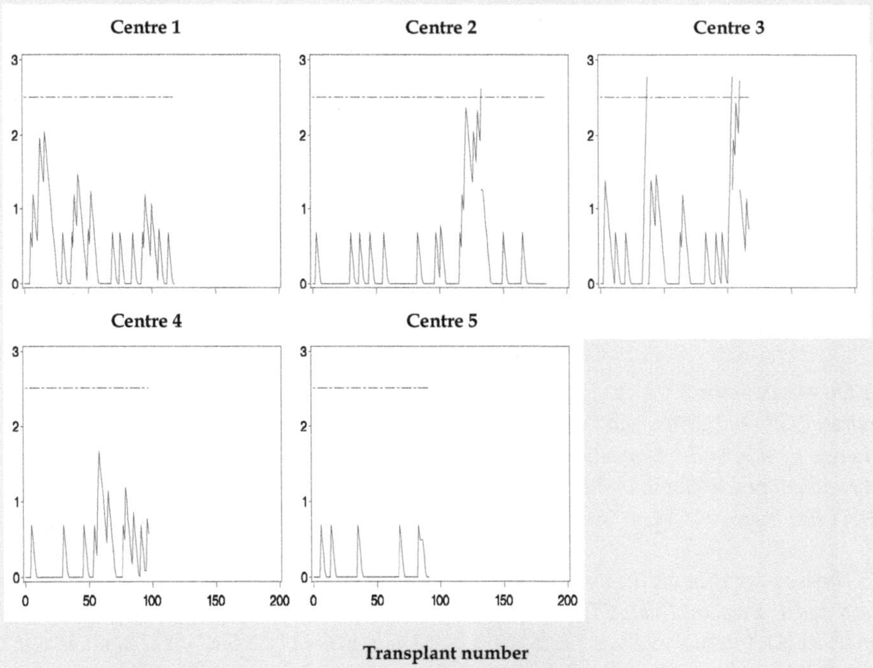

Fig. 5. Tabular CUSUM for 90-day mortality after adult heart transplant unadjusted for patient risk, January 2004 to March 2010 (reproduced from the RCS / NHSBT UK Cardiothoracic Transplant Audit, August 2010, (Rogers et al., 2010)).

Extracts as follows (Please note that all figures referred to have not been included in these extracts but are available in the full report available at http://www.specialisedservices.nhs.uk/document/review-recent-outcomes-in-heart-transplant-service-at-harefield-hospital). (NSCT, 2008)

NATIONAL COMMISSIONING GROUP (NCG)
REPORT OF THE EXTERNAL REVIEW OF RECENT OUTCOMES IN THE HEART TRANSPLANT SERVICE AT HAREFIELD HOSPITAL (2008)

1. INTRODUCTION

1.1 This report summarises an external review of a higher than expected number of deaths following heart transplants performed at Harefield Hospital in July and August 2008.

1.2 The review was an agreed joint approach between the National Specialised Commissioning Team (NSC Team) and the Healthcare Commission (HCC). It was also agreed with the Royal Brompton and Harefield NHS Trust (RBHT). The HCC has reviewed the findings of this report.

2. BACKGROUND

2.1 On 4 September 2008, the Director of Cardiothoracic Transplantation at Harefield Hospital, Professor Gilles Dreyfus, told the NSC Team that:
between 17 July and 3 September 2008 four consecutive heart transplant patients transplanted in July and August died within 30 days
RBHT had begun an urgent internal review of these events.

2.2 These consecutive deaths were enough for the monthly sequential analysis carried out by NHS Blood and Transplant (NHSBT) statisticians to signal a subsequent alert (see paragraph 3.12 and Appendix A). Internal audit prompted Professor Dreyfus to inform the NSC Team without delay prior to this analysis being reported.

2.3 The RBHT internal review investigated these four deaths and three other deaths beyond 30 days in patients transplanted earlier in 2008. Seven (47%) of the 15 heart patients transplanted this year have died. The Internal Review is considered later in this report.

2.4 These events followed a period of low 30- and 90-day heart transplant mortality in 2006 and 2007. A statistical analysis of heart transplant outcomes carried out by the UK Cardiothoracic Transplant Audit (UKCTA) is summarised below in Section 3 of this report.

2.5 Early mortality following lung transplant has been low at Harefield this year: one death in 21 patients transplanted in 2008 (4.8%).

2.6 In 2005, the National Specialist Commissioning Advisory Group (NSCAG) undertook an external review of the Harefield service because of an above expected early mortality following both heart and lung transplants. In contrast to the present situation, this review followed a gradual but non-statistically significant increase in early mortality compared to other transplant centres. The 2005 review found no single explanation but considered the outcomes in 2005 were linked to system and process problems in donor assessment, organ retrieval and intra-operative care. Harefield implemented a series of actions recommended by its own internal review and the external review.

2.7 Following completion of the RBHT internal review of deaths in 2008, the Trust, NSC Team and HCC agreed that an external review should be completed within one month by a heart transplant surgeon and a transplant cardiologist from other centres. If a suitable donor heart were to become available during the course of the review, the transplant team at Harefield would consult with the external reviewers before undertaking a transplant.

3. MORTALITY AFTER HEART TRANSPLANT: STATISTICAL ANALYSIS

3.1 The NSC Team commissioned a specific review of mortality after heart transplants carried out at Harefield between 1 January 2006 and 31 August 2008. This was compiled by members of the Audit Project Group of the Cardiothoracic Transplant Audit (UKCTA). The findings of the UKCTA report are summarised below. (see Appendix A for its executive summary and the limitations of statistical analysis – ***this is available in the full report****)*

Mortality within 30 days
3.2 30-day mortality at Harefield for the whole period (1 January 2006 to 31 August 2008) was similar to other UK centres: 10.3% (95% CI 3.9%-21.2%) compared to 12.3% (95% CI 8.3%-17.3%) elsewhere. Although the 30-day mortality of 26.7% (95% CI 7.8%-55.1%) at Harefield in 2008 was more than double the expected rate, the number of transplants was low and the difference from other centres was not statistically significant.

Mortality within 90 days
3.3 90-day mortality was not significantly different from other centres for the period 1 January 2006 to 30 June 2008: 9.6% (95% CI 3.2%-21%) at Harefield compared to 13.1% (8.9%-18.4%) elsewhere. Similarly, the difference in 90-day mortality for the nine transplants done between 1 January 2008 and 30 June 2008 was not statistically significant: 22.2% (95% CI 2.8%-60%) compared to 5.4% (95% CI 0.6%- 18.2%) elsewhere. But further analysis, when 90 days have elapsed after all the transplants undertaken up to 31 August 2008, will include the patients transplanted after 30 June and this will affect the estimate of statistical significance.

Mortality rates by donor organ retrieval centre
3.4 There was no evidence that donor hearts retrieved by Harefield were associated with higher mortality than those retrieved by other UK centres (p=0.11). However, nationally in the last three years, the 30-day mortality was significantly higher for donor hearts retrieved by any one centre and then transplanted in a different centre (p=0.006). The UKCTA report gives evidence that this was not the case before 2006.

Post-operative adverse events (PAE)
3.5 The rate of PAEs 7 within 30 days was significantly higher at Harefield than other UK centres: 67.2% (95% CI 53.7%-79%) for the whole period compared to 44.9% (38.3%-51.7%) elsewhere. In 2008, the difference was more marked: 93.3% (95 CI 68-99.8%) at Harefield and 42% (28.1%-56.8%) elsewhere. The UKCTA report commented that the high PAE rate "may be due, at least in part, to the risk profile of patients transplanted" (see paragraphs 3.7-3.11 below).

Ischaemic time
3.6 The median total ischaemia time for the whole period was similar but slightly lower at Harefield than elsewhere: 196 minutes (interquartile range 175-218) compared to 220 minutes (190-251) for the other centres combined. The corresponding figures for 2008 were 213 (160-229) and 227 (192-263). Transport and implant times were also slightly lower at Harefield. These times were stable at Harefield during 1 January 2006 - 31 August 2008.

Risk profile of heart transplant patients
3.7 The risk profile of heart transplant patients at Harefield was higher in 2008 than in 2007 and 2006 (Figure 1). The risk model has been developed by the UKCTA from a dataset that extends back 13 years and is used to adjust for factors found to be associated with an increased risk of early death after heart transplant. The risk factors are diabetes, reduced creatinine clearance (renal function), previous open heart operation, older donor age and longer ischaemic times.

3.8 Figure 2 shows that the proportion of transplant patients with individual risk factors (except for ischaemic time) was higher in 2008 than the previous two years.

3.9 The proportion of patients, who at the time of transplant had been receiving inotrope drugs to improve heart contraction or mechanical circulatory support by ventricular assist devices (VADs), extracorporeal membrane oxygenation (ECMO) and/or intra-aortic balloon pump (IABP), was significantly higher at Harefield than at other centres: 93% compared to 45% (p=0.002). These factors are not included in the UKCTA risk model.

3.10 The UKCTA report commented that "the data reported to the audit suggests that the majority of patients who underwent transplantation were high risk; only one of the patients transplanted this calendar year was not on inotropes, a VAD, ECMO or IABP at transplant".

Risk-adjusted mortality
3.11 Risk adjustment using the UKCTA risk model reduced the difference between the observed and expected number of deaths within 30 days at Harefield and at other UK centres in 2008. The centre effect estimate for Harefield reduced by more than 50% with risk adjustment and the UKCTA analysis found that "although mortality at Harefield remained 52% higher than expected using the risk model, the number of cases was low and Harefield was not identified as significantly divergent."

Sequential monitoring of mortality
3.12 The sequence of deaths in July and August 2008 was enough to cause the more sensitive technique of sequential monitoring using cumulative sum (CUSUM) method to signal an alert for

30-day mortality at Harefield. The signal occurred after Harefield had contacted the NSC Team as the charts are produced on a monthly basis when the 30-day follow-up point has passed.

Conclusion of the UKCTA report
3.13 "The number of operations reviewed is small as [heart] transplantation in the UK is a low volume procedure, with only around 288 transplants carried out nationally over the 32 months of the review. As a consequence differences and changes in mortality, which may appear large, are not necessarily identified as significant from a statistical perspective. Nonetheless, the rise in 30-day mortality at the end of the series was sufficient to trigger an alarm using the tabular CUSUM methodology. The rise in early mortality seen at Harefield can be explained, at least in part, by the risk profile of the patients, the majority of whom were high risk."

The additional statistical analyses were able to inform the review process and highlight the issues when basing analyses on very small numbers. They also highlight the importance of robust and appropriate case-mix adjustment which is yet another challenge we face in highly complex services that involve small numbers of cases.

3. Extracorporeal Membrane Oxygenation (ECMO)

Monitoring of the outcomes from extracorporeal membrane oxygenation (ECMO) is via the annual reporting of each centres activity and outcomes as submitted to the international voluntary Extracorporeal Life Support Organisation (ELSO). Membership of ELSO is a requirement of each centre as part of the national service and ensures that the data collected on outcomes are consistent internationally, thus allowing benchmarking of outcomes across organisations.

3.1 Extracorporeal membrane oxygenation (ECMO) for adults and children with potentially reversible severe respiratory failure

Extracorporeal Membrane Oxygenation (ECMO) for adults and children with potentially reversible severe respiratory failure has been nationally commissioned in England since 1997. Currently ECMO is provided by the current hospital Trusts:

- The Newcastle upon Tyne Hospitals NHS Foundation Trust (children only)
- Great Ormond Street Hospital for Children NHS Trust (children only)
- University Hospitals of Leicester NHS Trust (adults and children)

There is also a children's ECMO service in provided at Yorkhill Hospital, Glasgow, that is commissioned by National Services Division Scotland. The four providers of ECMO for children with potentially reversible severe respiratory failure work in collaboratively to ensure the needs of the UK are met.

All providers of the national ECMO programme (adult and / or paediatric) are registered with the Extracorporeal Life Support Organisation (ELSO) which is the international registry recording the outcomes for patients receiving ECMO. All centres provide their anonymised activity and outcome data on an annual basis to the National Specialised Commissioning Team as part of the end of year review visits to each centre.

This data collection and presentation is supplemented by an annual meeting of all the UK centres along with representatives from the ECMO service at the Karolinska Institute,

Stockholm, where each centre's anonymised activity and outcomes are presented along with agreed educational topics relating to recent experience or anticipated innovation. Again, this facilitates joint learning and service improvement in a very open and transparent setting.

National commissioning of the adult ECMO service enabled the definitive trial of ECMO in adults with potentially reversible severe respiratory failure to be commissioned jointly with the National Coordinating Centre for Health Technology Assessment (now part of the National Institute for Health Research Evaluation, Trials and Studies Coordinating Centre). The results of this trial were published in the Lancet in September 2009 (Peek et al., 2009) and as a NIHR Health Technology Assessment Monograph in 2010 (Peek et al., 2010).

4. Ventricular Assist Device (VAD) for bridging to heart transplantation

The provision of Ventricular Assist Devices (VADs) as a bridge to heart transplantation has been available at Papworth Hospital NHS Foundation Trust, the Royal Brompton and Harefield NHS Trust and The Newcastle upon Tyne Hospitals NHS Foundation Trust since 2002, and more recently at the other cardiothoracic transplant centres in the UK. Data on implantation, explantation, death and ongoing survival are recorded by NHSBT as part of the cardiothoracic transplant database.

NHSBT provide monthly reports to the National Specialised Commissioning Team on VAD activity and outcomes for each of the national centres. These data are shared with all centres at twice yearly meetings of the National VAD Forum convened and chaired by the National Specialised Commissioning Team and where representatives from each of the national cardiothoracic transplant centres are present. This allows an open and transparent forum for shared learning and has been the vehicle for developing the commissioning policy for expansion of the VAD service within the national cardiothoracic transplant programme.

Additionally, the UK Cardiothoracic Transplant Audit publishes the 30-day, 90-day, 1-year, 2-year and 3-year mortality for those individuals receiving short-term and long-term VADs as a bridge to transplantation, and highlights the survival experience with these devices. The audit also presents data on those VADs used to mechanically support a recently transplanted heart where primary graft failure is experienced, once again informing the development of the service and supporting quality improvement. These data are reviewed at the twice yearly National VAD Forum meetings.

A recent innovation is development of a much more comprehensive and bespoke VAD Database overseen by NHSBT that will allow much greater understanding of the experience with long-term VADs and provide a rich repository for research. The three early providers of long-term VADs (Papworth Hospital NHS Foundation Trust, the Royal Brompton and Harefield NHS Trust and The Newcastle upon Tyne Hospitals NHS Foundation Trust) are completing the population of the database with all historical cases receiving a long-term VAD, whilst all current providers are contributing to data entry on all prospective cases receiving a VAD.

This will provide anonymised data on the entire national cohort of patients receiving VADs and is expected to enable research to help further develop the evidence base in this rapidly changing technology.

5. Pulmonary endarterectomy – Introducing a new technology into the NHS

Chronic thromboembolic pulmonary hypertension (CTEPH) is a form of pulmonary hypertension that occurs as a result of chronic pulmonary embolic blood clots occluding the arteries to the lungs. Over time these emboli build up in the pulmonary arteries causing occlusion and scarring with narrowing of the vessels which eventually leads to reduced blood flow, pulmonary arterial hypertension and right sided heart failure.

Pulmonary endarterectomy (PEA, and previously known as PTE or pulmonary thromboendarterectomy) is a complex cardiac surgical procedure used to remove the blood clots and scarred elements of the vessel walls and restore blood flow through the lungs. It is used as a surgical treatment of CTEPH in those patients where this is appropriate (not all patients with CTEPH are surgical candidates).

This is technically difficult surgery which was introduced into the NHS in 2000 (through national commissioning) at a single centre in the UK at Papworth Hospital NHS Foundation Trust. This allowed the necessary expertise to be developed and outcomes were monitored using the established monitoring and reporting mechanisms established for adult heart and lung transplantation, and with which Papworth Hospital NHS Foundation Trust were already contributing to as an adult cardiothoracic transplant centre.

The concentration of expertise in this single centre aligned to real-time monitoring of mortality outcomes for all patients undergoing PEA has resulted in the outcome data (30-day mortality) at Papworth Hospital NHS Foundation Trust now being consistent with the best in the world.

The effectiveness of this approach will also be highlighted using the example of setting up routine systems for monitoring early mortality in pulmonary endarterectomy to monitor introduction of a new surgical technique into the UK in a single centre. The benefit of experience and systems that allow the development of expertise are shown in the learning curve attached to introducing this technique. Data are emerging that show that the international results are strongly linked to volume.

6. References

Kenny, T. Jessop, E. Gutteridge, W. (2008) Monitoring clinical quality in rare disease services - experience in England. *Orphanet Journal of Rare Diseases,* 2008, 3:23 Available from < http://www.ojrd.com/content/3/1/23>

Klein, G. (1998) *Sources of Power: How people make decisions,* MIT Press, 0-262-61146-5, London

Peek GJ, Mugford M, Tiruvoipati R et al. (2009) Efficacy and economic assessment of conventional ventilatory support versus extracorporeal membrane oxygenation for severe adult respiratory failure (CESAR): a multicentre randomised controlled trial. *Lancet* 2009; 374(9698):1351-1363.

Peek GJ, Elbourne D, Mugford M et al. (2010) Randomised controlled trial and parallel economic evaluation of conventional ventilatory support versus extracorporeal membrane oxygenation for severe adult respiratory failure (CESAR). *Health Technol Assess* 2010;14(35).

Rogers C, Emin A, Thomas H et al. (2010) The Royal College of Surgeons of England Clinical Effectiveness Unit and NHS Blood and Transplant UK Cardiothoracic Audit End of Year Report from the Audit Steering Group to the National Commissioning Group (August 2010). Available from

<www.rcseng.ac.uk/surgical_research_units/ceu/docs.html>
NHS Blood and Transplant. (2011) Available from<www.nhsbt.nhs.uk/about/index>
NSCT (2008) Report of the external review of recent outcomes in the heart transplant service at Harefield Hospital. Available from <http://www.specialisedservices.nhs.uk/document/review-recent-outcomes-in-heart-transplant-service-at-harefield-hospital>

7

Early Postoperative Care After Cardiac Surgery

Paul M. H. J. Roekaerts[1] and John H. Heijmans[2]
[1]*Department of Intensive Care*
[2]*Department of Anaesthesiology*
University Hospital Maasticht, Maastricht
The Netherlands

1. Introduction

The early postoperative course for most patients after cardiac surgery is characterized by a typical pattern of pathophysiologic derangements that benefits form standardized care. Multimodal, multidisciplinary standardization of the care process has been shown to improve use of resources, efficiency, quality, safety and patient satisfaction.

The initial management in the postoperative care after routine cardiac surgery has fundamentally shifted during the past two decades towards a more efficient use of limited postoperative care facilities, early extubation and rapid discharge. The fast-track protocol became feasible after cardiac surgery due to improvements in perioperative anaesthesia management, new surgical techniques, better myocardial protection and cardiopulmonary bypass techniques and to better management of bleeding using point-of-care testing and new hemostatic drugs.

This chapter will briefly discuss the major pathophysiologic derangements and their management during the first 24 hours after surgery. It will than summarize the postoperative care to more specific procedures. Finally, the management of common postoperative complications will be discussed.

2. Pathophysiology during the early postoperative period

Arrival in the intensive care unit

Upon arrival in the ICU, an efficient transfer of care from operation room staff to ICU staff is mandated, while at the same time vital signs are to be maintained stable.

The initial goals in postoperative cardiac recovery are sufficient analgesia, normothermia, adequate oxygenation and ventilation, control of bleeding, restoration of intravascular volume, optimization of blood pressure and cardiac output to maintain organ perfusion and metabolic stabilization.

Hypothermia

Hypothermic cardiopulmonary bypass is usually terminated after the patient has rewarmed to a core body temperature of at least 36 °C. (1) However, patients usually arrive in the ICU with lower core temperatures. This drop in temperature from end of CPB until arrival in the ICU is due to the cool ambient temperatures in the operation room, poor peripheral perfusion and anesthesia-induced inhibition of normal themoregulation. Even patients operated under normothermic CPB, have a tendency to significantly cool down before conclusion of surgery.

Hypothermia has many potential adverse effects. (2) It increases the systemic vascular resistance (SVR) which increases myocardial afterload and myocardial oxygen demand. This compensatory mechanism to provide core warming may contribute to slow warming of peripheral tissues. Drugs that provide vasodilation may improve peripheral perfusion. To prevent hypotension, warmed infusions should be administered concomitantly. Peripheral vasodilation augments heat loss, and core hypothermia may therefore persist.

Hypothermia also precipitates shivering, thereby increasing CO2 production and oxygen consumption, and predisposes to ventricular arrhythmias and coagulation cascade impairments. (3,4)

Therefore, warming should be hastened by forced-air warming blankets, heated humidifiers in the ventilator circuit and warmed infusion fluids. The use of other types of warming blankets or radiant heading hoods can also be considered. (5)

After cardiac surgery, patients may rapidly rewarm and occasionally overwarm to higher temperatures. This phenomenon is attributed to the resetting of the central thermoregulation system.

Blood loss after cardiac surgery

Careful hemostasis in the operation room is the cornerstone in reducing postoperative blood loss. However, bleeding can also be medical and determing the cause of bleeding is often difficult. Although the clinical situation must be individualized for each patient, bleeding in general should not exceed 400 mL/hr during the first hour, 200 mL/hr for each of the first 2 hours, or 100 mL/hr over the first four hours. (6)

There are numerous medical causes for bleeding following cardiac surgery. Residual heparinization is common post cardiac surgery and usually occurs when insufficient protamine is used or heparined pump blood is transfused following CPB.

Platelet dysfunction is also common following cardiac surgery. The CPB circuit itself leads to contact activation and degranulation of platelets, resulting in their dysfunction. Fibrinolysis frequently occurs after CPB, caused by activation of inflammatory or coagulation pathways.

Coagulation factors may decrease from activation and dilution in the CPB circuit.

There has been a dramatic increase in the iatrogenic use of heparin and newer antiplatelet, antithrombotic and thrombolytic drugs during (interventional) treatment of acute cornary syndromes. If revascularization surgery is warranted immediately after these treatments, the anticoagulant effect of these drugs is notable in the postoperative period.

Conventional coagulation tests are helpful to identify the coagulation abnormality contributing to the bleeding. Common laboratory testing includes Hb, platelet count, aPTT, INR, and fibrinogen level. Thromboelastography is also commonly used and has been demonstrated to reduce transfusion requirements.

The most basis principles of the management of postoperative bleeding are:

1. Diagnose underlying medical cause by coagulation tests;
2. Rule out surgical bleeding;
3. Restore clotting parameters to normal by means of medications , transfusion of blood products or clotting factors, and restore normothermia;
4. Monitor for stability of clotting parameters.

Most cardiac surgical centers use the antifibrinolytic lysine analogues, tranexaminic acid and aminocaproic acid, to reduce intraoperative bleeding. These drugs significantly reduce allogeneic blood transfusion after cardiac surgery.

Although rescue therapy with recombinant factor VII can be life-saving in massive bleeding after cardiac surgery, its safety has been questioned. A recent meta-analysis (N = 4468 from 35 studies) demonstrated that this therapy significantly increased the rate of arterial but not venous thromboembolic events. Given its cost and arterial thrombotic risk, it is likely that this hemostatic intervention will continue to be reserved for life-saving therapy of massive coagulopathy after cardiac surgery.(7)

Blood transfusion management

Although there are guidelines for blood transfusion in cardiac surgery, considerable variability has persisted in clinical practice. This variability also exists in anticoagulation and coagulation management.

A recent randomized controlled trial has already demonstrated that restrictive perioperative transfusion does not result in inferior clinical outcome after cardiac surgery. (8) Transfusion burden may in the future be interpreted as a quality indicator in cardiac surgery that must balance risks and benefits to achieve cost-effective optimal clinical outcomes. (9,10)

Perioperative transfusion algorithms for the administration of blood products, coagulation factors and pro-coagulant drugs should assist in preserving resources with improvement in patient safety. (11)

Fluid resuscitation

Cardiac surgery and CPB elicit a systemic inflammatory response which produces a capillary leak. Therefore, fluid resuscitation with cristalloids and/or colloids is necessary to offset the hemodynamic consequences of the capillary leak and the vasodilation that occurs from rewarming and vasodilating drugs. However, the maintenance of intravascular volume in the leakage phase occurs at the expense of expansion of the interstitial space. (12,13)

After the capillairy leak has ceased and hemodynamics have stabilized, diuretics are often used to eliminate the excessive salt and water administered during surgey and the early postoperative phase. This forced diuresis may beneficially affect pulmonary function and early successful extubation.

Several intraoperative measures that have been implemented throughout the years caused a reduction in the inflammatory response and may have contributed to the faster recovery times currently observed after cardiac surgery. The measures include the use of membrane oxygenation, centrifugal pumps, anti-fibrinolytic drugs and steroids, leukocyte filters and coated CPB tubings. (14,15)

Perioperative cardiovascular dysfunction

Adequacy of organ perfusion and tissue oxygenation is the primary goal of hemodynamic management in the postoperative cardiac surgical patient. Preload, afterload and contractility should therefore be maintained at their optimal level. This commonly requires atrial or atrioventricular pacing.

Approximately 20 % of cardiac surgical patients develop cardiovascular dysfunction in the perioperative period, resulting in an inability to pump sufficient blood at normal end-diastolic pressures. There are three distinct clinical scenarios of cardiac impairment in the perioperative period of cardiac surgery - precardiotomy, failure to wean and postcardiotomy - differing from each other substantially concerning diagnosis, monitoring and management.

Precardiotomy heart failure

Myocardial ischaemia is one of the most frequent causes of precardiotomy low output syndrome. The dysfunctional myocardium may not be irreversibly damaged and possibly only 'stunned'or 'hibernating'. Revascularization of the reversibly injured heart areas may result in improved cardiac performance. The first priority should therefore be prompt surgery avoiding further alterations in myocardial contractility, possibly by introducing an IABP preoperatively. However, inadequate myocardial protection during cardiac surgery may exacerbate ischaemic injury in some patients. Patients with longer standing previous poor preoperative cardiac function or with recently irreversibly injured ischaemic heart areas, will of course continue to have poor ventricular performance postoperatively.

Failure to wean

For the successful therapeutic approach of failure to wean, a correct diagnosis of the underlying cause is necessary. The heart failure may be procedure related or patient specific and includes inadequate myocardial protection, reperfusion injury, ischaemia, infarction, incomplete revascularization, metabolic, uncorrected pathology, mechanical issues, conduction issues, pulmonary hypertension and right ventricular failure.

Postcardiotomy heart failure

The priority is to preserve end organ function. Preload and heart rhytm should be optimized, and positive inotropic and/or vasopressor drugs are often used to maintain adequate cardiac output and blood pressure. Although this strategy will restore haemodynamics in most patients, mechanical circulatory support may be indicated.

Monitoring and assessing volume status

Heart failure cannot be ascertained unless the volume status is optimal. However, it is difficult to ascertain volume loading using single haemodynamic measures. Pressure estimates such as pulmonary capillary wedge pressure and central venous pressure are generally unreliable indicators of LV and RV preload. Uncoupling between PCWP and LVEDP frequently occurs as a consequence of elevated pulmonary vascular resistance, pulmonary venoconstriction, mitral stenosis and reduction in transmural cardiac compliance.

Volumetric estimates by echocardiography or transpulmonary thermal dilution techniques are more predictive of preload. In predicting fluid responsiveness in ICU patients, it is preferable to use more reliable dynamic indicators reflecting hypovolaemia, such as stroke volume variation, than static parameters. (16) Several devices are now being used to assess cardiac function based on pulse contour analysis of an arterial waveform. (17)

Echocardiography is of great value in the perioperative cardiac surgical setting. It not only is helpfull in assessing the optimal volume status, but may also immediately identify causes of cardiovascular failure, including valvular problems, cardiac tamponade, systolic anterior motion of the anterior mitral valve leaflet and pulmonary embolism. Echocardiography may differentiate between acute right, left and global heart failure as well as between systolic and diastolic dysfunction.

If there are echocardiographic signs of RV failure, a pulmonary artery catheter (PAC) preferably with continuous SvO_2 measurement should be introduced. PACs can differentiate between pulmonary hypertension and RV ischaemia, which necessitates a reduction of RV afterload. PAC and TEE are complementary to each other for diagnosis and treatment of the cardiac surgical patient. Indications for the use of a PAC are, high risk and/or complex cardiac surgery, hemodynamic instability, low cardiac output syndrome, pulmonary hypertension, differentiating between severe right and left ventriclular dysfunction, vasodilation/vasoconstriction, hypovolemia. SvO_2 in combination with lactate concentration was used postoperative as a goal-oriented hemodynamic therapy to improve outcome.(18,19)

Risk stratification

Risk stratification is increasingly used in open-heart surgery to help adjust resources to predicted outcome. According to all scoring systems major clinical risks include heart failure, unstable coronary syndromes, significant arrhythmias and severe valvular disease. The euroSCORE is mostly used to calculate operative risk, although updating its sensitivity is warranted. (20,21)
In addition to scoring systems, levels at hospital admission of B-type natriuretic peptide (BNP) and the amino-terminal fragment of pro-BNP (NT pro-BNP) are powerful predictors of outcome with regard to in-hospital mortality and rehospitalisation in heart failure patients. (22)

Perioperative myocardial protection

The ultimate goal of perioperative myocardial protection is to limit the extent and consequences of myocardial ischaemia-reperfusion injury. This injury is caused by free radical formation, calcium overload and impairment of the coronary vasculature. Protective measures include the use of free radical oxygen scavengers, inhibitors of the complement system and neutrophil activation, modulation of intracellular gradients and maintenance of sufficient myocardial high energy phosphate stores. Drugs affecting the complement-inflammation pathways, adenosine modulators, cardioplegia solution adjuvants, Na^+/H^+ exchange inhibitors, K_{ATP} channel openers such as volatile anaesthetics and levosimendan, and anti-apoptotic agents are all used for this purpose. (23,24)

Pharmacologic support of myocardial dysfunction

Pharmacological treatment of low cardiac output and reduced oxygen delivery to vital organs is often required in the perioperative cardiac surgical setting. Inadequate treatment may lead to multiple organ failure, one of the main causes of prolonged hospital stay, postoperative morbidity and mortality. Optimal use of inotropes and vasopressors is still controversial and needs further large multinational randomized controlled trials.
However, some recommendations can be made:

- Norepinephrine should be used in case of low blood pressure due to vasoplegia to maintain an adequate perfusion pressure. Preload should be assessed regularly to avoid hypovolemia under vasopressors.
- All catecholamines have positive inotropic and chronotropic effects. There is evidence that dobutamine better preserves the myocardial oxygen balance as compared to the other commonly used drugs. Dobutamine increases stroke volume and heart rate while PCWP is moderately decreased. If blood pressures are low, the combination dobutamine-norepinephrine is frequently used.
- Phosphodiesterase III inhibitors are potent vasodilators and cause less tachyarrhythmias as compared to dobutamine. They also have a more favourable effect on the myocardial oxygen balance as compared to the catecholamines.
- Levosimendan, a calcium sensitizer, has recently been introduced for the treatment of low cardiac output in the perioperative period with success. (25,26,27,28)

Mechanical circulatory support

The intra-aortic balloon pump (IABP) is recommended in the case of heart dysfunction with suspected coronary hypoperfusion. It's main mechanism of action is a reduction of afterload

and diastolic coronary perfusion pressure. The IABP reduces heart work and myocardial oxygen consumption, favourably modifying the balance of oxygen supply/demand.
Extra-corporeal membrane oxygenation (ECMO) is increasingly used for temporary mechanical circulatory support. Advantages of the system include low cost, availability in all cardiac surgical centers and versatile use for cardiac, pulmonary and renal support. ECMO is used as a bridge to recovery, to transplantation, to long-term assist-device and to decision making.
Ventricular assist devices are used today as an established option for patients with end-stage heart failure to obtain a level of functionality that results in an acceptable quality of life for the patient.

Cardiac arrhythmias

Temporary pacing

Two temporary right atrial and two right ventricular epicardial pacing wire electrodes are usually placed at the conclusion of cardiac surgery. Atrial pacing wires can be used diagnostically to record atrial activity. These recordings, obtained simultaneously with standard limb leads, can distinguish among atrial and junctional arrhythmias and differentiate them from more life-threatening ventricular arrhythmias. (6)
The use of pacing is often required in the per- and postoperative period to increase heart rate. Atrial or AV pacing will nearly always demonstrate superior haemodynamics to ventricular pacing. Reentrant rhytms can be terminated by rapid pacing.

Arrhythmias after cardiac surgery

The development of cardiac arrhythmias following open-heart surgery is fairly common and related to altered impulse formation and conduction. An understanding of these mechanisms and the electrophysiologic effects of antiarrhythmic drugs provides a rational basis for the treatment of the different rhythm disturbances.

Atrial fibrillation

Despite various prophylactic measures, atrial fibrillation and flutter occur in about 35 % of all cardiac surgical patients, most commonly on the second and third postoperative day. Etiologic factors include atrial distension, pericardial inflammation, enhanced sympathetic activity, surgical trauma and poor atrial preservation.
To prevent atrial fibrillation, ß-blockers with or without class III (Sotalol) antiarrhythmic properties, are commonly administered orally in the perioperative phase. Dual site atrial pacing and numerous other medications (amiodarone, magnesium sulphate, triodothyronine, digoxin, steroids, procainamide, verapamil, diltiazem) have all been reported to have some favourable effect on the incidence of atrial fibrillation after cardiac surgery.
Treatment consists of cardioversion in the haemodynamically unstable patient. For the stable patient, rate control and attempts to achieve conversion are usually initiated. Drugs used for rate control include calcium-channel blockers (diltiazem, verapamil), ß-blockers (esmolol, metoprolol), magnesium sufate and digoxin. For conversion to sinus rhythm, magnesium sulphate, IA medications (procainamide, quinidine) , IC (propafenone) or III antiarrhythmics (Ibutilide, Amiodarone) are commonly used. (29,30,31)

Ventilation management

Pulmonary complications following cardiac surgery are common, even in patients with healthy lungs, and include diminished functional residual capacity (FRC) following general anaesthesia and muscle relaxants, reductions in vital capacity (VC) following median sternotomy and intrathoracic manipulation, atelactasis, increased intravascular lung water, and increased capillary leakage and extravascular lung water due to the inflammatory response to CPB and surgery. Multiple blood product transfusions and excessive fluid loading may further compromise lung functioning. Acute FRC reduction results in arterial hypoxemia due to ventilation-perfusion mismatch and shunting. In the early postoperative phase, restoration of FRC and maintenance of adequate gas exchange in the face of rising VO_2 and VCO_2 are the primary goals. This can be achieved by a lung-protective ventilation strategy with adequate levels of PEEP. (32,33,34)

For several decades, the medical care of the cardiac surgical patients in the perioperative setting consisted of high-dose opioid stress-free anaesthesia and prolonged mechanical ventilation in the ICU. In recent years, the concepts of Fast-Track Cardiac Anesthesia, Early Extubation and Short-Stay Intensive Care became the backbone of modern perioperative care. Indeed, several randomized trials have shown the safety of fast-tracking. (35,36,37,38,39)

Alterations in anaesthetic protocols using short-acting sedatives-hypnotics and analgesics, less invasive surgical and perfusion techniques, improved perioperative haemostasis management, fluid restriction, preservation of normothermia and reduction of the inflammatory response were all crucial steps in the development of fast-track cardiac surgery. As the number of elderly people is growing fast and cardiac surgery is now an accepted practice in these older patients, fast-tracking makes it possible to more efficiently use the limited facilities and resources. (40)

The debate regarding the optimal extubation time, the window of opportunity, is still ongoing. (41) There are several studies on outcome after extubation in the operation room, which show that it is feasible with good results.(42, 43) However, the nadir of ventricular function occurs about 4 hours following cardiopulmonary bypass. Also, the first few hours after cardiac surgery are characterized by periods of haemodynamic instability, temperature dysregulation, increased mediastinal blood loss and other homeostatic disturbances. Patients can rapidly deteriorate in this early postoperative phase and we believe that instabilities can be best anticipated and treated in an ICU setting in sedated and ventilated patients. The window of opportunity for extubation is therefore between 2 and 6 hours postoperatively.

Weaning strategies should be protocolized.(44) In table 1 is shown a nurse-driven weaning protocol which includes the criteria for the start of the weaning procedure, adequate breathing criteria and the extubation criteria. Only three steps in this protocol may mandate the consultation of the ward doctor.

After ventilatory weaning, the next step in the postoperative ICU management is the discharge of the patient to a step-down unit. This is usually accomplished within 8 hours after arrival in the ICU. Intensive Care discharge criteria are shown in Table 2.

The postoperative (intensive) care unit

The advent of Fast-Track Cardiac Anaesthesia and Short-Stay Intensive Care after Cardiac Surgery also started the discussion whether or not these patients should be treated in a conventional ICU setting. Can adequate and safe postoperative care be given to these patients in parallel "special-care units" such as a dedicated Cardiac Recovery Area (CRA). If a hospital has such a highly-equipped special care unit with a competent and qualified ICU doctor on the ward, adequate nurse-patient ratio and immediate access to ICU-OR facilities, then special care may be feasible. Several institutions reported safe and adequate care in these special units. (45,46) However, in the early postoperative phase, the clinical condition of the patient may

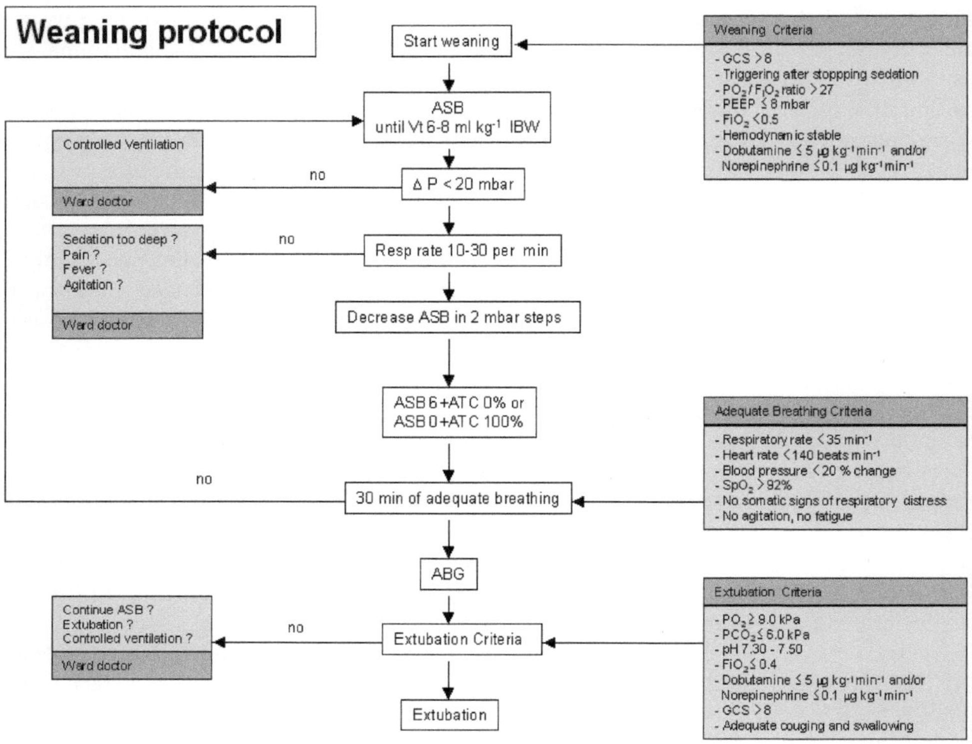

Table 1. Weaning protocol

ICU Discharge Criteria

Pulmonary	Extubation > 30 min Oxygen < 5 L min -1 nasally Respiratory rate > 10 min and < 25 min PaO2 > 9 kPa and PCO2 < 6.5 Kpa
Cardiac	No myocardial ischaemia or ongoing infarction No haemodynamically significant dysrhythmias
Fluid balance	Chest tube drainage < 100 mL hr -1 Diuresis > 0.5 mL Kg -1 hr –1
Neurologic	No signs/symptoms of major neurologic complications
Haemodynamic	No iv vasoactive drugs Except dobutamine 2 g Kg -1 min –1 and/or nitroglycerine 0.5 g Kg -1 min –1 No IABP Cardiac Index > 2 L min –1 m –2

Table 2. ICU Discharge Criteria

deteriorate extremely rapidly. Therefore, continuous adequate monitoring and maximal acute treatment or intervention should always be readily possible for these patients in the early postoperative period. We believe that currently in most hospitals, the ICU setting is the safest and best place to recover from cardiac surgery. In the integrated model, in which all patients are admitted to the ICU, the postoperative management such as nursing-to-patient ratio is variable based on patient requirements. The goal is thus a postoperative unit that allows variable levels of monitoring and care based on patient need. In this model, discharge to a step-down unit as soon as possible after extubation and stabilization of vital parameters should be strived after for every single patient.

Postoperative anticoagulation

After *coronary artery surgery*, antiplatelet therapy has been shown to inhibit platelet deposition on vein grafts and may delay or attenuate the development of fibrointimal hyperplasia and atherosclerosis. Aspirin should therefore be started after CABG surgery and continued indefinitely because of its beneficial effects in patients with native coronary disease. (47)

After tissue *aortic valve surgery*, there is some evidence that short-term anticoagulation may reduce the incidence of thromboembolism. Therefore, anticoagulation is generally recommended for 3 months in younger patients or those with no contraindication for anticoagulation, and is then converted to aspirin. If anticoagulation is not used, aspirin is given. (48,49)

After mechanical aortic valve surgery, all patients should receive anticoagulation indefinitely to achieve an INR of 2.5 – 3.5 for tilting and bileaflet valves.

After mitral tissue valve or mitral ring implantation, anticoagulation should be given for 3 months to achieve an INR of 2.0 – 3.0 and should then be converted to aspirin if the patient is in sinus rhythm. Anticoagulation should be continued indefinitely in patients with atrial fibrillation, an enlarged left atrium (> 50 mm in diameter), or a history of thromboembolism. After mechanical mitral valve insertion, anticoagulation is given to achieve an INR of 2.5 – 3.5. The addition of aspirin is safe and may further reduce the thromboembolic risk. (50,51)

Echocardiography

During the past few decades, the effect of perioperative transoesophageal echocardiography's (TEE) influence on perioperative cardiac surgical decision making has become increasingly more appreciated. Data from several clinical investigations have consistently implicated an important, clinically significant, and cost-effective role for TEE as a safe and valuable haemodynamic monitor in identifying high-risk patients, in assessing in the determination of the definitive surgical approach, and in providing a timely post-cardiopulmonary bypass evaluation of the procedure, thereby allowing for the opportunity to immediately re-intervene or to at least triage patients appropriately. In addition, perioperative TEE has been instrumental in diagnosing cardiac and associated great vessel pathology and in identifying structural abnormalities, aortic disease, intracardiac masses, and pericardial disease. TEE is perhaps most useful for the perioperative evaluation of cardiac valvular disease, especially during surgical procedures involving the mitral valve.

In the intra- and early postoperative period of cardiac surgery, an experienced echocardiographer remains an indispensable clinical team member. Increasing numbers of cardiac anaesthesiologists and intensivists are now being trained and certified as perioperative echocardiographers. (52,53,54)

Analgesia and sedation

An essential element of postoperative care is the provision of adequate analgesia and sedation. In the patient in whom delayed extubation is anticipated, the residual effects of anesthetics and midazolam in combination with a narcotic are generally accepted.
With the trend toward earlier extubation, short-acting narcotics and analgesics are administered during surgery. This requires early postoperative administration of short-acting medications for pain relief and sedation. We prefer to give low dose continuous infusions of morphine in combination with propofol in the ICU. This usually produces adequate sedation and pain relief without respiratory depression and allows for fairly early extubation.

3. Management after specific cardiac surgical procedures

Coronary Artery Bypass Grafting

Treatment of coronary artery disease can be medical or interventional. Catheterization procedures include balloon angioplasty, cardiac stenting and drug-eluding stents, which release drugs capable of preventing stenosis. Surgery includes CABG with the use of the cardiopulmonary bypass machine and OPCAB without the use of the CPB machine. OPCAB surgery may include sternotomy, thoracotomy (MIDCAB) or robotically assisted thoracotomy.
With increasing number of treatment options, it is crucial to establish for each patient which option is superior with regard to angina recurrence, graft patency, and long term survival with the least morbidity at the lowest costs. Several studies address this important issue. Analysis of individual patient data from ten randomized trials including 7812 patients concluded that long-term mortality after CABG and PCI in most patient subgroups with multivessel CAD is similar. (55) CABG versus PCI had lower mortality in diabetes and patients older than 65 years. The SYNTAX investigators concluded from their study that in low and intermediate risk patients with multivessel CAD, PCI and CABG have similar outcomes. In high risk patients with multivessel CAD, CABG is preferred. (56)
Although the COURAGE study, which provided optimal medical therapy (OMT) to all patients and demonstrated no incremental advantage of PCI on outcomes other than angina-related quality of life in stable CAD, a recent analysis by Borden et al reported that among patients with stable CAD undergoing PCI, less than half were receiving OMT before PCI and approximately two-thirds were receiving OMT at discharge following PCI. (57,58)
A number of randomized controlled studies comparing OPCAB to on pump CABG have been completed. Although outcomes have been largely comparable, the evidence of benefits of OPCAB from these trials has not been as convincing as was first anticipated. A large adequately powered RCT of OPCAB versus on pump CABG in high risk patients is needed to determine whether this undeniably harder technique is here to stay. (59,60,61)

Aortic Valve Surgery

Aortic valve replacement surgery may be complicated by heart block because the conduction system lies adjacent to the base of the right coronary cusp. If AV pacing is necessary for more than 4 to 5 days, during which time edema or hemorrhage should subside, placement of a permanent DDD pacemaker is necessary because the conduction system then probably has been damaged by sutures or débridement.

The hypertrophied, noncompliant left ventricle in aortic stenosis depends on adequate preload and on atrial contractions. Loss of sinus rhythm is associated with a 30 % reduction in stroke volume and requires AV pacing.

In aortic regurgitation, the left ventricle is volume and pressure overloaded resulting in a dilated and often hypertrophied chamber. Aortic valve repair for aortic regurgitation is evolving into a standard of care. The systematic classification of aortic regurgitation based on leaflet mobility within the functional aortic annulus makes it possible to study outcomes of the specific interventions. (62,63)

A recent RCT showed that transcatheter aortic valve implantation (TAVI) is significantly superior to medical management of severe aortic stenosis in patients judged to be at excessive risk for conventional aortic valve replacement. (64) TAVI significantly reduced all-cause 1-year mortality. Recent studies have documented rates of cerebral embolism of 70-80 %. (65) Future trials should focus on interventions for stroke reduction after TAVI, including cerebral embolic protection. Techniques for reduction of embolic load may also improve renal dysfunction after TAVI. Although the short and medium term durability of the TAVI valve with preserved hemodynamic performance has been established, further studies are required to elucidate the long term effects. (66,67,68) To this term, guidelines for standardized endpoints in TAVI trials have been published.(69)

Mitral valve surgery

Patients with chronic mitral stenosis often have pulmonary hypertension and usually are diuretic-dependent. They have a small left ventricular cavity with preserved LV function. Common postoperative problems are a low cardiac output syndrome associated with the small LV end-diastolic and end-systolic volumes, RV dysfunction and ventilatory failure due to the pulmonary hypertension, cachexia and fluid overload.

Due to the systolic unloading in patients with mitral valve regurgitation reducing LV wall stress, greater systolic wall stress is required after surgery to achieve adequate cardiac output. Therefore, the use of inotropic support and afterload reduction is often indicated.

In the postoperative period, cardiovascular management is often directed toward increasing filling pressures to above 15-20 mmHg, reduction of pulmonary hypertension and improvement of RV and LV failure. Guiding hemodynamic support with the use of a pulmonary artery catheter may be very helpfull. When atrial fibrillation has been present for more than 1 year or when LA dimension exceeds 50 mm, it is very unlikey to maintain sinus rhythm in the postoperative period. AV pacing is often possible after surgery and may improve cardiac performance. (6)

Diseases of the thoracic aorta

Multidisciplinary guidelines for thoracic aortic diseases were published in 2010. (70) We will highlight some concerns that concern the perioperative setting.

Ascending aortic *dilatation* should be carefully measured in patients with a bicuspid aortic valve presenting for surgery. Earlier surgical intervention is warranted to avoid rupture or dissection.

In aortic arch *aneurysm* surgery, hybrid repair has emerged as low risk aortic repair in high-risk patients. Type I repairs have adequate proximal and distal landing zones: after off-pump anastomosis of the brachiocephalic vessels to the ascending aorta, an endovascular stent is deployed for complete arch repair. Type II repairs have adequate distal landing zone but insufficient ascending aorta to serve as a proximal stent landing zone: after ascending aortic replacement with aortic arch debranching, an endovascular stent is deployed for

complete arch repair with the ascending aortic graft serving as proximal landing zone. Type III repairs have inadequate proximal and distal landing zones: after total arch replacement with a distal elephant trunk, the descending thoracic aortic repair is completed by endovascular stentingwith the elephant trunk serving as the proximal landing zone.
Concerning aortic *dissection*, the Penn classification of a type A dissection integrates type of clinical presentation with dissection extent to stratify perioperative outcome and facilitate decision-making about the type of surgical repair. (71)
The American Heart Association recently published a position paper on the integrated management of decending thoracic aortic disease that complements the recent guidelines from the Society of Thoracic surgeons. (72) These guidelines together summarize the paradigm shift in the management of descending thoracic aortic pathologies due to endovascular therapies. In Stanford type B aortic dissection, the conservative management of refractory pain and hypertension is associated with significant short-term mortality. Therefore, although a survival advantage has not been demonstrated yet, endovascular intervention of these type B dissections is now more often applied.
Depending on the type of organ protection applied during aortic surgery (deep hypothermic circulatory arrest, selective perfusion of brain and kidneys) coagulopathies and neurologic deficit may occur. Brain damage may be due to ischemia or embolisation and paraplegia may result from crossclamping of the descending aorta. Careful neurologic evaluation before and after surgery are important.
Also, the hypotensive regimen used in the early postoperative period must reduce systolic blood pressure and the force of cardiac contraction. The most common regimens include the use of beta-blockers.

4. Management of complications

Atrial fibrillation

Atrial fibrillation following cardiac surgery is common and occurs in up to 35 % of patients. While the cause of AF is not completely understood, it is associated with an increase in mortality, stroke, and prolonged hospital stay. AF has been discussed in Section I of this chapter.

Low cardiac output syndrome

A low cardiac output state may result from decreased left ventricular preload (hypovolemia, cardiac tamponade, vasoplegia), decreased contractility (myocardial stunning, ischemia or infarction related to poor intraoperative myocardial protection, incomplete myocardial revascularization, anastomotic stenosis, or coronary artery spasm), arrhythmias, increased afterload or diastolic dysfunction.
Transoesophageal echocardiography can help define whether a low cardiac output state is related to left ventricular systolic or diastolic dysfunction, right ventricular dysfunction or cardiac tamponade. The management of low cardiac output has been discussed in Section I of this chapter.
Right ventricular dysfunction produces inadequate filling of the left heart resulting in a low cardiac output state. It may be attributable to poor myocardial protection, prolonged ischemic times, coronary embolism, hypotension, RV pressure overload (pulmonary disease, ARDS, pulmonary embolism) or acute pulmonary hypertension due to vasoactive substances, LV dysfunction, protamine or hypoxia and acidosis.

Right coronary artery disease, right ventricular infarction and pulmonary hypertension associated with mitral/aortic disease predispose to RV failure after cardiac surgery.
PAC's and TEE are very helpful in assessing the status of the RV function. In the absence of LV dysfunction, a high RA/PCWP pressure ratio is suggestive for RV dysfunction. The goals of treatment are to optimize RV preload, maintain systemic perfusion pressure, improve RV contractility, and reduce RV afterload by reducing pulmonary vascular resistance. (27)
Diastolic dysfunction , defined as increased resistance to filling of one or both cardiac chambers, is a common finding after cardiac surgery, especially after cardioplegic arrest. Echocardiography has greatly improved the knowledge of diastole by showing the real-time activities in the heart, as related to filling pressures, shape and relaxation. Failure of the RV can contribute to left-sided diastolic dysfunction by increasing cardiac pressures, which causes decreased relaxation of the myocardium yielding decreased myocardial distensibility. Factors responsible for increased chamber stiffness include fibrosis, cellular disarray, and hypertrophy. Factors responsible for decreased relaxation include asynchrony, abnormal loading, ischemia, abnormal calcium ion flux and hypertrophy. Note that ventricular hypertrophy affects both stiffness and relaxation, increasing the risk of diastolic dysfunction. (73)

Cardiac tamponade

Cardiac tamponade is primarily the result of impaired filling of one or more of the cardiac chambers and leads to low cardiac output. Adrenergic and endocrine mechanisms are activated resulting in tachycardia and vasoconstriction.
The diagnosis of cardiac tamponade depends on a high degree of suspicion. Tamponade after cardiac surgery is different from a medical tamponade due to compressing fluid within an intact pericardium. In the setting of cardiac surgery, the pericardial space is often left open and in open communication with one or both the pleural spaces, and the compressing blood is at least in part clotted and able to cause localized compression of the heart. Serious suspicion for tamponade should rise in patients with deteriorating haemodynamics or gradually increasing requirements for inotropic drugs. The classic signs of elevated CVP or equalization of CVP and PAOP are often absent. Cardiac tamponade is difficult to distinguish from biventricular failure. A useful clue may be the pronounced respiratory variation of blood pressure in association with high filling pressures and low cardiac output. TEE may be helpful in diagnosing cardiac tamponade. Echolucent crescents between the RV wall and the pericardium or the posterior LV wall are discernible. A classic sign is diastolic collapse of the right atrium or RV.
A rule of thumb in the acute management of cardiac tamponade is to keep the patient *Full, Fast* and *Thight*. Full, the delivery of volume expansion in order to achieve an adequate preload. Fast, using pacing or medication to increase the heart rate to maintain cardiac output since the strokevolume is compromised. Tight, applying vasopressor therapy to increase preload, maintain bloodpressure and coronary perfusion pressure.
The definitive treatment of tamponade is surgical exploration with evacuation of hematoma.

Renal insufficiency

No clear definition exists as to what constitutes renal impairment or failure following CPB. Renal failure requiring dialysis is infrequent following CPB, although reductions in creatinine clearance are more frequent. There are several risk factors for postoperative renal

failure, including postoperative low cardiac output, repeat cardiac surgery, valve surgery, age greater than 65, and diabetes.
The primary cause may be prerenal (low pressure, low output, ACE, NSAID's), renal (Acute Kidney Injury) from ischaemic insult or interstitial drug-related nephritis or postrenal.
Management of these patients consists of supportive treatment ensuring adequate cardiac ouput, perfusion pressure and volume status and of determining the primary cause, and then directing specific treatment as necessary such as discontinuing the offending drug.
If patients do require dialysis, continuous dialysis may be better than intermittent dialysis. (6,74,75,76)

Impediments to weaning and extubation

The most important factors limiting weaning and extubation in the early postoperative period after cardiac surgery include:

1. neurologic dysfunction
   - agitation, restlessness and disorientation may occur after discontinuation of the sedative medication. The ethiology of this syndrome is multifactorial and includes patient characteristics, perioperative psychotropic drugs used for anaesthesia, pain relief and sedation, and brain ischaemia and inflammation. Initial management consists of reassurance and orientation of the patient and control of pain with opioids. Resedation for a period or the use of haloperidol may be usefull until the patient is oriented and tranquil.
   - diaphragmatic paralysis may complicate cardiac surgery, especially after reoperations, due to surgical lesion of the phrenic nerve in fibrotic pericardial tissue. The phrenic nerve can also be injured or transected during dissection of the internal mammary arteries or during mobilization of the heart in redo surgery. Transient diaphragmatic paralysis can also occur secondary to cold injury by the cold cardioplegic solutions to the phrenic nerve. (6)

     The diagnosis of diaphragmatic paralysis should be considered whenever a patient fails to wean from mechanical ventilation and can be documented by observing paradoxical movement of the diaphragm during inspiration.
2. unstable haemodynamics

   Postoperative cardiac surgical patients with unstable haemodynamics and/or low cardiac output syndromes may not well tolerate the extra work of breathing associated with weaning. Weaning is difficult and may further deteriorate the already compromised myocardium.

   Weaning affects cardiac output due to changes in pulmonary vascular resistance. Increased pulmonary vascular resistance (PVR) leads to septal shifts and reduced efficiency of biventricular function. It is therefore better to keep the patient sedated on full ventilator support until the cardiac problem is resolved. (77)
3. fluid overload

   Cardiac surgery and CPB result in a systemic inflammatory response syndrome which produces a capillary leak. The duration and severity of this syndrome include factors related to the patient characteristics, severity of the surgical trauma, administration of blood products and CPB management. The use of heparin-coated tubings, membrane oxygenator, centrifugal pumps, steroids and leukocyte filters may reduce the SIRS. The capillary leak syndrome is usually most predominant the first 6 to 8 hours after the termination of CPB.

During this period, fluid resuscitation is necessary to offset the capillary leak syndrome and the vasodilation secondary to medications and rewarming. Crystalloid and colloid infusions are used to maintain intravascular volume, although this usually occurs at the expense of expansion of the interstitial space. After the capillary leak has ceased and haemodynamics are stable, diuretics contribute to a faster recovery from surgery.

Succesfull early extubation is compromised by fluid overload. Optimal monitoring and adequate measures should therefore be taken in the operation room and in the intensive care to minimize the positive fluid balance while maintaining adequate tissue perfusion. (78)

Central nervous system dysfunction

Neurologic complications are dreaded sequelae of cardiac surgery. Notwithstanding a progressive decrease in cardiac surgical mortality over the past decades, the incidence of postoperative neurological complications remains relatively unchanged.

Focal neurologic complications

Focal neurologic events complicate approximately 2 % of cardiac procedures requiring CPB, but may increase as more patients with advanced age and diffuse vascular disease undergo cardiac surgery. Focal deficits may include hemiparesis or hemiplegia, aphasia, dysarthria, hand incoordination and visual field deficits.

Preoperative risk factors include increasing age (risk of up to 10 % in patients older than age 75), pre-existing cerebrovascular disease, hypertension, peripheral vascular disease, and poor LV function. Intraoperative and postoperative risk factors include: ascending aortic atherosclerosis and calcification, LV mural thrombus, complex surgery and prolonged bypass and haemodynamic instabilities.

The mechanisms for neurologic injury include some combination of cerebral embolism, hypoperfusion, and inflammation; associated vascular disease and cerebral autoregulatory dysfunction make the brain more susceptible to injury. Particulate embolism due to atherosclerotic plaque, blood thrombus embolus, and air and platelet-fibrin debris is the most common cause of stroke. Cerebral hypoperfusion may be the result of systemic hypotension or impaired regional cerebral blood flow. Although cerebral autoregulation should protect the brain during CPB, hypothermia, blood gas regulation, diabetes and pre-existing hypertension may affect the adequacy of cerebral autoregulation. (6,79,80,81)

In the prevention of focal neurologic complications, preoperative evaluation for extracranial carotid disease should be considered in any patient with neurologic symptoms. Symptomatic carotid disease warrants carotid endarterectomy(CE) prior or at the time of cardiac surgery. Asymptomatic carotid disease in the presence of a carotid bruit should be evaluated by non-invasive testing. There is a trend toward performance of combined CABG-CE in these patient groups. (82)

Intraoperative echocardiograhic scanning of the ascending aorta to identify atherosclerosis might alter cannulation sites and clamping - and manipulation techniques of this diseased aorta. Techniques to avoid embolic load include the use of membrane oxygenators, arterial filters in the CPB circuit, meticulous débridement and irrigation of valves, removal of LV thrombi and of air after intracardiac procedures.

In general, in patients with hypertension or intracranial vascular disease, blood pressure during CPB should be maintained at a higher level.

In the treatment of embolic stroke, heparin is recommended when there is no evidence of intracranial hemorrhage on the CT scan. Heparin prevents propagation of intracardiac thrombus and improves cerebral microcirculation, but is of unclear benefit in preventing further atheroembolism from dislodged plaque.

Encephalopathy

Encephalopathy is fairly common after cardiac surgery and is usually manifested by disorientation and confusion, lethargy or agiation, and paranoia and hallucinations.
The ethiology of this syndrome is multifactorial. It may be related to brain inflammation, cerebral hypoperfusion or microemboli from the CPB circuit. Other factors include patient characteristics, hypoxia, metabolic disturbaces, perioperative psychotropic drugs used for anaesthesia, pain relief and sedation, and drug or alcohol withdrawal.
Initial management consists of reassurance and orientation of the patient and control of pain with opioids. Resedation for a period or the use of haloperidol may be usefull until the patient is oriented and tranquil. The encephalopathy has a fluctuating course but is usually transient. (79,81)

5. References

[1] Ho K.M. and J.A. Tan. Benefitis and Risks of Maintaining Normothermia During Cardiopulmonary Bypass in Adlut Cardiac Surgery: A Systemic Review. Cardiovasc Ther 2009; 29: 260-279.
[2] Sessler D.I.. Complications and Treatment of Mild Hypothermia. Anesthesiology 2001; 95: 531-543.
[3] Crossley A.W.. Peri-operative Shivering. Anaesthesia 1992; 47:193-195.
[4] Rajagopalan S., E. Mascha, J. Na, and D.I. Sessler. The Effectis of Mild Perioperative Hypothermia on Blood Loss and Transfusion Requirement. Anesthesiology 2008;108: 71-77.
[5] Frank S.M., L.A. Fleisher, M.J. Breslow, M.S. Higgins, K.F. Olson, S. Kelly, and C. Beattie. Perioperative Maintenance of Normothermia Reduces the Incidence of Morbid Cardiac Events. A Randomized Clinical Trial. JAMA 1997; 277:1127-1134.
[6] Bojar R.M.. Manual of Perioperative Care in Adult Cardiac Surgery. 2011 Wiley-Blackwell. ISBN: 978-1-4443-3143-1.
[7] Levi M., J.H. Levy, H.F. Andersen, and D. Truloff. Safety of Recombinant Activated Factor VII in Randomized Clinical Trials. N Engl J Med 2010; 363: 1791-1800.
[8] Hajjar L.A., JL. Vincent, F.R.B.G. Galas, R..E. Nakamura, C.M.P. Silva, M.H. Santos, J. Fukushima, R.K. Filho, D.B. Sierra, N.H. Lopes, T. Mauad, A.C. Roquim, M.R. Sundin, W.C. Leao, J.P. Almeida, P.M. Pomerantzeff, L.O. Dallan, F.B. Jatene, N.A.G. Stolf, and J.O.C. Auler Jr.. Transfusion Requirements After Cardiac surgery. The TRACS Randomized Controlled Trial. JAMA 2010; 304: 1559-1567.
[9] Shander A.S. and L.T. Goodnough. Blood Transfusion as a Quality Indicator in Cardiac Surgery. JAMA 2010; 304: 1610-1611.
[10] Varghese R., and M.L. Myers. Blood Conservation in Cardiac Surgery: Let's Get Restrictive. Semin Thoracic Surg 2010; 22: 121-126.
[11] 2011 Update to The Society of Thoracic Surgeons and the Society of Cardiovascular Anesthesiologists Blood Conservation Clinical Practice Guidelines. The Society of Thoracic Surgeons Blood Conservation Guidelines Task Force: Ferraris V.A., J.R. Brown, G.J. Despotis, J.W. Hammon, B. Reece, S.P. Saha, H.K. Song, and E.R. Clough. The Society of Cardiovascular Anesthesiologists Special Task Force on

Blood Transfusion: Shore-Lesserson L.J., L.T. Goodnough, D. Mazer, A. Shander, M. Stafford-Smith, and J. Waters. The International Consortium for Evidence Based Perfusion: Baker R.A., T.A. Dicksinson, D.J. FitzGerald, D.S. Likosky, and K.G. Shann. Ann Thorac Surg 2011; 91: 944-982.

[12] Vincent JL. Fluid Resuscitation: Colloids vs Crystalloids. Acta Clin Bel, Suppl, 2007; 2: 408-411.

[13] Bundgaard-Nielsen M., N.H. Secher, and H. Kehlet. 'Liberal' vs. 'Restrictive' Perioperative Fluid Therapy – A Critical Assessment of the Evidence. Acta Anaesthesiol Scand 2009; 53: 843-851.

[14] Dieleman J.M., J. van Paassen, D. van Dijk, M.S. Arbous, C.J. Kalkman, J.P. Vandenbroucke, G.J. van der Heijden, and O.M. Dekkers. Prophylactic Corticosteroids for Cardiopulmonary Bypass in Adults (Review). Cochrane Database of Systematic Reviews 2011, Issue 5. Art. No.: CD005566.

[15] Henry D.A., P.A. Carless, A.J. Moxey, D. O'Connell, B.J. Stokes, D.A. Fergusson, and K. Ker. Anti-fibrinolytic use for Minimising Perioperative Allogeneic Blood Transfusion (Review). Cochrane Database of Systematic Reviews 2011, Issue 3. Art. No.: CD001886.

[16] Renner J., J. Scholz, and B. Bein. Monitoring Fluid Therapy. B Prac Res Clin Anaesth 2009; 23: 159-171.

[17] Heijmans J.H., Y.M. Ganushchak, M.S. Theunissen, J.G. Maessen, and P.M.H.J. Roekaerts. Predictors of Cardiac Responsiveness to Fluid Therapy after Cardiac Surgery. Acta Anaesth Belg 2010; 16:151-158.

[18] Carl M., A. Alms, J. Braun, A. Dongas, J. Erb, A. Goetz, M. Goepfert, W. Gogarten, J. Grosse, A.R. Heller, M. Heringlake, M. Kastrup, A. Kroener, S.A. Loer, G. Marggraf, A. Markewitz, D. Reuter, D.V. Schmitt, U. Schirmer, C. Wiesenack, B. Zwissler, and C. Spies. S3 Guidelines for Intensive Care in Cardiac Surgery Patients: Hemodynamic Monitoring and Cardiocirculary System. GMS Ger Med Sci. 2010; 8:Doc 12.

[19] Polonen P., E. Ruokonen, M. Hippelainen, M. Poyhonen, and J. Takala. A Prospective, Randomized Study of Goal-Oriented Hemodynamic Therapy in Cardiac Surgical Patients. Anesth Analg 2000; 90: 1052-1059.

[20] Heijmans J.H., J.G. Maessen, and P.M.H.J. Roekaerts. Risk Stratification for Adverse Outcome in Cardiac Surgery. European J Anesth 2003 ; 20 : 515-527.

[21] Nashef S.A., F. Roques, P. Michel, E. Gauducheau, S. Lemeshow, R. Salamon. European System for Cardiac Operative Risk Evaluation (EuroSCORE). Eur J Cardiothorac Surg 1999; 16: 9-13.

[22] Lainchbury J.G., R.W. Troughton, K.M. Strangman, C.M. Frampton, A. Pilbrow, T.G. Yandle, A.K. Hamid, M.G. Nicholls, and A.M. Richards. N-Termed Pro-B-type Natriuretic Peptide-Guided Treatment for Chronic Heart Failure. J Am Coll Cardiol 2010; 55: 53-60.

[23] Warren O.J., A.J. Smith, C. Alexiou, P.L.B. Rogers, N. Jawad, C. Vincent, A.W. Darzi, and T. Athanasiou. The Inflammatory Response to Cardiopulmonary Bypass: Part 1 – Mechanisms of Pathogenesis. J Cardiothorac Vasc Anesth 2009; 23: 223-231.

[24] Warren O.J., A.L. Watret, K.L. de Wit, C. Alexiou, C. Vincent, A.W. Darzi, and T. Athanasiou. The Inflammatory Response to Cardiopulmonary Bypass: Part 2 –

Antiinflammatory Therapeutic Strategies. J Cardiothorac Vasc Anesth 2009; 23: 384-393.

[25] Duranteau J., P. Sitbon, JL. Teboul, E. Vicaut, N. Anguel, C. Richard and K. Samii. Effects of Epinephrine, Norepinephrine, or the Combination of Norepinephrine and Dobutamine on Gastric Mucosa in Septic Shock. Crit Care Med 1999; 27: 893-900.

[26] Mebazaa A., A.A. Pitsis, A. Rudiger, W. Toller, D. Longrois, SE. Ricksten, I. Bobek, S. De Hert, G. Wieselthaler, U. Schirmer, L.K. von Segesser, M. Sander, D. Poldermans, M. Ranucci, P. C. J. Karpati, P. Wouters, M. Seeberger, E. R. Schmid, W. Weder, and F. Follath. Clinical Review: Practical Recommendations on the Management of Perioperative Heart Failure in Cardiac Surgery. Critical Care 2010; 14: 201. Epub 2010 April 28.

[27] Mebazaa A., P. Karpati, E. Renaud, and L. Algotsson. Acute Right Ventricle Failure - from Pathophysiology to New Treatments. Int Care Med 2004; 30: 185-196.

[28] Lahtinen P., O. Pitkanen, P. Polonen, A. Turpeinen, V. Kiviniemi, and A. Uusaro. Levosimendan Reduces Heart Failure after Cardiac Surgery - A Prospective, Randomized, Placebo - Controlled Trial. Crit Care Med 2011;Jun 9 (Epub ahead of print).

[29] Bradley D., L.L. Creswell, C.W. Hogue Jr., A.E. Epstein, E.N. Prystowsky, and E.G. Daoud. American College of Chest Physicians Guidelines for the Prevention and Management of Postoperative Atrial Fibrillation After Cardiac Surgery. Chest 2005; 128, Suppl: 39S-47S.

[30] Koniari I., E. Apostolakis, C. Rogkakou, N.G. Baikoussis, and D. Dougenis. Pharmacologic Prophylaxis for Arial Fibrillation Following Cardiac Surgery: A Systemic Review. J Cardiothorac Surg 2010; 5: 121.

[31] Mitchell L.B., and the CCS Atrial Fibrillation Guidelines Committee. Canadian Cardiovascular Society Atrial Fibrillation Guidelines 2010: Prevention and Treatment of Atrial Fibrillation Following Cardiac Surgery. Can J Cardiol 2011; 27: 91-97.

[32] Apostolakis E.E., E.N. Koletsis, N.G. Baikoussis, S.N. Siminelakis, and G.S. Papadopoulos. Strategies to Prevent Intraoperative Lung Injury During Cardiopulmonary Bypass. J Cardiothorac surg 2010; 5: 1.

[33] Kilpatrick B., and P. Singer. Lung Protective Strategies in Anaesthesia. Brit J Anaesthesia 2010;105: i108/i116.

[34] The Acute Respiratory Distress Syndrome Network. Ventilation with Lower Tidal Volumes as Compared with Traditional Tidal Volumes for Acute Lung Injury and the Acute Respiratory Distress Syndrome. N Eng J Med 2000; 342: 1301-1308.

[35] Cheng D.C.H., J. Karski, C. Peniston, B. Asokumar, G. Raveendran, J. Carroll, H. Nierenberg, S. Roger, D. Mickle, J. Tong, J. Zelovitsky, T. David, and A. Sandler. Morbidity Outcome in Early versus Conventional Tracheal Extubation After Coronary Artery Bypass Grafting: A Prospective Randomized Controlled Trial. J Thorac Cardiovasc Surg 1996;112: 755-764.

[36] Hawkes C.A., S. Dhileepan, and D. Foxcroft. Ealry Extubation for Adult Cardiac Surgical Patients. Cochrane Database of Systematic Reviews. 2003;(4): CD003587.

[37] Myles P.S., and D.McIlroy. Fast-Track Cardiac Anesthesia: Choise of Anesthetic Agent and Techniques. Sem Cardiothorac Vasc Anesth 2005: 9: 5-16.

[38] Mastrigt van G.A.P.G., J. Heijmans, J.L. Severens, E.J. Fransen, P. Roekaerts, G. Voss, and J.G. Maessen. Short-Stay Intensive Care After coronary Artery Bypass Surgery: Randomized Clinical Trial on Safety and Cost-Effectiveness. Crit Care Med 2006; 34: 65-75.
[39] Svircevic V., A.P. Nierich, K.G.M. Moons, G.J. Brandon Bravo Bruinsma, C.J. Kalkman, and D. van Dijk. Fast-Track Anesthesia and Cardiac Surgery: a Retrospective Cohort Study of 7989 Patients. Anesth Analg 2009;108: 727-733.
[40] Paone G., R.S.D. Higgins, S.L. Havestad, and N.A. Silverman. Does Age Limit the Effectiveness of Clinical Pathways After Coronary Artery Bypass Graft Surgery? Circulation 1998; 98: II-41 - II-45.
[41] Higgins T.L. Safety Issues Regarding Early Extubation After Coronary Artery Bypass Surgery. J Cardiothorac Vasc Anesth 1995; 9: 24-29.
[42] Lee T.W.R., and E. Jacobsohn. Pro: Tracheal Extubation Should Occur Routinely in the Operating Room After Cardiac Surgery. J Cardiothorac Vasc Anesth 2000; 14: 603-610.
[43] Djaiani G.N., M. Ali, L. Heinrich, J. Bruce, J. Carroll, J. Karski, R.J. Cusimano, and D.C. Cheng. Ultra-Fast-Track Anesthetic Techniques Facilitates Operating Room Extubation in Patients Undergoing Off-pump Coronary Revascularisation Surgery. J Cardiothorac Vasc Anesth 2001;15: 152-157.
[44] Van Mastrigt G.A.P.G., J.G. Maessen, J. Heijmans, J.L. Severens, and M.H. Prins. Does Fast-track Treatment Lead to a Decrease of Intensive Care Unit and Hospital Length of Stay in Coronary Artery Bypass Patients ? A Meta-regression of Randomized Clinical Trials. Crit Care Med 2006; 34: 1624-1634.
[45] Flynn M., S. Reddy, W. Shepherd, C. Holmes, D. Armstrong, C. Lunn, K. Khan, and S. Kendall. Fast-tracking Revised: Routine Cardiac Surgical Patients Need Minimal Intensive Care. Eur J Cardiothorac Surg 2004; 25: 116-122, 2004.
[46] Ender J., M.A. Borger, M. Scholz, AK. Funkat, N. Anwar, M. Sommer, F.W. Mohr, and J.F. Fassl. Cardiac Surgery Fast-track Treatment in a Postanesthetic Care Unit. Six-month Results of the Leipzig Fast-track Concept. Anesthesiology 2008; 109: 61-68.
[47] Zimmerman N., E. Gams, and T. Hohlfeld. Aspirin in Coronary Artery Bypass Surgery: New Aspects of and Alternatives for an Old Antithrombotic Agent. Review. Eur J Cardiothorac Surg 2008; 34: 93-108.
[48] Brueck M., W. Kramer, P. Vogt, N. Steinert, P. Roth, G. Gorlach, M. Schonburg, and M.C. Heidt. Antiplatelet Therapy Early After Bioprosthetic Aortic Valve Replacement is Unnecessary in Patients Without Thromboembolick Risk Factors. Eur J Cardiothorac Surg 2007; 32: 108-112.
[49] Colli A., JP. Verhoye, R. Heijmen, J.T. Strauch, J.A.J. Hyde, D. Pagano, M. Antunes, H. Koertke, S.K. Ohri, D.H.L. Bail, P. Leprince, B.H.M. Van Straten, T. Gherli, on behalf of ACTION Registry Invetigators. Antithrombotic Therapy After Bioprosthetic Aortic Valve Replacement: ACTION Registry Survey Results. Eur J Cardiothorac Surg 2008; 33: 531-536.
[50] Kulik A., F.D. Rubens, P.S. Wells, C. Kearon, T.G. Mesana, J. van Berkom, and BK. Lam. Early Postoperative Anticoagulation After Mechanical Valv Replacement: A systematic Review. Ann Thrac Surg 2006; 81: 770-781.
[51] Dunning J., M. Versteegh, A. Fabbri, A. Pavie, P. Kolh, U. Lockowandt, S.A.M. Nashef, on behalf of the EACTS Audit and Guidelines Committee. Guideline on

Antiiplatelet and Anticoagulation Management in Cardiac Surgery. Euro J Cardiothorac Surg 2008; 34: 73-92.
[52] Couture P., A.Y. Denault, S. McKenty, D. Boudreault, F. Plante, R. Perron, D. Babin, L. Normandin, and N. Poirier. Impact of Routine use of Intraoperative Transesophageal Echocardiography during Cardiac Surgery. Can J Anesth 2000; 47: 20-26.
[53] Fox J., K. Glas, M. Swaminathan, and S. Shernan. The Impact of Intraoperative Echocardiography on Clinical Outcome Following Adult Cardiac surgery. Sem Cardiothorac Vasc Anesth 2005; 9: 25-40.
[54] Shernan S.K.. Perioperative Transesophageal Echocardiographic Evaluation of the Native Mitral Valve. Crit Care Med 2007; 35: 8 (suppl): S372-S383.
[55] Hlatky M.A., D.B. Boothroyd, D.M. Bravata, E. Boersma, J. Booth, M.M. Brooks, D. Carrie, T.C. Clayton, N. Danchin, M. Flather, C.W. Hamm, W.A. Hueb, J. Kahler, S.F. Kelsey, S.B. King, A.S. Kosinski, N. Lopes, K.M. McDonald, A. Rodriguez, P. Serruys, U. Sigwart, R.H. Stables, D.K. Owens, and S.J. Pocock. Coronary Artery Bypass Surgery Compared With Percutaneous Coronary Interventions for Multivessel Disease: A Collaborative Analysis of Individual Patient Data from Ten Randomized Trials. Lancet 2009; 373: 1190-1197.
[56] Kappetein A.P., T.E. Feldman, M.J. Mack, MC. Morice, D.R. Holmes, E. Stahle, K.D. Dawkins, F.W. Mohr, P.W. Serruys, and A. Colombo. Comparison of Coronary Bypass Surgery with Drug-eluting Stenting for the Treatment of Left Main and/or Three-vessel Disease: 3-year Follow-up of the SYNTAX trial. Eur Heart J 2011; doi:10.1093/eurheartj/ehr213
[57] Boden W.E., R.A. O'Rourke, K.K. Teo, P.M. Hartigan, D.J. Maron, W.J. Kostuk, M. Knudtson, M. Dada, P. Casperson, C.L. Harris, B.R. Chaitman, L. Shaw, G. Gosselin, S. Nawaz, L.M. Title, G. Gau, A.S. Blaustein, D.C. Booth, E.R. Bates, J.A. Spertus, D.S. Berman, J. Mancini, and W.S. Weintraub for the COURAGE Trial Research Group. N Engl J Med 2007; 356: 1503 – 1516.
[58] Borden W.B., R.F. Redberg, A.I. Mushlin, D. Dai, L.A. Kaltenbach, and J.A. Spertus. Patterns and Intensity of Medical Therapy in Patients Undergoing Percutaneous Coronary Intervention. JAMA 2011; 305: 1882-1889.
[59] Khan N.E., A. De Souza, R. Mister, M. Flather, J. Clague, S. Davies, P. Collins, D. Wang, U. Sigward, and J. Pepper. A Randomized Comparison of Off-pump and On-pump Multivessel Coronary-artery Bypass Surgery. N Engl J Med 2004; 350: 21-28.
[60] Louagie Y.A.G., J. Jamart, and A.Gruslin. Do Coronary Bypass Graft Flows Differ Between On-Pump and off-Pump Operations ? Ann thorac Surg 2005; 79: 2004-2012.
[61] Shroyer A.L., F.L. Grover, B. Hattler, J.F. Collins, G.O. McDonald, E. Kozora, J.C. Lucke, J.H. Baltz, and D. Novitzky for the Veterans Affairs Randomized On/Off Bypass (ROOBY) Study Group. N Engl J Med 2009; 361: 1827-1837.
[62] Augoustites J.G.T., W.Y. Szeto, and J.E. Bavaria. Advances in Aortic Valve Repair; Focus on Functional Approach, Clinical Outcomes, and Central Role of Echocardiography. Expert Review. J Cardiothorac Vasc Anesth 2010; 24: 1016-1020.
[63] Boodhwani M., L. de Kerckhove, D. Glineur, J. Rubay, JL. Vanoverschelde, P. Noirhomme, and G. El Khoury. Repair of Regurgitant Bicuspid Aortic Valves: A Sytematic Approch. J Thorac Cardiovasc Surg 2010; 140: 276-284.

[64] Leon M.B., G.R. Smith, M. Mack, C. Miller, J.W. Moses, L.G.Svensson, M. Tuzcu, J.G. Webb, G.P. Fontana, R.R. Makkar, D.L. Brown, P.C. Block, R.A. Guyton, AD. Pichard, J.E. Bavaria, H.C. Herrmann, P.S. Douglas, J.L. Petersen, J.J. Akin, W.N. Anderson, D. Wang, and S. Pocock for the PARTNER Trial Investigators. Transcatheter Aortic-valve Implantation for Aortic Stenosis in Patients who Cannot Undergo Surgery. N Engl J Med 2010; 363: 1597-1607.

[65] Ghanem A., A. Muller, C.P. Nahle, J. Kocurek, N. Werner, C. Hammerstingl, H.H. Schild, J.O. Schwab, F. Mellert, R. Fimmers, G. Nickenig, and D. Thomas. Risk and Rate of Cerebral Embolism After Transfemoral Aortic Valve Implantation. J Am Coll Cardiol 2010; 55: 427-432.

[66] Gotzmann M., W. Bojara, M. Lindstaedt, A. Ewers, L. Bosche, A. Germing, T. Lawo, M. Bechtel, A. Laczkovics, and A. Mugge. One-Year of Transcatheter Aortic Valve Implantation in Severe Symptomatic Aortic Valve Stenosis. Am J Cardiol 2011; 107: 1687-1692.

[67] Kodali S.K. W.W. O'Neill, J.W. Moses, M. Williams, C.R. Smith, M. Tuzcu, L.G. Svensson, S. Kapadia, G. Hanzel, A.J. Kirtane, and M.B. Leon. Early and Late (OneYear) Outcomes Following Transcatheter Aortic Vlave Implantation in Patients With Severe Aortic Stenosis (from the United States REVIVAL Trila). Am J Cardiol 2011; 107: 1058-1064.

[68] Gurvitch R., D.A. Wood, E.L. Tay, J. Leipsic, J. Ye, S.V. Lichtenstein, C.R. Thompson, R.G. Carere, N. Wijesinghe, F. Nietlispach, R.H. Boone, S. Lauck, A. Cheung, and J.G. Webb. Transcatheter Aortic Valve Implantation. Durability of Clinical and Hemodynamic Outcomes Beyond 3 Years in a Large Patient Cohort. Circulation 2010; 122: 1319-1327.

[69] Leon M.B., N. Piazza, E. Nikolsky, E.H. Blackstone, D.E. Cutlip, A.P. Kappetein, M.W. Krucoff, M. Mack, R. Mehran, C. Miller, MA. Morel, J. Petersen, J.J. Popma, J.J.M. Takkenberg, A. Vahanianm, GA. Van Es, P. Vranckx, J.G. Webb, S. Windecker and P.W. Serruys. Standardized Endpoint Definitions for Transcatheter Aortic Valve Implantation Clinical Trial: A Consensus Report from th Valve Academic research Consortium. Eur Heart J 2011; 32: 205-217.

[70] Hiratzka L.F., G.L. Bakris, J.A. Beckman, R.M. Bersin, V.F. Carr, D.E. Casey Jr, K.A. Eagle, L.K. Hermann, E.M. Isselbacher, E.A. Kazerooni, N.T. Kouchoukos, B.W. Lytle, D.M. Milewicz, D.L. Reich, S. Sen, J.A. Shin, L.G. Svensson, and D.M. Williams. ACCF/AHA/AATS/ACR/ASA/SCA/SIR/STS/SVM Guidelines for the Diagnosis and Management of Patients with Thoracic Aortic Disease. J Am Coll Cardiol 2010; 55: 27-129.

[71] Augustides J.G.T., W.Y. Szeto, N.D. Desai, A. Pochettino, A.T. Cheung, J.S. Savino, and J.E. Bavaria. Classification of Acute Type A Dissection: Focus on Clinical Presentation and Extent. Review. Eur J Cardiothorac Surg 2011; 39: 519-522.

[72] Coady M.A., J.S. Ikonomidis, A.T. Cheung, A.H. Matsumoto, M.D. Dake, E.L. Chaikof, R.P. Cambria, C.T. Mora-Mangano, T.M. Sundt and F.W. Sellk; On behalf of the American Heart Association Council on Cardiovascular Surgery and Anesthesia and Council on Peripheral Vascular Disease. Surgical Management of Descending Thoracic Aortic Disease: Open and Endovascular Approaches: A Scientific Statement From the American Heart Association. Circulation 2010 ;121: 2780-2804.

[73] Bernard F., A. Denault, D. Babin, C. Goyer, P. Couture, A. Couturier, and J. Buithieu. Diastolic Dysfunction is Predictive of Difficult Weaning from Cardiopulmonary Bypass. Anesth Analg 2001; 92: 291-298.

[74] Landoni G., T. Bove, M. Crivellari, D. Poli, O. Fochi, C. Marchetti, A. Romano, G. Marino, and A. Zangrillo. Acute Renal Failure After Isolated CABG Surgery : Six Years of Experience. Minerva Anesthesiol 2007; 73: 559-563.

[75] Bove T., M.G. Calabro, G. Landoni, G. Aletti, G. Marino, G. Crescenzi, C. Rosica, and A. Zangrillo.The Incidence and Risk of Acute Renal Failure after Cardiac Surgery. J Cardiothorac Vasc Anesth 2004; 18: 442-445.

[76] Schwann N.M., J. C. Horrow, M.D. Strong III, D. Chachad, A. Guerraty and A.S. Wechsler. Does Off-Pump Coronary Artery Bypass Reduce the Incidence of Clinical Evident Renal Dysfunction after Multivessel Myocardial Revascularisation ? Anesth Analg 2004; 99: 959-964.

[77] Andre A.C.St., and A. DelRossi. Hemodynamic Management of Patients in the First 24 Hours After Cardiac Surgery. Crit Care Med 2005; 33; 202-2093.

[78] Pradeep A., S. Rajagopalam, H.K. Kolli, N. Patel, R. Venuto, J. Lohr, and N.D. Nader. High Volumes of Intravenous Fluid During Cardiac surgery are Associated with Increased Mortality. HSR Proceedings in Intensive Care and Cardiovascular Anesthesia 2010: 2: 287-296.

[79] McKhann G.M., M.A. Grega, L.M. Borowicz, W.A. Baumgartner, and O.A. Selnes. Stroke and Encephalopathy After Cardiac Surgery. An Update. Stroke 2006; 37: 562-571.

[80] Van Eijk M.M.J., and A.J.C. Slooter. Delirium in Intensive Care Unit Patients. Sem Cardiothrac Vasc Anesth 2010; 14: 141-147.

[81] Mehta Y., and R. Singh. Cognitive Dysfunction After Cardiac Surgery. Review. J Alzheim Dis 2010; 22: S115-S120.

[82] Gopaldas R.R., D. Chu, T.K. Dao, J. Huh, S.A. LeMaire, P. Lin, J.S. Coselli, and F.G. Bakaeen. Staged Versus Synchronous Carotid Endarterectomy and Coronary Artery Bypass Grafting: Analysis of 10-Year Nationwide Outcomes. Ann Thorac Surg 2011; 91: 1323-1329.

8

Hemotherapy in Cardiac Surgery

Robert Wagner
Centre for Cardiovascular and Transplant Surgery,
St Anne's University Hospital,
Masaryk University, Brno
Czech Republic

1. Introduction

Demands for allogeneic blood transfusion in cardiac surgery were still high two decades ago. Today there is a gradual decline in transfusion requirements owing to recent advances in cardiac surgery and related specialties that have together developed techniques for peri-operative blood salvage and its autotransfusion; this trend continues to progress towards bloodless surgery. Its milestones have included a refinement of surgical methods, a better understanding of bleeding pathology related to extracorporeal circulation and an introduction of coagulation monitoring during surgery, using point-of-care testing [1,2,3,4,5]. A significant advancement in extracorporeal circulation came with the development of less aggressive, more biocompatible and miniature-circuit systems [6, 7]. As a result, allogeneic blood transfusion is currently not needed in over 50% of all surgical procedures and in almost 100 % of coronary heart operations [8,9]. However, over 40 % of patients undergoing cardiac surgery still require allogeneic blood transfusion; of them, 5-7 % show an excessive blood loss (more than a normal circulating blood volume), 10-15 % have a large blood loss (more than 2000 ml) and about 15-20 % have a moderate blood loss (1000 ml to 2000 ml) during the day of surgery up to 7 am next day. The average transfusion requirement ranges between 2 and 4 units of packed red blood cells (PRBC) per adult patient, depending on the centre. Cardiac surgery centers commonly utilize 10 to 15 % of the RBCs production of the regional blood bank centers [10].

In the last two decades, the efforts to develop techniques for refinements of surgical methods and peri-operative blood salvage have intensified because of an increase in the number of reoperations and surgery on elderly, polymorbid patients with preoperative anemia. These are the major components of a multi-modality strategy that involves the pre-operative preparation of a patient, surgical procedures, drug administration and homeostatic maintenance (Table 1).

2. Autotransfusion

Autotransfusion in cardiac surgery can be divided into three steps according to collection time and the method used, namely, pre-operative autologous blood donation, intra-operative blood collection and post-operative blood salvage.

Modality	Intervetion
Preoperative erythrocyte maximizing and/or blood conservation	Fe supplementation, vitamines (C, folates, B12), short-course erythropoietin, Autologous blood donation of 1-3 units: a: blood bank center collection b: perioperative isovolemic hemodiloution
Bleeding minimization	Sophisticated technology of incision (argon atmosphere, laser scalpel,...) Refinements of surgical methods Topical hemostatic agents Peroperative blood recuperation Postoperative blood salvage Early revision for surgical bleeding
Hemodilution minimization during CPB	Low priming volume and retrograde priming after starting CPB Ultrafiltration Minicircuits
Homeostasis optimization	Controlled hemostasis (blood fluidity) Controlled hemodynamics (blood pressure) Normothermia Internal environment (pH, blood gases, ionts, glycaemia)
Adherence to basic rule of transfusion	Complying with lowest and safe level of anemia for a given clinical case STS recommended transfusion point: Hb 7 ± 1 g/dl .

Table 1. Policy for limitation of blood bank transfusion in cardiac surgery

2.1 Pre-operative autologous blood donation

The efficacy of pre-operative blood donation varies according to the time between blood collection and cardiac surgery. The current storage and preservation techniques allow us to collect and maintain 2 to 4 units of full blood or PRBCs. This efficacy can be enhanced by stimulation of erythropoiesis during blood donation, but this is used only selectively because of the potential of thrombotic cardiovascular events and costs [11, 12]. The use of erythropoietin is also limited by the necessity of starting its administration 3 weeks before surgery [13]. A short course erythropoietin was also used several days before cardiac operation in anemic patients (haemoglobin < 13 g/dl) without autologous predonation [14, 15]. In cardiac patients, there are certain contraindications for participation in autologous blood donation programmes; in addition to anaemia (haematocrit below 33%), they include critical aortic stenosis, idiopathic subaortal stenosis, ischaemic heart disease with unstable angina or with left main coronary artery stenosis, chronic NYHA class IV heart failure, ventricular rhythm disturbances on the day of blood collection and an acute heart attack. This all narrows the selection of candidates for autologous blood donation in cardiac surgery. The proportion of patients meeting the criteria for autotransfusion varies from 10% to 30%; however, some centres can indicate more patients in relation to the range of surgical procedures done and according to experience of the blood collection team.

Intra-operative isovolaemic haemodilution

Blood collection performed immediately before cardiac surgery for the purpose of acute isovolaemic haemodilution is also included in an autologous blood donation programme, thus permitting participation of the patients otherwise contraindicated for a standard programme [16]. A 500- to 1000-ml amount of blood is collected via a central venous catheter or an arterial line and is replaced by a colloid or crystalloid solution before cardiopulmonary bypass (CPB) surgery is commenced. For calculation of the final haematocrit (HCT) value, it is necessary to take the CPB dilutional effect (minimum of 1.3 l) into consideration. Usually, a dilution of 25% to 20 % HCT is used, which is also recommended because of a lower risk of damage to blood elements during extracorporeal perfusion. In some centres, 15% HCT is an accepted transfusion trigger in the patients who do not tolerate allogeneic blood transfusion [17, 18].

The advantage of intra-operative haemodilution is in that the lost blood contains lower red blood cell counts and a transfusion of fresh autologous blood supplies functional platelets. The only contraindication for intra-operative isovolaemic haemodilution is anaemia and haemodynamic instability. Patients with a cardiac disease and a haemoglobin level below 130 g/l may not be able to compensate for a temporary decrease in erythrocyte counts and may show signs of tissue hypoxia or symptoms of cardiac disease. This approach can be combined with blood processing by apheresis.

Intra-operative apheresis

It was first used in thoracic surgery in 1987. It is a medical technology in which the blood of a patient is passed through an apparatus that separates out plasma and platelets and returns the reminder to the circulation. The separated components are then ready for use at the time needed to complete their deficiency. During cardiac surgery with extracorporeal circulation, this technology can also salvage part of the platelets which are otherwise absorbed onto the inner surface of the extracorporeal tubing or can end as platelet-leukocytes micro-aggregates in the capillary beds. The anaesthesiologist can decide between plasma with platelets or a platelet concentrate requiring a slowly rocking shaker for short-term maintenance. Similarly to many blood recuperation devices, the apheresis technique is based on centrifugal force. The proportion of platelets in plasma depends on the spin rate (2400-3600 revolutions per min). The amount of plasma safely collected is related to the patient's clinical condition and usually equals to 20 % of the calculated plasma volume or 12 ml/kg body weight. The procedure design for replenishing intravascular volume, which differs from centre to centre, involves crystalloids and starch derivatives or albumin. When a larger amount of blood is collected, it is necessary to check the ionogram, pH value and free calcium and magnesium levels. The efficiency of both plasmapheresis and thrombopheresis has been evaluated in many studies. Some have reported lower requirements for allogeneic blood transfusion [19, 20, 21] as well as lower post-operative blood losses [22]. A positive effect of pre-operative plasmapheresis has been demonstrated by low tendency to pathological fibrinolysis [23]. On the other hand, other authors described a low efficacy of pre-operative apheresis in cardiac surgery [24] and related it to the pre-operative administration of an anticoagulation and platelet anti-aggregation therapy. The patients who, before surgery, have received coumarin derivatives, heparin and non-steroidal anti-phlogistic drugs do not benefit from plasmapheresis [25].

2.2 Intra-operative blood salvage

The collection of blood shed from the wound is an integral part of CPB surgery. The procedure consists of two steps, namely, cardiotomy suction carried out during CPB with standard heparinisation and blood recuperation during normocoagulation.

Cardiotomy suction

The system is usually composed of two suction lines, two pumps and a cardiotomy reservoir with filters. Blood is retrieved not only from some heart and aorta sections, but also directly from the operative field which continually fills with blood coming from the open sternum and the mediastinum, and from around the cannulae connecting the circuit. The shed blood is aspirated and collected in the reservoir, passes through a filter and is returned via an oxygenator into the circulation. The patient can thus be re-infused with several litres of blood. However, during this process blood is exposed to air in the operative wound and to synthetic surfaces of tubing, which activates a non-specific inflammatory response including coagulation. Suction-produced mechanical stress results in damage to erythrocytes and contributes to haemolysis. An improvement could be achieved by processing shed mediastinal blood in an autotransfusion device that would separate viable erythrocytes from the rest of activated blood with cellular detritus, fat and vasoactive mediators. A good effect on pulmonary function and haemodynamics has been shown in patients receiving processed blood [26]. This technique, however, is not much used because of technical problems with processing large volumes of blood and the necessity of plasma and platelet substitution.

Blood recuperation

The processing of blood drained from the operative wound is carried out at the time the patient is not fully heparinised, i.e., before the beginning or after the end of extracorporeal perfusion. If, after the termination of perfusion, a large volume of blood with low HCT is left in the reservoir, its recuperation is advisable, particularly when problems with renal function are expected. A large reservoir blood volume can be avoided by inserting a haemofiltration coil in the CPB system. The approach, however, removes only water and low-molecular-weight substances.

From the clinical point of view, the patient always benefits from blood recuperation because no or only few blood products are necessary [27]. In terms of costs, the situation depends on the degree of bleeding. With current blood products prices on the one hand and the costs of a recuperation set on the other, the results are equal if at least two PRBC units are obtained. It means that recuperation is cost-effective in patients with excessive blood loss; the costs of both approaches are equal in patients with large blood loss and, in patients with low blood loss, recuperation comes at an increased cost to the institution [28]. This medico-economic analysis would be right on the assumption that transfusion of allogeneic PRBCs is as valuable as fresh autologous blood transfusion. The present-day evidence suggests that this is not true, although the major risks of allogeneic blood transfusion, such as infection or immunomodulation, are minimal. Packed red blood cells are more suitable for correcting severe chronic anaemia than for an acute large blood loss. Transfused banked erythrocytes are not capable of immediate oxygen release for tissue supply, and their accumulation in the pulmonary vascular bed may do acute damage to the lung tissue, causing right-sided pulmonary failure and paradoxically making circulatory shock worse. Nonetheless, for a patient with excessive blood loss, allogeneic blood transfusion is the only possible choice. Because of increasing awareness of these facts, blood recuperation is becoming a routine method in a growing number of centres for cardiac surgery and is currently used in about 50% and 60 % of these institutions in the EU and North America, respectively.

2.3 Post-operative blood salvage

The method of collection and re-infusion of mediastinal blood shed during surgery and drained in the early post-operative period has been used in cardiac surgery since 1978 [29]. The blood is collected into a special auto-transfusion device, or the cardiotomy reservoir of a CPB system can be used when it is connected to mediastinal drainage and a vacuum generator and with anti-coagulation citrate solution added. The cardiotomy reservoir involves a 40-μ filter, but insertion of an additional 20-μ filter in the outlet line is recommended. The salvaged blood has 20-25% HCT, a small number of platelets, free haemoglobin and no fibrinogen. It also contains fibrin-degradation products, cardiac enzymes and other inflammatory factors which may adversely affect biochemical tests and clinical outcomes [30, 31]. In spite of the disadvantages, this is a safe technique which can reduce demands for blood transfusion particularly in patients with blood loss exceeding 500 ml in the first two hours [32]. Doubts concerning the quality of salvaged erythrocytes were challenged by Schmidt et al. who did not find any differences in survival between the red blood cells of shed mediastinal blood and those of circulating blood [33]. At present the use of a recuperation technique for mediastinal blood is preferred because it reduces the organism's burden by free haemoglobin and inflammation mediators [34]. It is usually carried out in continuation of intra-operative recuperation and is regarded as a safe method up to 8 hours of the patient's transfer to an intensive care unit [35].

3. Blood bank products

A rational therapy with blood products and derivatives requires that their administration be based on a documented deficiency or dysfunction. However, surgical bleeding may be associated with additional haemostatic risk factors. A prolonged hypovolaemia with subsequent shock can initiate consumption coagulopathy and the substitution with crystalloids and colloids will result in clotting factor dilution. With the exception of patients with serious vascular disease or very old persons, the majority of patients can tolerate anaemia with a haemoglobin concentration of 7 g/dl or 24% HCT. However, in the early phase of circulatory and haemostatic homeostasis, it is advisable to increase Hb concentration to 8g/dl in order to spare the compensatory capacity of myocardium (increased cardiac output) and to utilise a possibility to regulate systemic blood pressure by blood viscosity. In patients with serious peripheral arterial disease, it is reasonable to increase the transfusion trigger. Transfusion should be administered only after the patient's medical history and their actual health status have been taken into consideration [36, 37].

3.1 Allogenic blood transfusion

In cardiac surgery, blood transfusion is indicated to correct severe anaemia due to excessive bleeding caused by vessel disruption during surgical exposure and dissection or by coagulopathy. Severe anaemia is characterised by a decrease in Hb concentration which leads to diffuse or localised tissue ischaemia. The attitudes to indications for transfusion have developed under the influence of diverse subjective views, ranging from a miraculous remedy to an absolute refusal, as well as on evidence-based information. Patients can greatly benefit from blood transfusion, if it is life-saving, or be severely harmed if a serious infection is transferred. The risk of viral infection transfer has recently decreased so much (HIV or HCV transfer is one per million transfusions) that it should no longer be a limiting factor in blood transfusion [37].

Transfusion can also induce immunomodulation in the recipient, i.e., stimulation or inhibition of immune responses.. The former involves the production of antibodies (alloimmunisation) against the surface antigens including HLA, which has several adverse effects. The latter, immune depression, involves a decrease in the ratio of circulating T-lymphocyte subpopulations (CD4+/CD8+) and impaired function of natural killer cells and antibody production by lymphocytes. The development of immunomodulation is associated with donor leukocytes; their removal can by half reduce the incidence of adverse conditions, such as transfusion-related acute lung injury (TRALI) [38]. In addition, immunomodulation can enhance susceptibility to infection, as suggested by a strong association found between transfusion and post-operative infection in a retrospective study on 15 000 patients surgically treated for ischaemic heart disease in Cleveland in 2006 [39].

Blood transfusion offers three advantages: it increases blood oxygen-carrying capacity, provides volume to support cardiac output and improves homeostasis; however, only the first one is the indication criterion. Which situation, therefore, requires an increase in oxygen-binding capacity of the blood by means of transfusion? A defined threshold Hb concentration is not the answer, because the capacity of blood to transport oxygen depends on other parameters such as cardiac output, pulmonary oxygenation, and haemoglobin ability to bind and release oxygen. Nevertheless, based on studies and expert opinions, a consensus has been reached that transfusion is beneficial to patients with an Hb concentration below 7 g/dl while it brings no benefits to patients with an Hb level above 10 g/dl. Moreover, an increase in oxygen-carrying capacity by transfusion is not accompanied by an immediate increase in oxygen delivery to tissues, because stored erythrocytes are depleted of 2, 3-diphosphoglycerate and nitric oxide concentrations, which markedly reduces their ability to offload oxygen. To recover this ability takes several hours, and blood bank transfusion thus only adds to haemodilution of functional haemoglobin and a transient drop in oxygen supply.

In healthy individuals, an acute anaemic state no longer manageable by compensatory mechanisms and leading to a switch to anaerobic metabolism occurs at Hb levels between 3 and 4 g/dl. This is associated with venous haemoglobin oxygen saturation of 56%, which equals to a tissue supply of 333 ml oxygen/min/m^2. The major compensatory mechanisms include increased cardiac output, an increase in oxygen extraction and an increase in capillary erythrocyte transit time. Patients with coronary heart disease may develop acute anaemia at an Hb level of about 6 g/dl. These limit values have been obtained in animal experiments and confirmed by cardiac surgery in several thousands of Jehovah's Witness patients. The level of evidence, defined as C and D, allows us to accept the fact that, in certain clinical situations, patients can tolerate an Hb concentration of about 6 g/dl. The range of clinical conditions is very broad and, in the present-day ageing polymorbid population, there are not many patients who would tolerate acute anaemia with threshold Hb values 6 g/dl.

3.2 Fresh frozen plasma (FFP)

Full blood collected from donors is treated by plasmapheresis or centrifugation to obtain plasma which is frozen within 6 hours of collection. Although FFP is indicated for documented either isolated or multiple coagulation factor deficiencies (II, V, VII, IX, X, XII), it has formerly been used as volume replacement and in the prophylaxis of potential coagulopathy in relation to massive transfusions and extracorporeal circulation. At the 1984 conference on FFP it was concluded that such indications for FFP administration are not justified and this conclusion has so far been accepted [40,10]. Prophylactic FFP administration on the basis of massive transfusion (more than 10 red blood cell mass units) and abnormal laboratory tests (PT and aPTT) in the absence of clinically apparent bleeding is not supported by evidence either. Abnormal PT and aPTT results are often found even after five administrations of blood transfusion. Their positive predictive value is only about 30%. However, patients in whom the blood transfusion volume exceeds the total blood volume will always require either platelet substitution or FFP, or both products. A correlation between the volume of lost plus transfusion blood and the occurrence of coagulopathy is not a simple one. On the other hand, there is a strong correlation between the occurrence of coagulopathy and the duration of hypotension and/or hypothermia. Patients with no or only a short period of hypotension, even if they receive massive transfusion, will not have coagulopathy while those exposed to one hour of hypotension will often develop a serious form of it. Similarly, hypothermia plays an important role; its avoidance is a decisive factor in the prevention of coagulopathy after massive transfusion Patients undergoing cardiac surgery with extracorporeal circulation experience a drop in coagulation factor levels by 30 to 40 %, but only few of them show clinical bleeding. Excessive bleeding after cardiac surgery, if not due to surgical reasons, results from platelet dysfunction or their deficiency, and/or is caused by hypothermia, prolonged hypotension (circulatory shock) or residual heparinisation. Because of the lack of scientific evidence for clinical efficacy, indication criteria for the use of FFP are largely based on cardiac surgeons' expertise. They include: 1) substitution therapy in isolated or multiple coagulation factor deficiencies.; 2) need to reverse over-warfarinisation, in that case two units are administered in the non-bleeding patient and six units in the bleeding one; 3) treatment of pathological bleeding due to a transfusion volume being larger than the patient's total blood volume.

3.3 Thrombocyte concentrate (TC)

Thrombocyte concentrates are transfusion products obtained from full blood by centrifugation. A pooled-donor TC is derived from four to six blood donors to give one therapeutic thrombocyte transfusion unit for an adult patient. A single-donor TC is obtained by apheresis using a platelet separator. Both products contain over 200 x 10^9 platelets in a 250- to 350-ml plasma volume. The TCs are stored in special storage bags allowing gas exchange on a shaking apparatus at 20-24°C for up to 5 days. In TC infusion, the ABO-blood group/Rhesus factor of the patient must be respected. If a TC of the required blood group is not available, thrombocytes suspended in plasma ABO compatible with the recipient's erythrocytes can be administered. Other options include a TC from an O-blood group donor who has a low titre of anti-A and anti-B agglutinins or the use of platelets resuspended in a plasma substitute. An Rh-positive donor can receive a TC from an Rh-negative donor, but not vice versa [41].

In major surgical procedures, it is recommended to maintain the platelet count above 50 x10^9/l because of a risk for microvascular bleeding. In cardiac surgery with cardiopulmonary bypass, where platelet-related defects are the most frequent cause of haemostatic abnormality, the recommended platelet count is 50-100 x10^9/l [42]. An increase above this level is justified only in severe platelet dysfunction. Platelet concentrates should not be administered routinely in cardiac surgery because it has been associated with increase in multi-organ failure and death [43, 44]. One therapeutic TC unit in an adult patient increases the platelet count by 10-20 x10^9/l. The therapeutic efficacy is assessed by clinical signs (decrease of bleeding) or laboratory evidence of increased platelet counts.

An insufficient increase in platelet counts can be due to reasons such as low TC quality or higher requirements for platelet counts in patients with trauma or disseminated intravascular coagulation. However, the most serious cause involves immune destruction of platelets by alloantibodies or autoantibodies, and this is suspected when other causes are excluded.

4. Blood bank transfusion for urgent procedures

In transfusion practice safety requires that allogeneic blood be cross-matched with the recipient's blood; the test takes about 60 min. In emergency live-saving procedures or unexpected massive blood losses, it is possible to perform transfusion after a minor cross-match test or without it, or to administer ABO/Rh compatible blood or O-type blood.

If immediate transfusion is necessary and the recipient's blood group is not known, then it is justified to use uncrossmatched type-O packed red blood cells (UORBC) that lack A and B surface antigens. For potential expecting mothers, the UORBCs should always be Rh negative to avoid sensibilisation and damage to the foetus in case the mother is Rh-negative. The patients should be given no more that 10 UORBC units and subsequently receive transfusion with standard blood testing.

If there is time to do blood group testing, ABO-compatible PRBCs are administered without a cross-match test.

In about 3 % of the human population, serum contains anti-erythrocyte antibodies which in a great majority (85 %) are of one type only. The magnitude of risk for a post-transfusion reaction is equal to this frequency, but the results from trauma centres show that it is in fact even lower. Gervin et al. have recorded no reaction in 875 transfusions without cross-matching in 160 patients [45].

When more time is available (about 20 min), a minor cross-match test is done which reveals most of the donor uncommon anti-erythrocyte antibodies. It fails to detect abnormal antibodies in only 0.04% of the patients and this makes the probability of post-transfusion reaction extremely low.

It can be concluded that, seen in a historical perspective, the needs for blood transfusion in cardiac surgery have varied, but are still high. With advances in cardiac surgery during the last 50 years, a significant decrease was recorded in the average blood product requirement per patient, but this trend has recently had declining tendency. The reason lies in increasing numbers of reoperations and surgery on very old and polymorbid patients with preoperative anemia. Our conclusion suggests a multi-modality blood-saving strategy ranging from patient pre-operative preparation, over surgical and autotransfusion techniques and drug intervention to homeostatic maintenance. So far this strategy has brought about results in the form of an increasing number of operations not requiring transfusion; this is currently more than 50 % of all cardiac surgery procedures. Despite its risks, allogenic blood transfusion still remains an important supportive and life-saving measure in ultimate situations.

5. References

[1] Buxton B, Frazier OH, Westaby S: Ischemic heart disease surgical management. Mosby International ltd.1999.

[2] Cohn LH, Edmunds LH. Cardiac Surgery in the Adults. McGraw-Hill Companies,Inc. Third ed.2008.

[3] Franco KL, Verrier ED: Advanced therapy in cardiac surgery. BC Decker Inc. 1999.

[4] Pleym H, Wahba A, Videm V, et al. Increased fibrinolysis and platelet activation in elderly patients undergoing coronary bypass surgery. Anesth Analg 2006;102:660-67.

[5] Spiess BD, Tuman KJ, McCarthy RJ, et al: Thromboelastography as an indicator of post-cardiopulmonary bypass coagulopathies. J Clin Monit 1987;3:25-30.

[6] Utley JR: Cardiopulmonary bypass. Cardiovasc Engineering 1996;1:7-26.

[7] Beholz S, Zheng L, Kessler M, Rusche M, Konertz W. A new PRECiSe (priming reduced extracorporeal circulation setup) minimizes the need for blood transfusions: first clinical results in coronary artery bypass grafting. Heart Surg Forum 2005;8: E132-5.

[8] Mehta RH, Sheng S, O Brien SM, et al. Reoperation for bleeding in patients undergoing coronary artery bypass surgery: incidence, risk factors, time trends and outcomes. Citc Cardiovasc Qual Outcomes 2009;2:583-90.

[9] Helm RE, Rosengart TK, Klemperer JD, et al: Comprehensive multimodality blood conservation: 100 consecutive CABG operations without transfusion. Ann Thorac Surg 1998; 65:125-36.

[10] Frerraris VA, Brown JR, Despotis GJ, et al. 2011 Update to the Society of thoracic surgeons and the Society of cardiovascular anesthesiologists blood conservation clinical practice guidelines. Ann Thorac Surg 2011;91:944/82.

[11] Helm RE, Gold JP, Rosengard TK, et al. Erythropoietin in cardiac surgery. J Card Surg 1993; 8:579-06.
[12] Schmoeckel M, Nollert G, Mempel M, Mempel W, Reichard: Effects of recombinant human erythropoietin on autologous blood donation before open heart surgery. J Thorac Cardiovasc Surg 1994;41:364-68.
[13] Yazicioglu L, Eryilmaz S, Sirlak M, Bahadir M, et al. Recombinant human erythropoietin administration in cardiac surgery. Thorac Cardiovasc Surg 2001;122:741-45.
[14] Sowade O, Warnke H, Scigalla P, et al. Avoidance of allogenic blood transfusions by treatment with epoetin beta [recombinant human erythropoietin] in patients undergoing open-heart surgery. Blood 1997;89:411-18.
[15] Weltert L, D'Alessandro S, Nardella S, Girola F, et al. Preoperative very short-term, high-dose erythropoietin administration diminishes blood transfusion rate in off-pump coronary artery bypass: A randomized blind controlled study. J Thorac Cardiovasc Surg 2010;139:621-27.
[16] Robblee JA, Starr NJ: Blood harvested before cardiopulmonary bypass decreases postoperative blood loss. J Cardiothorac Vasc Anesth 1990;4:519-25.
[17] Fang WC, Helm RE, Krieger KH, et al: The impact of low hematocrit during cardiopulmonary bypass on outcome in patients undergoing coronary artery surgery. Circulation 1996;94(Suppl I):I-170.
[18] Toraman F, Karabulut H, Alham C. Is it the patient or the physician who cannot tolerate anemia? A prospective analysis in 1854 nontransfused coronary artery surgery patients. Perfusion 2009;24(6):373-80.
[19] Jones JW, McCoy TA, Rawitscher RE, et al: Effects of intraoperative plasmapheresis on blood loss in cardiac surgery. Ann Thorac Surg 1990;49:585.
[20] Stammers AH, Kratz J, Johnson T, et al: Hematological assessment of patients undergoing plasmapheresis during cardiac surgery. J Extracorpol Technol 1993;(1):6-14.
[21] Li S, Ji H, Lin J, et al. Combination of acute preoperative plateletpheresis, cell salvage, and aprotinin minimizes blood loss and requirement during cardiac surgery. J Extracorpor Technol 2005;37:9-14.
[22] Boldt J, von Borman B, Kling D, et al: Preoparative plasmapheresis in patients undergoing cardiac surgery. Anesthesiology 1990;72:282-88.
[23] Stammers AH, Rasmussen CR, Kratz JM: The effects of platelet-rich plasma on postcardiopulmonary bypass fibrinolysis. J Extracorpor Technol 1993;25:122.
[24] Tobe CE, Vocelka C, Sepulvada R, et al: Infusion of autologous platelet-rich-plasma does not reduce blood loss and product use after coronary artery bypass. J Thorac Cardiovasc Surg 1993;105:1007-13.
[25] Wong CA, Franklin ML, Wade LD: Coagulation tests, blood loss, and transfusion requirements in platelet-rich plasmapheresed versus nonpheresed cardiac surgery patients. Anesth Analg 1994;78:29.
[26] Boodhwani M, Nathan HJ, Mesana TG, Rubens FD. Effects of shed mediastinal blood on cardiovascular and pulmonary function: a randomized, double-blind study. Ann Thorac Surg 2008;86:1167-73.

[27] Wang G, Bainbridge D, Martin J, Cheng D. The efficacy of an intraoperative cell saver during cardiac surgery: a metaanalysis of randomized trials. Anesth Analg 2009;109(2):320-30.
[28] Klein AA, Nashef SAM, Sharples L, Bottrill F, et.al. A randomized controlled trial of cell salvage in routine cardiac surgery. Anesth Analg 2008;107(5):1487-95.
[29] Schaff HV, Hauer J, Gardner TJ, et al: Routine use of autotransfusion following cardiac surgery: Experience in 700 patients. Ann Thorac Surg 1978;27:49.
[30] Wahl GW, Feins RH, Alfieres Ghixby K: Reinfusion of shed blood after coronary operations causes elevations of cardiac enzyme levels. Ann Thorac Surg 1999;53:625.
[31] Bland LA, Villarino ME, Arduino MJ, et al: Bacteriologic and endotoxin analysis of salvaged blood used in autologous transfusions during cardiac operations. J Thorac Cardiovasc Surg 1992;103:82.
[32] Morris JJ, Tan YS: Autotransfusion: is there a benefit in a current practice of aggressive blood conservation? Ann Thorac Surg 1994;58:502.
[33] Schmidt H, Lung JO, Nielson SL: Autotransfused shed mediastinal blood has normal erythrocyte survival. Ann Thorac Surg 1996;62:105.
[34] Griffith LD, Billman GF, Daily PO, et al: Apparent coagulopathy caused by infusion of shed mediastinal blood and its prevention by washing of the infusate. Ann Thorac Surg 1989;47:400.
[35] Murphy GJ, Allen SM, Unsworth-White J, Lewis CT, et al. Safety and efficacy of perioperative cell salvage and autotransfusion after coronary artery bypass grafting: a randomized trial. Ann Thorac Surg 2004;77:1553-59.
[36] Crosby ET. Perioperative hemotherapy: I. Indications for blood component transfusion. Review article. Can J Anaesth, 1992, 39: 7, 659.
[37] Ferraris VA, Ferraris SP, Spiess BD, et al. Perioperative blood transfusion and blood conservation in cardiac surgery: clinical practice guideline. Ann Thorac Surg 2007;83:S27-S86.
[38] Watkins TR, Rubenfeld GD, Martin TR, et.al. Effects of leukoreduced blood on acute lung injury trauma: a randomized controlled trial.Crit Care Med 2008;36:1493-99.
[39] Banbury MK, Brizzio ME, Rajeswaran J, et al. Transfusion increases the risk of postoperative infection after cardiovascular surgery. J *Am Coll Surg* 2006;202:131-138.
[40] Consensus Conference: Fresh Frozen Plasma. Indications and risks. JAMA, 1985, 253: 551.
[41] Stroncek DF, Rebulla P, et.al. Transfusion medicine 2 Platelet transfusions. Lancet 2007;370:427-38.
[42] Slichter SJ. Evidence-based platelet transfusions guidelines. Hematology Am Soc Hematol Educ program 2007;: 172-78.
[43] Simon TL, Akl BF, Murphy W. Controlled trial of routine administration of platelet concentrates in cardiopulmonary bypass surgery. Ann Thorac Surg 1984;37:359-64.
[44] Mangano DT. Aspirin and mortality from coronary bypass surgery. NEJM 2002;347:1309-17.

[45] Gervin AS, Fischer RP. Resuscitation of trauma patiens with type-specific uncrossmatched blood. J Trauma, 1984, 24:327.

9

Cardiac Surgery and Allogeneic Blood Transfusions

Yavuz M. Bilgin
Department of Hematology,
Erasmus Medical Center Rotterdam
The Netherlands

1. Introduction

Coronary artery bypass graft (CABG) surgery is a frequently performed intervention for re-vascularization of the myocardium. Worldwide approximately 1,000,000 patients are undergoing cardiac surgery annually. Nowadays more older patients with more comorbidities are operated, which is possible due to more advanced techniques. Herewith allogeneic blood transfusions play a crucial role in performing of these more complicated treatments. Until the discovery of the AB0-bloodgroups in the early 1900s allogeneic blood transfusions were a high-risk procedure: more than 50% of the recipients of blood died. The discovery of the blood groups followed by the development of citrate as anticoagulant to prevent clotting of blood enabled the start of safer transfusion medicine. Both World Wars and other disasters in the 20th century had a large impact on further development and structural organization of transfusion medicine. Before the introduction of centrifugation techniques in the 1960s whole blood transfusions were used. Since transfusion of red blood cells, platelet concentrates and plasma became possible over time, treatment of more diseases and opportunities for surgical interventions raised. Nowadays due to stringent donor selection and advanced preparation techniques transfusions of blood components became gradually considered as a safe therapy. From the blood components, red blood cells are used for blood loss and other causes of anemia, while plasma and platelets are transfused to treat or as prophylaxis for bleeding disorders. However unexpected adverse effects leading to more transfusion-related complications are the reasons of serious concerns, which resulted in more evidence-based research aiming to reduce the risks of allogeneic blood transfusions. Nowadays in the Western World every year about 50-70 per 1,000 patients receive a blood transfusion (Cobain et al., 2007), while at the age of 80 years approximately one in five persons has been transfused (Kamper-Jorgensen et al., 2009). Per year 75 millions of blood units are collected and transfused worldwide, thereby yearly saving thousands of lives, facilitating more complex surgery as cardiac surgery and making transfusion of different blood components indispensable for treatment of many diseases. The development of modern transfusion medicine represents one of the greatest achievements of medicine in the 20th century. However the safety of allogeneic blood transfusions is high, there are still risks leading to higher morbidity and mortality associated with blood transfusions. Many clinical and laboratory studies are performed in the past years to decrease the risks of allogeneic blood transfusions.

2. Clinical effects of anemia in cardiac surgery

Anemia is frequently found in patients undergoing cardiac surgery and is associated with postoperative adverse outcome. Cohort studies in patients with cardiovascular diseases, documented that anemia was associated with an increase in mortality. In a large cohort of 78,974 patients older than 65 years with acute myocardial infarction, patients with lower hematocrit (Ht) levels had a higher 30-day mortality rate and red blood cell (RBC) transfusions significantly reduced the mortality rate in patients with a Ht level of less than 30% at admission (Wu et al., 2001). In contrast, a post hoc analysis derived from three large cardiovascular studies showed that patients with an acute coronary syndrome who had received RBCs during the acute phase had (after adjustment for other predictive factors) significant higher 30-day mortality than non-transfused patients (Rao et al, 2004).
In cardiac surgery preoperative as well as postoperative anemia are important prognostic factors for outcome. One study showed that preoperative hemoglobin (Hb) level below 6.2 mmol/l (10.0 g/dl) is associated with higher mortality rate compared to patients with higher Hb values (Kulier et al., 2007). Furthermore, it has been observed that preoperative anemia is associated with increased risk of stroke or kidney failure (Karkouti et al., 2009). The preoperative anemia was also an independent predictor for renal and cerebral complications in patients with a low EuroSCORE; whereas in patients with high EuroSCORE all cardiac and non-cardiac postoperative adverse events were significantly higher in anemic patients. This proves that anemia is less tolerated in patients with higher comorbidities and preoperative anemia should be taken into account in the preoperative preparations (Murphy et al., 2007). Anemic patients had a higher early and late mortality than non-anemic patients undergoing cardiac surgery and not only preoperative anemia also the nadir of the Hb concentration during cardiac surgery is related with worse adverse outcome (van Straten et al., 2009). Furthermore blood loss is a common problem in cardiac surgery, which requires some re-interventions, while massive blood loss (the replacement by transfusion of more than 50 percent of a patient's blood volume) is associated with an 8-fold increase in mortality (Karkouti et al., 2004). These studies in homogenous patient population with high number of blood transfusions show that pre-and postoperative anemia in cardiac surgery are both predictive in early and late mortality.

3. Clinical effects of red blood cell transfusions in cardiac surgery

Due to a more critical oxygen delivery to the myocardium, patients with cardiovascular diseases are less tolerant to anemia than others. Blood transfusions for anemic patients with ischemic heart disease are intended to improve the patient survival. Patients undergoing cardiac surgery consumes a large proportion of RBC transfusions, estimated approximately 20% of the total blood supply (Snyder-Ramos et al., 2008). The transfusion rates for CABG show great variability between hospitals with a mean number of transfused units varying between 0.4 to 6.3 units per patient (Stover et al., 1998). Several observational studies showed that not anemia was associated with increased morbidity and mortality. Also the peroperative administration of RBCs was an important factor associated with mortality and morbidity, which was dose-dependently associated with postoperative infections and higher mortality (Chelemer et al., 2002, Leal-Noval et al., 2001). In a prospective study in cardiac surgery, 4.8% of patients who did not receive RBCs suffered from postoperative infections, contrasting with 29% in patients who received 6 or more RBC units (Koch et al.,

2006). Also uncomplicated cardiac surgery patients who received preoperative blood transfusions had higher morbidity and mortality (Mohnle et al., 2011). Patients who received RBC transfusions had a lower heart output and cause more congestive heart failure (Surgenor et al., 2006). Besides short-term (30-and 90-days) mortality, also long-term mortality (1-year, 5-and 10-years) was influenced by transfusion of RBCs negatively (Kuduvalli et al., 2005, Engoren et al., 2002, Koch et al., 2006). Especially in patients undergoing combined valve operations with CABG allogeneic blood transfusions played a deleterious role in the long-term outcome. However all these studies in cardiac surgery were retrospectively designed and provide by no means proof of a causal role of allogeneic RBC transfusions on postoperative morbidity and mortality, where many other factors, such as age and duration of surgery influence the outcome. The clinical effects of red blood cell transfusions in cardiac surgery have also been discussed very intensively in several RCTs. We discuss in this chapter the effects of blood transfusions in patients undergoing cardiac surgery. Hereby we focus on studies in cardiac surgery published in the last years that investigated the clinical effects of transfusion triggers of RBCs, storage of RBCs and the immunomodulatory effects of RBC transfusions.

3.1 Effects of transfusion triggers of red blood cells

For decade's a hemoglobin (Hb) level of 10 gr/dl (6.2 mmol/l) was considered as an appropriate trigger for red blood cell (RBC) transfusions. A randomized controlled trial (RCT) performed in the 1990s changed the classical transfusion policy for RBCs drastically (Hebert et al., 1999); resulting in a tendency for lower Hb triggers. In this large RCT in 838 patients, staying at an intensive care unit (ICU), patients were either transfused to maintain the Hb value between 7 and 9 g/dl (restrictive) or above 10 g/dl (liberal). Patients assigned to a restrictive trigger received an average of 2.6 units of RBCs compared with 5.6 units in the liberal group. Mortality at 30 days, the primary outcome measure, was not significantly different between the groups: 18.7% versus 23.3% (p=0.11) in favour of the restrictive trigger arm. In subgroups of patients younger than 55 years of age and those with a lower APACHE (Acute Physiology And Chronic Health Evaluation) risk score, mortality was significantly lower in the restrictive group than in the liberal group: 5.7% versus 13% (p=0.02) and 8.7% versus 16.1% (p=0.03), respectively. This study investigated all ICU-patients with different diseases. Recently, in cardiac surgery one randomized controlled trial in 502 patients suggested that a more restrictive RBC strategy aiming for a hematocrit of 24% is as safe as a liberal RBC strategy aiming for a hematocrit of 30%; the 30-day mortality and severe morbidity was approximately 10% in both groups (Haijar et al., 2010). Several trigger protocols are available developed in the last years aiming to reduce transfusions of RBCs in cardiac surgery. However since the implementation of universal leukodepletion of red blood cells in several countries, two observational studies showed that blood transfusions were not associated with higher mortality rates, instead higher Hb concentrations and receipt of blood transfusions were associated with lower hospital mortality (Vincent et al., 2008 and Sakr et al., 2010). These studies suggest that leukoreduction of RBCs could have beneficial effects. Although, in the last years older patients with more comorbidities are operated, who need more allogeneic blood transfusions. Therefore it seems that sicker patients are undergoing cardiac surgery and they receive more blood transfusions, which make difficult to analyze the exact effects of blood transfusions.

3.2 Effects of storage of red blood cells

Blood collected from voluntary donors is stored according to the protocols of the blood banks. During storage red blood cells show a number of structural and functional alterations, referred to as storage lesions. Changes in shape, rigidity, depletion of 2,3-diphosphoglycerate (2,3 DPG) and nitric oxide scavenging are presumed to result in impaired perfusion and oxygen delivery (Ho et al., 2003). The clinical effects of storage times have only been evaluated in observational studies with unequivocal conclusions in different clinical settings. In cardiac surgery several retrospective studies investigated the storage time of RBCs (Vamvakas and Carven, 1999, Yap et al., 2008, van de Watering et al., 2006 and van Straten et al., 2011), although these studies revealed controversial conclusions. Recently an observational study investigated the effects of peri-operatively transfusion of RBCs either stored more or less than 14 days in cardiac surgery (Koch et al., 2008). In this study one-year mortality was higher in patients receiving RBCs stored more than 14 days; however this association between storage time and mortality was only reported as an unadjusted analysis. Identifying confounders were not adjusted for the storage time of RBCs. Factors as publication bias and correction for confounders play an important role in the differences. Also the most associations between storage of red blood cells and outcomes were reported in North-America and none in European countries. This suggests that a difference in blood products and storage conditions between North America and most countries in Europe can cause the intercontinental difference. Recently an observational study from Denmark suggests that there is indeed an association between RBCs stored longer than 14 days and postoperative infections (Andersen et al., 2011). Because different blood products and storage times are used, meta-analysis cannot be used to formulate a reliable consensus on possible associations between storage time of RBCs and morbidity and mortality. Therefore results from prospective, if possible intercontinental, studies have to be awaited.

3.3 Clinical effects of allogeneic leukocytes red blood cells

Allogeneic RBC transfusions have profound effects on the recipient's immune system. This immunomodulatory effect of blood transfusions, presumed to result from allogeneic leukocytes, was recognized in the 1970s of the last century in patients receiving a kidney allograft in which pre-transplant blood transfusions improved the subsequent allograft survival (Opelz et al., 1971). In the 1980s it has been suggested that such immune suppression could enhance cancer recurrence and postoperative infections (Gantt, 1981). These possible adverse effects of blood transfusions are referred to as transfusion-related immunomodulation (TRIM). The existence and possible mechanisms of TRIM are hitherto not understood. Many clinical and laboratory studies investigated the possible immunomodulatory effects and mechanisms of TRIM. Several factors have been suggested to play a role. Most suspected factors are: allogeneic mononuclear cells, soluble biological response modifiers circulating in plasma and leukocyte-derived mediators. Allogeneic leukocytes or soluble factors released by leukocytes during storage have been most extensively studied in the last years (Vamvakas and Blajchman, 2007). Because allogeneic leukocytes are the most important factor held responsible for the clinical effects of TRIM; RCTs investigating their role are indispensable.

Before the 2000s only selected patients received leukodepleted (or leukoreduced) transfusions for the prevention of HLA-allo-immunization, cytomegalo-virus (CMV)-transmission (or reactivation) or febrile non-hemolytic transfusion reactions (FNHTR) due to cytokines or leukocyte antibodies present in the patient. Since 2002 in the Netherlands all patients who need blood receive leukodepleted blood transfusions. Last years more countries implemented universal leukodepletion for RBCs. If countries that did not convert to universal leukodepletion have to be made a new policy; their decisions should be based on the data of the available RCTs. Or new RCTs should be performed in countries that did not implemented universal leukoreduction to their patients.

To investigate the clinical effects of TRIM several studies were performed comparing leukocyte-containing with leukodepleted blood products in different clinical settings. In cardiac surgery more patients receive allogeneic blood transfusions on average than in other clinical settings. Therefore the role of TRIM in cardiac surgery is important to investigate aiming to understand the effects of allogeneic leukocytes on postoperative complications and outcome.

Six RCTs are performed in cardiac surgery; four of them are published as full articles (van de Watering et al.; 1998, Wallis et al., 2002, Bilgin et al., 2004, Connery et al., 2005). Two other studies in cardiac surgery are still available only as abstracts, mentioning limited data (Bracey et al., 2002 and Boshkov et al., 2006). Two of these trials randomised the patients for three different blood products. The main methods and results are mentioned in Table 1.

From these studies, one study compared buffy-coat-depleted (BCD)-RBCs with two filtered RBCs: fresh filtered RBCs before storage (FF) or stored filtered RBCs (SF) (van de Watering et al., 1998). There was a higher mortality in 60 days (7.8%) in the group who -received BCD-RBCs as compared with 3.6 % and 3.3 % in those receiving FF or SF products respectively (p=0.015). This suggests that soluble mediators, still present in the SF products, caused no more adverse effects than FF-RBC, lacking leukocyte-derived soluble factors. In a subgroup analysis, the difference in mortality was present only in patients who received more than three RBC units. A second study (Wallis et al., 2002) using three types of blood products, assigned patients to filtered whole blood (stored < 7 days before filtration), BCD-RBC or plasma-reduced RBCs. Postoperative mortality in 3 months was 0.5%, 2.9 % and 2.5% respectively (p=0.2), indicating no additional deleterious role of a higher number of leukocytes present in plasma-reduced RBCs as compared to BCD-RBCs. In the study of van de Watering the incidence of multiple-organ-dysfunction-syndrome (MODS) was not registered, however mortality due to MODS was the major cause of excess deaths after standard BCD-RBC transfusions. Another study was conducted in more complex cardiac valve surgery with a higher probability of multiple RBC transfusions and higher risk for postoperative complications. The aim was to explore the relationship with leukocyte-containing transfusions on MODS and mortality (Bilgin et al., 2004). The primary endpoint (90-day mortality) was (not significantly) reduced approximately with 33% in the patient group receiving leukocyte-depleted RBCs compared with BCD-RBCs (12.7 versus 8.4%, p=0.16). And hospital mortality was almost half in the patient group receiving leukocyte-depleted RBCs compared with BCD-RBCs (5.5% versus 10.1%, p=0.05). Surprisingly, in this study the incidence of MODS (20%) was similar in the groups receiving standard BCD-RBC or pre-storage filtered RBC; however MODS as a cause of death occurred more often in patients who received BCD-RBC. Subgroup analysis showed that only patients who received more than 3 units suffered higher mortality in the group receiving BCD-RBC (17.6% versus 8.3%, p=0.02). A fourth small study in 69 low-risk CABG patients compared bedside-filtered RBCs (containing soluble leukocyte-produced factors) with the same unfiltered RBC product (Connery et al., 2005). There was no difference in mortality between both randomization arms. This study was preliminary stopped because interim analysis showed less respiratory tract infections in the filtered group (p=0.048); although the total

Author; year	No. patients (% transfused)	No. RBCs mean ± SD or median	Main endpoints	Results (LD vs BCD)
van de Watering et al.; 1998	914 (95)	FF 5.3 ± 4.1 SF 5.5 ± 5.6 BCD 5.4 ± 5.1	1) Infections 2) 60-day mortality	1) 16.9 vs 17.9 vs 23.0% 2) 3.6 vs 3.3 vs 7.8%[b]
Bracey et al.; 2002[a]	357 (83)	LD 3 BCD 3	1) Infections 2) Mortality 3) ICU-/Hospital-stay	1) ns; data ND 2) 5.9 vs 7.5% 3) ns; data ND
Wallis et al.; 2002	597 (69)	WBF 3.9 ± 3.9 BCD 3.5 ± 2.6 PR 2.9 ± 1.8	1) Infections 2) 90-day mortality	1) 11.3 vs 10.8 vs 17.7% 2) 0.5 vs 2.9 vs 2.5%
Bilgin et al.; 2004	474 (91)	LD 6.2 ± 7.1 BCD 5.9 ± 6.1	1) Infections 2) MODS 3) Hospital mortality 4) 90-day mortality	1) 22.6 vs 31.6%[b] 2) 20.4 vs 20.7% 3) 5.5 vs 10.1%[b] 4) 8.4 vs 12.7%
Connery et al.; 2005	98 (70)	LD 5.6 ± 13 BCD 5.6 ± 10	1) Infections 2) 30-day mortality	1) 13.2 vs 25.8% 2) 2.6 vs 3.2%
Boshkov et al.; 2006[a]	1227 (46)	ND	1) Serious infections 2) 60-day mortality	1) ns; data ND 2) 4.9 vs 9.7%

[a] *Published as an abstract*
[b]*Statistically significant (p≤0.05; compared between leukocyte-depleted and leukocyte-containing RBCs)*
Abbreviations: LD=Leukodepleted RBCs; FF=Fresh filtered RBCs; SF=Stored filtered RBCs; BCD=Buffy-coat depleted RBCs; WBF=White blood cell filtered; PR=Plasma-reduced; ND=Not documented; PTI=Pulmonary tract infections.

Table 1. Summary of RCTs in cardiac surgery investigating the effects of leukocyte-depleted RBCs

infections rate was not different (p=0.22). When the results of RCTs conducted in cardiac surgery are combined in a meta-analysis, the mortality rate was increased with 72% in patients who received leukocyte-containing RBCs (OR=1.72; 95% CI: 1.05-2.81, p=0.01) (37). This difference between both blood products was mainly due to the two studies from the Netherlands (van de Watering et al. 1998 and Bilgin et al. 2004). It should be noted that these large studies were comparable and were conducted in patients with higher risk for postoperative complications and receive larger number of RBC transfusions. Because not all studies are published since their presentation as an abstract, only limited data are present (Boshkov et al., 2004 and Bracey et al., 2002). Therefore some (undocumented) differences in use and preparation of the blood products and in the endpoints could be influenced the differences between the studies.

In cardiac surgery six RCTs were performed investigating postoperative infections, which revealed different outcomes (Table 1). Two RCTs showed a transfusion-dose dependent beneficial effect of leukocyte-depleted RBCs (van de Watering et al., 1998 and Bilgin et al. 2004). Three RCTs did not show benefit of leukocyte-depleted RBCs (Wallis et al, 2002, Bracey et al, 2002, Boshkov et al, 2004) and one RCT only in the development of pneumonia (Connery et al., 2005). The characteristics and main results of these studies in cardiac surgery are mentioned in Table 1. The definitions of postoperative infections are not mentioned in the studies published only as abstracts, although this was not different in the full published studies. These results revealed that patients at risk for high numbers of blood transfusions have a benefit when transfused with leukocyte-depleted RBCs.

The observation that not the soluble mediators released by leukocytes during storage, nor the leukocyte load per transfusion, but rather the number of units transfused that entails the worse outcome, suggests that sicker patients in cardiac surgery requiring more RBC transfusions and are more susceptible to TRIM. We analysed in more detail the causes of death in two RCTs in cardiac surgery from the Netherlands (van de Watering et al., 1998 and Bilgin et al. 2004). This revealed that patients who received standard buffy-coat-poor RBCs, compared with before storage filtered leukodepleted RBCs, excessively died from a combination of infection and MODS (OR 2.92; 95% CI 1.22-6.97; p=0.02). Short-term mortality (60-day) from infections alone and from MODS without infections or from bleeding or surgical complications was equal in both transfusion arms (Bilgin et al., 2007). Although in cardiac surgery the long-term survival is negatively influenced by allogeneic blood transfusions as compared to non-transfused patients (Engoren et al., 2009). The long-term effect of allogeneic leukocytes in RBCs after cardiac surgery is not known and should be investigated in the future studies.

The filtration of the RBC products results in higher costs. However analyses on cost-effectiveness of leukodepletion are scarce and are mainly derived from observational data. In cardiac surgery cost-effectiveness was only analyzed with data derived from the two studies performed in the Netherlands (van de Watering et al., 1998 and Bilgin et al. 2004). The results revealed that leukodepletion of red blood cells have indeed benefits on the total hospital costs. In CABG patients the benefit of leukodepletion of RBCs was between 220-310 US Dollars per life-year gained (Postma et al., 2003) and in cardiac valve surgery on average 214 US Dollars per patient (van Hulst et al., 2005).

Because in most of Western World universal leukodepletion is implemented, no new randomized controlled trials from these countries are expected. Therefore observational studies were performed, that compared the incidence of complications before and after this implementation. One large multicenter study in critically ill patients from Canada (that included also cardiac surgery patients) reported reduced hospital mortality, decreased occurrence of fever and use of antibiotics after the implementation of universal leukoreduction (Hebert et al., 2003). Another "before-after study" observed a decrease in postoperative hospital-stay after cardiac surgery in patients who received leukoreduced blood transfusions (Fung et al., 2004). Despite a lot of publications; the controversy on the clinical effects of leukocyte-containing RBCs remains. However there are sufficient data showing that transfusion of leukodepleted red blood cells are beneficial in cardiac surgery.

3.4 Laboratory effects of allogeneic leukocytes in cardiac surgery

Cardiac surgery is associated with tissue trauma, ischemia-reperfusion injury and blood surface contact. These conditions induce systemic effects and release of inflammatory mediators, which are presumed to play a role in the development of postoperative complications such as systemic inflammatory response syndrome (SIRS), multiple-organ-dysfunction-syndrome (MODS) and infections. Moderate SIRS often develops after cardiac surgery and usually resolves with supportive care. However severe SIRS can evolve to MODS, which cause higher morbidity and mortality after cardiac surgery. Shear stress, surface-contact of the CPB and re-oxygenation of the myocardium results in an inflammatory response leading to activation of leukocytes. These responses lead to production and release of several pro-and anti-inflammatory responses during and after cardiac surgery. Imbalance of concentration of cytokines can play a pivotal role in a balanced equilibrium after cardiac surgery. Cytokines are low molecular weight polypeptides, which are produced by many cells, such as macrophages, monocytes, neutrophils and platelets. They are divided into two groups: pro-inflammatory cytokines as interleukin-1 (IL-1), IL-2, IL-8 and IL-12 and anti-inflammatory cytokines as IL-4, IL-5 and IL-10. While IL-6 has both pro-and anti-inflammatory properties. Directly in the postoperative period an anti-inflammatory response is important to further limit the post-surgical inflammatory response.

The production and release of the inflammatory mediators could be predictive in the development of postoperative complications after cardiac surgery. In one study (Sablotzki et al., 1997) the cytokine pattern were measured up to 48 hours after CABG surgery in 24 patients who all recovered uneventfully. After the start of bypass, soluble IL-2 receptor, IL-2 and IL-12 decrease and incompletely restore themselves, respectively 6-48 hours after surgery. The levels of IL-6 and IL-10, undetectable before surgery, increase at the end of bypass and reperfusion. The very high IL-10 peak fades away after 6 hours, while IL-6 remains high up to 48 hours. Such a cytokine pattern shows that cardiac surgery immediately evokes a biphasic cytokine response. Few studies investigated the possible mechanisms of allogeneic leukocyte-containing blood products on the cytokine balance. One a small study in 24 burn trauma patients showed an increase in IL-6 in patients receiving leukocyte-containing RBC transfusions (Nielsen et al., 1999). A larger study found in 114 patients an association after cardiac surgery between peri-operative allogeneic RBC transfusions and postoperative increase of concentrations of the inflammatory mediators bactericidal permeability increasing protein (BPI), as a marker of neutrophil activation, and IL-6 (Fransen et al., 1999). While another study found an increase in IL-6, but not in TNF-alpha, in patients undergoing cardiac surgery who received blood transfusions (Senay et al., 2009). However none of these studies investigated the combined relationships between the type of blood products, inflammatory mediators and the outcome after cardiac surgery. Therefore the exact effects of blood transfusions in cardiac surgery could not be determined. We were able to investigate profiles of some inflammatory mediators in 346 patients participating in our RCT comparing leukodepekted with leukocyte-containing (buffy-coat depleted) red blood cells. Pre-and post-surgical blood samples were available and the concentrations of inflammatory markers were measured (Bilgin et al., 2010). We selected four key mediators that represent the inflammatory response after surgery. The pro-inflammatory cytokine IL-6 has been shown to be an early predictor for mortality in cardiac surgery. IL-10, an anti-inflammatory cytokine, has been found to be increased after per-operative allogeneic blood transfusions in orthopaedic surgery in association with prolonged hospital stay (Kirkley et al., 1998). IL-12 reflects activation and proliferation of lymphocytes and natural killer cells, which are relevant for the defense against nosocomial infections. The concentration of procalcitonin on the first postoperative day after cardiac surgery has been shown to be an early marker for organ dysfunction with severe outcome (Falcoz et al., 2005). In patients who would develop infections, MODS or eventually die from these complications had higher pro-inflammatory cytokine concentrations in the group that received leukocyte-containing RBC and lower anti-inflammatory cytokine IL-10 in the group that received leukocyte-depleted RBC (Bilgin et al., 2010). In both study arms the concentration of procalcitonin was not influenced by RBC transfusions. In patients staying longer at ICU the concentration of IL-10 had decreased already on arrival at ICU. The increase of IL-6 and IL-12 peaked later and for IL-6 a higher peak level was measured in the group that received leukocyte-containing RBC than in the group that received leukocyte-depleted RBC. The concentrations of cytokines are shown in Figure 1.

These findings of this study support that leukocyte-containing blood transfusions amplify an inflammatory response in addition to an ongoing systemic inflammatory response induced by cardiac surgery. This may lead to a more profound counteractive anti-inflammatory response as well to explain enhanced susceptibility for postoperative infections. This inflammatory response can be reduced by transfusion of leukocyte-depleted blood transfusions. One study observed that the cytokine gene expression was altered by transfusion of allogeneic RBCs in patients who developed MODS after cardiac surgery (Sitniakowsky et al., 2011). Furthermore, soluble CD40 ligand which could be accumulated during storage of blood products and could induce the production and release of proinflammatory mediators, was higher in patients who received blood transfusions (Khan et al., 2006). Moreover, recently one study showed higher levels of IL-8, tumor necrosing factor (TNF)-alpha and thrombin-antithrombin-complex (TATc) levels in bronchoalveolar lavage fluid of patients who received perioperative multiple blood transfusions. This study suggests that not only the inflammation system is activated after cardiac surgery, but also the coagulation system is activated (Tuinman et al., 2011). These studies resulted in several hypothesis that investigated the possible relationship between allogeneic (leukocyte-containing) blood transfusions and complications after cardiac surgery.

4. The inflammatory response and allogeneic leukocytes in cardiac surgery

During cardiac surgery blood is exposed to the extra-corporeal circuit, hypothermia, ischemia/reperfusion injury and many inflammatory responses are activated. These responses lead to post-perfusion systemic inflammatory response syndrome (SIRS). SIRS is defined by a body temperature less than 36^{0}C or more than 38^{0}C, heart rate more than 90/min, tachypnea with breaths more than 20/min or pCO_2 less than 4.4 kPa (32 mm Hg) and leukocyte count less than $4x10^9/l$ or more than $12x10^9/l$. SIRS can be diagnosed when two or more criteria are present (Bone et al., 1992). SIRS is a subset of cytokine storm with an abnormal regulation of cytokines and is immediately counteracted by a compensatory anti-inflammatory response syndrome (CARS) (Bone, 1996). An overwhelming SIRS causes a dormant state of cell metabolism, referred to as MODS; SIRS usually resolves with adequate supportive therapy and most of the patients recover. However overwhelming SIRS can dominate CARS and progress to MODS, which may lead to mortality. Previous studies support that leukocyte-containing blood transfusions amplify an inflammatory response in addition to an ongoing systemic inflammatory response induced by cardiac surgery. This may lead to a more profound counteractive anti-inflammatory response as well to explain enhanced susceptibility for postoperative infections. We presume that leukocyte-containing RBC transfusions to patients with an activated inflammatory response (as after cardiac

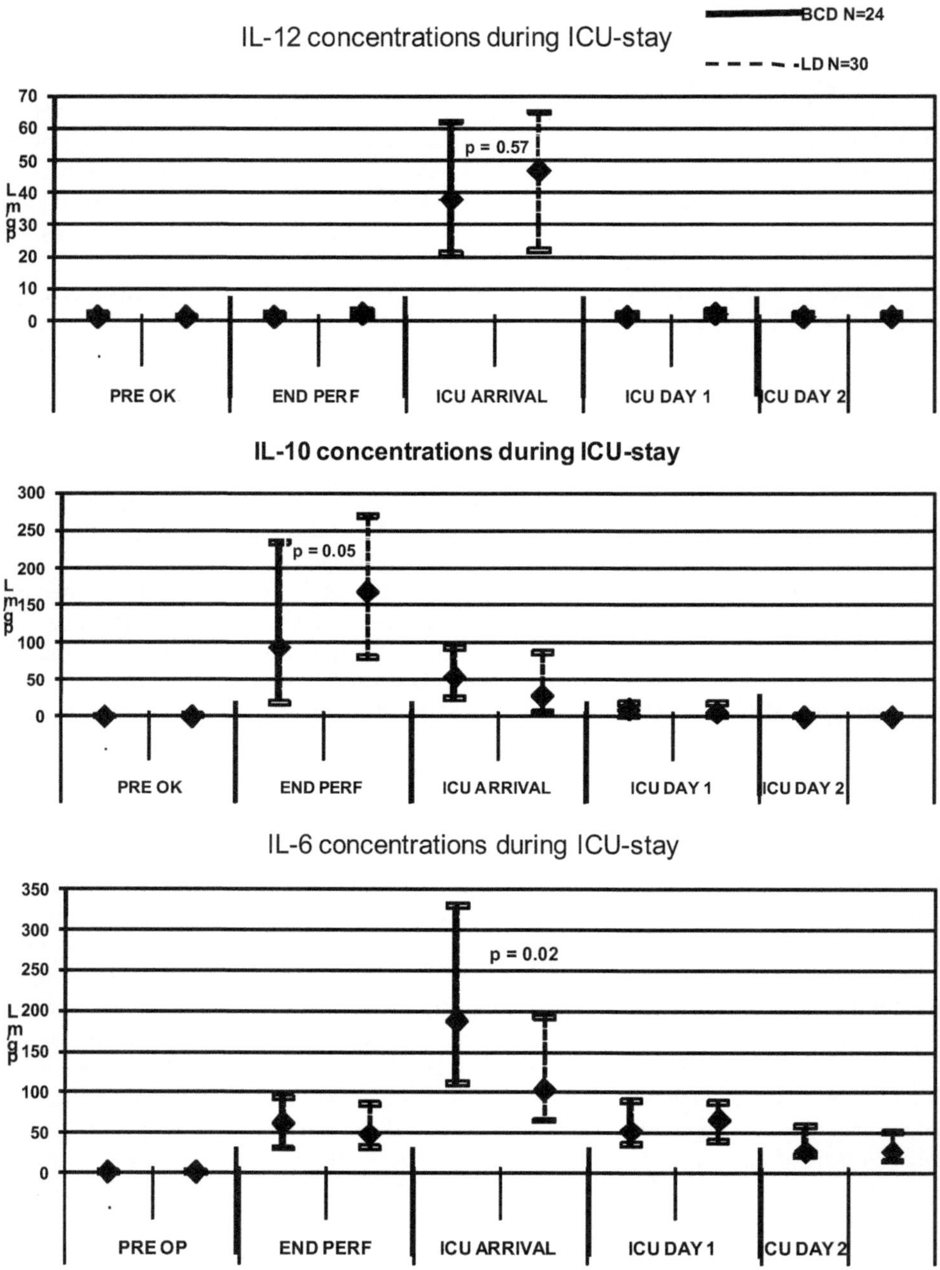

Fig. 1. Pre-operative (PRE OP), at end of perfusion (END PERF), at arrival at ICU (ICU ARRIVAL) and at days 1 and 2 (ICU DAY 1 and 2) the concentrations of cytokines (IL-6, IL-10 and IL-12) (Bilgin et al., 2010).

surgery) could further imbalances the postoperative SIRS-CARS equilibrium initially in favour of SIRS; this second-hit response induced by allogeneic leukocytes may be in combination with infections the cause of a more severe MODS (Bilgin and Brand, 2008). This interaction is shown in Figure 2.

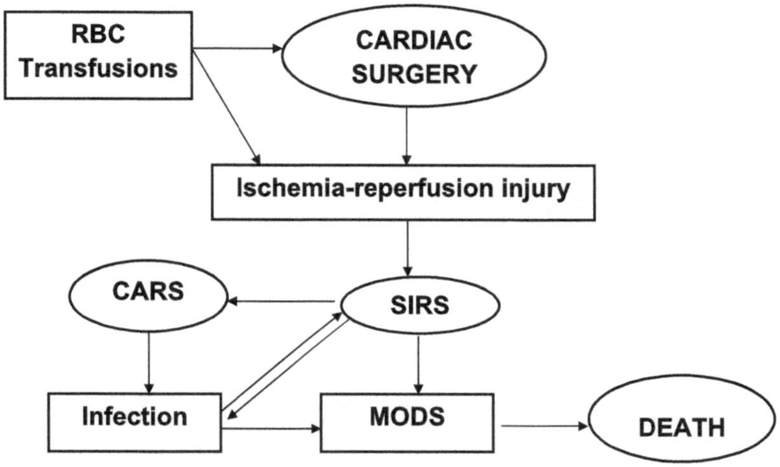

Fig. 2.

This hypothesis initiated a discussion whether allogeneic leukocytes are the substrate for postoperative infections or for MODS. From our RCT we investigated the time-interval in patients who developed MODS and infections in the postoperative period. We found that twice more patients developed MODS after postoperative infections in the group that received leukocyte-containing (buffy-coat depleted) RBCs compared with leukocyte-depleted RBCs. While patients who developed first MODS followed by postoperative infections was comparable in both groups. The difference in deaths between both types of blood products was due to more deaths in patients that developed MODS after postoperative infections and received leukocyte-containing (buffy-coat depleted) RBCs. Deaths in patients with MODS followed by postoperative infections was also not different between both blood products (Figure 3). This suggests that allogeneic blood transfusions initiate first an inflammatory response, which is more pronounced and results more in MODS after transfusion of leukocyte-containing RBCs.

As an explanation for the development of MODS, we found in a laboratory analysis in patients with low mannose-binding lectin (MBL) levels is a risk factor in the development of multiple-organ-dysfunction-syndrome (MODS); when they were transfused with plasma units (Bilgin et al, 2008). The lectin pathway can be triggered by binding of carbohydrates exposed on a wide range of micro-organisms to mannose-binding lectin (MBL) (Neth et al, 2000). Polymorphisms in the MBL gene result in a wide range of functional MBL levels. Roughly 30% of the Caucasian population has reduced levels of MBL, due to single nucleotide polymorphisms in exon 1 of the *MBL2* gene, and approximately 5-10 % has a functional MBL deficiency. MBL deficiency in itself does not lead to clinical problems, but several studies have shown that MBL deficiency confers an increased susceptibility for infections in immune-compromised patients (Bouwman et al, 2005, Peterslund et al., 2001,

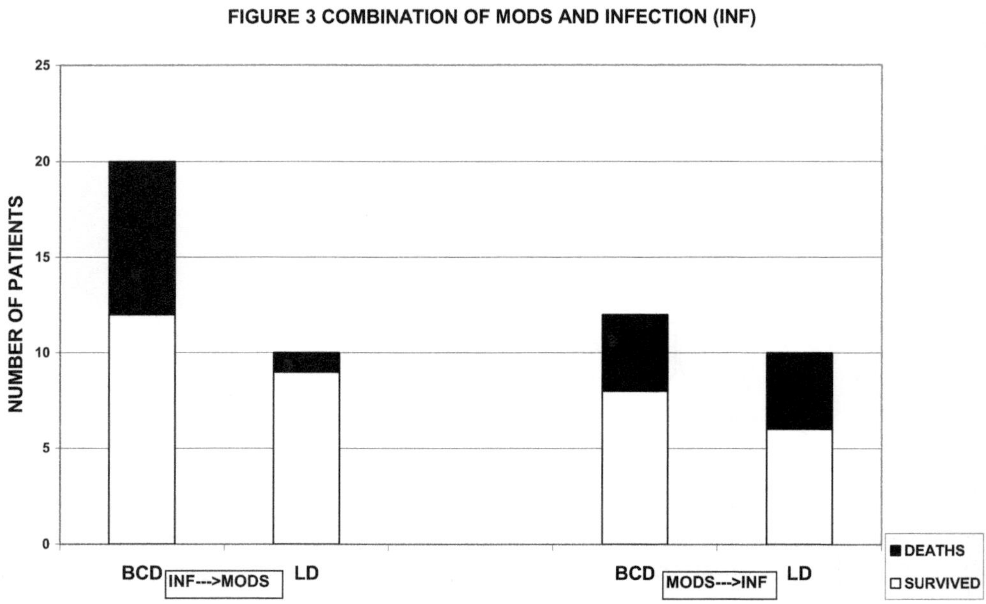

Fig. 3. Relation between allogeneic blood transfusions and MODS combined with infections and survival Abbreviations: LD=Leukodepleted RBCs; BCD=Buffy-coat depleted RBCs

Garred et al., 2003). The role of MBL deficiency on the development and outcome of SIRS and sepsis syndrome is controversial. Worse outcome in patients with sepsis is described (Fidler et al., 2004). Cardiac surgery is associated with MBL consumption, independent of the transfusion of allogeneic leukocytes. We found that patients with MBL-deficiency develop no MODS, unless they have been transfused with FFP, which is associated with MBL reconstitution. Therefore, sustained MBL deficiency may be a favourable status for patients undergoing cardiac surgery (Bilgin et al, 2008). Probably MBL-deficiency plays an protective role in the development of MODS, until patients are transfused with plasma. Furthermore platelet units contain bioactive mediators. Increased CD40 ligand (CD40L or CD154) present in platelet units can induce production and release of pro-inflammatory markers. Besides leukocyte-containing RBCs, plasma and also platelet transfusions could thus aggravate an existing inflammatory reaction impairing the outcome after cardiac surgery. More investigations are needed on the possible causal roles of transfusion of different blood components. Several factors play a role in the inflammatory response after cardiac surgery. One of them is transfusion of allogeneic RBCs, especially leukocyte-containing RBCs. However these factors are not the only one and the exact mechanisms are unravelled until now.

5. Clinical effects of plasma and platelet transfusions in cardiac surgery

Not only RBCs are transfused during cardiac surgery. Patients undergoing cardiac surgery are at increased risk for bleeding, because of thrombocytopenia secondary to hemodilution, platelet dysfunction and consumption of platelets in the extracorporal circuit. In addition, intra-operatively anticoagulant medication is administered to these patients. To improve hemostasis, platelets and fresh-frozen plasma (FFP) are often transfused in the peri-operative and postoperative periods. Plasma transfusions can contribute to adverse outcome by causing transfusion-related acute lung injury (TRALI), a serious life-threatening condition and an underreported complication of allogeneic blood transfusions. The pathophysiology of TRALI has not been clarified yet, while all plasma-containing blood products could be involved in the development of TRALI (Silliman, 2006). According to an international agreed definition, the onset of TRALI is within 6 hours after blood transfusion. The pathophysiology of TRALI has not been completely clarified yet and is the final result of a cascade of neutrophil priming, activation and endothelial damage. One of the causes is passively transfused anti-leukocyte antibodies in the donor's plasma, which bind to antigens on patient's neutrophils and initiate priming and activation with release of cytokines, proteases and free oxygen radicals. Neutrophil sequestration in the lung is finally leading to endothelial damage and capillary leakage (Silliman et al., 2009). Furthermore it has been suggested that platelet transfusions in cardiac surgery could be associated with postoperative complications. Whether platelet and plasma transfusions contribute to such postoperative complications, or are just a surrogate marker for the need for a higher number of RBC transfusions, is controversial. A predominant role of plasma transfusions on outcome after cardiac surgery is suggested (Ranucci et al., 2008). However other studies that focused on plasma transfusions reported contradictory findings (Banbury et al, 2006 and Sreeram et al, 2005). On the other hand, some studies found that platelet transfusions in cardiac surgery were not been independently associated with mortality (Karkouti et al., 2006 and McGrath et al., 2008), while other studies which applied no correction for concomitant RBC and plasma transfusions (Spiess et al., 2004 and Mangano, 2002). Data from two randomized controlled studies (van de Watering et al., 1998 and Bilgin et al., 2004) were combined to analyze the effects of platelet and/or plasma transfusions on postoperative infections, length of stay in the intensive care unit (ICU), all-cause mortality and mortality in the presence or absence of infections in the postoperative period. This retrospective analysis revealed that the number of transfused plasma units was independently associated with all-cause mortality. Although leukocyte-containing RBCs were associated with mortality, the number of transfused RBC units was not. The number of transfused RBC units, but not the number of transfused plasma units or the receipt of platelet transfusion, was associated with the development of postoperative infections and with the stay in the ICU for 4 or more days. Transfusion of platelet units was associated with mortality with postoperative infections developed during the hospital-stay (Bilgin et al., 2011). Because patients, who receive RBC transfusions, receive also plasma and platelet transfusions, it is difficult to determine whether plasma and platelet transfusions could be independently associated with postoperative complications. This study suggests that plasma transfusions are associated with all-cause mortality, probably by volume overload and transmission of plasma-derived factors. And that platelets and leukocyte-containing RBCs are associated with mortality in the presence of infections, suggesting that both influence the inflammatory response after cardiac surgery. However, only few retrospective studies have considered the effects of plasma and platelet transfusions, which predominantly are transfused to patients who also received RBC transfusions. Our findings underscore the need for further studies to investigate the aggregate effects of all the various blood components transfused in cardiac surgery.

6. Possible relation between blood transfusions and thrombosis

The inflammatory response and pro-inflammatory cytokines also lead to activation of the coagulation system and down-regulate the anticoagulant systems (Levi et al., 2003) Activation of the coagulation factors can in turn activate inflammation. This may enhance the development of infections and microvascular thrombi. Both thrombi and infection play a central role in the development and worse outcome of MODS (Gando, 2010). This could occur by increasing the circulating RBC mass and vascular rheologic deformations by RBC transfusions. Activated platelets (during storage) may contribute to thrombosis in patients at risk. It has recently been shown that leukocyte-containing RBCs and platelets contain prothrombotic soluble mediators, which interact with leukocytes preceding the apoptosis and death of leukocytes, subsequently producing microparticles with procoagulant activity (Keating et al., 2010). Leukocyte-containing RBCs contain prothrombotic soluble mediators, such as CD40L, which induce the synthesis of proinflammatory mediators that can further activate the coagulation system (Blumberg et al., 2006). Observational studies showed an association between allogeneic blood transfusions and the development of venous thromboembolism (Nilsson et al, 2007 and Khorana et al., 2008). The possible association between allogeneic blood transfusions and the formation of thrombosis, as a factor aggravating MODS and having a role in increased mortality due to MODS, is a new subject and should be investigated further. Recently one study found that not only inflammatory mediators were increased in bronchoalveolar lavage fluid after cardiac surgery, also coagulation was activated (Tuinman et al, 2011). This study supports that allogeneic blood transfusions could result in both activation of the inflammatory and coagulation systems.

7. Conclusions

Transfusion of allogeneic blood components is commonly used in cardiac surgery. Several observational and randomized studies found higher morbidity and mortality if patients were transfused with allogeneic blood products. In the last years the clinical effects of transfusion triggers, the storage times and the presence of allogeneic leukocytes in red blood cells were investigated intensively. In cardiac surgery it has been found that allogeneic blood transfusions could increase postoperative complications, which is controversial in the last years. Clinical effects of storage of RBCs are discussed intensively and until now there is no clear evidence that older RBCs are deleterious in cardiac surgery. It has been found that mainly leukocyte-containing blood products play a crucial role in the development of postoperative complications in cardiac surgery. To understand the differences between leukocyte-containing and leukocyte-depleted RBC transfusions we described in this review several possible causal mechanisms. Soluble mediators derived from deteriorating leukocytes during storage of RBC are unlikely to play a role. The complement activation by lectin pathway may be relevant to explore as a causal deleterious effect of plasma transfusions, although does not explain excess death by MODS in association with allogeneic leukocytes. An acute phase reaction represented by procalcitonin could be excluded as a mediator induced by allogeneic leukocytes. A difference in cytokine responses in the recipient was the only significant factor that could be identified as playing a possible causal role. In most countries of the Western World transfusion of leukodepleted blood components is standard practice. Although the final conclusion on this issue is not made yet. Furthermore other factors, such as plasma and platelet transfusions (due to activation or storage lesions) and the (possible) activation of the coagulation system by the allogeneic blood transfusions, may remain to play important roles in the development of transfusion-associated complications and are input for further improvement of transfusion management in cardiac surgery. Thus many residual questions have still to be answered in the future.

8. References

Andersen, J.J.; Dethlefsen, C.; Modrau, I.S.; Baech. J.; Schonheyder, H.C.; Moeller, J.K. & Johnsen, S.P. (2011). Storage time of allogeneic red blood cells is associated with risk of severe postoeprative infection after coronary artery bypass grafting. *Eur J Cardiothorac Surg*, Vol 39, pp 329-334

Banbury, M.K.; Brizzio, M.E.; Rajeswaran, J.; Lytle, B.W. & Blackstone, E.H. (2006). Transfusion increases the risk of postoperative infection after cardiac surgery. *J Am Coll Surg*, Vol 202, pp. 131-138

Bilgin, Y.M.; van de Watering, L.M.G.; Eijsman, L.; Versteegh, M.I.M.; Brand, R.; van Oers, M.H.J. & Brand, A. (2004). Double-blind randomized controlled trial on the effect of leukocyte-depleted erythrocyte transfusions in cardiac valve surgery. *Circulation*, Vol. 109, pp. 2755-2760

Bilgin, Y.M.; van de Watering, L.M.G.; Eijsman, L.; Versteegh, M.I.M.; van Oers, M.H.J. & Brand, A. (2007). Is increased mortality associated with postoperative infections after leukocytes containing red blood cell transfusions in cardiac surgery? *Transf Med*, Vol. 17, pp. 304-311

Bilgin ,Y.M.; Brand, A.; Berger, S.P.; Daha, M.R. & Roos, A. (2008). Mannose-binding lectin is involved in multiple organ dysfunction syndrome after cardiac surgery: effects of blood transfusions. *Transfusion*, Vol. 48, pp. 601-608

Bilgin, Y.M. & Brand, A. (2008). Transfusion-related immunomodulation: a second hit in an inflammatory cascade? *Vox Sang* Vol. 95, pp. 261-271

Bilgin, Y.M.; van de Watering, L.M.G.; Versteegh, M.I.M.; van Oers, M.H.J. & Brand, A. (2010). The effects of allogeneic leukocytes in blood transfusions during cardiac surgery on inflammatory mediators and postoperative complications. *Crit Care Med*, Vol. 38, pp. 546-552.

Bilgin, Y.M.; van de Watering, L.M.G.; Versteegh, M.I.M.; van Oers, M.H.J. & Brand, A. (2011). Postoperative complications associated with transfusion of platelets and plasma in cardiac surgery. *Transfusion*, in press.

Blumberg, N.; Gettings, K.F.; Turner, C.; Heal, J.M. & Phipps, R.P. (2006). An association of soluble CD40 ligand (CD154) with adverse reactions to platelet transfusions. *Transfusion*, Vol. 46, pp. 1813-1821

Bone, R.C.; Balk, R.A.; Cerra, F.B.; Dellinger, R.P.; Fein, A.M.; Knaus, W.A.; Schein, R.M. & Sibbald, W.J. (1992). Definitions for sepsis and organ failure and guidelines for the use of innovative therapies in sepsis. The ACCP/SCCM Consensus Conference Committee. American College of Chest Physicians/Society of Critical Care Medicine. *Chest*, Vol. 101, pp. 1644-1655

Bone, R.C. (1996). Sepsis, SIRS and CARS. *Crit Care Med*, Vol. 24, pp. 1125-1128

Boshkov, L.K.; Chien , G.; VanWinkle, D.; Furnary, A.P.; Wu, Y.; Grunkemeirer, G.L. & Morris, C.D. (2006). Prestorage leukoreduction of transfused packed red cells is associated with significant ongoing 1-12 month survival benefit cardiac surgery patients. *Blood*, Vol. 108, pp. 578

Bouwman, L.H.; Roos, A.; Terpstra, O.T.; de Knijff, P.; van Hoek, B.; Verspaget, H.W.; Berger, S.P.; Daha, M.R.; Frölich, M.; van der Slik, A.R.; Doxiadis, I.I.; Roep, B.O. & Schaapherder, A.F. (2005). Mannose binding lectin gene polymorphisms confer a major risk for severe infections after liver transplantation. *Gastroenterology,* Vol. 129, pp. 408-14

Bracey, A.W.; Radovancevic, R. & Nussmeier, N.A. (2002). Leukocyte-depleted blood in open-heart surgery patients: effects on outcome. *Transfusion,* Vol. 42 (Suppl), pp. 5S

Chelemer, S.B.; Prato, S.; Cox, P.M.; O'Connor, G.T. & Morton, J.R. (2002). Association of bacterial infection and red blood cell transfusion after CABG. *Ann Thorac Surg,* Vol. 73, pp. 138-142

Cobain, T.J.; Vamvakas, E.C.; Wells, A. & Titlestad, K. (2007). A survey of the demographics of blood use. *Transf Med,* Vol. 17, pp. 1-15

Connery, C.P.; Toumpoulis, I.K.; Anagnostopoulis, C.E.; Hillei, Z.; Rahman, F.G.; Katritsis, D. & Swistel, D.G. (2005). Does leukofiltration reduce pulmonary infections in CABG patients? A prospective, randomised study with early results and mid-term survival. *Acta Cardiol,* Vol. 60, pp. 285-293

Engoren, M.C.; Habib, R.H.; Zacharias, A.; Schwann, T.A.; Riordan, C.J. & Durham, S.J. (2002). Effect of blood transfusion on long-term survival after cardiac operation. *Ann Thorac Surg,* Vol. 74, pp. 1180-1186

Engoren, M.C.; Habib, R.H.; Hadaway, J.; Zacharias, A.; Schwann, T.A.; Riordan, C.J.; Durham, S.J. & Shah, A. (2009). The effect on long-term survival of erythrocyte transfusion given for cardiac valve operations. *Ann Thorac Surg,* Vol. 88, pp. 95-100

Falcoz, P.E.; Laluc, F.; Toubin, M.M.; Puyraveau, M.; Clement, F.; Mercier, M.; Chocron, S. & Etievent, J.P. (2005). Usefulness of procalcitonin in the early detection of infection after thoracic surgery. *Eur J Cardiothorac Surg,* Vol. 27, pp. 1074-1078

Fidler, K.J.; Wilson, P.; Davies, J.C.; Turner, M.W.; Peters, M.J. & Klein, N.J. (2004). Increased incidence and severity of the systemic inflammatory response syndrome in patients deficient in mannose-binding lectin. *Intensive Care Med,* Vol. 30, pp. 1438-1445

Fransen, E.; Maessen, J.; Dentener, M.; Senden, N. & Buurman, W. (1999). Impact of blood transfusions on inflammatory mediator release in patients undergoing cardiac surgery. *Chest,* Vol. 116, pp. 1233-1239

Fung, M.K.; Rao, N.; Rice, J.; Ridenour, M.; Mook, W. & Triulzi, D.J. (2004). Leukoreduction in the setting of open heart surgery: a prospective cohort-controlled study. *Transfusion,* Vol. 44, pp. 30-35

Gando, S. (2010). Microvascular thrombosis and multiple organ dysfunction syndrome. *Crit Care Med* Vol. 38, pp. S35-S42

Gangireddy, C.; Rectenwald, J.R.; Upchurch, G.R.; Wakefield, T.W.; Khuri, S.; Henderson, W.G. & Henke, P.K. (2007). Risk factors and clinical impact of postoperative symptomatic venous thromboembolism. *J Vasc Surg,* Vol. 45, pp. 335-342

Gantt, CL. (1981). Red blood cells for cancer patients. *Lancet,* Vol. 2, p. 363

Garred, P.J.; Madsen, H.O.; Balslev, U.; Hofmann, B.; Pedersen, C.; Gerstoft, J. & Svejgaard, A. (1997). Suspectibility to HIV infection and progression of AIDS in relation to variant alleles of mannose-binding lectin. *Lancet,* Vol. 349, pp. 236-240

Garred, P.J.; Strom, J.J; Quist, L.; Taaning, E. & Madsen, H.O. (2003). Association mannose-binding lectin polymorphisms with sepsis and fatal outcome in patients with systemic inflammatory response syndrome. *J Infect Dis,* Vol. 188, pp. 1394-1403

Hajjar, L.A.; Vincent, J.L.; Galas, F.R.G.B.; Nakamura, R.E.; Silva, C.M.; Santos, M.H.; Fukushima, J.; Kalil Filho, R.; Sierra, D.B.; Lopes, N.H.; Mauad, T.; Roquim, A.C.; Sundin, M.R.; Leão, W.C.; Almeida, J.P.; Pomerantzeff, P.M.; Dallan, L.O.; Jatene, F.B.; Stolf, N.A. & Auler, J.O. (2010). Transfusion requirements after cardiac surgery. *JAMA,* Vol. 304, pp. 1559-1567

Hebert, P.C.; Wells, G.; Blajchman, M.A.; Marshall, J.; Martin, C.; Pagliarello, G.; Tweeddale, M.; Schweitzer, I. & Yetisir, E. on behalf of the Canadian TRIC investigators. (1999). A multicenter randomised, controlled clinical trial of transfusion requirements in critical care. *New Engl J Med,* Vol. 340, pp. 409-417

Hebert, P.C.; Fergusson, D.; Blajchman, M.A.; Wells, G.A.; Kmetic, A.; Coyle, D.; Heddle, N.; Germain, M.; Goldman, M.; Toye, B.; Schweitzer, I.; vanWalraven, C.; Devine, D. & Sher, G.D. on behalf of the Leukoreduction Study Investigators. (2003). Clinical outcomes following institution of the Canadian universal leukoreduction program for red blood cell transfusions. *JAMA,* Vol. 289, pp. 1941-1949

Ho, J.; Sibbald, W.J. & Chin-Yee, I.H. (2003). Effects of storage on efficacy of red cell transfusion: when is it not safe? *Crit Care Med,* Vol. 31, pp. S687-S697

Kamper-Jorgensen, M.; Edgren, G.; Rostgaard, K.; Biggar, R.J.; Nyrén, O.; Reilly, M.; Titlestad, K.; Shanwell, A.; Melbye, M. & Hjalgrim, H. (2009). Blood transfusion exposure in Denmark and Sweden. *Transfusion,* Vol. 49, pp. 888-894

Karkouti,, K.; Wijeysundera, D.N.; Yau, T.M.; Beattie, W.S.; Abdelnaem, E.; McCluskey, S.A.; Ghannam, M.; Yeo, E.; Djaiani, G. & Karski, J. (2004). The independent association of massive blood loss with mortality in cardiac surgery. *Transfusion,* 2004; 44:1453-1462.

Karkouti, K.; Wijeysundera, D.N.; Yau, T.M.; Callum, J.L.; Meineri, M.; Wasowicz, M.; McCluskey, S.A. & Beattie, W.S. (2006). Platelet transfusions are not associated with increased morbidity or mortality in cardiac surgery. *Can J Anesth,* Vol. 53, pp. 279-287

Karkouti, K.; Wijeysundera, N. & Beattie, W.S. (2008). Risk associated with preoperative anemia in cardiac surgery: a cohort study. *Circulation* Vol. 117, pp. 478-484

Karkouti, K.; Wijeysundera, D.N.; Yau, T.M.; McCluskey, S.A.; van Rensburg. A. & Beattie. W.S. (2008). The influence of baseline hemoglobin concentration on tolerance of anemia in cardiac surgery. *Transfusion,* Vol. 48, pp. 666-672

Karkouti, K.; Wijeysundera, D.N.; Yau, T.M.; Callum, J.L.; Cheng, D.C.; Crowther, M.; Dupuis, J.Y.; Fremes, S.E.; Kent, B.; Laflamme, C.; Lamy, A.; Legare, J.F.; Mazer, C.D.; McCluskey, S.A.; Rubens, F.D.; Sawchuk, C. & Beattie, W.S. (2009). Acute kidney injury after cardiac surgery: Focus on modifiable risk factors. *Circulation,* Vol. 119, pp. 495–502

Keating, F.K.; Butenas, S.; Fung, M.K. & Schneider, D.J. (2010). Platelet-white blood cell (WBC) interaction, WBC apoptosis and procoagulant activity in stored red blood cells. *Transfusion,* 2010; in press.

Khorana, A.A.; Francis, C.W.; Blumberg, N.; Culakova, E.; Refaai, M.A. & Lyman, G.H. (2008). Blood transfusions, thrombosis and mortality in hospitalized patients with cancer. *Arch Intern Med,* Vol. 168, pp. 2377-2381

Kirkley, S.A.; Cowles, J.; Pellegrini, V.D.; Harris, C.M.; Boyd, A.D. & Blumberg, N. (1998). Blood transfusion and total joint replacement: T helper 2 cytokine secretion and clinical outcome. *Transf Med,* 1998 Vol. 8, pp. 195-204

Koch, C.G.; Li, L.; Duncan, A.I.; Mihaljevic, T.; Cosgrove, D.M.; Loop, F.D.; Starr, N.J. & Blackstone, E.H. (2006). Morbidity and mortality risk associated with red blood cell and blood-component transfusion in isolated coronary artery bypass grafting. *Crit Care Med*, Vol. 34, pp. 1608-1616

Koch, C.G.; Li L.; Duncan, A.I.; Loop, F.D.; Starr, N.J. & Blackstone, E.H. (2006). Transfusion in coronary artery bypass grafting is associated with reduced long-term survival. *Ann Thorac Surg,* Vol. 81, pp. 1650-1657

Koch, C.G.; Li, L.; Sessler, D.I.; Figueroa, P.; Hoeltge, G.A.; Mihaljevic, T. & Blackstone, E.H. (2008). Duration of red-cell storage and compliactions after cardiac surgery. *N Engl J Med,* Vol. 358, pp. 1229-1239

Kuduvalli, M.; Oo, A.Y.; Newall, N.; Jackson, M.; Desmond, M.J.; Fabri, B.M. & Rashid, A. (2005). Effect of peri-operative red blood cell transfusion on 30-day and 1-year mortality following coronary artery bypass grafting. *Eur J Cardio-thorac Surgery,* Vol. 27, pp. 592-598

Kulier, A.; Levin, J.; Moser, R.; Rumpold-Seitlinger, G.; Tudor, I.C.; Snyder-Ramos, S.A.; Moehnle, P. & Mangano, D.T. (2007). Impact of preoperative anemia on outcome in patients undergoing coronary artery bypass graft surgery. *Circulation,* Vol. 116, pp. 471-479

Leal-Noval, S.R.; Rincon-Ferrari, M.D.; Garcia-Curiel, A.; Herruzo-Avilés, A.; Camacho-Larana, P.; Garnacho-Montero, J. & Amaya-Villar, R. (2001). Transfusion of blood components and postoperative infection in patients undergoing cardiac surgery. *Chest,* Vol; 119, pp. 1461-1468

Levi, M.; Cromheecke, M.E.; de Jonge, E.; Prins, M.H.; de Mol, B.J.; Briet, E. & Buller, HR. (1999). Pharmacological strategies to decrease excessive blood loss in cardiac surgery: a meta-analysis of clinically relevant endpoints. *Lancet,* Vol. 354, pp. 1940-1947

Levi, M.; Keller, T.T.; van Gorp, E. & ten Cate, H. (2003). Infection and inflammation and the coagulation system. *Cardiovasc Res,* Vol. 60, pp. 23-29

Mangano, D.T. for the multicenter study of perioperative ischemia research group. Aspirin and mortality from coronary bypass surgery. *N Engl J Med,* Vol. 347, pp. 1309-1317

McGrath, T.; Koch, C.G.; Xu, M.; Li, L.; Mihaljevic, T.; Figueroa, P. & Blackstone, E.H. (2008). Platelet transfusion in cardiac surgery does not confer increased risk for adverse morbid outcomes. *Ann Thorac Surg,* Vol.86, pp. 543-553.

Moehnle, P.; Snyder-Ramos, S.A.; Miao, Y.; Kulier, A.; Bottiger, B.W.; Levin, J. & Mangano, D.T. (2011). Postoperative red blood cell transfusion and morbid outcome in uncomplicated cardiac surgery. *Intensive Care,* Vol. 37, pp. 97-109

Mullighan, C.G.; Heatley, S.; Doherty, K.; Szabo, F.; Grigg, A.; Hughes, T.P.; Schwarer, A.P.; Szer, J.; Tait, B.D.; Bik To, L. & Bardy P.G. (2002). Mannose-binding lectin gene polymorphisms are associated with major infection following allogeneic hemopoietic stem cell transplantation. *Blood,* Vol. 10, pp 3524-3529

Murphy, G.J.; Reeves, B.C.; Rogers, C.A.; Rizvi, S.I.A.; Culliford, L. & Angelini, G.D. (2007). Increased mortality, postoperative morbidity and cost after red blood cell transfusion in patients having cardiac surgery. *Circulation,* Vol. 116, pp. 2544-2552

Neth, O.; Jack, D.L.; Dodds, A.W.; Holzel, H.; Klein, N.J. & Turner, M.W. (2000). Mannose-binding lectin binds to a range of clinically relevant microorganisms and promotes complement deposition. *Infection and immunity,* Vol. 68, pp. 688-693

Nielsen, H.J.; Hammer, J.H.; Krarup, A.L.; Nielsen, L.M.; Reimert, C.M.; Pedersen, A.N.; Dybkjaer, E.; Partoft, S. & Alsbjørn, B. (1999). Prestorage leukocyte filtration may reduce leukocyte-derived bioactive substances accumulation in patients operated for burn trauma. *Burns,* Vol. 25, pp. 162-170

Nilsson, K.R.; Berenholtz, S.M.; Garrett-Mayer, E.; Dorman, T.; Klag, M.J. & Pronovost, P.J. (2007). Association between venous thromboembolism and perioperative allogeneic transfusion. *Arch Surg,* Vol. 142, pp. 126-132

Opelz, G.; Sengar, D.D.S.; Mickey, M.R. & Terasaki, P.I. Effect of blood transfusions on subsequent kidney transplants. *Transplant Proc,* Vol. 5, pp. 253-259

Peterslund, N.A.; Koch, C.; Jensenius, J.C. & Thiel, S. (2001). Association between deficiency of mannose-binding lectin and severe infections after chemotherapy. *Lancet,* Vol. 358, pp. 637-638

Postma, M.J.; van de Watering, L.M.G.; de Vries, R.; Versmoren, D.; van Hulst, M.; Tobi, H.; van der Poel, C.L. & Brand, A. (2003). Cost-effectiveness of leucocyte depletion of red-cell transfusions for patients undergoing cardiac surgery. *Vox Sang,* Vol. 84, pp. 65-67

Ranucci, M.; Pazzaglia, A.; Bianchini, C.; Bozzetti, G. & Isgro, G. (2008). Body size, gender, and transfusions as determinants of outcome after coronary operations. *Ann Thorac Surg,* Vol. 85, pp. 481-487

Rao, S.V.; Jollis, J.G.; Harrington, R.A.; Granger, C.B.; Newby, L.K.; Armstrong, P.W.; Moliterno, D.J.; Lindblad, L.; Pieper, K.; Topol, E.J.; Stamler, J.S. & Califf, R.M. (2004). Relationship of blood transfusion and clinical outcomes in patients with acute coronary syndromes. *JAMA,* Vol. 292, pp. 1555-1562

Sablotzki, A.; Dehne, M.G.; Welters, I.; Menges, T. & Lehman. N. (1997). Alterations of the cytokine network in patients undergoing cardiopulmonary bypass. *Perfusion,* Vol. 12, pp. 393-403

Sakr, Y.; Lobo, S.; Knuepfer, S.; Esser, E.; Bauer, M.; Settmacher, U.; Barz, D. & Reinhart, K. (2010). Anemia and blood transfusion in a surgical intensive care unit. *Crit Care* Vol. 14, R92

Senay, S.; Toraman, F.; Gunaydin, S.; Kilercik, M.; Karabulut, H. & Alhan, C. (2009). The impact of allogeneic red cell transfusion and coated bypass circuit on the inflammatory response during cardiopulmonary bypass: a randomized study. *Interactive Cardiovascular and Thoracic Surgery,* Vol. 8, pp. 93-99

Silliman, C.C. (2006). The two-event model of TRALI. *Crit Care Med,* Vol. 34, pp. S124-S131

Silliman, C.C.; Fung, Y.L; Ball, J.B. & Khan, S.Y. (2009). Transfusion-related acute lung injury (TRALI): current concepts and misconceptions. *Blood reviews,* Vol. 23, pp 245-255

Sitniakowsky, L.S.; Later, A.F.L.; van de Watering, L.M.G.; Bogaerts, M.; Brand, A.; Klautz, R.J.M.; Smit, N.P.M. & van Hilten, J.A. (2011). The effect of RBC transfusions on cytokine gene expression after cardiac surgery in patients developing post-operative multiple organ failure. Transfusion Medicine, in press.

Snyder-Ramos, S.A.; Moehnle, P.; Weng, Y.S.; Bottiger, B.W.; Kulier, A.; Levin, J. & Mangano, D.T. (2008). The ongoing variability in blood transfusion practices in cardiac surgery. *Transfusion,* Vol. 48, pp. 1284-1299

Spiess, B.D.; Royston, D.; Levy, J.H.; Fitch, J.; Dietrich, W.; Body, S.; Murkin, J. & Nadel, A. (2004). Platelet transfusions during CABG surgery are associated with serious adverse outcomes. *Transfusion,* Vol. 44, pp. 1143-1148

Sreeram, G.M.; Welsby, I.J.; Sharma, A.D.; Philips-Bute, B.; Smith, P.K. & Slaughter, T.F. (2005). Infectious complications after cardiac surgery: lack of association with FFP or platelet transfusions. *J Cardiothoracic Vasc Anesthesia,* Vol.19, pp. 430-434

Stover, E.P.; Siegel, L.C.; Parks, R.; Levin, J.; Body, S.C.; Maddi, R.; D'Ambra, M.N.; Mangano, D.T. & Spiess, B.D. (1998). Variability in transfusion practice for coronary artery bypass surgery despite national consensus guidelines. *Anesthesiology,* Vol. 88, pp. 327-333

Surgenor S.D.; DeFoe G.R.; Fillinger M.P.; Likosky D.S.; Groom R.C.; Clark C.; Helm R.E.; Kramer R.S.; Leavitt B.J.; Klemperer .J.D.; Krumholz C.F.; Westbrook B.M.; Galatis D.J.; Frumiento C.; Ross C.S.; Olmstead E.M.; & O'Connor G.T. Intraoperative red blood cell transfusion during coronary artery bypass graft surgery increases the risk of postoperative low-output heart failure. *Circulation* Vol. 114, pp. I-43-I-48.

Tuinman, P.R.;. Vlaar, A.P.; Cornet, A.D.; Hofstra, J.J.; Levi, M.; Meijers, J.C.M.; Beishuizen, A.; Schultz, M.J.; Groeneveld, A.B.J. & Juffermans, N.P. (2011). Blood transfusion during cardiac surgery is associated with inflammation and coagulation in the lung: a case control study. *Crit Care,* Vol. 15, pp. R59

Vamvakas, E.C. & Carven, J.H. (1999). Transfusion and postoperative pneumonia in coronary artery bypass graft surgery: effect of the length of storage of transfused red cells. *Transfusion,* Vol. 39, pp. 701-710

Vamvakas, E.C. & Blajchman, M.A. (2007). Transfusion-related immunomodulation (TRIM): an update. *Blood reviews,* Vol. 21, pp. 327-348

van Hulst, M.; Bilgin, Y.M.; van de Watering, L.M.G.; de Vries, R.; van Oers, M.H.J.; Brand, A. & Postma, M.J. (2005). Cost-effectiveness of leucocyte-depleted erythrocyte transfusion in cardiac valve surgery. *Transf Med,*Vol. 15, pp. 209-217

van Straten, A.H.M.; Soliman Hamad, M.A.; Tan, M.E.; de Wolf, A.M.; Scharnhorst, V. & van Zundert, A.A. (2011). Effect of duration of red blood cell storage on early and late mortality after CABG. *J Thorac Cardiovasc Surg,* Vol. 141, pp. 238-243

van de Watering, L.M.; Hermans, J.; Houbiers, J.G.; van den Broek, P.J.; Bouter, H.; Boer, F.; Harvey, M.S.; Huysmans, H.A. & Brand, A. (1998). Beneficial effects of leukocyte depletion of transfused blood on postoperative complications in patients undergoing cardiac surgery: a randomized clinical trial. *Circulation,* Vol. 97, pp. 562-568

van de Watering, L.; Lorinser, J.; Versteegh, M.; Westendord, R. & Brand, A. (2006). Effects of storage time of red blood cell transfusions on the prognosis of coronary artery bypass graft patients. *Transfusion,* Vol. 46, pp. 1712-1718

Vincent, J.L., Sakr, Y.; Sprung, C.; Harboe. S. & Damas, P. (2008). Are blood transfusions associated with greater mortality rates? Results of the Sepsis Occurrence in Acutely Ill Patients study. *Anesthesiology,* Vol. 108, pp. 31-39

Wallis, J.P.; Chapman, C.E.; Orr, K.E.; Clark, S.C. & Forty, J.R. (2002). Effect of WBC reduction of transfused RBCs on postoperative infection rates in cardiac surgery. *Transfusion,* Vol. 42, pp. 1127-1134

Wu, W.C.; Rathore, S.S.; Wang, Y.; Radford, M.J. & Krumholz, H.M. (2001). Blood transfusion in elderly patients with acute myocardial infarction. *N Engl J Med,* Vol. 345, pp. 1230-1236

Yap, C.H.; Lau, L.; Krishnaswamy, M.; Gaskell, M. & Yii, M. (2008). Age of transfused red cells and early outcomes after cardiac surgery. *Ann Thorac Surg,* 86:554-559

10

Glycemic Control in Cardiac Surgery

Martín Martínez Rosas[1], Eduardo Wilfrido Goicoechea-Turcott[2], Pastor Luna Ortiz[3], Alberto Salazar[4] and Benito Antón Palma[4]

[1]*Physiology Department, National Institute of Cardiology "Ignacio Chavez", Mexico, D.F*

[2]*Faculty of Medicine, National Autonomous University of Mexico (UNAM), Mexico, D.F*

[3]*Pharmacology Department, National Institute of Cardiology "Ignacio Chavez", Mexico, D.F*

[4]*Laboratory of Molecular Neurobiology, National Institute of Psychiatry "Ramón de la Fuente", Mexico, D.F*

Mexico

1. Introduction

In cardiac surgery, hyperglycemia is a common occurrence in patients with and without diabetes (1,2). For many years, stress-induced hyperglycemia was considered an adaptive and beneficial response of the organism. However, both human and animal studies suggest that it is not a benign condition and, in contrast, it is associated with a high risk of morbidity and mortality. Stress hyperglycemia is defined as an elevation of plasma glucose levels (above 126 mg/dl in fasting condition or 200 mg/dl at any time) in critically ill or hospitalized patients, with or without history of diabetes (3). More specifically, elevated values of blood glucose in presence of normal levels of glycosylated hemoglobin (HbA1c), regardless of diabetes status, may be considered a stress response; this kind of hyperglycemia is developed during any physiological reaction to a situation of high metabolic demand or injury, in which diverse mechanisms become active for maintaining homeostasis, for example: major burns, severe trauma, hemorrhage, septicemia, and major surgery, in which it is very common for blood sugar to reach levels up to 370 mg/dl (4). It was the French physiologist Claude Bernard who first described this phenomenon in dogs subjected to hemorrhagic shock in 1885 (5); since then, this finding has been extensively studied, especially in recent decades because of it´s impact on outcomes of critically ill patients.

Hyperglycemia is a well recognized condition that increases the overall hospital morbidity and mortality of any patient admitted for any reason. In addition, it also increases the rate of complications in diabetic and non-diabetic patients undergoing major surgeries; besides this condition is associated with a longer hospital-stay and higher costs (1). Considering the strong association between hyperglycemia and general morbidity and mortality in surgery, there has been great interest for developing protocols to control blood-glucose levels during the perioperative period in order to prevent hyperglycemia, to achieve euglycemia and to reduce episodes of hypoglycemia, aiming the improvement of patient outcomes. In particular, the glycemic control in cardiac surgery has become a very important matter in

the full standard care as a mean of reducing infections and further complications, and in consequence, the patient's improvement.
This chapter reviews the mechanisms of stress hyperglycemia, the evidence of the association between hyperglycemia and adverse outcomes in surgical patients particularly in cardiac surgery. Besides, it offers a general overview about discordant reports found in the literature on the strict glycemic control during the peri-operative period of a cardiac surgery. In addition to, it also recommends common approaches to control the glycemia in surgical intensive care unit (ICU) and post-surgical cardiovascular patients based on the best performed randomized controlled trials.

2. Mechanisms of stress hyperglycemia

Stress Hyperglycemia, also called stress-induced diabetes, diabetes (6), is a multifact metabolic disorder that is characterized by the presence of hyperglycemia with hyperinsulinemia, peripheral resistance to insulin and an over-production of glucose by different mechanisms that result in incremented glycogenolysis and increased gluconeogenesis. Figure 1 shows how endogenous and exogenous predisposing factors may trigger the development of stress hyperglycemia, particularly during a cardiac surgery. The most important trigger is the surgical stress itself that conduces to a catabolic state that results in high levels of blood-glucose; the appearance of stress-hormones and a diminished peripheral response to insulin, cause hyperglycemia, and raises even more previous glycemia breeding an abnormal immune response (3, 6-9.). Stress hyperglycemia is caused mainly by the effects of counter-regulatory hormones (catecholamines, growth hormone, and cortisol) and by depletion of the functional reserve of the beta-cells in the Langerhans islets of the pancreas (7). During perioperative period of major surgeries, the counter-regulatory hormones and the inflammatory response induced by surgical stress are the most important triggers of hyperglycemia (10). The degree of insulin resistance has been related to the magnitude and endurance of surgical stress. In addition, it has been reported that in the perioperative period, increased glucose reabsorption or decreased renal glucose clearance may enhance this phenomena that contribute to hyperglycemia (11).

Predisposing factors

Although stress hyperglycemia is mainly caused by six events: severe trauma, bleeding, hypothermia, septicemia, severe burns and great-magnitude surgeries, there are several factors that may contribute to this alteration, which could and should be explored in the preoperative examinations (Table 1). All of these predisposing factors can be divided in endogenous and exogenous factors.

a. Endogenous factors

The first and most important predisposing factor for developing stress hyperglycemia is to be previously diagnosed with Diabetes Mellitus; in this case glucose blood-levels after cardiac surgery may reach even 20 mmol/l (370mg/dl) or more, compared with non-diabetic patients which might reach 15 mmol/l (270 mg/ml) (12-14). With a previous diagnosis of diabetes, it is not just more likely to develop stress hyperglycemia, but this one is more severe.
Other endogenous factor is acute pain which inhibits the suppression of endogenous glucose by insulin; in addition, it releases diverse acute-stress hormones that contribute hyperglycemia, such as cortisol, glucagon, growth hormone, etc. (15). It has been impossible

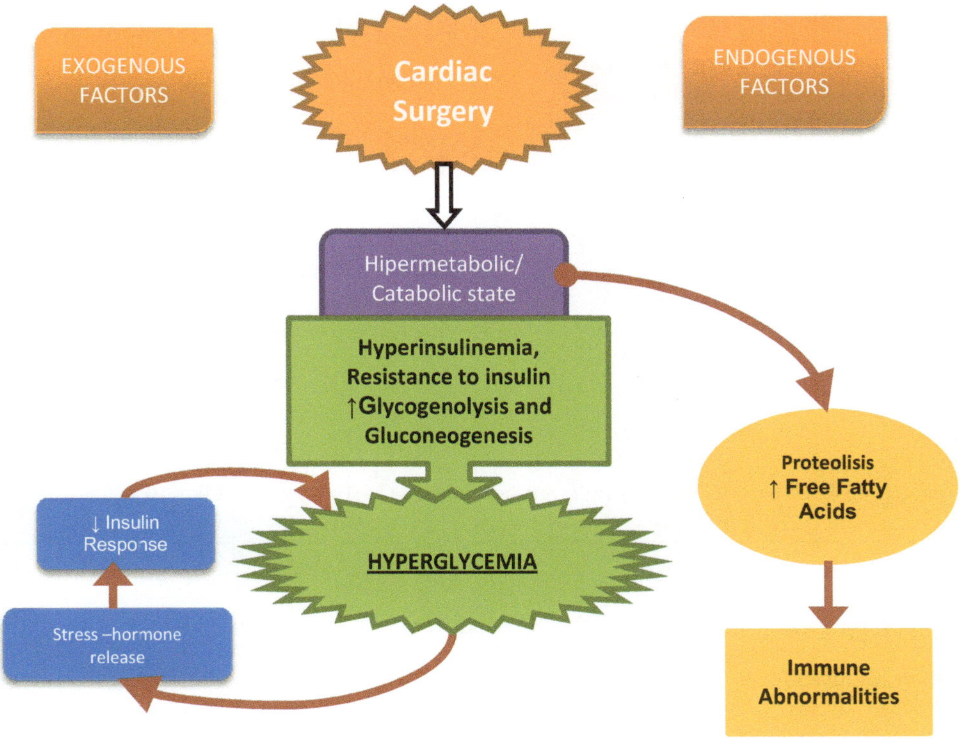

Fig. 1. It is showed how endogenous and exogenous predisposing factors may trigger the developing of stress hyperglycemia, adding cardiac surgery's aggression. Physiological-stress triggers a catabolic state that results in stress hyperglycemia; the appearance of stress-released hormones and a diminished peripheral response to insulin augment glycemia, and condition the release of proteins and free fatty acids that in addition to hyperglycemia entail an abnormal immune response.

to quantify the real affection caused by pain in the glucose-metabolism, but the tendency of an aggressive-pain management might be helpful for decreasing the peripheral resistance to insulin (16).

Elderly patients represent an important group that undergoes cardiac surgeries; it is well known that insulin secretion is diminished in this group of age. This is reinforced by different studies; the comparison between patients over 60 years versus younger people shows incidence-reduction of hyperglycemia up to 38% in young adults (17). So, elderliness is a very important factor for elevated blood glucose levels (18).

b. Exogenous factors

Hypothermia, especially present in coronary bypass surgery due to cardioplegic solutions, provokes hyperglycemia by inhibiting the negative-feedback of the insulin response (19). Also, desaturation and arterial hypoxemia, increase a sympathetic autonomous response that favors glucagon release by an alpha-receptor action (20).

Many drugs commonly used with inpatient care might modify glucose metabolism. Some of them are well known as 'diabetogenic' medications such as glucocorticoids and opiates;

Action	Factor
Insulin deficiency (relative or absolute)/Insulin resistance	Diabetes mellitus
Higher counterregulatory hormone levels	Acute Pain Elevated Acute Physiology and Chronic Health Evaluation (APACHE) score
Insulin Peripheral resistance	Catecholamine-Infusion Glucocorticoid treatment Overweight Septicemia/Sepsis/Septic Shock Uremia Bed rest Fasting
Insulin impaired secretion	Elderly Hypothermia Hypoxemia

Modified from ref. 29: McCowen KC, Malhotra A, Bistrian BR. Stress-induced hyperglycemia. *Crit Care Clin* 2001; 17: 107-24.

Table 1. Predisposing factors for developing stress hyperglycemia

others are used for treating hypertension such as calcium channel blockers, clortalidone, and prazosin. Every synthetic catecholamine or catecholamine-agonist or blocker (such as epinephrine, norepinephrine, salbutamol, metoprolol, propanolol) and tricyclic anti-depressants, might elevate glucose levels. Particularly, catecholamine-infusion during cardiac surgery contributes greatly to this metabolic state during surgery, as well as in the early postoperative period; it might also overlap and/or worsen stress response. Even alcohol and salicylates raise glycemia. All volatile anesthetic agents, including halothane, enflurane, and isoflurane, inhibit the insulin response to glucose in a dose dependent manner in vitro (21). The hyperglycemic response during inhaled anesthesia with isoflurane is a consequence of both impaired glucose clearance and increased glucose production (22,23).

Other factor that contributes to augment glycemia is bed resting. This condition reduces the sensitivity of the skeletal muscle to insulin, and in consequence increases fasting plasma insulin concentration as well as oral glucose challenge; insulin clamp studies showed no insulin secretion deficiency during repose. This response is mainly because of proteolysis that reduces total muscle mass and decreases the total number of transporters (24).

Other exogenous factor is the preoperative fasting. Fasting is a routinely action taken before undergoing a programmed cardiac surgery; fasting before surgery diminishes the glycogen reserve, induces protein breakdown (that releases alanine) and might disrupt insulin action and the stress responsiveness (25).

An underappreciated cause of hyperglycemia in critically ill patients is the provision of dextrose in excessive of amounts that can be easily oxidized or stored. In addition to hyperglycemia, other complications may result from the administration of dextrose over the rate of 4 mg/kg/min, inducing lipogenesis and increased carbon dioxide production (26).

The role of the glucose transporters

Stress-induced diabetes seems to be supported mainly by peripheral resistance to insulin, i.e. the inability of skeletal muscles and adipocytes to uptake glucose. This condition appears because of the affection of the glucose transporter type 4, called GLUT4 which is dependent of insulin. This very important hexose-transporter is located in skeletal-muscle, cardiac muscle and adipocytes (27). This protein is member of a family of transmembranal proteins that are responsible for uptaking glucose in different cells which depend of insulin for their action. These transporters are responsible of plenty of physiological phenomena that maintain glucose homeostasis (28,29). The physiological stress inhibits -by different mechanisms- the insulin's action on the GLUT4, mainly by impairing the phosphorylation of several molecules of the intracellular signaling pathway of insulin (30); the result is a decreased function of the transporter and therefore, a diminution of insulin-mediated glucose uptake. Additionally, the transporters GLUT1 (present in endothelial and non-skeletal muscle cells) and GLUT3 (present in neurons) are affected –as well as GLUT4 -by diverse cytokines such as IL-1, IL-6 and C-Reactive Protein which are augmented in surgical stress (29, 31,32).

Non-glucosydic substrates used during stress hyperglycemia

The carbohydrate metabolism during periods of stress uses different non-glucosydic substrates for gluconeogenesis such as glycerol, alanine, pyruvate and lactate. The last two mentioned molecules are generated when aerobic glucolysis and Kreb's cycle is impaired (23). In particular, lactate is produced because of inhibition of the pyruvate-dehydrogenase enzyme, mainly by IL-1, IL-6 and Tumoral Necrosis Factor-alpha (TNF-α) (33,34). The aminoacids alanine and glutamine are substrate for gluconeogenesis of critical illness. They are derived from proteolysis of skeletal muscle (33). The alanine is converted to glucose via Cori´s cycle (29). Glycerol is a product of lypolisis, and might be elevated because of the action of several counter-regulatory hormones (29), glycerol is used as a substrate of 20% of hepatic-derived glucose (29).

The role of the counterregulatory hormones

Hyperglycemia severity is directly correlated with the intensity of the inflammatory response (6). It is well known that inflammation produces an endocrine response that releases the so called "stress hormones" that raise glucose plasma levels. A wide variety of both hormones and cytokines affect glucose homeostasis by different pathways, including the promotion of gluconeogenesis or provoking insulin resistance; when hypoglycemia becomes present (less than 70 mg/dl, 3.9 mmol/l) there is a correlation with the initial threshold for releasing counterregulatory hormones and cytokines (35,36).

In healthy people, when gluconeogenesis is augmented, glucagon production is inhibited and insulin is released to the circulation; in the post-operated patient, there is an inflammatory response in which endogenous –or exogenous- cytokines and cathecolamines may interfere with this negative-feedback system and allow a hyperglycemic state by augmenting hepatic gluconeogenesis and glycogenolysis (34).

Although adrenaline, noradrenaline and cortisol are the best-studied hormones in the metabolic response to trauma, the most important stress hormone in postsurgical stress is the Growth Hormone (37). In other hand, adrenaline and noradrenalin are cathecolamines that greatly impair carbohydrates' metabolism. Adrenaline has shown to increase hepatic gluconeogenesis (29, 38), favors glycogenolysis in skeletal muscle and impairs glucose uptake in peripheral tissues, and via the β-3 adrenergic receptor, elevates free fatty acids (FFAs) in plasma (39). Likewise, noradrenaline may promote gluconeogenesis because its lipolytical effects and the marked glycerol supply to the liver (40). The glucogenolytic state mediated by these cathecolamines lasts no more than 36 hours (29). Additionally, cortisol is a major insulin counterregulatory hormone, which stimulates hepatic glucose production and enhances renal glucose production through glyconeogenesis, favors the presence of FFAs in plasma (34,41).

Growth Hormone is a very well known "diabetogenic" hormone and is the most important counterregulatory hormone present in surgical stress. It inhibits the insulin signaling cascade and it has been demonstrated in experimental animals to reduce the number of insulin receptors, as well as it reduces the phosphorylation on tyrosine residues triggered by insulin (42). Growth hormone also raises FFAs into plasma, and greatly affects the GLUT-1 and GLUT-4 activity (43). The Insulin-like Growth Factor (IGF-1 and -2) characterizes hepatic resistance to insulin's action, it has been proved that it keeps a direct association with mortality (44). There is not a clear relationship between every individual hormonal response that may result in a common phenomenon: hyperglycemia. More research is needed for augmenting our knowledge about hormonal regulation of this phenomenon, and also for understanding the role and importance of each one of these endocrine signals. Figure 2 shows how stress hormones might disrupt glucose metabolism by causing resistance to insulin's action and starting the usage of non-glucosydic substrates that contribute to raise glycemia.

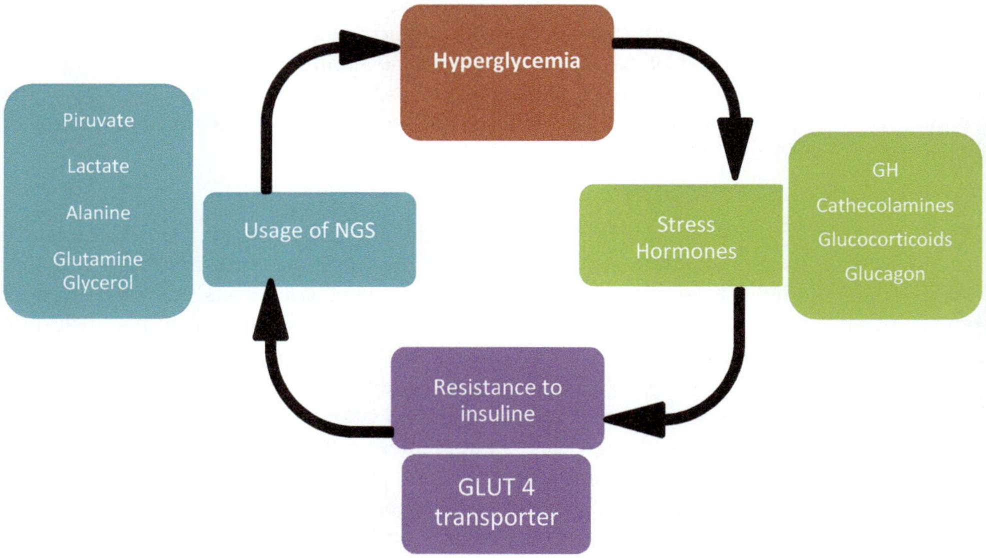

Fig. 2. The release of stress hormones produces gluconeogenesis and peripheral resistance to insulin. Stress hormones might disrupt glucose metabolism by causing resistance to insulin's action in the GLUT-4 transporter and originates the usage of non-glucosydic substrates, that contribute to raise glycemia. GH: Growth Hormone. NGS: non glucosydic substrates.

The role of the inflammatory response

Surgical stress establishes an acute inflammatory response that promotes the release of different cytokines –specifically TNF-α, IL-1, IL6- from mononuclear cells, this contributes to insulin resistance (29) and raising glucose levels in blood; at the same time, induces the production of diverse pro-inflammatory and mitogen cytokines like the nuclear factor kappa-B (NF-kB), the Early Growth Response-1 gene, the Plasminogen Activator Inhibitor-1 (PAI-1), Intracellular Adhesion Molecule-1 (iCAM-1), Monocyte Chemotactic Protein-1 (MCP-1) and matrix metalloproteinases-1, -2 and -9.

The mechanism whereby TNF-α mediates stress hyperglycemia has been well studied. This cytokine causes insulin resistance in both liver and skeletal muscle (6) most likely through the modification of signaling properties of insulin receptor substrates. In particular, endotoxin derived from cell wall of Gram-negative bacterial is also a potent stimulant of secondary production of TNF-α and various proximate interleukins, mainly IL-1 and -6 which disrupt both the insulin post-receptor signaling and the phosphorylation of molecules associated to the tyrosine-kinase receptor that lastly affects GLUT's activity, and glucose uptake (32, 45).

The Nuclear Factor kappa-B (NF-kB) is a pleiotropic transcription factor that is present in almost all cell types and is involved in many biological processes such as inflammation, immunity, cell differentiation, growth and apoptosis, and carcinogenesis. The early growth respone-1 gene is a nuclear protein that functions as a transcriptional regulator that favors cell differentiation and mitogenesis. The intracellular Adhesion Molecule-1 (iCAM-1) favors leucocyte adhesion, and metalloproteinases help in extracellular matrix remodeling (46-48).

Hyperglycemia affects immune cellular responsiveness by reducing neutrophyle activation, chemotactism, fagocytosis, and diminishing bactericidal activity of the reactive oxygen species (ROS). Humoral-cell response is affected by immunoglobulin glycosylation and altered synthesis of IL-6 and TNF-α (6,9). As mentioned, hyperglycemia has been associated to an altered immune response, an enhanced proinflammatory response, endothelial dysfunction, a hypercogulability state as well as neural damage with an augmented oxidative stress and secondary release of ROS from leucocytes (8,49).

All conditions above mentioned make up a not favorable setting for the surgical patient and represent a challenge to reach out a condition of stable normoglycemia. Figure 3 shows the relationship in between the abnormal glucose usage and how does physiological stress modifies the carbohydrate metabolism, leading to a deleterious non-homeostatic condition.

3. The stress hyperglycemia and adverse outcomes in surgical patients

The hyperglycemic response to acute stress induced by surgery was initially considered a beneficial-adaptive response, being the raised blood glucose a ready "source of fuel" for several tissues including the neural and cardiac-muscle cells. However, retrospective studies in patients undergoing cardiac surgery have suggested that perioperative hyperglycemia was associated with an increased risk of post-operative infections and an increased mortality (50-52). Furthermore, these studies suggested that control of blood glucose reduced these complications. The severity of hyperglycemia depends on many factors as showed in Table 1. There are different mechanisms in which a variety of risk factors affect the glucose metabolism and insulin responsiveness (53). Specifically, on surgery-invasiveness: the more invasive the surgery, the more intense the hyperglycemia (11, 54). Stress hyperglycemia has many deleterious effects, including vasodilatation, impaired

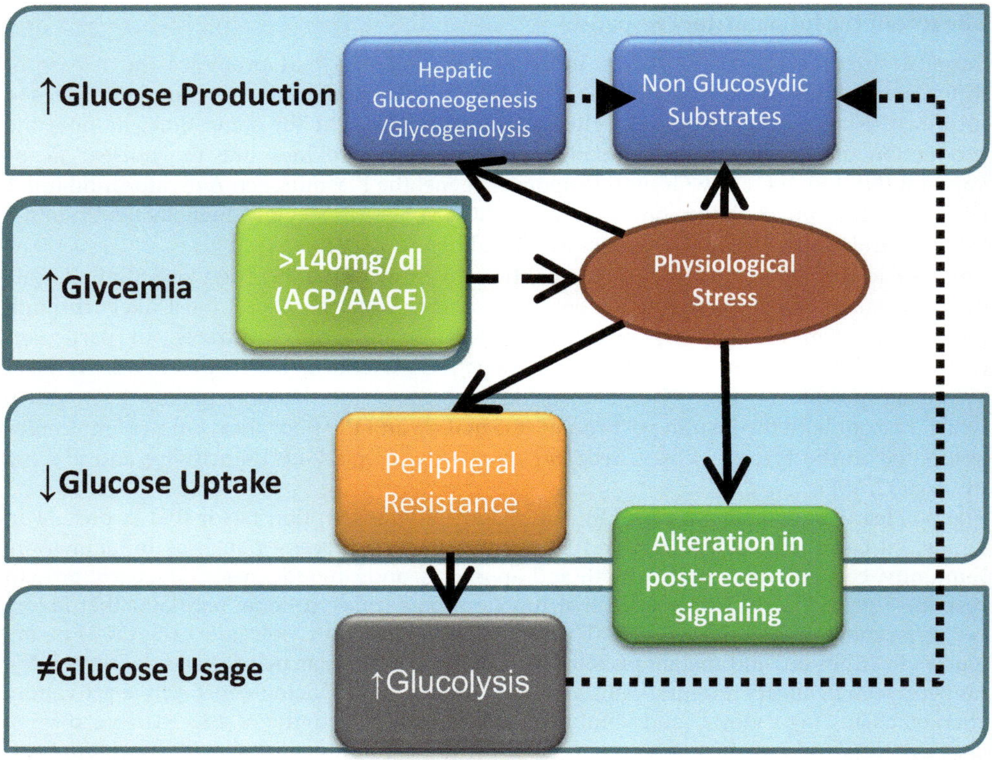

Fig. 3. The relationship between the abnormal glucose usage and physiological stress is exposed. Stress modifies the carbohydrate metabolism, the augmented glucose production and a diminished glucose uptake raises blood glucose levels, as well as the glucose intracellular metabolism is deviated.

reactive endothelial nitric oxide generation, decreased complement function, increased expression of leukocyte and endothelial adhesion molecules, increased cytokine levels, and impaired neutrophyle chemotaxis and phagocytosis, leading to increased inflammatory state and infection-vulnerability, and multiorgan system dysfunction (55). Others effects of excessive glucose levels include the impairment in hepatic functions, abolishment of ischemic preconditioning, and protein glycosylation (56).

Cardiac Surgery has been traditionally considered a highly-invasive procedure (57, 58) and taking in account that the hyperglycemic response is increased by anesthetics and the preoperative emotional stress (59), this major surgery, induces the release of several counter-regulatory hormones and deeply modifies the metabolism of carbohydrates, causing increased hepatic gluconeogenesis, insulin resistance in various peripheral tissues, and the relative insulin production deficiency (60,61). This insulin resistance has been related to an increased risk of postoperative complications in cardiac surgery, regardless of the patient´s diabetic status (62).

These metabolic and physiological responses to surgical stress often cause maintaining euglycemia during a cardiac surgery, to become a very difficult goal. Nevertheless, the reports about association of hyperglycemia and adverse outcomes in cardiac surgery make the glycemic control, something indispensable. Cardiac surgery mortality, tightly correlated to glucose blood levels, becomes significant lower when glycemia reaches less than 150 mg/dl (63) and it raises to even 17% with every 1 mmole/l (18 mg/dl) over 6.8 mmole/l (110 mg/dl) (61,64). Hyperglycemia during cardiac procedures and pulmonary bypass is severe, particularly in diabetic patients - who comprise a significant percentage of the patient population that undergo cardiac surgery. As it was commented, this impairment in glucose metabolism is related considerably to the metabolic response to surgical trauma, but it is associated mostly to specific aspects of cardiopulmonary bypass, such as heparinization, hypothermia, and rewarming (65, 66).

Independently of controversy about the reports on tight control of glycemia during perioperative period, is well known than poor perioperative glycemic control is associated with an increased morbidity and mortality.

4. Approaches on glycemic control during the perioperative period in cardiac surgery

In 2001, van den Berghe and coworkers (67) published a "landmark study" named "The Leuven Intensive Insulin Therapy Trial". In this study, they demonstrated that in critically-ill patients -the majority of them undergoing cardiac surgery- the Tight Glycemic Control (TGC) (blood glucose between 80-110 mg/dl) using intensive insulin therapy (IIT), improved the general clinical outcome (significant reduction in mortality; 42%) (67). After this study was published, TGC became rapidly adopted as the reference standard of care in surgical ICUs throughout the world (63, 68). The publication of new randomized controlled trials has diminished the initial enthusiasm on TGC because it has also been linked with increased morbidity and mortality. In last decade, there have been reports about the IIT has led to an increased iatrogenic rate of hypoglycemia episodes, emerging as an important risk factor for mortality exceeding, in some cases, the mortality-risk associated with hyperglycemia. In fact, even moderate and short hypoglycemia events in the ICU can produce permanent brain damage (69). After van den Berghe's work, two multicenter-randomized European studies were prematurely discontinued due to an alarmingly high rate of hypoglycemia in the TGC arm, showing no mortality benefits (70, 71). Two additional single centers, randomized studies showed a trend towards a higher mortality in the TGC arm (72, 73). TGC is strongly associated with an even sixfold-increase in episodes of severe hypoglycemia (glucose levels < 2.2 mmole/l, 40 mg/dl) (20) and, as mentioned before, this state can have dramatically adverse effects such as coma or even death (74). The recent NICE-SUGAR study showed that an intensive glucose control increased mortality among ICU adults, and that an 81-108 mg/dl target was too ambitious and potentially dangerous (12).

On the other hand, glucose variability has emerged as another important factor associated with mortality (75). Glucose profiles from patients are characterized by important fluctuations, even during continuous intravenous insulin infusion. However, many of the reported trials have evaluated the effects of IIT based on the absolute glucose levels, although clinical effects of IIT should be interpreted using temporal courses (76, 77). From this point of view, we should consider simultaneously the combined and independent clinical impact of glycemia's sudden fluctuations, glycemia temporal trends, and glycemia variability during hospitalization. In this way of thought, in a study including over 7,000 critically ill patients was demonstrated that the standard deviation of glucose concentration is a significant independent predictor of ICU and hospital mortality (78). Recently, it has been reported a relationship between ICU mortality and glucose variability in a cohort of 5,728 patients managed with IIT (79).

Although there is agreement that both hyperglycemia and hypoglycemia are deleterious, and that we should consider the fluctuations in blood glucose levels, there is no a consensus on the target glucose values to enhance desirable clinical outcomes. In this regard, relatively recent guidelines have been published from different international study-groups, like the American College of Physicians (ACP), American Diabetes Association (ADA), American Association of Clinical Endocrinologists (AACE) and the European Society of Cardiology (ESC) (80,81). The next section is related with recommendations about management of hyperglycemia in both patients with and without diabetes undergoing cardiac surgical, and the procedures that should be taken into account during the perioperative period, obtained from the Society of Thoracic Surgeons (STS) Practice Guideline series (81), which is derived in turns from evidence-based recommendations. We consider these guidelines as the most important work on the glucose management in cardiac surgery and we mention several paragraphs textually.

In summary, these useful guidelines offer some central ideas about the management of glycemia during cardiac surgery. The first of them is about detrimental effects of hyperglycemia in perioperative period, and they highlight that poor perioperative glycemic control is associated with increased morbidity and mortality, quoting the guidelines: "Collectively, these studies strongly suggest that increased fasting glucose levels during and immediately after cardiac surgery, are predictive of increased perioperative morbidity and mortality in patients with and without diabetes" (81). In this regard, the following central idea is about the beneficial effects of glycemic control on clinical outcomes during cardiac surgery, and afterwards, it recommends - after a review of the most important randomized trials - a glycemic control <180 mg/dl, mainly in patients with diabetes during cardiac surgery.

In the following paragraph, guidelines are focused about glycemic control in patients without diabetes during cardiac surgery, and they point –after analyzing several randomized trials of good quality- that "intraoperative glycemic control using intravenous insulin infusions is not necessary in cardiac surgery patients without diabetes, as well as glucose values remain < 180 mg/dl. This previous conclusion was obtained from the comparison between groups with TGC using IIT and without insulin finding no difference in the primary outcome, which consisted of the composite incidence of death, sternal wound infections, prolonged ventilation, cardiac arrhythmias, strokes, and renal failure within 30 days of surgery (82). There was also no difference in ICU or hospital stay between the groups. There was a tendency for more deaths (p=0.06) and strokes (p=0.02) in the IIT".

In the next section, the guidelines point to management of hyperglycemia using insulin protocols in the perioperative period considering that intravenous insulin therapy is the preferred method of insulin delivery during this period. It is used an evidence-based recommendations, depending on the procedure it is classified as beneficial, useful and effective (table 3; ref. 81). The recommendations class I are based on when glycemic control is best achieved with continuous insulin infusions rather than intermittent subcutaneous insulin injections or intermittent intravenous insulin boluses (level of evidence A). In addition, all patients with diabetes undergoing cardiac surgical procedures should receive an insulin infusion in the operating room, and for at least 24 hours postoperatively to maintain serum glucose levels ≤180 mg/dl (level of evidence=B; table 3).

Following the recommendations of the guidelines, the next part refers to the perioperative management and assessment for patients with diabetes. The next recommendations are classified after an exhaustive analysis of several trials with this kind of patients. Thus, we

Action	Factor
Lypolisis	Adrenaline Noradrenaline Growth Hormone
Enhanced Gluconeogenesis	Glucagon Glucocorticoids Growth Hormone
Supression of Insulin Secretion	Adrenaline Glucocorticoids (Cortisol)
Glucogenolysis	Adrenaline Glucagon
Peripheral Insulin Resistance	Tumoral Necrosis Factor alpha Adrenaline Glucocorticoids (Cortisol) Growth Hormone
Hepatic Insulin Impairment	Tumoral Necrosis Factor alpha

Modified from ref. 29: McCowen KC, Malhotra A, Bistrian BR. Stress-induced hyperglycemia. *Crit Care Clin* 2001; 17: 107-24.

Table 2. Major actions of counterregulatory hormones and cytokines in stress hyperglycemia

Class I: Conditions for which there is evidence for and/or general agreement that the procedure is beneficial, useful, and effective.
Class II: Conditions for which there is conflicting evidence and/or a divergence of opinion about the usefulness/efficacy of a procedure or treatment
Class IIA: Weight of evidence/opinion is in favor of usefulness/efficacy
Class IIB: Usefulness/efficacy is less well-established by evidence/opinion
Class III: Conditions for which there is evidence or general agreement that the procedure/treatment is not useful/effective, or both, and in some cases may be harmful
Level of Evidence – A: Data derived from multiple randomized clinical trials
Level of Evidence – B: Data derived from a single randomized trial or nonrandomized studies
Level of Evidence – C: Only consensus opinion of experts, case studies, or standard- of-care

Modified from ref. 81: Lazar. *Ann Thorac Surg* 2009; 87: 663-669.

Table 3. Classification system used for evidence based recommendations from society of thoracic surgeons practice guidelines

have summarized the experience of these trials. Class I: a) "patients taking insulin should hold their nutritional insulin after dinner the evening prior to surgery (level of evidence=B). b) Scheduled insulin therapy, using a combination of long-acting and short-acting subcutaneous insulin, or an insulin infusion protocol, should be initiated to achieve glycemic control for in-hospital patients awaiting surgery (level of evidence=C; table 3). c) All oral hypoglycemic agents and noninsulin diabetes medications should be held for 24 hours prior to surgery (level of evidence=C). d) The hemoglobin A1c (HbA1c) level should be obtained prior to surgery in patients with diabetes or those patients at risk for postoperative hyperglycemia to characterize the level of preoperative glycemic control" (level of evidence=C; table 3). Class IIA. Prior to surgery, it is reasonable to maintain blood glucose concentration ≤ 180 mg/dl (level of evidence=C; table 3). Efforts should be made to optimize glucose control prior to surgery, because poor preoperative glycemic control has been associated with increased mortality, including a higher incidence of deep sternal wound infections and prolonged postoperative length of stay. In general, all oral diabetes medications should be withheld within 24 hours prior to surgery, especially sulfonylureas (eg, glipizide) and glinides (eg, nateglinide or repaglinide). These drugs can induce hypoglycemia in the absence of food. Patients who are taking insulin and who are admitted on the day of surgery should be instructed to continue their basal insulin dose (eg, glargina, determir or NPH) and hold their nutritional insulin (eg, lispro, aspart, glulisine, or regular) unless instructed otherwise by their primary physician. The NPH insulin may be reduced by one half or one third of the dose prior to surgery to avoid hypoglycemia.

"To achieve rapid control in hospitalized patient with hyperglycemia (glucose > 180 mg/dl for more than 12 hours before surgery), insulin therapy -either with intravenous variable-rate continuous infusion or subcutaneous basal plus rapid-acting insulin- should be used depending on the availability of either therapy. For the hyperglycemic patient in the preoperative area, on the day of surgery, IV insulin therapy is an effective way to achieve immediate control. Patients with a known history of diabetes (either type 1 or type 2) can be started immediately on IV therapy in the preoperative area. All preoperative medications should be reviewed to determine the potential for insulin resistance. These include steroids, protease inhibitors, and anti-psychotic drugs. Finally, patients with renal insufficiency should be identified, because insulin clearance is impaired and the risk for hypoglycemia is increased".

Next section is the "intraoperative control recommendations". Above recommendations are classified upon the level of evidence and quality of trials. Class I. a) Glucose levels > 180 mg/dl that occur in patients without diabetes only during cardiopulmonary bypass may be treated initially with a single or intermittent dose of IV insulin as long as levels remain ≤ 180 mg/dl. However, in those patients with persistently elevated serum glucose (> 180 mg/dl) after cardiopulmonary bypass, a continuous insulin drip should be instituted, and an endocrinology consult should be obtained (level of evidence = B; table 3). b) If an intravenous insulin infusion is initiated in the preoperative period, it should be continued throughout the intraoperative and early postoperative period according to institutional protocols to maintain serum glucose ≤ 180 mg/dl (level of evidence = C; table 3).

Concerning glycemic control in the ICU, guidelines recommend the following procedures: Recommendation Class I. a) Patients with and without diabetes with persistently elevated serum glucose (> 180 mg/dl) should receive IV insulin infusion to maintain serum glucose < 180 mg/dl for the duration of their ICU care (level of evidence = A; table 3). b) All patients who require ≥ 3 days in the ICU because of ventilatory dependency or requiring the need for inotropes, intra-aortic balloon pump, or left ventricular assist device support, anti-arrhythmics, dialysis, or continuous veno-venous hemofiltration should have a continuous insulin infusion to keep blood glucose ≤ 150 mg/dl, regardless of diabetic status (level of evidence =B; table 3). b) Before intravenous insulin infusions are discontinued, patients should be transitioned to a subcutaneous insulin schedule using institutional protocols (level of evidence=B; table 3).

Finally, the Glycemic control in the stepdown units and on the floor recommendations is the last part of the guidelines. Class I. a) A target blood glucose level < 180 mg/dl should be achieved in the peak postprandial state (level of evidence = B; table 3). b) A target blood glucose level ≤ 110 mg/dl should be achieved in the fasting and pre-meal states after transfer to the floor (level of evidence = C; table 3). c) Oral hypoglycemic medications should be re-started in patients who have achieved target blood glucose levels if there are no contraindications. Insulin dosages should be reduced accordingly (level of evidence = C; table 3). d) According to the AACE, a reasonable goal for a noncritically ill patient on a regular hospital ward is < 110 mg/dl and< 180 mg/dl postprandial or randomly (83). The best method to realize this control is with scheduled subcutaneous basal and, or bolus insulin therapy, such as glargine or determir (basal) and lispro, aspart, or glulisine (bolus). Patients with type 2 diabetes who have used oral diabetes medications preoperatively can be restarted on those medications once they have reached their targeted glucose goals and are eating a regular diet. Metformin should not be restarted until stable renal function has been documented. In relation to preparation for hospital discharge, the guidelines recommend that prior to discharge, all patients with diabetes and those who have started a new glycemic control regimen, should receive in-patient education regarding glucose monitoring, medication administration (including subcutaneous insulin injection if necessary), nutrition, and lifestyle modification (level of evidence = C, table 3). Upon discharge, changes in therapy for glycemic control should be communicated to primary care physicians, and follow up appointments should be arranged with an endocrinologist when appropriate (level of evidence = C, table 3). All patients with hyperglycemia after cardiac surgery should be assessed by an inpatient diabetes team to decide on a glycemic control program after discharge.

The conditions that are important to consider are, in summary: avoidance of deep hypothermia, excessive blood losses, a prolonged preoperative fasting period and prolonged immobilization, because all these conditions augment perioperative insulin resistance. In addition, considering that most anesthetic agents cause hyperglycemia, the choice of anesthetic agent will be influenced by the severity of systemic diseases, such as coronary artery disease, nephropathy (with the concomitant risk of hyper/hypokalemia and other hidroelectrolytic disorders), and hypertension, and the choice of neuromuscular blocking agent will be affected by renal function.

5. Conclusion

Although reports differ, and not enough data are available to allow specifying optimal treatment goals or the best approach to perioperative management of glycemia, it is clear that surgical outcomes are improved in patients who are maintained in good metabolic control. Physicians must be cognizant of patients´ preoperative control, in diabetic patients, their relative need for insulin, and any factors that may be likely to increase insulin requirements. The guidelines presented here represent just an approximate approach based in evidence with different qualities. So, the administration of adequate glucose in conjunction with the judicious use of insulin will prevent hypoglycemia. However, diabetic ketoacidosis or hyperosmolar states, which may result from inadequate dosing of insulin, are not so easily managed. The key to success of any perioperative management plan is frequent monitoring of glucose, electrolyte, and fluid levels, and acid-base status. Prevention of surgical complications as a result of hyperglycemia is possible with meticulous perioperative glucose management. Finally, we need further research to be done to provide definitive answers on the benefits of tight glycemic control for cardiac surgery patients.

6. References

[1] Umpierrez GE, Isaacs SD, Bazargan N, You X, Thaler LM, Kitabchi AE. Hyperglycemia: an independent marker of in-hospital mortality in patients with undiagnosed diabetes. J Clin Endocrinol Metab. 2002;87:978-982

[2] Levetan CS, Passaro M, Jablonski K, Kass M, Ratner RE. Unrecognized diabetes among hospitalized patients. Diabetes Care. 1998;21:246-9.

[3] Fahy BG, Sheehy AM, Coursin DB. Glucose control in the intensive care unit. Crit Care Med. 2009; 31:1769–76.

[4] Luna-Ortiz P, Carbó R, Rojas E, de Micheli A, Pastelin G, Martínez M. Strict control of glycemia and cardioprotection. Rev Mex Anest 2008; 31:298-310.

[5] Bernard C. Lecons de physiologie experimentale appliqué a la medicine. Vol. 1. Balliere, Paris 1855; 1:296-313

[6] Collier B, Dossett LA, May AK, Dı´az JJ. Glucose control and the inflammatory response. Nutr Clin Pract. 2008;23:3–15.

[7] Sakharova OV, Inzucchi SE. Endocrine assessments during critical illness. Crit Care Clin. 2007;23:467–90.

[8] Langouche L, Vanhorebeek I, Van den Berghe G. Therapy insight: The effect of tight glycemic control in acute illness. Nat Clin Pract Endocrinol Metab. 2007;3:270–8.

[9] Van den Berghe G, Wouters PJ, Bouillon R, Weekers F, Verwaest C, Schetz M, et al. Outcome benefit of intensive insulin therapy in the critically ill: Insulin dose versus glycemic control. Crit Care Med. 2003;31:359–66.

[10] Bagry HS, Raghavendran S, Carli F: Metabolic syndrome and insulin resistance: Perioperative considerations. ANESTHESIOLOGY 2008; 108:506–23.

[11] Sicardi Salomo´n Z, Rodhe P, Hahn RG: Progressive decrease in glucose clearance during surgery. Acta Anaesthesiol Scand 2006; 50:848 –54.

[12] NICE-SUGAR Study Investigators, Finfer S, Chittock DR, Su SY, Blair D, Foster D, Dhingra V, Bellomo R, Cook D, Dodek P, Henderson WR, Hébert PC, Heritier S, Heyland DK, McArthur C, McDonald E, Mitchell I, Myburgh JA, Norton R, Potter J, Robinson BG, Ronco JJ. Intensive versus conventional glucose control in critically ill patients. N Engl J Med 2009;360 (13):1283–1297.

[13] Mills NL, Beaudet RL, Isom OW, Spencer FC. Hyperglycemia during cardiopulmonary bypass. Ann Surg 1973;177(2):203–205.

[14] Chaney MA, Nikolov MP, Blakeman BP. Attempting to maintain normoglycemia during cardiopulmonary bypass with insulin may initiate postoperative hypoglycemia. Anesth Analg 1999;89:1091-1095.

[15] Greisen J, Juhl CB, Grofte T, Vilstrup H. Acute pain induces insulin resistance in humans. Anesthesiology 2001;95:578-84.

[16] Carli F, Phil M, Benneth GJ. Pain and postoperative recovery. Anesthesiology 2001;95:573-4.

[17] Frankenfield D, Cooney RN, Smith JS, et al: Age-related differences in the metabolic response to injury. J Trauma 48:49-56, 2000.

[18] Desai D, March R, Watters JM: Hyperglycemia after trauma increases with age. J Trauma 29:719-723, 1989.
[19] Werb MR, Zinman B, Teasdale SJ, et al: Hormonal and metabolic responses during coronary artery bypass surgery: Role of infused glucose. J Clin Endocrinol Metab 69:1010-1018, 1989.
[20] Baum D, Porte D Jr: Stress hyperglycemia and the adrenergic regulation of pancreatic hormones in hypoxia. Metabolism 29:1176-1185, 1980
[21] Desborough JP, Jones PM, Persaud SJ, Landon MJ, Howell SL. Isoflurane inhibits insulin secretion in isolated rat pancreatic islets of Langerhans. Br J Anaesth. 1993;71: 873-876.
[22] Lattermann R, Schricker T, Wachter U, Georgieff M, Goertz A. Understanding the mechanisms by which isoflurane modifies the hyperglycemic response to surgery. Anesthesia Analgesia. 2001;93:121-127.
[23] Tanaka K, Kawano T, Tomino T, Kawano H, Okada T, Oshita S, Takahashi A, Nakaya Y: Mechanisms of impaired glucose tolerance and insulin secretion during isoflurane anesthesia. ANESTHESIOLOGY 2009; 111:1044 –51.
[24] Stuart CA, Shangraw RE, Prince MJ, et al: Bed-rest-induced insulin resistance occurs primarily in muscle. Metabolism 37:802-806, 1988.
[25] Planas M, García de Lorenzo A, López Martínez J, Montejo JC. ¿Es bueno el ayuno en el paciente crítico? Nutr Hosp 1999;14:53-6.
[26] Guenst JM, Nelson LD: Predictors of total parenteral nutrition-induced lipogenesis. Chest 105:553-559, 1994.
[27] Goodyear LJ, Hirshman MF, Napoli R, Calles J. Glucose ingestion causes GLUT-4 translocation in human skeletal muscle. Diabetes 1996;45:1051-6.
[28] García de Lorenzo, A. Longarela, A., Olarra, J., Suárez, L. Rodríguez-Montes, JA. "Hiperglucemia Postagresión Quirúgica. Fisiopatología y Prevención". Cir Esp. 2004;75:167-70.
[29] McCowen KC, Malhotra A, Bistrian BR. "Stress-Induced Hyperglycemia". Critic Care Clinics 17,1: 107-124. 2001.
[30] Flakoll PJ, Hill JO, Abumrad NN: Acute hyperglycemia enhances proteolysis in normal man. Am J Physiol 265:E715-E721, 1993.
[31] Jeschke MG, Klein D, Herndon DN. Insulin treatment improves the systemic inflammatory reaction to severe trauma. Ann Surg. 2004;239:553–60.
[32] Yu WK, Li WQ, Li A, Li JS. Influence of acute hyperglycemia in human sepsis on inflammatory cytokine and contra-regulatory hormone concentrations. World J Gastroenterol. 2003;9:1824–7.
[33] Vary TC: Sepsis-induced alterations in pyruvate dehydrogenase complex activity in rat skeletal muscle: effects on plasma lactate. Shock 6:89-94, 1996.
[34] Manzanaer W., Aramendi I. "Hiperglucemia de estrés y su control con Insulina en el paciente crítico: Evidencia Actual". Med Intensiva.2010;34(4):273–281.
[35] Egi M, Bellomo R, Stachowski E, French CJ, Hart GK, Hegarty C, et al. Blood glucose concentration and outcome of critical illness: The impact of diabetes. Crit Care Med. 2008; 36: 2249–55.
[36] Yendamuri S, Fulda GJ, Tinkoff GH. Admission hyperglycemia as a prognostic indicator in trauma. J Trauma. 2003;55:33–8.

[37] Strömmer L, Permert J, Arnelo U, Koehler C. Skeletal muscle insulin resistance after trauma: insulin signaling and glucose transport. Am J Physiol 1998;275:E351-8.
[38] Sherwin RS, Sacca L. Effect of epinephrine on glucose metabolism in humans: contribution of the liver. Am J Physiol 247:E157-E165, 1984
[39] Bessey PQ, Brooks DC, Black PR, et al: Epinephrine acutely mediates skeletal muscle insulin resistance. Surgery 94:172-179, 1983
[40] Connolly CC, Steiner KE, Stevenson RW, et al: Regulation of glucose metabolism by norepinephrine in conscious dogs. Am J Physiol 1991;261:E764-E772.
[41] Dresner A, Laurent D, Marcucci M, et al: Effects of free fatty acids on glucose transport and IRS-1-associated phosphatidylinositol 3-kinase activity. J Clin Invest 1999; 103:253-259.
[42] Dominici FP, Cifone D, Bartke A, et al: Alterations in the early steps of the insulin-signaling system in skeletal muscle of GH-transgenic mice. Am J Physiol 277:E447-E454, 1999.
[43] Smith TR, Elmendorf JS, David TS, et al: Growth hormone-induced insulin resistance: Role of the insulin receptor, IRS-1, GLUT-1, and GLUT-4. Am J Physiol 1997; 272:E107-E109.
[44] Van den Berghe G. How does blood glucose control with insulin save lives in intensive care? J Clin Invest. 2004;114: 1187–95
[45] Jeschke MG, Klein D, Herndon DN. Insulin treatment improves the systemic inflammatory reaction to severe trauma. AnnSurg.2004;239:553–60.
[46] Umpierrez GE, Kitabchi AE. ICU Care for Patients with Diabetes. *Current Opinions Endocrinol* 2004; 11: 75-81.
[47] Mizock BA. Blood glucose management during critical illness. *Rev Endocr Metab Disord* 2003; 4: 187-94.
[48] Garber AJ, Moghissi ES, Bransome ED, Jr., et al. American College of Endocrinology position statement on inpatient diabetes and metabolic control. *Endocr Pract* 2004; 10: 4-9.
[49] Kitabchi AE, Freire AX, Umpierrez GE. Evidence for strict inpatient blood glucose control: time to revise glycemic goals in hospitalized patients. *Metabolism* 2008; 57:116-20.
[50] Furnary AP, Wu Y. Clinical effects of hyperglycemia in the cardiac surgery population: the Portland Diabetic Project. Endocr Prac 2006; 12 Suppl 3:22-26.
[51] Furnary AP, Wu Y. Eliminating the diabetic disadvantage: the Portland Diabetic Project. Semin Thorac Cardiovasc Surg 2006; 18:302-308.
[52] Zerr KJ, Furnary AP, Grunkemeier GL, Bookin S, Kanhere V, Starr A. Glucose control lowers the risk of wound infection in diabetics after open heart operations. Ann Thorac Surg 1997; 63:356-361.
[53] Oswald GA, Smith CC, Betteridge DJ, et al: Determinants and importance of stress hyperglycaemia in non-diabetic patients with myocardial infarction. Br Med J (Clin Res Ed) 293:917-922, 1986
[54] Schricker T, Lattermann R, Schreiber M. The hyperglycemic response to surgery: Pathophysiology, clinical implications and modification by the anaesthetic technique. Clin Intens Care 1998;9:118-128.
[55] Turina M, Fry DE, Polk HC Jr: Acute hyperglycemia and the innate immune system: Clinical, cellular, and molecular aspects. Crit Care Med 2005; 33:1624–33.

[56] Amour J, Brzezinska AK, Jager Z, Sullivan C, Weihrauch D, Du J, Vladic N, Shi Y, Warltier DC, Pratt PF Jr, Kersten JR: Hyperglycemia adversely modulates endothelial nitric oxide synthase during anesthetic preconditioning through tetrahydrobiopterin-and heat shock protein 90-mediated mechanisms. Anesthesiology 2010; 112:576 – 85.
[57] Fleisher L. Preoperative cardiac evaluation of the patient undergoing major vascular surgery. Anesthesiol Clin North Am 1995; 13:53
[58] Goldman L, Caldera D, Nussbaum S, et al. Multifactorial index of cardiac risk in non-cardiac surgical procedures. N Eng J Med 1977; 197:845.
[59] Schricker T, Lattermann R, Schreiber M. The hyperglycemic response to surgery: Pathophysiology, clinical implications and modification by the anaesthetic technique. Clin Intens Care 1998;9:118-128.
[60] Soop M, Nygren J, Thorell A, Ljungqvist O. Stress-induced insulin resistance: recent developments. Curr Opin Clin Nutr Metab Care 2007;10:181-186.
[61] Anderson R, Brismar K, Barr G, Ivert T. Effects of cardiopulmonary bypass on glucose homeostasis after coronary bypass surgery. Eur J Cardiothoracic Surg 2005; 28: 425-30.
[62] Sato H, Carvalho G, Sato T, Lattermann R, Matsukawa T, Schricker T: The association of preoperative glycemic control, intraoperative insulin sensitivity, and outcomes after cardiac surgery. J Clin Endocrinol Metab 2010; 95:4338 – 44
[63] Furnary A, Gao G, Grunkeimer GL. Continuous insulin infusion reduces mortality in patients with diabetes undergoing coronary artery bypass grafting. J Thorac Cardiovasc Surg 2003;125:1007-1021.
[64] McAlister FA, Man J, Bistritz L. Diabetes and coronary artery bypass surgery: An examination of perioperative glycemic control and outcomes. Diabetes Care 2003;26:1518-1524.
[65] Kuntschen FR, Galletti PM, Mahn C. Glucose-insulin interactions during cardiopulmonary bypass. Hypothermia versus normothermia. J Thorac Cardiovasc Surg 1986; 91: 451-459.
[66] Kuntschen FR, Galletti PM, Han C, Arnulf JJ, Isetta C, Dor V. Alterations of insulin and glucose metabolism during cardiopulmonary bypass under normothermia. J Thorac Cardiovascular Surg 1985; 89: 97-106
[67] Van den Berghe G, Wouters P, Weekers F, et al. Intensive Insulin Therapy in the Critically ill Patients. N Engl J Med 2001; 345: 1359-67.
[68] Ouattara A, Lecomte P, Le Manach Y, Landi M, Jacqueminet S, Platonov I, Bonnet N, Riou B, Coriat P. Poor intraoperative blood glucose control is associated with a worsened hospital outcome after cardiac surgery in diabetic patients. Anesthesiology 2005;103:687—94.
[69] Duning T, Ellger B. Is hypoglycemia dangerous? Best Pract Res Clin Anaesthesiol 2009; 23:473-485.
[70] Devos P, Preiser JC, Melot C. Impact of tight glycemic control by intensive insulin therapy on ICU mortality and the rate of hypoglycemia: final results of the Glucontrol Study. Intensive Care Med 2007; 33 Suppl2: S189.
[71] Brunkhorst FM et al. Intensive Insulin therapy and pentasarch resuscitation in severe sepsis. N. Engl J Med 2008; 358: 125-139.

[72] De la Rosa G del C et al. Strict glycemic control in patients hospitalized in a mixed medical and surgical intensive care unit: a randomized clinical trial. Crit Care 2008; 12: R120.

[73] Arabi YM, Dabbaqh OC, Tamim HM, Al-Shimemeri AA, Memish ZA, Haddad SH, Syed SJ, Giridhar HR, Rishu AH, Al-Daker MO, Kahoul SH, Brittis RJ, Sakkijha MH. Intensive versus conventional insulin therapy: a randomized controlled trial in medical and surgical critically ill patients. Crit Care Med 2008; 36:3190-97.

[74] Kovalaske GY. Glycemic control in the medical intensive care unit. J Diabetes Sci. Technol 2009 3:1330-1341.

[75] Ouattara A, Grimaldi A, Riou B. Blood glucose variability: a new paradigm in critical care? Anesthesiology 2006;105:233-234.

[76] M, Bellomo R. Reducing glycemic variability in intensive care unit patients: a new therapeutic target? J Diabetes Sci Technol 2009;3:1302—8.

[77] Meyfroidt G, Keenan DM, Wang X, Wouters PJ, Veldhuis JD, Van den Berghe G. Dynamic characteristics of blood glucose time series during the course of critical illness: effects of intensive insulin therapy and relative association with mortality. Crit Care Med 2010;38:1021—9.

[78] Polito A, Thiagarajan RR, Laussen PC, Gauvreau K, Agus MS, Scheurer MA, Pigula FA, Costello JM. Association between intraoperative and early postoperative glucose levels and adverse outcomes after complex congenital heart surgery. Circulation 2008;118:2235—42.

[79] Hermanides J, Vriesendorp TM, Bosman RJ, Zandstra DF, Hoekstra JB, Devries JH. Glucose variability is associated with intensive care unit mortality. Crit Care Med 2010;38:838—42.

[80] Qaseem et al. Use of Intensive Insulin Therapy for the Management of Glycemic Control in Hospitalized Patients: A Clinical Practice Guideline from the American College of Physicians. Ann Intern Med. 2011; 154: 260-267.

[81] Lazar HL, McDonnell M, Chipkin ST, Furnary AP, Engelman RM, Sadhu A, et al. The Society of thoracic Surgeons Practice Guidelines Series: Blood Glucose Management During Adult Cardiac Surgery. Ann Thorac Surg 2009; 87:663-669.

[82] Gandhi GY, Nuttall GA, Abel MD, et al. Intensive intraoperative insulin therapy versus conventional glucose management during cardiac surgery: a randomized trial. Ann Intern Med 2007; 146:233-243.

[83] American Association of Clinical Endocrinologists medical guidelines for clinical practice for the management of diabetes mellitus. Endocr Pract 2007; 13 (suppl 1):1-68.

11

Coagulation Measurement and Optimisation in Cardiac Surgery

Philip Johnson and Andrew Westbrook
Department of Anaesthesia, Intensive Care and Pain Medicine,
St Vincent's University Hospital, Elm Park, Dublin
Ireland

1. Introduction

Coagulation is a complex physiological balancing mechanism that maintains haemostasis when blood vessels are injured. A hypercoaguable state as seen in early sepsis, cancer or pregnancy can cause arterial and/or venous obstruction with disruption of blood-flow and end organ damage. Similarly a hypocoaguable state can cause catastrophic haemorrhage and lead to death.

Up to 20% of all blood transfusions in the USA are related to cardiac surgery (1). The pathogenesis of coagulopathy in this patient group is multifactorial: patients are older (2), and more complex and this is reflected in the number of redo surgeries and the concomitant use of agents such as clopidogrel, aspirin, coumarin anticoagulants and heparins. Also cardiopulmonary bypass activates the coagulation system with an initial hypercoaguable state and platelet activation, followed by factor and platelet consumption. Hypothermia, acidosis, hypocalcaemia and the dilutional effects of circuit priming all increase the risk of bleeding (3).

Platelet transfusion per se in the perioperative period has been associated with an increased risk of serious adverse events (4). Indeed both red cell and platelet transfusion have been shown to have a negative risk-adjusted effect on health-related quality of life after cardiac surgery (5). The haemostatic status of a patient undergoing cardiopulmonary bypass can change very quickly because of haemorrhage or the use of high dose heparin or protamine and as such blood component administration in cardiac surgery can often be empiric. This is compounded by the limited utility of the standard coagulation tests, which have a slow turnaround time in a setting where there can be rapid changes in coagulation status.

All patients presenting for cardiac surgery will be anticoagulated in the perioperative period, either for cardiac or non-cardiac reasons, and an appropriate balance needs to be struck between minimising perioperative blood loss and use of homologous blood products, and avoiding pathological thrombosis.

Coagulation status can be measured by means of laboratory tests or near-patient tests (also referred to as point-of-care tests). Effective use and interpretation of these tests can guide physicians and surgeons alike in the use of medications and homologous blood products and timely intervention of surgery to optimise patient outcomes. Indeed, the thromboelastogram (TEG), a point-of-care test, should discriminate "surgical" from "medical" causes of bleeding in this population thus reducing unnecessary transfusions and allowing timely return to the operating room for definitive treatment. The TEG will also facilitate targeted therapy in a "medically" bleeding patient by providing information about platelet function and degree of fibrinolysis as well as factors produced in the liver. Standard coagulation tests and point-of-care tests will be discussed in detail with reference to their individual utility in this group of patients.

2. Coagulation pathways

Coagulation requires complex interactions of cellular and molecular components, mainly involving platelets, plasma and red blood cells. The process was classically described as a cascade of 'Intrinsic', 'Extrinsic', and 'Common' pathways (see Figure 1). These pathways

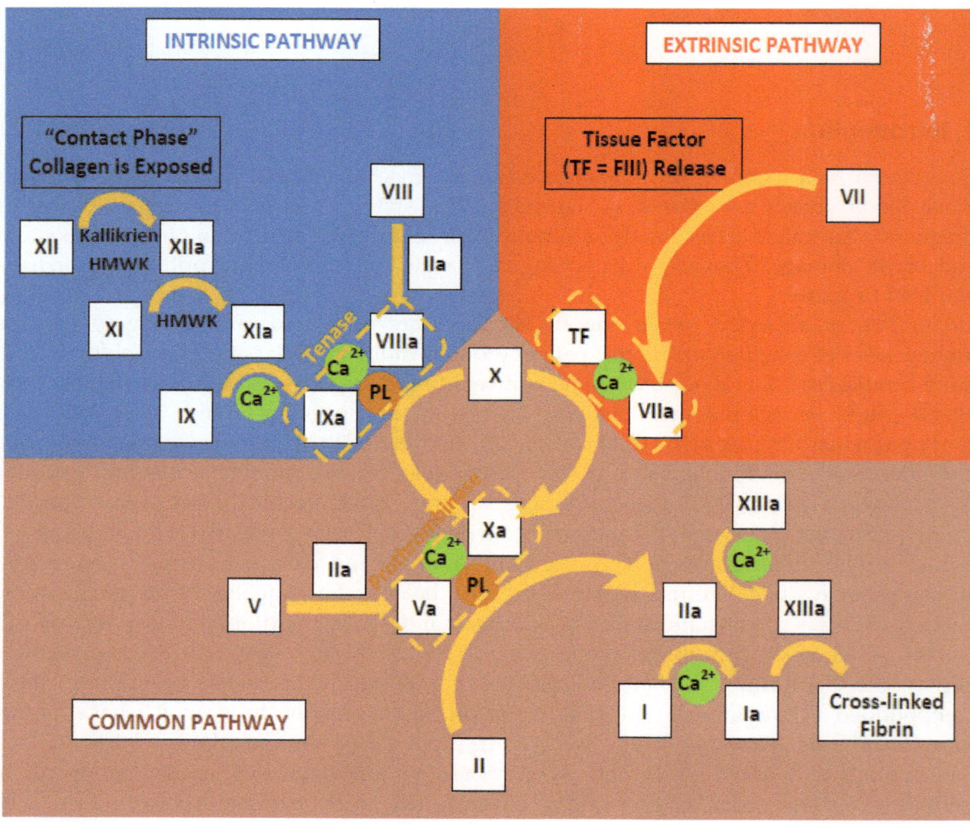

The Intrinsic Pathway is activated when FXII binds to exposed collagen of damaged endothelium. The cascade of activations occur as shown, and amplification also occurs (for example FXIIa converts prekallikrien to kallikrien and auto-activates more FXII). The resulting "Tenase" complex (shown in a dashed yellow line) activates FX. The Extrinsic Pathway is initiated by Tissue Factor, and results in a TF/FVIIa complex (in a dashed yellow line) that activates FX. The Common Pathway yields thrombin (FIIa), which not only activates Fibrinogen (FI) but also amplifies other stages of the cascade by activating FVIII, FV and FXIII. The ultimate result is a cross-linked Fibrin mesh. HMWK = High Molecular Weight Kininogen. PL = Phospholipid.

Fig. 1. The Classic Coagulation Cascade Model(6).

are useful in terms of interpreting some of the coagulation tests, but in vitro coagulation is less linear and occurs by a combination of these pathways. Current understanding of the coagulation process is best described by the cell-based model.

The coagulation factors were discovered in the 1940s and 1950s. They are proenzymes found in plasma, which are converted to active enzymes during the coagulation process. The factors were assigned roman numerals in the order they were discovered; each factor also has one or more names. The more commonly used ones are shown in the figure 2 (6). The numerals are prefixed by "F" for "factor", and the suffix "a" is used to indicate the activated form of the factor.

I	Fibrinogen
II	Prothrombin
IIa	Thrombin
III	Tissue Factor / Tissue Thromboplastin (sometimes excluded from the list of factors - not actually a plasma proenzyme, but an integral membrane protein, which is a receptor for FVII)
IV	Calcium ions
V	Labile Factor / Proaccelerin / accelerator (AC-) globulin
VI	Factor Va was once known as FVI
VII	Serum Factor / Stable Factor / Proconvertin / Serum Prothrombin Conversion Accelerator (SPCA) / Cothromboplastin / Autoprothrombin I
VIII	Haemophilia A factor / antihaemophiliac Factor / Plasma Thromboplastic Factor / Thromboplastinogen / Platelet Cofactor
IX	Haemophilia B Factor / Christmas Factor / Plasma Thromboplastin Component
X	
XI	Haemophilia C factor / Plasma Thromboplastin Antecedent (PTA)
XII	Hageman Factor / Contact Factor
XIII	Fibrin Stabilizing Factor

Fig. 2. Factor Numbers and Common name(s) – anomalies are shown in green

3. Intrinsic pathway

The "Intrinsic Pathway", so-called because its components are all present within whole blood, is initiated when blood comes in contact with a negatively charged surface such as glass or the surface of an activated platelet. It consists of a reaction cascade involving FXII, High Molecular Weight Kininogen (HMWK), prekallikrien, FXI, FIX, FIIa, FVIII, and Ca^{2+} and culminates in the activation of FX at the Common Pathway. The activated partial thromboplastin time (APTT) laboratory test measures the intrinsic pathway.

4. Extrinsic pathway

The "Extrinsic Pathway" is initiated when endothelial injury causes tissue factor (TF, or FIII) to come into contact with FVII. TF non-proteolytically activates FVII. The FVIIa/TF complex then activates FX. The extrinsic pathway can be measured by the Prothrombin Time (PT) laboratory test.

5. The common pathway

The intrinsic and extrinsic pathways both lead to activation of FX. FXa, FVa and Ca^{2+} activate prothrombin (FII) to form thrombin (FIIa). Thrombin has several actions: it activates fibrinogen (FI) to yield fibrin monomers; it amplifies the coagulation process by activating further prothrombin, FV and FVIII; it activates FXIII whose active form promotes cross-linking of fibrin monomers to form stable polymers; (as discussed later in the cell-based model, it also participates in processes that temper coagulation to avoid overwhelming pathological thrombosis.) The common pathway thus yields a mesh of covalently cross-linked fibrin strands and entrapped red blood cells, which form a stable blood clot. Disorders of the common pathway will affect tests of the intrinsic and extrinsic pathways.

6. The cell-based model

The five steps of this model are initiation, amplification, propagation, stabilisation and inhibition of further coagulation (7). In health, 1% of circulating FVII is in the active form.

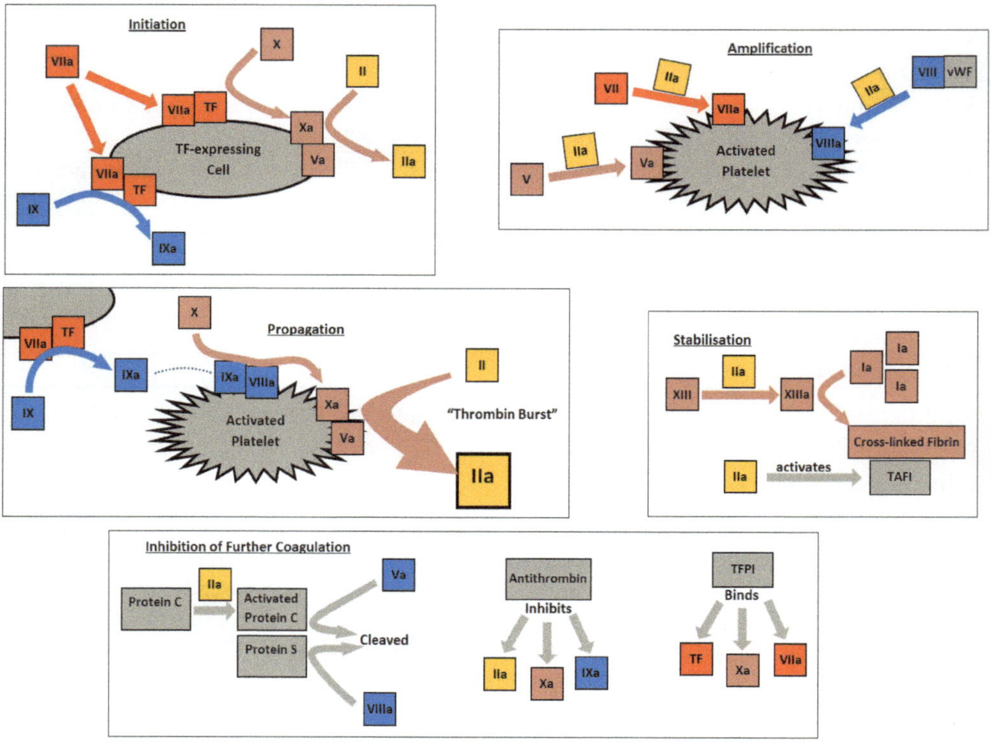

Blue, Red and Purple correspond respectively to Intrinsic, Extrinsic and Common Pathways of the Classic Coagulaton Cascade. Thrombin has a key role throughout, hence is shown in yellow. TF = Tissue Factor. vWF = von Willebrand Factor. TAFI = Thrombin Activated Thrombolysis Inhibitor. TFPI = Tissue Factor Pathway Inhibitor.

Fig. 3. The Cell-Based Model of Coagulation

- At 'initiation', TF binds to circulating FVIIa and acts with FV to generate FIXa and FXa. The FXa converts a small amount of FII to thrombin.
- During 'amplification' this thrombin triggers reactions on the surface of activated platelets, where more FVIIa is produced. Thrombin activates co-factors FV and FVIII. These active factors facilitate the sequence of thrombin-producing reactions.
- In 'propagation', the TF/FVIIa complex continues to activate FIX and the FIXa/FVIIIa ("tenase") complex generates more FXa to drive a continuous "thrombin burst".
- In 'stabilisation', FXIII is activated by high levels of thrombin and polymerises the fibrin monomers to complete the clot. Thrombin-activated Fibrinolysis Inhibitor contributes to clot stability.
- Pathological thrombosis is prevented by regulation of the coagulation process. 'Inhibition of further coagulation' occurs via activated protein C (aPC), protein S, tissue factor pathway inhibitor (TFPI) and antithrombin. Thrombin activates protein C, which cleaves FVa and FVIIIa with Protein S acting as a cofactor. TFPI binds TF/FVIIa and FXa in a quaternary complex. Antithrombin inhibits thrombin, FIXa and FXa. (8, 9)

7. Platelet function in haemostasis

Platelets respond to vascular wall damage by adhesion, aggregation, release of granule content and morphological changes. Von Willebrand Factor is a plasma protein that acts as a bridge between platelets and the exposed collagen of damaged tissue. The platelet binding site is the membrane glycoprotein GPIb-VIX. Von Willebrand Factor also acts as a carrier protein for, and stabiliser of FVIII, preventing premature proteolytic degradation by Protein C.

8. Coagulation pathology

Hypercoagulability / Thrombophilia

A hypercoagulable state can predispose a patient to deep vein thrombosis (DVT), pulmonary embolism (PE), stroke, and recurrent miscarriage. Causes include disorders of platelets, vessel walls, systemic disease and well as genetic and environmental factors (10).

Haemophiliae and other Bleeding Diatheses

Disorders of coagulation factors tend to present with haemarthroses and muscle haematomas. Patients with platelet disorders more commonly present with skin bruising, epistaxis or menorrhagia. Von Willebrand's Disease is the most common inherited coagulopathy; other forms are rare, apart from Haemophilia A and B. The most common acquired coagulation disorders are disseminated intravascular coagulation (DIC), liver disease and vitamin K deficiency although disorders discussed elsewhere in this chapter are more common in the setting of cardiac surgery.

9. Anticoagulant drugs

These drugs are used to prevent thrombus formation, or limit the extension of existing thrombus. Venous thrombus consists of a fibrin web with trapped platelets and erythrocytes and is more successfully treated or prevented with anticoagulants than arterial thrombus, which contains proportionally more platelets and less fibrin.

Source	Hypercoagulable risk factor (mechanism and notes in brackets)
Blood	Protein S and Protein C deficiencies (these normally regulate coagulation) Polycythaemia rubra vera, Thrombocytosis (blood is more viscous thus prone to stasis – treatment may include bone marrow suppression) Paroxysmal Nocturnal Haemoglobinuria (excessive RBC sensitivity to complement) Prothrombin 20210 mutation (leads to increased prothrombin levels) Heparin Induced Thrombocytopenia (heparin-associated antibodies develop) Antithrombin III deficiency (incidence 1 in 5000) Inherited dysfibrinogenaemia (rare) Leiden Factor V mutation - the most common hereditary cause of hypercoagulable state (anticoagulant effect of activated protein C is ineffective against mutated factor V) Thalassaemia Sickle Cell Disease
Systemic	Pregnancy / postpartum Iatrogenic Oestrogen (increases coagulation factors and reduces anticoagulant effect of antithrombin III) Sepsis (increased circulating tissue factor) Hyperhomocysteinaemia (genetic disorder, treated with folate, vitamin B_6 & vitamin B_{12}) Smoking (mechanisms include endothelial damage and platelet adhesion) Congestive Heart Failure (mechanisms include vascular endothelial dysfunction & increased fibrinogen) Antiphospholipid syndrome, including lupus anticoagulant (either primary or secondary to infection, drugs, malignancy) Uraemia (endothelial dysfunction, increased cytokines) Surgery (reduced risk with thromboprophylactic drugs perioperatively) Diabetes mellitus (increased platelet activation) Hyperlipidaemia Obesity Malignancy (tumour cells activate clotting cascade and inhibit fibrinolysis) Trauma/burns (release of tissue thromboplastin) Immobility (blood stasis) Hyperthyroidism (increase in circulating FX) Hypothyroidism (increased circulating fibrinogen, FVII)

Fig. 4. Causes of a Hypercoagulable State (11)

Inherited Bleeding Disorders	**Notes**
Von Willebrand Disease (vWD)	Autosomal dominant, affects 1% of population. Von Willebrand Factor (vWF) can be deficient, defective or completely absent. vWF allows platelets to adhere to damaged endothelium and also stabilises circulating FVIII. Severe vWD can therefore cause FVIII deficiency. Desmopressin raises vWF in mild disease, in more severe disease FVIII/vWF concentrate may be required.
Haemophilia A = FVIII deficiency	Inherited, X-linked recessive (affecting males). Severe coagulation disorder. FVIII concentrate is given prophylactically in profound deficiency, and as required in milder forms of the disease.
Haemophilia B = FIX deficiency	Severe coagulation disorder, also X-linked, clinically indistinguishable from Haemophilia A.
Thrombocytopenia	May be due to primary bone marrow dysfunction, autoimmune disease, or a consequence of other disease processes or drugs.
FXI deficiency	Patients exhibit a variable bleeding disorder
Factor V deficiency	
Structural problems with blood vessels	Disorders such as Haemorrhagic Telangiectasia and Ehlers-Danlos syndrome
Acquired Bleeding Disorders	**Notes**
DIC	Pathological activation of coagulation from triggers such as sepsis, malignancy, burns, or obstetric emergencies. Widespread microvascular thrombosis leads to consumption of clotting factors and platelets which is followed by bleeding. Increased Fibrin Degradation Products (FDPs) may also impair coagulation. High mortality, primarily from complications of microvascular thrombosis. Fresh frozen plasma and platelets are given whilst underlying trigger is addressed.
Liver Disease	Synthesis of coagulation factors is affected. Portal hypertension can also lead to splenomegaly with sequestration of platelets and resultant thrombocytopenia
Vitamin K Deficiency	Can occur with malabsorption of this fat-soluble vitamin in obstructive jaundice. Deficiency of FII, FVII, FIX, FX occurs
Thrombocytopenia	May be due to primary bone marrow dysfunction, autoimmune disease, or a consequence of other disease processes or drugs.
Platelet dysfunction	Disorders of platelet granules can occur in myelodysplastic disease, haematological malignancy, uraemia or liver disease. Antiplatelet drugs are also discussed in this chapter.
HELLP syndrome	A severe variant of preeclampsia characterised by **H**aemolysis, **E**levated **L**iver enzymes, and **L**ow **P**latelets
Allergic purpura	Inflammation of small blood vessels with leakage

10. Thrombin inhibitors

Thrombin (FIIa) is central to the coagulation process. It usually converts soluble fibrinogen to fibrin, stimulates platelets and activates FV, FVIII, FXI and FXIII. Thrombin inhibitors can work directly on FIIa, or indirectly by preventing activation of FII.

Heparin is long-established as an anticoagulant, which facilitates endogenous antithrombin to decrease activation of FII. The indirect mechanism has limited activity against thrombin that is bound to fibrin or fibrin degradation products (FDPs). In contrast, direct-acting thrombin inhibitors (DTIs) inhibit bound, as well as free, FIIa.

Heparin remains the most widely used drug in this class, but other agents are being investigated that may offer increased efficacy or a more favourable side-effect profile. Thrombin inhibitors may also have administrative advantages over heparin if they can be given orally and if anticoagulation monitoring is unnecessary.

Indirect thrombin inhibitors

Heparin

Heparin is found in the liver and mast cell granules. Commercial heparin is extracted from bovine or porcine sources and is a mixture of acid mucopolysaccharides with molecular weights ranging from 3000 to 60,000 daltons. It is available in this unfractionated form and also as various low-molecular weight preparations. Heparin reversibly binds to antithrombin III, thereby enhancing inhibition of FIX, FX, FXI, FXII, FXIII, thrombin and also plasmin. At high concentrations heparin also inhibits platelet aggregation.

Unfractionated heparin is given intravenously or subcutaneously and is also used to anticoagulate the cardiopulmonary bypass circuit in cardiac surgery. Intravenous doses are titrated to a target range of ACT or APTT. The biological half-life is 1hr at physiological temperature but longer at lower temperatures during cardiopulmonary bypass. Heparin effects are reversed by protamine, a base that forms a stable, inactive salt complex with the acidic heparin.

Low-molecular weight heparin preparations have an average molecular weight below 8000 daltons. They are more effective at inhibiting factor Xa than unfractionated heparin, with less of an effect on thrombin. Their longer half-life and more predictable pharmacokinetic profile make them suitable for once-daily subcutaneous dosing without routine coagulation monitoring. APTT is not altered by LMWH so if monitoring is needed, anti-Xa levels are measured; this is useful for patients with renal impairment or at extremes of weight. LMWH effects cannot be reversed with protamine.

Side-effects of heparin can include hyperkalaemia and Heparin-induced Thrombocytopaenia (HIT). HIT has a frequency of 2.6% when unfractionated heparin is used, and 0.2% with LMWH (12). The most severe form of HIT is immune-mediated and can be complicated by thrombosis. Platelet counts should therefore be monitored in patients receiving heparin. If HIT occurs, heparin should be discontinued and an alternative anticoagulant used to reduce the risk of thrombosis. Warfarin should not be given to patients with HIT because of the high risk of warfarin necrosis, so alternatives such as lepirudin or danaparoid are chosen. A screening test for antibodies is the initial investigation when HIT is suspected. Patients testing positive proceed to the more specific serotonin release assay.

For post-CPB reversal of heparin, protamine sulphate is used. 1 mg of protamine neutralises the effect of 100 i.u of unfractionated heparin, by combining with heparin to form an

inactive salt compound. Protamine acts within 5 minutes and can last for 2 hours. Effective protamine reversal is confirmed when the ACT returns to the baseline value.
Excess administration of protamine is undesirable, as it has its own intrinsic anticoagulant effect at high doses. It should be given slowly to minimise cardiovascular side-effects (systemic arterial vasodilatation and pulmonary arterial vasoconstriction), and the maximum administration rate in adults is 50mg per 10 minute period.
Protamine can only partially reverse the anticoagulant effect of LMWH.

Other indirect thrombin inhibitors

Warfarin reduces hepatic synthesis of FII. Factor Xa inhibitors will reduce activation of FII. These agents are considered by some sources to be indirect thrombin inhibitors and are covered elsewhere in this chapter.

Direct thrombin inhibitors

This class includes Dabigatran, Argatroban, Bivalirudin, the recombinant Hirudins (eg lepirudin and desirudin) and also Melagatran and its prodrug Ximelagatran.
Dabigatran is a direct thrombin inhibitor, taken orally, which is being increasingly used in prevention of thromboembolism following lower limb joint replacement surgery. Dabigatran is also gaining a role in prevention of embolic stroke in patients with atrial fibrillation. The predictable pharmacokinetic profile allows a fixed-dose regimen to be used without routine coagulation monitoring. Dabigatran cannot be reversed. It should be discontinued at least 24hrs before elective surgery. In the event of life-threatening haemorrhage, non-specific prohaemostatic agents such as recombinant factor VIIa and prothrombin concentrate complexes could be considered; accelerated clearance using haemofiltration or charcoal filtration has also been suggested (13).
Argatroban is given intravenously and has a role in prevention/treatment of thrombosis and during Percutaneous Coronoary Interventions (PCI) in patients with HIT. It is metabolised hepatically so may be more appropriate than Lepirudin for patients with renal impairment. Its effect can be monitored by APTT.
Hirudins are direct thrombin (FIIa) inhibitors derived from chemicals found in leech saliva. Lepirudin and Desirudin are recombinant agents. Lepirudin is used to anticoagulate patients with HIT. It is given intravenously, titrated according to APTT(14), and cleared renally. Desirudin can be given subcutaneously to prevent thromboembolism.
Bivalirudin is a hirudin analogue, and can be used in combination with antiplatelet agents for patients undergoing percutaneous coronary intervention (PCI). It can be titrated according to ACT(14). Thrombin function recovers to normal approximately 1hr after Bivalirudin infusion is discontinued.
Melagatran and its prodrug **Ximelagatran** were withdrawn from the market after the EXTEND trial found potential risk of severe liver injury (15).

11. Factor Xa inhibitors

The synthetic pentasaccharide Fondaparinux is an indirect FXa inhibitor, with structural similarities to heparin. It works by facilitating antithrombin III (AT) activity, and is therefore dependent on AT for its effect (16). Fondaparinux is given subcutaneously for prevention/treatment of venous thromboembolism, and for acute coronary syndrome. In patients with normal renal function, anticoagulation effects persist for 2-4 days after discontinuation of Fondaparinux. There is no antidote available to reverse the effect of

Fondaparinux. It does not affect PT, APTT or ACT. Although monitoring is not routinely required in healthy patients, it can be achieved by an anti-FXa assay.
Newer orally-administered drugs Rivaroxiban and Apixaban are direct FXa inhibitors. They have similar indications to Fondaparinux.

Heparinoids

Danaparoid is produced from the same porcine material as heparin, but all heparin and heparin fragments are extracted. It catalyses AT-mediated inhibition of FXa and, to a lesser extent, FIIa (17). It has been used to anticoagulate patients with HIT. There can be cross-reactivity so patients should continue to have platelet count monitored (18). Coagulation monitoring, if required, is by anti-Xa assay. It is not reversed by protamine.

Warfarin

This oral agent is used to minimise the risk of embolic stroke in patients with valvular heart disease or arrhythmia, and to prevent/treat venous thromboembolism. It inhibits the hepatic synthesis of vitamin K-dependent coagulation factors (FII, FVII, FIX, FX) as well as proteins C, S and Z (19). It takes at least 48hrs to develop the anticoagulant effect, during which time the inhibition of proteins C and S may paradoxically create a prothrombotic state, hence heparin is usually added during warfarin introduction. Warfarin effect is titrated using PT or INR tests with target ranges shown in the table. Additional or alternative agents may be recommended in valvular or structural heart disease (20).
Perioperatively, warfarin is only continued for certain procedures with low risk of bleeding. Warfarin is usually held 5 days prior to surgery with INR ≤1.5 confirmed immediately pre-op. A shorter-acting anticoagulant, such as LMWH, can be given as bridging anticoagulant therapy until shortly before surgery and continued once haemostasis has been obtained. The decreased risk of thrombosis or embolism by using bridging anticoagulation is weighed against the increased risk of haemorrhage. Decisions regarding perioperative anticoagulation are made on an individual patient basis (22).

Warfarin Indication	Target INR (+/- 0.5)
Atrial fibrillation, DVT, PE	2.5
Recurrent DVT/PE despite INR >2	3.5
For Cardioversion in Atrial Fibrillation	3.0 for ≥ 3 weeks prior, and 2.5 for ≥ 4 weeks post-Cardioversion
Mechanical Prosthetic Heart Valves: Individualised targets based on: (a) thrombogenic risk of the valve type and position, (b) patient-related risk factors for thrombosis and haemorrhage (20, 21).	Typically 3 for aortic valves, 3.5 for mitral valves.
Bioprosthetic Valves	2.5 for 3 months post-insertion, after which consider discontinuation if no other risk factors

INR = International Normalised Ratio, DVT = Deep Venous Thrombosis, PE = Pulmonary Embolism (22)

Fig. 5. INR targets.

In the event of major haemorrhage in a patient who is anticoagulated with warfarin, it may be necessary to discontinue warfarin, administer vitamin K 5-10mg (phytomenadione), and in some cases replace the deficient coagulation factors using prothrombin complex concentrate 30-50 units/kg (containing FII, FVII, FIX, FX) or fresh frozen plasma 10-15ml/kg.

Antiplatelet agents

These agents have a variety of mechanisms of action as shown in the table. Decisions regarding perioperative discontinuation of these medications are made on an individual patient basis. As with other anticoagulants, continuation increases perioperative bleeding but withholding the agent increases risk of thrombosis. The risk of withholding antiplatelet agents in the setting of acute coronary syndrome generally outweighs the benefits so they are usually continued in this context (23).

Prostacyclins

Epoprostenol is a prostacyclin that can be infused to treat pulmonary hypertension, or to inhibit platelet aggregation during renal dialysis.

Antifibrinolytic Agents

Aprotinin, tranexamic acid and aminocaproic acid are antifibrinolytic agents, which can be used to decrease peri-operative bleeding. Aprotinin is a naturally-occurring serine protease inhibitor, and the other two agents are lysine analogues. Studies have shown reduction in blood loss and transfusion requirements with the use of these agents, particularly in patients taking antiplatelet agents perioperatively (25, 26).

Aprotinin was associated with increased incidence of death, cerebrovascular accidents and renal events in an observational study of patients undergoing revascularisation surgery (27). These effects were not seen with tranexamic acid or ε aminocaproic acid. Indeed a prior meta-analysis of aprotinin use in patients undergoing cardiopulmonary bypass suggested it was safe (28). The current recommendation is to reserve aprotinin use for patients at the highest risk of bleeding complications (29).

12. Laboratory coagulation tests

Platelet count

The normal range is 150-400 $x10^9$ / L. Thrombocytopenia can occur as a result of decreased bone marrow production or excessive destruction. Typically, traumatic bleeding, purpura and easy bruising occur at platelet counts less than 50 $x10^9$/L; spontaneous bleeding may occur at platelet counts below $20x10^9$/L. There is not a strong evidence base for a transfusion trigger in thrombocytopaenia (30), however the consensus is that a platelet count of >50 $x10^9$ should be achieved prior to invasive procedures (31) with a higher target of >100 $x10^9$ prior to neurosurgery.

Platelet function

Platelet function can be impaired by low pH, hypothermia, myeloproliferative disease, uraemia, non-steroidal anti-inflammatory drugs and antiplatelet drugs. As well as having a sufficient number of platelets, adequate platelet function is also necessary for haemostasis. Platelet function is not measured in standard laboratory tests, but it is possible to measure platelet activity using methods such as aggregometry. Platelet function can be inferred from

Antiplatelet Drug Name	Mechanism of Action	Implications for Cardiac Surgery
Aspirin = Acetylsalicylic acid	Prevents Thromboxane A2 production (by irreversibly acetylating cyclooxygenase-1) therefore reducing platelet aggregation	Antithrombotic effect starts within 30min of oral loading dose and lasts for lifespan of the platelet (8–10 days). Is often continued perioperatively with some degree of platelet dysfunction expected.
Thienopyridine derivatives: Clopidogrel, Ticlopidine, Prasugrel	Their metabolites covalently bind to the P2Y12 receptor, the main platelet receptor responsible for ADP-induced platelet aggregation.	Active within 2hrs of oral loading dose. Lower risk of GI-bleeding than aspirin. Expect platelet dysfunction if not discontinued at least 7 days pre-operatively (23).
Direct-acting P2Y12 inhibitors: Cangrelor, Ticagrelor, Elinogrel	These agents change P2Y12 receptor conformation, causing a reversible, concentration-dependent receptor inhibition.	These are in phase 3 of development(24)
Dipyridamole	Inhibits phosphodiesterase, therefore increasing intraplatelet concentrations of cyclic AMP which reduces the activation of cytoplasmic second messengers. Also stimulates prostacyclin release and inhibits thromboxane 2A production	Short half-life so usually given as a slow-release preparation.
Glycoprotein IIb/IIIa receptor antagonists: Abciximab, Tirofiban, Eptifibatide	Compete with ligand binding of fibrinogen to glycoprotein IIb/IIIa receptor, therefore block the final common pathway for platelet aggregation. Given intravenously as loading bolus followed by infusion.	Platelet function can take 2 days to recover following discontinuation of Abciximab infusion. Strategies to reduce blood loss may include: 1) Delaying surgery for 12hrs post-abciximab, and 2hrs post-tirofiban or eptifibatide. 2) Platelet transfusion (less effective if given when free drug still in circulation) 3) Fibrinogen or antifibrinolytics may be of benefit

Fig. 6. Antiplatelet Agents, their mechanisms of action and implications for Cardiac Surgery

thromboelastography (see later section). Bearing in mind the lack of routine platelet function measurement prior to cardiac surgery, it is important to identify clinical clues to impaired platelet activity. A patient's medication history should be noted. Some patients are advised to stop antiplatelet agents in advance of elective surgery. In those taking clopidogrel up to the day of surgery, platelet dysfunction should be anticipated as should the need for platelet transfusion.

Prothrombin time (PT) and international normalized ratio (INR)

Blood is sampled into a tube containing EDTA or citrate, both of which chelate calcium and prevent the blood clotting en route to the laboratory. The sample is centrifuged in the lab to yield platelet-poor plasma. The test starts when calcium and thromboplastin (consisting of tissue factor and phospholipid) are added to the plasma, and is complete when fibrin strands are formed. The time taken is the PT. The INR puts the measured PT in context by comparing it with the PT of a standardised plasma sample. An INR of 1.0 is normal; higher INRs represent coagulation that is impaired secondary to pathology or drugs. PT and INR are considered to be tests of the extrinsic pathway, with FVII deficiency having the greatest impact on raising the INR/PT. Other causes of abnormal PT and INR are shown in the table. Of note, the large amount of TF used to trigger coagulation in this test negates the effect of TFPI and renders the test independent of FVIII, FIX and FXI, meaning patients with haemophilia can have normal PT and INR results.

Activated partial thromboplastin time (APTT) and aptt ratio (APTTR)

The blood sample for this test is prepared in the same way as that for the PT. The resultant platelet-poor plasma is triggered to coagulate by mixing it with the APTT reagent and replacing the chelated calcium. The APTT reagent consists of phospholipid (as a substitute for the platelet membrane) and negatively-charged particles that cause contact activation. The time taken for fibrin strands to form is the APTT. The APTT ratio is calculated in a similar manner to the INR, with normal APTTR being 1.0 and higher values representing coagulopathy. APTT is prolonged by deficiencies of the Intrinsic or Common pathways, meaning any procoagulant factor deficiency apart from FVII and FXIII will prolong the

Causes of Prolonged PT and INR	Notes
Decreased FVII	FVII deficiency has a greater impact on PT and INR than other factor deficiencies
Decreased FI, FII, FV, FX	
Liver disease	Decreased factor (including fibrinogen) synthesis
Vitamin K deficiency	Synthesis of FII, FVII, FIX, FX are vitamin K-dependent
Disseminated Intravascular Coagulation (DIC)	Widespread factor depletion due to consumption
High dose heparin	
Sample tube under-filled	Dilution artefact due to standard volume of citrate (or EDTA) mixing with lower volume of plasma
Raised Haematocrit	Thus lower percentage volume of plasma, also leads to dilution artefact

Fig. 7. Causes of Prolonged PT and INR

APTT. APTT is used to titrate unfractionated heparin anticoagulation. It is also a screening tool for Haemophilia A and B. Prolonged APTT does not necessarily predict clinical bleeding, for example FXII deficiency greatly prolongs APTT but is not associated with bleeding tendency.

Causes of Prolonged APTT and APTTR	Notes
Procoagulant factor deficiency (except FVII or FXIII)	FVII is not involved in the intrinsic pathway. Completion of the test does not require FXIII-dependent cross-linking of fibrin.
Specific Clotting Factor Inhibitors	eg. Factor VIII inhibitors develop in up to 10% of patients with haemophilia A
Contamination of sample with heparin	Sample drawn from vein upstream of heparin infusion, or contaminated by heparin in the pressure-bag of an arterial line
Lupus Anticoagulant	This is a non-specific inhibitor of the intrinsic pathway so prolongs APTT. Paradoxically, patients with lupus anticoagulant actually have a prothrombotic tendency.
Dilution artefact	Underfilling of the sample tube, or raised haematocrit will increase the proportion of citrate (or EDTA) to plasma

Thrombin clotting time (TT or TCT) and hemoclot®

TT measures the time taken for fibrin to form when thrombin is added to the plasma sample. Prolongation of TT suggests low fibrinogen levels, dysfibrinogenaemia or inhibition of thrombin. Thrombin can be inhibited by unfractionated heparin or direct thrombin inhibitors. Fibrin degradation products inhibit fibrin cross-linking; at high concentrations these can also prolong the TT.

Adding Protamine sulphate to the sample will negate the effect of heparin and FDPs. Adding Toluidine Blue will negate the effect of heparin but not FDPs. Another technique for samples containing heparin is to perform a "Reptilase Test", where a snake venon product 'Reptilase' is used to activate fibrinogen. Unlike thrombin, reptilase is not inhibited by heparin.

Hemoclot® is a sensitive, diluted TT assay.

These tests are used to assess the effectiveness of fibrinolytic therapy and may be useful in quantifying the effects of direct thrombin inhibitor drugs.

Ecarin clotting time (ECT)

This is a specific assay of thrombin generation. Ecarin comes from snake venom, and specifically activates prothrombin (FII). ECT can be used to monitor anticoagulation during Cardiopulmonary Bypass but is not widely utilised outside a research setting (13)

Fibrinogen

Fibrinogen (FI), the precursor of fibrin, is synthesised by hepatocytes and normal plasma concentration is 1.5-4.0g/L. Levels vary seasonally within an individual, and causes of abnormal fibrinogen level or function are shown in the tables below. Fibrinogen can be depleted by haemorrhage and consumed by coagulation during or after cardiac surgery, and is routinely quantified by the Clauss method in this setting. The PT-derived fibrinogen level (PT-Fg) is more convenient but less reliable. When investigating congenital fibrinogen defects, more complex and time-consuming tests are employed.

There is evidence that the low preoperative fibrinogen concentrations correlate with higher peri-operative blood loss in coronary artery bypass surgery (32, 33). Pre-operative prophylactic fibrinogen infusion may be beneficial, although larger trials are required to determine safety and efficacy of this practice (34). Pre-operative hyperfibrinogenaemia is associated with higher all-cause mortality (35), possibly because raised fibrinogen levels are a marker of inflammation, reflecting the presence of a systemic disorder (eg sepsis, acute coronary syndrome).

In major blood loss treated with packed red blood cells and crystalloid/colloid intravascular volume resuscitation, fibrinogen is the first coagulation factor to become depleted (36). It is therefore a useful marker for severity of haemorrhage (37).

Fibrinogen quality is assessed when thromboelastometry is performed in the presence of a platelet inhibitor, a test available commercially as "FIBTEM" (see ROTEM section).

A prolonged Thrombin Time will also detect low fibrinogen levels.

Options for replacing fibrinogen are fibrinogen concentrate reconstituted to 20g/L, Fresh Frozen Plasma containing 1.6-2g/L fibrinogen, or cryoprecipitate containing 17g/L. The traditional target of replacement of fibrinogen aimed for a level of 1g/L, but higher targets of 1.5-2g/L may be more appropriate in patients undergoing cardiac surgery (38).

It remains to be established whether it is better to administer fibrinogen concentrate prophylactically, or to reserve treatment only for patients who are bleeding. There is also debate regarding the most suitable goal for fibrinogen replacement, which may be fibrinogen quantity (eg Clauss assay) or fibrin quality (eg. FIBTEM).

The Clauss assay

A high concentration of thrombin is added to diluted plasma and the clotting time is measured. A reference curve has been plotted using plasma of known fibrinogen concentrations. The fibrinogen concentration of the test sample is determined by comparing the clotting time with the reference curve. The clotting time can be determined automatically using systems that detect changes in light scattering, or light absorption as fibrin is formed. Artefacts can occur when turbid or lipaemic plasma causes abnormal light scattering, and when free haemoglobin or bile cause abnormal light absorption. Heparin will affect clot formation, making the Clauss assay inaccurate, so every effort should be made to obtain a heparin-free sample (avoid sampling within 4 hours of low-molecular weight heparin administration, caution when sampling from arterial lines flushed with heparin). If a heparin-free sample cannot be obtained (eg during Cardiopulmonary Bypass) then ion-exchange resins or heparinase can be used to negate the heparin effect. Fibrin Degradation Products (FDPs) affect fibrinogen activity in vivo, and also affect the time taken to complete the Clauss assay, so this assay naturally reflects the any potential impact of FDPs.

PT-derived fibrinogen assays (PT-Fg)

This method indirectly measures fibrinogen by analysing the change in light scattering or optical density as fibrin is formed in the sample during the PT test. The advantage of this method is that it can give a measurement of fibrinogen any time the PT is tested without additional expense. The test may be inaccurate in samples with high fibrinogen and, of particular relevance to Cardiac Surgery, the test may be less reliable than Clauss in the investigation of bleeding diathesis. FDPs have less effect on the PT-Fg than on the Clauss

Causes of Elevated Plasma Fibrinogen Concentration	Notes
Increased age	
Female Sex	
Pregnancy and Oral Contraception	
Acute phase reaction	
Smoking	
Acute exercise	
Disseminated malignancy	
Seasonal change	Higher fibrinogen levels in winter
Genetic Polymorphism of the beta fibrinogen gene promoter (G-455A)	Occurs in 20% of population, leads to 7-10% higher fibrinogen levels than GG genotype (39)

Causes of Decreased Plasma Fibrinogen Concentration	Notes
Inherited Fibrinogen Defects (rare):	
Congenital Afibrinogenaemia	Grossly decreased fibrinogen synthesis, with low or undetectable plasma fibrinogen. Patients have haemorrhagic diathesis, prolonged clotting times and abnormal platelet function
Congenital Hypofibrinogenaemia	Mild-to-moderate reduction in circulating fibrinogen levels. Potential for haemorrhagic problems, but patient may be asymptomatic.
Congenital Dysfibrinogenaemia	Immunoassays may detect fibrinogen, but tests that depend on production of fibrin strands will give lower fibrinogen results. Patients may have haemorrhagic tendency, thrombophilia or be asymptomatic
Acquired hypofibrinogenaemia	
Decompensated liver disease	Hepatocellular failure leads to decreased fibrinogen synthesis. Excessive glycosylation of fibrinogen leads to an acquired dysfibrinogenaemia. Excess Fibrin Degradation Products (FDPs) also disrupt fibrinogen function.
Viral Hepatitis	
Disseminated Intravascular Coagulation (DIC)	Generalised fibrin formation throughout the microcirculation leads to consumption and depletion of fibrinogen. FDP concentration is also raised.
Haemodilution	From massive blood transfusion or fluid administration
Systemic Thrombolytic Therapy	Usually leads to gross reduction in fibrinogen levels and high risk of haemorrhage

assay; an adequate fibrinogen measurement using PT-Fg may not reflect adequate fibrinogen activity if there is a significant quantity of FDPs in circulation.

Clottable protein

This test is too time-consuming and labour-intensive to be used routinely, but does give very accurate results and can be used for reference assays.

Testing for specific coagulation factor abnormalities

Clinical or laboratory evidence of abnormal coagulation that is not explained by haemorrhage, known pathology, or iatrogenic causes may require investigation of specific factor abnormalities. Uncommonly, individuals may have a factor deficiency or a factor inhibitor (the most common example is lupus anticoagulant). Consultation with a haematologist followed by specialised laboratory tests may be indicated.

Other measurements in coagulopathy

For effective coagulation, supportive management to maintain homeostasis is required. Temperature <34°C, pH <7.1, ionised Calcium <0.9mmol/L and Haematocrit <30% have all been shown to adversely affect haemostasis (40).

In coagulopathy, hypocalcaemia should be corrected because of calcium's key role in the activation of FX, FII, FXIII and Fibrinogen. Both haemodilution and chelation of serum calcium by citrate in units of packed red blood cells can contribute to hypocalcaemia in massive transfusion. A value for ionised Calcium can be rapidly obtained from many blood gas analysis machines, and the reference range is 1.0 - 1.3 mmol/L (no correction calculation required). Total Calcium ranges from 2.1 - 2.7mmol/L (corrected for hypoalbuminaemia may be necessary).

Prevention of heat loss and active warming may be required to raise core temperature, acidotic patients may benefit from buffering, and haematocrit should be maintained with transfusion to optimise coagulation.

When transfusing Packed Red Cells it is preferable to use blood that has been stored for the minimum possible duration, ideally less than two weeks. Transfusion of older blood has been associated with greater incidence of complications and higher mortality (41).

13. Near patient coagulation tests

ACT and TEG are the two most common Near Patient Tests (NPT) used in cardiac surgery. The main value of NPT is the short turn-around time, which gives feedback to the treating physician/surgeon without delay. An ACT reading can be obtained generally within 4 minutes of test initialisation, and a TEG within 10 to 15 minutes. A conventional coagulation screen generally has a turn-around time of 30 minutes, during which time one or more interventions may already have taken place, making the result less valuable and potentially obsolete.

ACT (Activated Clotting Time)

This is generally performed at the bedside or in the operating room by a perfusionist or doctor who is actively managing the patient. A pre-heparin baseline value is obtained to assist interpretation of subsequent results. Anticoagulation whilst on cardiopulmonary bypass (CPB) is usually guided by ACT, and the test is also used to assess success of protamine reversal of heparin when CPB is over. After Protamine, an ACT that is prolonged beyond the baseline value suggests heparin reversal may be incomplete, but it offers no information regarding other potential causes of coagulopathy.

14. Thromboelastography

Thromboelastography was first described in 1948. Viscoelastic changes during coagulation are plotted against time(42). The abbreviation 'TEG' was used for this technique. TEG® is now a trademark for one manufacturer of thromboelastograph device, an alternative manufacturer uses the trademark ROTEM®. The principles are similar, described below.

15. The principles of the thromboelastography (TEG)

Samples for analysis are stored in a citrated tube and must be analysed within 4 hours. Kaolin (a clotting factor) is added to two separate cuvettes both containing sufficient calcium chloride to reverse the effect of the citrate. One of the cuvettes also contains a surface coating of heparinase to deactivate any heparin in the sample. Both cuvettes are loaded onto the analyser for simultaneous analysis.
Each cuvette sits on a platform that oscillates through an angle of 4°45′. The whole cycle lasts ten seconds including a 1 second rest period. A pin is freely suspended within the blood and is attached to a torsion wire which in turn is attached to a mechanical-electrical transducer. As the blood starts to clot within the cuvette, fibrin strands form between the blood and the pin and the torque is transmitted via the transducer to give a signal that is recorded by a computer (See figure 8).
The variables that are recorded are as follows: "r" (reaction time) is the period of time, in minutes, taken to form the initial fibrin strands after placement of blood in the TEG analyser.

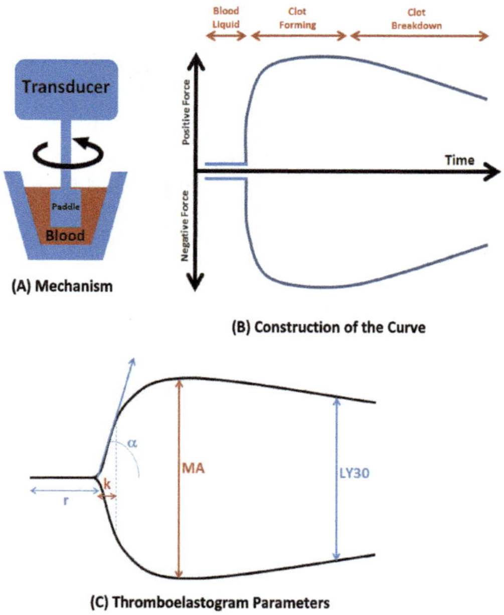

Fig. 8. This image represents the TEG diagrammatically. (A) Shows a cross-sectional view of the apparatus. (B) Demonstrates the construction of the curve. (C) Shows the final printout of the TEG

Before this happens, the liquid blood in the cuvette exerts very little torque on the pin and the signal remains effectively zero (see figure 8). It is prolonged by congenital or acquired deficiencies in hepatic coagulation factors and anticoagulants such as unfractionated heparin, the low molecular weight heparins and warfarin. The "K" (K time) is the time, in minutes, after clot formation begins and the clot itself is of sufficient strength to produce a 20mm divergence of the line. This reflects the speed of clot strengthening. The "K" is reduced by an elevated fibrinogen and by effective platelet function and is prolonged by the same factors that prolong the "r". The "α" (alpha angle), measured in degrees, is the slope of the TEG tracing with respect to the r line (the line drawn between r_1 and r_2). It reflects the speed at which the clot is formed and behaves very much like the "K". If the "K" is undefined (i.e. the signal generated by the computer never reaches an amplitude of 20mm) such as in hypocoaguable states then the "α" becomes more important. The "MA" (maximum amplitude) is a measure of the maximum strength developed by the clot. It is dependent on fibrin formation and platelet function. Percentage clot lysis is estimated at 30 (LY30) minutes or 60 (LY60) minutes after the "MA" is reached. The percentages are calculated by using the following formula: $LY30 = (MA - A_{30})/MA \times 100$ and $LY60 = (MA - A_{60})/MA \times 100$, where A_{30} is the amplitude of the trace 30 minutes after "MA" is reached and A_{60} the corresponding value after 60 minutes. If the LY30 or LY60 are high then fibrinolysis is high. Finally, "C.I." (coagulation index) can also be derived from "r", "K", "α" and "MA"by substitution into the following equation: $C.I. = 0.3258r - 0.1886K + 0.1224MA + 0.0759\alpha - 7.7922$. This equation has been derived after multiple regression of a large database of TEG tracings. The "C.I." reflects the patient's overall coagulation state and normal values range from – 3.0 to + 3.0 (43).

Platelet mapping with TEG

Platelet mapping studies measure the degree to which a patient's platelets can be activated by stimulation of either the thromboxane A2 (Txa2) receptor or the adenosine diphosphate (ADP) receptor. These receptors can be inhibited by aspirin and clopidogrel respectively, but the degree of inhibition varies between individuals. Thrombin activates platelets independent of the arachidonic acid and ADP receptors via the glycoprotein IIb/IIIa receptor.

In cardiac surgery, antiplatelet agents are often withheld to minimise bleeding complications, which can expose patients to increased risks of peri-operative myocardial ischaemia. Platelet mapping may have a role in determining the optimum time to operate, such that antiplatelet agents are withheld for long enough to decrease the bleeding risk, but no longer than necessary. In the medical management of coronary artery disease, this technique could potentially be used before antiplatelet therapy is commenced, to determine which antiplatelet agent is likely to be effective for an individual patient. It might also be used after antiplatelet therapy has been initiated to measure the response to therapy.

Platelet mapping can be assessed by the following method: 4 TEG channels (cups) are required. Cup 1 contains blood and kaolin (this activates the clotting cascade ex vivo) and the MA reflects thrombin activated platelets ($MA_{thrombin}$). Thrombin in the blood sample is produced by trauma during the blood sampling procedure. Since the direct effect of thrombin on the IIb/IIIa receptor is not dependent on stimulation of either the Txa2 or ADP receptors, $MA_{thrombin}$ is an indirect measure of platelet function even in the presence of aspirin or clopidogrel. In all other 3 cups heparin is added to inhibit thrombin thus eliminating its direct action on the IIb/IIIa receptor. To the second cup 10μL reptilase and activated factor XIII (Activator F) is added which convert fibrinogen to fibrin by generating a cross-linked fibrin clot thus isolating the contribution of fibrin to the clot strength.

Activator F has no effect on platelets so the "MA" reflects the action of fibrin only (MA_{fibrin}) (44). To the third cup 10µL Activator F and 10µL arachidonic acid (AA) are added and the MA_{AA} reflects platelet responsiveness to AA. To the fourth cup 10µL Activator F and 10µL ADP are added and the MA_{ADP} reflects platelet responsiveness to ADP. The relative response of platelets to either AA or ADP is calculated as follows with a normal reference value for each being above 80%:

$$\text{Relative response of platelets to AA} = (MA_{AA} - MA_{fibrin}) / (MA_{thrombin} - MA_{fibrin}) \times 100.$$

$$\text{Relative response of platelets to ADP} = (MA_{ADP} - MA_{fibrin}) / (MA_{thrombin} - MA_{fibrin}) \times 100.$$

The platelet inhibition in response to an agonist is calculated by subtracting the percentage aggregation from 100 (45).

Rotational Thromboelastometry (ROTEM®)

ROTEM is based on the same principles as thromboelastography. Citrated whole blood is mixed with reagents in a stationary cuvette, then a pin is placed vertically into the blood and alternating clockwise and anticlockwise forces are applied to the pin. As the blood clots the pin's oscillation is impeded, and when fibrinolysis occurs the pin will move more freely.
The device records the changes in oscillation against time, creating the 'thromboelastogram' (TEM). The zero line indicates free movement of the pin. An amplitude of 100mm would indicate no movement of the pin, meaning the clot has reached the maximum possible firmness measurable by ROTEM. Combinations of reagents can be used to produce a series of TEMs that measure different aspects of the coagulation and fibrinolysis processes.
The ROTEM machine has four channels, thus four TEMs can be generated simultaneously. By using combinations of coagulation triggers and coagulation inhibitors, a clearer understanding of the coagulation abnormalities can be obtained. The reference ranges for the parameters are not interchangeable between the different types of TEM, for example the MCF seen in the FIBTEM test will be significantly lower than that in INTEM or EXTEM, because clot firmness is due to the effect of fibrin only.

Parameters measured using the ROTEM are as follows:

ROTEM Parameter [Measured Variable]	Significance	Clinical Application
Clotting time (CT) [Delay from the start of the reaction to the start of clot formation. An amplitude of 2mm is taken to signify the start of clot formation.]	This represents: - the initiation of clotting - thrombin formation - the start of clot polymerisation Although not linearly related, CT is related to the PT for EXTEM, and the APTT for INTEM. Abnormalities that prolong the laboratory tests will prolong the CT in the comparable ROTEM test, but the endpoint for the laboratory test is fibrin formation, whereas in ROTEM a degree of fibrin stabilisation is required to attain 2mm amplitude.	Prolonged CT suggests anticoagulant drug activity or coagulation factor abnormalities. Consider: - Anticoagulant inhibitors such as protamine. - Replacement of coagulation factors (eg. specific factor concentrates, or fresh frozen plasma)

ROTEM Parameter [Measured Variable]	Significance	Clinical Application
Clot Formation Time (CFT) [Delay from start of the reaction (2mm) to formation of a 20mm clot.]	CFT represents fibrin polymerisation, and stabilisation of the clot by activated platelets and FXIII. Prolonged CFT signifies a hypocoagulable state, and a short CFT corresponds with a hypercoagulable state.	Prolonged CFT may represent: - deficiency of platelet quantity or function - low fibrinogen level - deficiency of fibrin polymerisation Consider: - fibrinogen replacement (fibrinogen concentrate, cryoprecipitate, fresh frozen plasma) - platelet transfusion
Alpha(α)-angle [Angle formed between the x axis and a line that forms a tangent with the temogram curve and crosses the x axis at the point where clotting starts (2mm)]	This describes the kinetics of clotting. A reduced α-angle will correspond with a prolonged CFT. Increased α-angle will be seen in a hypercoagulable state.	Reduced angle indicates a hypocoagulable state, consider the same causes and management as described for CFT.
A (x) values [This is the amplitude at time x after the clot has started to form. (eg the A10 value is the amplitude at 10 minutes after CT)]	Low values are caused by the same abnormalities that prolong CFT and decrease the α-angle (platelets, fibrinogen, FXIII)	Reduced A (x) Values indicate a hypocoagulable state, consider the same causes and management as described for CFT.
Maximum Clot Firmness (MCF) [The peak amplitude of the Temogram]	Low MCF indicates a soft clot with potential for haemorrhage. Inadequate clot quality can reflect an abnormality of platelets, fibrinogen or FXIII. It can also be caused by hyperfibrinolysis. High MCF suggests a hypercoagulable state.	With low MCF: - exclude hyperfibrinolysis - consider supplementing fibrinogen and/or platelets
Lysis Index at 30 minutes (LI30) [The amplitude 30 minutes after CT, given as a percentage of MCF (the % remaining clot firmness) (LI45 and LI60 can be used to quantify late fibrinolysis)]	In health, the high concentration of fibrinolysis inhibitors means there is negligible fibrinolysis and LI30 should be close to 100%	An abnormally low LI30 usually indicates hyperfibrinolysis, so antifibrinolytic drugs should be considered.

ROTEM Parameter [Measured Variable]	Significance	Clinical Application
Maximum Lysis (ML) [The decrease in amplitude (relative to the peak at MCF) that has occurred by the end of the measurement period given as a percentage of MCF. This is the % clot firmness lost.]	This value represents the inverse of LI (% remaining clot firmness + % clot firmness lost = 100%) This value will increase if an extended measurement period is used.	An abnormally high ML usually indicates hyperfibrinolysis, so antifibrinolytic drugs should be considered.

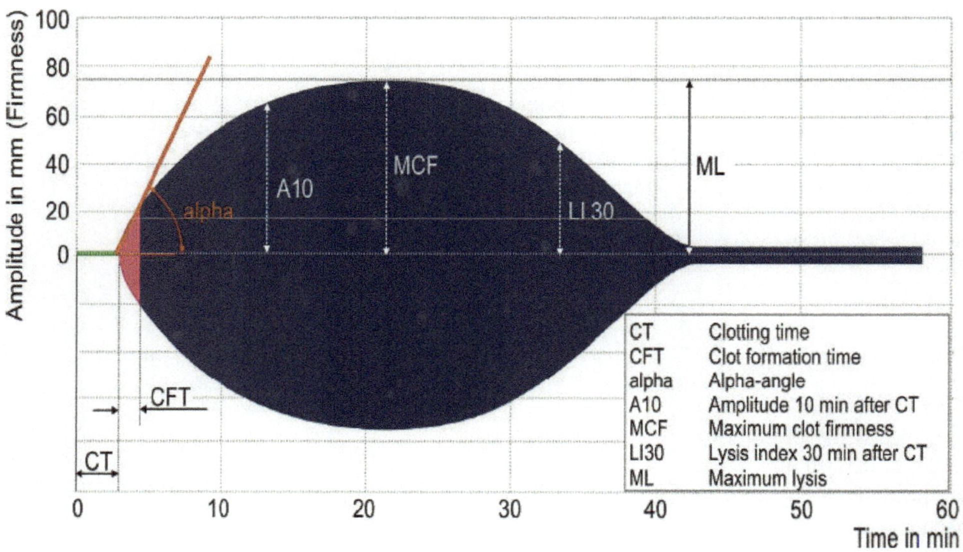

[Reproduced with permission of Tem International GmbH]

Fig. 9. ROTEM graph and basic parameters (a graph of an unstable clot has been chosen to enable illustration of the lysis parameters)

The available ROTEM tests are described below:

Name of Test [Test description]	Relevant Parameters [Considerations if parameters are abnormal]
INTEM [Mild intrinsic coagulation pathway activation]	**CT** [Factor deficiency (intrinsic pathway); Anticoagulant effects (heparin, thrombin inhibitors)] **MCF, A(x), CFT, α-angle** [Platelet contribution to clot firmness; Fibrinogen concentration; Fibrin polymerisation] **ML, LI(x)** [Hyperfibrinolysis]

Name of Test [Test description]	Relevant Parameters [Considerations if parameters are abnormal]
	MCF, A(x), ML, LI(x) [FXIII deficiency]
HEPTEM [Mild intrinsic pathway activation. Heparinase added to degrade any heparin present in the sample.]	If abnormal values seen on INTEM are corrected in the HEPTEM graph, these effects are attributable to heparin.
EXTEM [Mild extrinsic pathway activation]	**CT** [Factor deficiency (extrinsic pathway)] **MCF, A(x), CFT, α-angle** [Platelet contribution to clot firmness; Fibrinogen concentration; Fibrin polymerisation] **ML, LI(x)** [Hyperfibrinolysis] **MCF, A(x), ML, LI(x)** [FXIII deficiency]
FIBTEM [Mild extrinsic pathway activation. Platelet inhibitor (cytochalasin D) added, therefore the TEM represents only the fibrin component of the clot.]	**MCF, A(x), CFT, α-angle** [Fibrinogen concentration and Fibrin polymerisation] **ML, LI(x)** [Hyperfibrinolysis] **MCF, A(x), ML, LI(x)** [FXIII deficiency] When compared with EXTEM, FIBTEM gives an indirect evaluation of the platelet contribution to clot
APTEM [Mild extrinsic pathway activator. Fibrinolysis inhibitor (aprotinin)]	If abnormalities of EXTEM are corrected on APTEM they are attributable to hyperfibrinolysis and may be correctable with antifibrinolytic drugs.

A suitable combination of TEMs for a patient undergoing cardiac surgery would be INTEM, FIBTEM and HEPTEM. The INTEM is performed to look at CT (prolonged in consumptive coagulopathy and the heparin effect on the intrinsic pathway) and also the α-angle and MCF (to assess whether fibrinogen or platelet supplementation is needed). The HEPTEM is compared with INTEM to determine the degree of Heparin effect. FIBTEM is performed to define the fibrinogen contribution to the haemostatic plug.

As recommended at the European ROTEM meeting 2007, a minimum of 3 sets of ROTEM should be performed; a baseline, a set whilst on CPB, and one after CPB. Further sets are to be performed if the patient is still bleeding. These tests can be performed quickly and interpreted safely between 10-15 minutes from the start of the tests.

The FIBTEM test is used clinically to guide administration of fibrinogen (46), but evidence for the treatment trigger or therapeutic target has not been conclusively established. It has been suggested that a FIBTEM MCF of 7mm is adequate for haemostasis in orthopaedic surgery, but a higher target of 22mm has been discussed for cardiac surgery.

Caveats for ROTEM use:

The INTEM and EXTEM are not very sensitive to mild coagulation factor deficiencies, and are insensitive to defects of primary haemostasis (platelet aggregation). The EXTEM test may still be normal when INR is as high as 4, and may show pathological values with very high heparin levels.

Thromboelastography (TEG) versus Rotational Thromboelastometry (ROTEM)

As discussed above, the techniques have a common origin. Both systems generate graphs of clot firmness between a cuvette and pin versus time. In the TEG system the cuvette oscillates around a pin throughout the clotting process, whilst in the ROTEM system the cuvette is fixed and the pin rotates.
By convention, the parameters obtained from the graphs have been given different names in the two tests. A comparison of the nomenclature is given in the table below from an article by Luddington (42).

Instrumentation	TEG®	ROTEM®
Measurement period	–	RT
Clot time (period to 2 mm amplitude)	*r*	CT
Period from 2 to 20 mm amplitude	*k*	CFT
Alpha angle	α (slope between *r* and *k*)	α (angle of tangent at 2 mm amplitude)
Maximum angle	–	CFR
Maximum strength	MA	MCF
Time to maximum strength	TMA	MCF-t
Amplitude (at set time)	A (A30, A60)	(A5, A10...)
Clot elasticity	G	MCE
Maximum lysis	–	ML
Lysis at a fixed time	CL30, CL60	LY30, LY45, LY60
Time to lysis	TTL (2 mm drop from MA)	CLT (10% from MCF)
Maximum lysis	–	CLR (maximum tangent post-MCF)

Fig. 10. Nomenclature of TEG and ROTEM

Clinical application of near patient test results and evidence base for decision-making

There are several studies in the literature that highlight the usefulness of the TEG in cardiac surgery. Shore-Lesserson et al demonstrated in a prospective randomized controlled trial of high risk cardiac surgical patients (n=105) that fewer patients randomized to the TEG arm were transfused fresh frozen plasma ($p < 0.002$) or platelets ($p < 0.05$) compared to those patients managed by standard coagulation tests in the post-operative period (47). Total blood product transfusion was less in the TEG arm and this reached statistical significance. TEG was used to guide protamine, platelet, FFP and antifibrinolytic therapy. The authors concluded that TEG -based transfusion algorithm reduced transfusion requirements.
Spiess et al assessed the usefulness of TEG in predicting postoperative haemorrhage and need for reoperation. They found that TEG was a better predictor (87% accuracy) than coagulation profile (51%) or activated clotting time (30%) (48). Another study by the same author concluded that costs and risks associated with allogenic blood transfusions could be reduced with the introduction of a TEG based haemostasis protocol in cardiac surgery (49). Tuman found that TEG predicted postoperative haemorrhage more accurately than routine coagulation tests (88% versus 33% respectively) (50).

Avidan et al (51) showed in a prospective randomised comparison trial that following algorithms based on point of care tests or on structured clinical practice with standard laboratory tests did not decrease blood loss, but did reduce the transfusion of all blood components ($p < 0.05$) after routine cardiac surgery, when compared with clinician discretion.

Finally, Westbrook et al showed in a prospective randomised controlled study a non-statistically significant trend toward less blood product usage in a strict protocol utilizing TEG compared to physician's choice based on clinical experience and standard laboratory coagulation tests. The study also demonstrated a cost saving benefit (52).

Use of an automated protamine titration system, such as the commercially available point-of-care Hepcon®, has been shown to be associated with higher heparin and lower protamine doses. This can potentially decrease activation of the coagulation and inflammatory cascades, with possible advantages of decreased postoperative bleeding and blood product requirement.(23)

Blood product administration in cardiac surgery and the cardiothoracic ICU

If a patient bleeds in the postoperative period, it is important to distinguish between 'surgical' and 'medical' bleeding. A 'medical bleed' from the microvasculature occurs due to a coagulation abnormality, and this abnormality must be detected and corrected with blood products or pharmacological agents to halt the bleeding. In contrast a 'surgical bleed' is from a cardiac or large vessel injury and will often require resternotomy to re-establish haemostasis surgically. Misdiagnosis of 'surgical bleeding' can lead to unnecessary resternotomy, whilst failure to diagnose a 'surgical bleed' may lead to delay and futile use of blood products. A progressive, untreated 'surgical bleed' will lead to a combined 'medical' AND 'surgical' bleed. Likewise, a 'medical bleed' that is not correctly treated may result in a pericardial tamponade that needs surgical intervention.

Factors to be considered in post-operative haemorrhage include:

- Complexity of surgery and adequacy of surgical haemostasis at end of operation
- Baseline coagulation status (APTT, PT, platelet count, ACT or TEG) compared with post-operative measurements
- Anticoagulation therapy pre-operatively (Antiplatelet therapy, Warfarin, Heparins, FXa or thrombin inhibitors)
- Intraoperative blood loss and blood product replacement
- CPB duration
- Intra-operative anticoagulant use and reversal
- Pump blood usage (this contains additional heparin, thus may require further protamine reversal).
- Core temperature
- Blood pH
- Ionised calcium level

Where possible, administration of blood products should be minimised(53). With donor screening and testing of donated blood, the risk of blood-borne disease transmission has decreased. Uncertainties regarding prion-related disease transmission remain, and there is also evidence that blood transfusion during cardiac procedures is associated with worse short- and long-term outcomes (41, 54). The measures below are adapted from the 2011 Blood Conservation Clinical Guidelines published by the Society of Thoracic Surgeons and the Society of Cardiovascular Anaesthesiologists.(55)

General Measures for Blood Conservation

- If allogenic transfusion required, use leukodepleted red blood cells.
- Routine blood salvage with centrifugation is useful. Intra-op autotransfusion, either direct or following centrifugation is useful
- Blood salvage may be considered in malignancy, as the risk may be less than that associated with allogenic blood transfusion.
- Multidisciplinary blood management teams can limit transfusion and peri-operative bleeding whilst maintaining safe outcomes.
- Minimise volume taken for blood sampling
- Do not transfuse if Hb≥10g/dL unless specifically indicated
- Non-red cell haemostatic products ideally guided by point-of-care tests
- DDAVP (Desmopressin) considered if platelet dysfunction likely to respond (eg uraemia, type I von Willebrand's Disease)
- Consider FIX in Haemophilia B

Pre-op Measures

- Identify high risk patients and utilise all available measures to conserve blood in this setting (ie. increased age, pre-op anaemia, small body size, non-CABG or urgent surgery, pre-op antithrombotic drugs, acquired/congenital clotting abnormality, multiple comorbidities, thrombocytopenia or abnormal platelet function)
- Erythropoietin (EPO) and iron to correct anaemia, or for patients at high risk of developing anaemia
- If possible, stop platelet P2Y12 inhibitors [thienopyridine pro-drugs (ticlopidine, clopidogrel, prasugrel), direct-acting P2Y12 inhibitors (cangrelor, ticagrelor)] and delay surgery until effect has subsided
- Point-of-care testing of ADP-responsiveness may identify clopidogrel-non-responders who do not require delay

Intra-op Measures

Medical

- Lysine analogues (E-aminocaproic acid, tranexamic acid) reduce blood loss.
- Risk/benefit ratio does not favour aprotinin use in adults

Perfusion

- Post-CPB pump salvage with reinfusion of pump blood is reasonable. Centrifugation is reasonable. Modified ultrafiltration is indicated.
- Mini-CPB-circuits, vacuum-assisted venous drainage and retrograde autologous CPB circuit priming may reduce transfusion requirements.
- Microplegia may reduce haemodilution associated with larger volumes of crystalloid cardioplegia solution
- During CPB with moderate hypothermia, Hb≥6g/dL may be adequate, but higher transfusion trigger may be appropriate for patients at greater risk of critical non-cardiac end-organ ischaemia
- Open venous reservoir membrane oxygenator systems during CPB may decrease blood loss and improve safety
- If CPB ≥2hrs, higher and/or patient-specific heparin concentrations may reduce consumption of platelets and coagulation factors
- Protamine titration or empiric low-dose regimen post-CPB may decrease blood loss

Blood Products • Use safer fractionated products if possible, but plasma transfusion reasonable if multiple factor deficiencies and serious bleeding • Prothrombin Concentrate Complex (PCC) preferable to plasma for warfarin reversal provided PCC contains adequate FVII • Plasma transfusion considered as part of massive transfusion algorithm. • Intra-op platelet plasmapheresis for platelet salvage considered in high risk patients • Antithrombin III (AT) concentrate considered in patients with AT-mediated heparin resistance pre-CPB **Surgical** • TEVAR (thoracic endovascular aortic repair) may reduce blood loss compared with open procedure • Off-pump CABG may reduce blood loss compared with CPB approach • Topical haemostatic devices to aid anastomotic closure and topical antifibrinolytic agents may decrease blood loss.
Post-op Measures • Routine dual antiplatelet therapy not indicated - only for patients with acute coronary syndrome or recent drug-eluting coronary artery stents • Consider FXIII for clot stabilisation if bleeding persists despite routine blood conservation measures • Consider FVIIa for intractable non-surgical bleeding unresponsive to routine haemostatic management • Mediastinal shed blood reinfusion, following washing and centrifugation, can be considered (direct reinfusion not recommended) • Therapeutic PEEP trial to decrease post-op bleeding is not well established

Choice of fluid for intravascular volume replacement can also affect coagulation. Colloidal plasma substitutes may interfere with haemostasis in non-specific or specific ways. Non-specific effects relate to haemodilution, with decreased circulating concentrations of coagulation factors, platelets and red blood cells. Specific effects are discussed by colloid type.

Albumin inhibits platelet aggregation directly (56), and may affect fibrin polymerisation, but in vitro is considered not to affect haemostasis (57).

Dextrans are not widely used due to potential allergic, renal and haemostatic side effects. They cause platelet dysfunction by decreasing vWF, possibly by adsorption. Dextrans also accelerate activation of fibrinogen, facilitate fibrinolysis, and may coat endothelium and platelets thus decreasing platelet adhesion.

Gelatins can impair platelet coagulation (58) and decrease vWF, but are generally accepted not to influence perioperative bleeding (57).

Hydroxyethyl starches (HES) induce platelet dysfunction through effects on GPIIb-IIIa expression and on vWF and FVIII levels. HES can also favour fibrinolysis. Haemorrhagic complications have been reported more frequently with high molecular weight (Mw) HES than with lower Mw.

Use of colloids outside the context of clinical studies has recently been questioned as well (59). When using crystalloid alternatives, a balanced salt solution may offer less disruption of haemostasis than saline, possibly due to maintenance of plasma calcium concentrations.

16. Conclusion

Perioperative management of coagulation needs to be tailored to the needs of the individual patient and delivered within the available resources of the Cardiac Surgery Centre. Appropriate use of medication and blood products can minimise perioperative thrombosis and bleeding, limit exposure to potentially harmful blood products and thus maximise quality of patient care.

17. Acknowledgement

Supported by St. Vincent's Anaesthesia Foundation.

18. References

[1] Shander A, Moskowitz D, Rijhwani TS. The safety and efficacy of "bloodless" cardiac surgery. Semin Cardiothorac Vasc Anesth. 2005;9(1):53-63. Epub 2005/03/01.

[2] Boldt J, Haisch G, Kumle B, Brosch C, Lehmann A, Werling C. Does coagulation differ between elderly and younger patients undergoing cardiac surgery? Intensive Care Med. 2002;28(4):466-71. Epub 2002/04/23.

[3] Prisco D, Paniccia R. Point-of-Care Testing of Hemostasis in Cardiac Surgery. Thromb J. 2003;1(1):1. Epub 2003/08/09.

[4] Spiess BD, Royston D, Levy JH, Fitch J, Dietrich W, Body S, et al. Platelet transfusions during coronary artery bypass graft surgery are associated with serious adverse outcomes. Transfusion. 2004;44(8):1143-8. Epub 2004/07/22.

[5] Koch CG, Khandwala F, Li L, Estafanous FG, Loop FD, Blackstone EH. Persistent effect of red cell transfusion on health-related quality of life after cardiac surgery. The Annals of thoracic surgery. 2006;82(1):13-20. Epub 2006/06/27.

[6] Monroe DM, Hoffman M, Roberts HR. Fathers of modern coagulation. Thrombosis and haemostasis. 2007;98(1):3-5. Epub 2007/06/29.

[7] Riddel JP, Jr., Aouizerat BE, Miaskowski C, Lillicrap DP. Theories of blood coagulation. Journal of pediatric oncology nursing : official journal of the Association of Pediatric Oncology Nurses. 2007;24(3):123-31. Epub 2007/05/04.

[8] Curry AN, Pierce JT. Conventional and near-patient tests of coagulation. Continuing Education in Anaesthesia, Critical Care & Pain. 2007;7(2):45-50.

[9] Bombeli T, Spahn DR. Updates in perioperative coagulation: physiology and management of thromboembolism and haemorrhage. British journal of anaesthesia. 2004;93(2):275-87. Epub 2004/06/29.

[10] Chan MY, Andreotti F, Becker RC. Hypercoagulable states in cardiovascular disease. Circulation. 2008;118(22):2286-97. Epub 2008/11/26.

[11] Platt A. Can you recognize a patient at risk for a hypercoagulable state? JAAPA : official journal of the American Academy of Physician Assistants. 2008;21(12):20-6. Epub 2009/03/04.

[12] Martel N, Lee J, Wells PS. Risk for heparin-induced thrombocytopenia with unfractionated and low-molecular-weight heparin thromboprophylaxis: a meta-analysis. Blood. 2005;106(8):2710-5. Epub 2005/06/30.

[13] van Ryn J, Stangier J, Haertter S, Liesenfeld KH, Wienen W, Feuring M, et al. Dabigatran etexilate--a novel, reversible, oral direct thrombin inhibitor:

interpretation of coagulation assays and reversal of anticoagulant activity. Thrombosis and haemostasis. 2010;103(6):1116-27. Epub 2010/03/31.
[14] Di Nisio M, Middeldorp S, Buller HR. Direct thrombin inhibitors. The New England journal of medicine. 2005;353(10):1028-40. Epub 2005/09/09.
[15] Agnelli G, Eriksson BI, Cohen AT, Bergqvist D, Dahl OE, Lassen MR, et al. Safety assessment of new antithrombotic agents: lessons from the EXTEND study on ximelagatran. Thrombosis research. 2009;123(3):488-97. Epub 2008/05/20.
[16] Walenga JM, Jeske WP, Samama MM, Frapaise FX, Bick RL, Fareed J. Fondaparinux: a synthetic heparin pentasaccharide as a new antithrombotic agent. Expert opinion on investigational drugs. 2002;11(3):397-407. Epub 2002/02/28.
[17] Acostamadiedo JM, Iyer UG, Owen J. Danaparoid sodium. Expert opinion on pharmacotherapy. 2000;1(4):803-14. Epub 2001/03/16.
[18] Magnani HN, Gallus A. Heparin-induced thrombocytopenia (HIT). A report of 1,478 clinical outcomes of patients treated with danaparoid (Orgaran) from 1982 to mid-2004. Thrombosis and haemostasis. 2006;95(6):967-81. Epub 2006/05/30.
[19] Ansell J, Hirsh J, Poller L, Bussey H, Jacobson A, Hylek E. The pharmacology and management of the vitamin K antagonists: the Seventh ACCP Conference on Antithrombotic and Thrombolytic Therapy. Chest. 2004;126(3 Suppl):204S-33S. Epub 2004/09/24.
[20] Salem DN, O'Gara PT, Madias C, Pauker SG. Valvular and structural heart disease: American College of Chest Physicians Evidence-Based Clinical Practice Guidelines (8th Edition). Chest. 2008;133(6 Suppl):593S-629S. Epub 2008/07/24.
[21] Vahanian A, Baumgartner H, Bax J, Butchart E, Dion R, Filippatos G, et al. Guidelines on the management of valvular heart disease: The Task Force on the Management of Valvular Heart Disease of the European Society of Cardiology. European heart journal. 2007;28(2):230-68. Epub 2007/01/30.
[22] Keeling D, Baglin T, Tait C, Watson H, Perry D, Baglin C, et al. Guidelines on oral anticoagulation with warfarin - fourth edition. British journal of haematology. 2011. Epub 2011/06/16.
[23] Dunning J, Versteegh M, Fabbri A, Pavie A, Kolh P, Lockowandt U, et al. Guideline on antiplatelet and anticoagulation management in cardiac surgery. European journal of cardio-thoracic surgery : official journal of the European Association for Cardio-thoracic Surgery. 2008;34(1):73-92. Epub 2008/04/01.
[24] Storey RF. Pharmacology and clinical trials of reversibly-binding P2Y12 inhibitors. Thrombosis and haemostasis. 2011;105 Suppl 1:S75-81. Epub 2011/04/12.
[25] Landymore RW, Murphy JT, Lummis H, Carter C. The use of low-dose aprotinin, epsilon-aminocaproic acid or tranexamic acid for prevention of mediastinal bleeding in patients receiving aspirin before coronary artery bypass operations. European journal of cardio-thoracic surgery : official journal of the European Association for Cardio-thoracic Surgery. 1997;11(4):798-800. Epub 1997/04/01.
[26] Bidstrup BP, Hunt BJ, Sheikh S, Parratt RN, Bidstrup JM, Sapsford RN. Amelioration of the bleeding tendency of preoperative aspirin after aortocoronary bypass grafting. The Annals of thoracic surgery. 2000;69(2):541-7. Epub 2000/03/29.
[27] Mangano DT, Tudor IC, Dietzel C. The risk associated with aprotinin in cardiac surgery. The New England journal of medicine. 2006;354(4):353-65. Epub 2006/01/27.

[28] Sedrakyan A, Treasure T, Elefteriades JA. Effect of aprotinin on clinical outcomes in coronary artery bypass graft surgery: a systematic review and meta-analysis of randomized clinical trials. The Journal of thoracic and cardiovascular surgery. 2004;128(3):442-8. Epub 2004/09/09.

[29] Henry D, Carless P, Fergusson D, Laupacis A. The safety of aprotinin and lysine-derived antifibrinolytic drugs in cardiac surgery: a meta-analysis. CMAJ : Canadian Medical Association journal = journal de l'Association medicale canadienne. 2009;180(2):183-93. Epub 2008/12/04.

[30] Slichter SJ. Evidence-based platelet transfusion guidelines. Hematology / the Education Program of the American Society of Hematology American Society of Hematology Education Program. 2007:172-8. Epub 2007/11/21.

[31] Wall MH, Prielipp RC. Transfusion in the operating room and the intensive care unit: current practice and future directions. International anesthesiology clinics. 2000;38(4):149-69. Epub 2000/12/02.

[32] Karlsson M, Ternstrom L, Hyllner M, Baghaei F, Nilsson S, Jeppsson A. Plasma fibrinogen level, bleeding, and transfusion after on-pump coronary artery bypass grafting surgery: a prospective observational study. Transfusion. 2008;48(10):2152-8. Epub 2008/07/29.

[33] Ucar HI, Oc M, Tok M, Dogan OF, Oc B, Aydin A, et al. Preoperative fibrinogen levels as a predictor of postoperative bleeding after open heart surgery. The heart surgery forum. 2007;10(5):E392-6. Epub 2007/09/15.

[34] Karlsson M, Ternstrom L, Hyllner M, Baghaei F, Flinck A, Skrtic S, et al. Prophylactic fibrinogen infusion reduces bleeding after coronary artery bypass surgery. A prospective randomised pilot study. Thrombosis and haemostasis. 2009;102(1):137-44. Epub 2009/07/03.

[35] Volzke H, Robinson DM, Kleine V, Hertwig S, Schwahn C, Grimm R, et al. Preoperative plasma fibrinogen levels predict mortality after coronary artery bypass grafting. Thrombosis and haemostasis. 2003;89(5):885-91. Epub 2003/04/30.

[36] Fries D, Martini WZ. Role of fibrinogen in trauma-induced coagulopathy. British journal of anaesthesia. 2010;105(2):116-21. Epub 2010/07/16.

[37] Hiippala ST, Myllyla GJ, Vahtera EM. Hemostatic factors and replacement of major blood loss with plasma-poor red cell concentrates. Anesthesia and analgesia. 1995;81(2):360-5. Epub 1995/08/01.

[38] Rahe-Meyer N, Pichlmaier M, Haverich A, Solomon C, Winterhalter M, Piepenbrock S, et al. Bleeding management with fibrinogen concentrate targeting a high-normal plasma fibrinogen level: a pilot study. British journal of anaesthesia. 2009;102(6):785-92. Epub 2009/05/05.

[39] Humphries SE, Luong LA, Montgomery HE, Day IN, Mohamed-Ali V, Yudkin JS. Gene-environment interaction in the determination of levels of plasma fibrinogen. Thrombosis and haemostasis. 1999;82(2):818-25. Epub 1999/12/22.

[40] Lier H, Krep H, Schroeder S, Stuber F. Preconditions of hemostasis in trauma: a review. The influence of acidosis, hypocalcemia, anemia, and hypothermia on functional hemostasis in trauma. The Journal of trauma. 2008;65(4):951-60. Epub 2008/10/14.

[41] Koch CG, Li L, Sessler DI, Figueroa P, Hoeltge GA, Mihaljevic T, et al. Duration of red-cell storage and complications after cardiac surgery. The New England journal of medicine. 2008;358(12):1229-39. Epub 2008/03/21.

[42] Luddington RJ. Thrombelastography/thromboelastometry. Clinical and laboratory haematology. 2005;27(2):81-90. Epub 2005/03/24.
[43] Srinivasa V, Gilbertson LI, Bhavani-Shankar K. Thromboelastography: where is it and where is it heading? Int Anesthesiol Clin. 2001;39(1):35-49. Epub 2001/04/05.
[44] Craft RM, Chavez JJ, Bresee SJ, Wortham DC, Cohen E, Carroll RC. A novel modification of the Thrombelastograph assay, isolating platelet function, correlates with optical platelet aggregation. J Lab Clin Med. 2004;143(5):301-9. Epub 2004/05/04.
[45] Bochsen L, Wiinberg B, Kjelgaard-Hansen M, Steinbruchel DA, Johansson PI. Evaluation of the TEG platelet mapping assay in blood donors. Thromb J. 2007;5:3. Epub 2007/02/22.
[46] Solomon C, Pichlmaier U, Schoechl H, Hagl C, Raymondos K, Scheinichen D, et al. Recovery of fibrinogen after administration of fibrinogen concentrate to patients with severe bleeding after cardiopulmonary bypass surgery. British journal of anaesthesia. 2010;104(5):555-62. Epub 2010/03/30.
[47] Shore-Lesserson L, Manspeizer HE, DePerio M, Francis S, Vela-Cantos F, Ergin MA. Thromboelastography-guided transfusion algorithm reduces transfusions in complex cardiac surgery. Anesth Analg. 1999;88(2):312-9. Epub 1999/02/11.
[48] Spiess BD, Tuman KJ, McCarthy RJ, DeLaria GA, Schillo R, Ivankovich AD. Thromboelastography as an indicator of post-cardiopulmonary bypass coagulopathies. J Clin Monit. 1987;3(1):25-30. Epub 1987/01/01.
[49] Spiess BD, Gillies BS, Chandler W, Verrier E. Changes in transfusion therapy and reexploration rate after institution of a blood management program in cardiac surgical patients. J Cardiothorac Vasc Anesth. 1995;9(2):168-73. Epub 1995/04/01.
[50] Tuman KJ, Spiess BD, McCarthy RJ, Ivankovich AD. Comparison of viscoelastic measures of coagulation after cardiopulmonary bypass. Anesth Analg. 1989;69(1):69-75. Epub 1989/07/01.
[51] Avidan MS, Alcock EL, Da Fonseca J, Ponte J, Desai JB, Despotis GJ, et al. Comparison of structured use of routine laboratory tests or near-patient assessment with clinical judgement in the management of bleeding after cardiac surgery. Br J Anaesth. 2004;92(2):178-86. Epub 2004/01/15.
[52] Westbrook AJ, Olsen, J., Bailey, M., Bates, J., Scully, M., Salamonsen, R.F. Protocol based on thromboelastograph (TEG) out-performs physician preference using laboratory coagulation tests to guide blood replacement during and after cardiac surgery: a pilot study. Heart Lung and Circulation {Manuscript number: HLC-D-08-00027R1 Heart Lung and Circulation (in press)}. 2008.
[53] Marik PE, Corwin HL. Efficacy of red blood cell transfusion in the critically ill: a systematic review of the literature. Critical care medicine. 2008;36(9):2667-74. Epub 2008/08/06.
[54] Engoren MC, Habib RH, Zacharias A, Schwann TA, Riordan CJ, Durham SJ. Effect of blood transfusion on long-term survival after cardiac operation. The Annals of thoracic surgery. 2002;74(4):1180-6. Epub 2002/10/29.
[55] Ferraris VA, Brown JR, Despotis GJ, Hammon JW, Reece TB, Saha SP, et al. 2011 update to the Society of Thoracic Surgeons and the Society of Cardiovascular Anesthesiologists blood conservation clinical practice guidelines. The Annals of thoracic surgery. 2011;91(3):944-82. Epub 2011/03/01.

[56] de Jonge E, Levi M. Effects of different plasma substitutes on blood coagulation: a comparative review. Critical care medicine. 2001;29(6):1261-7. Epub 2001/06/08.
[57] Van der Linden P, Ickx BE. The effects of colloid solutions on hemostasis. Canadian journal of anaesthesia = Journal canadien d'anesthesie. 2006;53(6 Suppl):S30-9. Epub 2006/06/13.
[58] de Jonge E, Levi M, Berends F, van der Ende AE, ten Cate JW, Stoutenbeek CP. Impaired haemostasis by intravenous administration of a gelatin-based plasma expander in human subjects. Thrombosis and haemostasis. 1998;79(2):286-90. Epub 1998/03/11.
[59] Hartog CS, Bauer M, Reinhart K. The efficacy and safety of colloid resuscitation in the critically ill. Anesthesia and analgesia. 2011;112(1):156-64. Epub 2010/12/04.

12

Heparin Induced Thrombocytopenia: Its Significance in Cardiac Surgical Patient

Marcin Wąsowicz
Department of Anesthesia and Pain Management, Toronto General Hospital
Cardiovascular Intensive Care Unit, Toronto General Hospital
Department of Anesthesia, University of Toronto
Canada

1. Introduction

Intravenous heparin remains main stem therapy during cardiac and vascular surgical procedures. Heparin therapy is often continued after surgery as part of prophylactic treatment (deep venous thrombosis) or bridging therapy (for atrial fibrillation, prosthetic valve(s) or Dacron grafts implanted in the heart) until INR levels reach therapeutic levels with warfarin therapy.

Complications resulting from the use of heparin are relatively rare. Among the most common are bleeding initiated by excessive inhibition of thrombin and other clotting factors and thrombosis caused by inadequate anticoagulation. Heparin Induced Thrombocytopenia (HIT) is a rare but potentially life-threatening complication. The literature, which is describing HIT is still somewhat confusing since it uses a variety for terms for HIT. Type I HIT, sometimes called non-immune heparin-associated thrombocytopenia, is a benign process and presents as a mild thrombocytopenia with the platelet count rarely decreasing below 100.000/ml. Type I HIT develops early after heparin exposure, typically within 2-3 days. It probably results from a direct effect of heparin on platelets and occurs in about 10%–30% of patients receiving heparin (1).

In contrast, and of greater clinical concern, is type II HIT - and immune mediated syndrome associated with platelet activation, increased thrombin production and thrombogenesis leading to thrombo-embolic complications.

The following chapter will briefly discuss the epidemiology, pathogenesis and management options for ICU and cardiac surgical patients diagnosed with true HIT.

2. Epidemiology and pathogenesis

HIT is a rare complication of heparin therapy primarily affecting the surgical population. It occurs in 1-2% of cardiovascular surgery patients, 3%-10% of orthopaedic surgery patients and in less than 1% of obstetrical patients. It is higher in the orthopaedic population since they usually require prolonged treatment with heparin for DVT prophylaxis following surgery. Within the cardiac surgical population, patients who require implantation of a left ventricular assist device are at very high risk of developing HIT (> 10%). The incidence of HIT in patients treated in medical wards is usually very low (< 0.25%).

HIT develops primarily in patients treated with unfractionated heparin (UFH) but it can also develop in patients treated with low molecular weight heparins (LMWH) however the probability is significantly lower. The classical presentation of HIT might be confusing since the thrombocytopenia is usually not severe (a drop of 50-60% when compared to pre-op values) and the dominating clinical symptoms are usually related to thrombo-embolic complications. The final diagnosis can be confirmed only by additional, relatively complicated laboratory tests, which usually take several days to complete. In the meantime, if HIT is suspected, treatment should be initiated based on strong clinical indications.
HIT is an immune reaction associated with the formation of antibodies directed against heparin-Platelet Factor 4 (PF-4) complexes. Once heparin is administered to a patient, platelets release PF-4, which binds heparin. The heparin-PF-4 complex is highly immunogenic and initiates formation of antibodies, which belong to many subgroups (IgG, IgM and IgA). Among these classes of immunoglobulins, only IgG is capable of triggering the reaction responsible for HIT. The immune system of the patient develops sensitivity (memory) to complexes of heparin-PF-4. When a second dose of heparin is given (even a small amount) it causes platelet degranulation and release of PF-4. Antibodies then bind to the complexes (Fab fragment) and to the surface of platelets (Fc fragment) initiating a cascade of events that result in further platelet activation and release of large amounts of PF-4 along with further platelet aggregation and thrombin generation. Strong activation of thrombin leads to clot formation and subsequent thrombo-embolic events. PF-4 can also bind to other substances, which are chemicaly similar to heparin. They belong to a group of molecules called glycosaminoglycans (GAGs). Many GAGs are present on the surface of the endothelial cells. This interaction amplifies the reaction leading to further platelet activation and aggregation, inflammation and propagates clot formation. The above described sequence of events presents clinically as thrombocytopenia accompanied by thrombotic complications. 80% of embolic events take place in the venous system while the remaining 20% occur in the arterial system. Rarely, HIT presents as a systemic reaction, for example disseminated intravascular coagulation (DIC). Therefore, HIT should be considered as a pro-thrombotic disorder leading to venous or major arterial thrombosis with potentially life-threatening consequences.
Antibodies against heparin-PF-4 are usually detectable for up to 3 months after the last heparin exposure. After the antibodies disappear the patient can be safely treated with heparin again.

3. Diagnosis

Usually the first clinical suspicion of HIT occurs when the platelet count drops in a patient being treated with heparin. Thrombocytopenia is usually not severe (40-60,000) or more than 50% of baseline value and it very rarely reaches a level that would cause spontaneous bleeding. The incidence of thrombocytopenia usually has a predictable time pattern. There are 3 possible clinical scenarios.

1. Thrombocytopenia occurring 5-10 days after initiating therapy with heparin. This is the most common clinical scenario.
2. Thrombocytopenia occurring within 24 h after initiating heparin therapy (so-called acute or rapid-onset HIT). This scenario usually occurs in patients who received heparin before surgery, for example as a treatment of unstable angina
3. Thrombocytopenia with delayed onset. In this scenario the platelet drop occurs many days after discontinuing the heparin therapy, usually after the patient is being

discharged from hospital. There are some cases of super-acute HIT, which occurs almost immediately after a second dose of heparin and presents in the form systemic syndrome with dramatic picture of disseminated intravascular coagulation (DIC).

Among patients who develop thrombocytopenia caused by HIT, 30-50 % have thrombotic complications (Table 1). For many clinicians this is a paradoxical phenomenon since heparin is supposed to prevent thrombosis. Venous thrombosis commonly occurs in the lower extremities frequently leading to pulmonary embolism (PE) or venous gangrene with distal necrosis of the limb.

Vasculature	Venous	Arterial
Lower extremities	DVT	Ischemia
Upper extremities	Often with venous catheters	
Adrenal veins	Adrenal insufficiency	
Mesenteric or portal	Liver dysfunction	Bowel or renal
Cerebral venous sinus	Neurological impairment	Stroke
Coronary artery/graft		Ischemia or MI

Table 1. Thrombosis occurring in HIT.

HIT may also present as a systemic reaction. With the injection of the second dose of heparin (i.e. subcutaneous heparin used for DVT prophylaxis), the patient can develop several systemic symptoms, for example skin necrosis, seizures, shivering, hypo- or hypertension and tachycardia, or an anaphylactic reaction. As mentioned before the most severe form of HIT with systemic presentation is DIC. These symptoms are most likely related to a massive release of platelet contents including PF-4 but also histamine, serotonin and other vasoactive substances. Additionally, it has been suggested that systemic presentation of HIT includes extensive endothelial involvement (PF4 binds to GAGs). Various skin lesions at injection sites (erythema induratum, localized or diffuse urticaria, diffuse exanthema) can be also suggestive of HIT in 20% of cases. Livedo reticularis is observed in some patients and is associated with microangiopathy and microvascular thrombosis of the dermis. Lesions are painful, spread centrifugally, and may appear like necrotic purpura with a hemorrhagic bullous course, and central necrosis. 75% of patients showing cutaneous symptoms do not have any notable thrombocytopenia.

Basic laboratory tests reveal thrombocytopenia, and sometimes the blood film can show fragmentation of destroyed erythrocytes. Severe thrombocytopenia (< 20,000) usually indicates that diagnosis of HIT is unlikely. At the same time we need to rule out the most common causes of thrombocytopenia in patients being treated in the ICU (massive blood loss, sepsis, other drug-induced thrombocytopenia, i.e. vancomycin,). Among other less common syndromes causing thrombocytopenia, which should be included in differential diagnosis are: antiphospholipid syndrome, disseminated intravascular coagulation caused by other precipitating factor, thrombotic thrombocytopenic purpura and post-transfusion purpura.

One of the most popular schemes of assessment and clinical diagnosis of HIT was developed by Warkentin and called 'four T' (Table 2). T stands for thrombocytopenia, timing, thrombosis and other causes. For each category the patient receives 0, 1 or 2 points. For a score of 0-3 points, the diagnosis of HIT is unlikely, 4-5 points requires laboratory testing to confirm the diagnosis but in most cases does not require treatment, however, if patients receive a score of ≥ 6 points treatment should be initiated immediately.

Criteria	2 points	1 point	0 points
Timing (of thrombo-cytopenia)	5-10 days after heparin or during 1st day of therapy if heparin within previous 30 days	> 10 days after heparin or during 1st days of therapy if heparin used before (31-100 days)	No previous use of heparin
Thrombocytopenia (Platelet count)	< 50% of baseline value or > 20,000	30-50% of baseline value or 10-20,000	< 30% of baseline value or < 10,000
Thrombosis	New incident of thrombosis or skin necrosis in injection site or systemic reaction during dosing of heparin	Progressing or recurrent thrombosis or suspicion of thrombosis without proven diagnosis	No thrombo-embolic complications
Other explanations of thrombocytopenia	No other causes	Potential causes	Confirmed other causes
≥ 6 points mandates initiation of HIT therapy prior to receiving laboratory results confirming the diagnosis.			

Table 2. Table describes scoring system used for clinical diagnosis of HIT.

As mentioned before HIT can be only confirmed by a specific laboratory tests. First, a screening test is performed to detect HIT antibodies. This screening test detects all classes of immunoglobulins but as mentioned earlier, only IgG can trigger HIT. For example, in the case of cardiac surgical patients 20-40% of them develop antibodies, but only 1-2% are truly HIT-positive. On the other hand, if the screening test does not detect any immunoglobulins the presence of HIT can be ruled out. In the case of a positive HIT screen we need further confirmation to be able to show that these (detected) antibodies can trigger platelet activation. The most popular assay used is the Serotonin Release Assay (SRA), which uses plasma obtained from the patient, heparin and specially prepared, radio-labeled platelets. If the patient's plasma activates platelets (ie: causes release of serotonin) the patient can be diagnosed as having HIT (positive). Unfortunately, SRA is performed in only a few centers and thus the results of the test are usually not available for several days. An alternative to the SRA performed by some laboratories is the heparin-induced platelet aggregation assay (HIPA), which also demonstrates the presence of a clinically relevant antibody. In the meantime, the medical team needs to initiate treatment based on the clinical symptoms and probability of a positive diagnosis of HIT (>6 points in scale proposed by Warkentin).

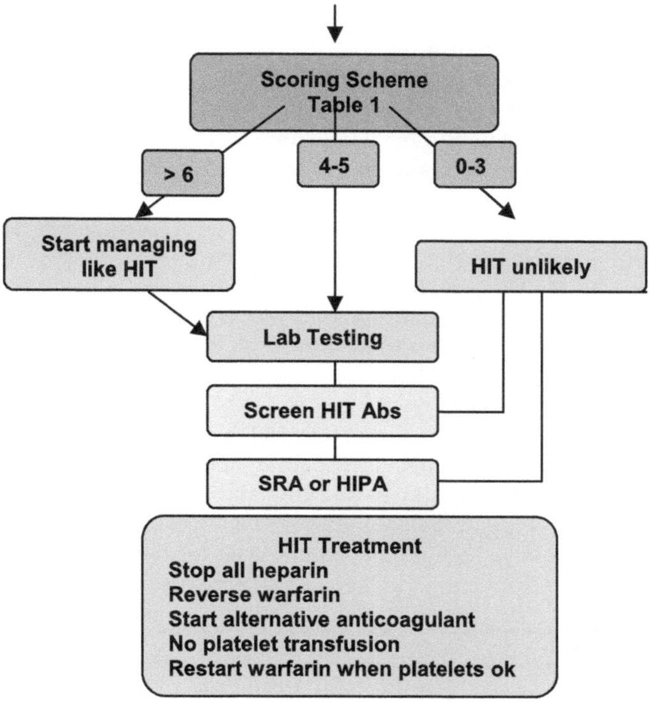

Fig. 1.

4. Management

Principles of treatment for patient diagnosed with HIT can be outlined in the following points.

1. Discontinue all forms of heparin including line flushes, LMWH or lines coated with heparin (i.e. heparin-bound Swan-Ganz catheter). Even tiny amounts of heparin can precipitate HIT.
2. Do not transfuse platelets to treat thrombocytopenia. Transfusion may precipitate further thrombotic events because HIT antibodies will activate transfused platelets.
3. Initiate treatment with heparin alternatives, the most commonly used drugs belong to 2 classes of anticoagulants: long acting, antithrombin III (ATIII) dependent factor Xa inhibiting oligosaccahrides or direct thrombin inhibitors (DTI).
4. If patient is already receiving warfarin it should be reversed with vitamin K. During the early stages of warfarin therapy, levels of protein C (a natural anticoagulant) will drop before the rest of the coagulation factors are inhibited and this can make the patient even more pro-thrombotic at the initial stages of warfarin therapy.
5. Warfarin therapy may be re-instituted when the platelets recover back to the baseline level. Warfarin derivatives must overlap for 4-5 days with anti Xa inhibitors or DTI therapy.

It should be stressed that stopping heparin without initiating anti- Xa inhibitors or DTI therapy is not sufficient for prevention of thrombotic complications.

The fundamental difference between heparin and Xa inhibitors or DTIs lies in the mechanism of their action. Heparin requires a cofactor, which is called antithrombin- III (ATIII), additionally it can not bind to thrombin, which is already attached to a fibrin network. A long half-life and a stable level of anticoagulation characterize indirect factor Xa inhibitors, similar to heparin since they also require ATIII. The pharmacokinetic profile of anti-Xa inhibitors makes them favorable to use in the ICU setting (one dose a day). On the other hand, the fact that they do not have antidote may complicate clinical management in case patient requires surgical intervention. Specific assays are available to measure drug levels.

The second group of medications DTIs bind and inhibit thrombin directly by connecting to 2 active exosites. They have a short half-life and may interfere with the thrombin-induced protein C pathway. Similar to indirect Xa inhibitors, DTIs do not have an antidote, therefore their action cannot be reversed. All these agents can be safely used in patients with thrombocytopenia.

Currently there are five main drugs used for HIT therapy: danaparoid, fondaparinux, bivalirudin, argatroban and hirudins. Danaparoid and fondaparinux belong to ATIII-dependent anti-Xa inhibitors, lepirudin, bavalirudin and argatroban belong to group of DTI. Danaparoid, lepirudin and argatroban are approved for treatment of HIT, bivalirudin and fondaparinux are not but have high rationale to be used for HIT therapy. Those five agents will be discussed below; additionally their brief characteristics are presented in Table 3.

Non-thrombin Inhibitors			
	Danaparoid		Ancrod
T1/2 Elimination	7-25 hrs		3-5 hrs, >24 hr
Monitoring	Anti Xa levels		Fibrinogen
Reversal	incomplete with protamine		FFP, cryo
Direct Thrombin Inhibitors			
	r-hirudin	Argatroban	Bivalirudin
Thrombin binding	Irreversible	Reversible	Reversible
Metabolism	Renal	Hepatic	Plasma, renal
T1/2 Elimination	40-120 min	25-50 min	25 min
Monitoring	aPTT, ECT	aPTT, ACT	ECT, kACT

Table 3. Short description of pharmacokinetic properties of alternative anticoagulants used in treatment of HIT

Danaparoid. Danaparoid is a mixture of several glycoaminoglycans, mainly haparan sufate. It has both anti-thrombin and anti- Xa properties but later predominates. It can be given as subcutaneous or intravenous injection and has long half-life (25h). Danaparoid has a unique property; in therapeutic concentration it can inhibit platelet activation caused by HIT antibodies, stopping vicious circle of thrombotic complications. It is usually administered once a day and first dose should be given intravenously to rapidly achieve therapeutic concentration. Similar to other agents used for treatment of HIT Danaparoid has no antidote.

Fondaparinux. Fondaparinux also belongs to group of indirect anti-Xa inhibitors but when compared to Danaparoid it does not have anti-thrombin properties. Half-life of Fondaparinux is 17 h. Paradoxically, Fondaparinux can trigger formation of HIT antibodies but its use is still considered to be very effective treatment of HIT.
R-Hirudins. Currently, there are two formulations of r-Hirudins available on the market: lepirudin and desirudin. Hirudins belong to DTI and have very high affinity to thrombin including molecules bonded to fibrin. This high affinity makes binding practically irreversible. Half-life of R-Hirudins is 80 min., they are eliminated almost exclusively by kidneys. In patients with kidney dysfunction half-life of r-Hirudins is totally unpredictable. R-hirudins are highly efficacious but treatment is complicated by high incidence of hemorrhagic complications (15%). Literature reports on several cases of lethal anaphylactic reactions complicating re-exposure to Hirudins.
Argatroban. When compared to Hirudins, Argatroban bindings to thrombin are reversible. Drug is primarily metabolized and excreted by liver therefore is recommended for use in patients with kidney dysfunction or failure. Frequency of major bleeding complicating argatroban therapy is 8%, more over patients treated with Argatroban have high incidence of limb amputation. Most likely it is related to difficulties in achieving therapeutic level and fact that Argatroban artificially elevates values of INR. It may compromise safe overlap and transition from Argatroban therapy to Coumadin. Experience with Argatroban used for cardiac surgical procedures is highly unfavorable.
Bivalirudin. Bivalirudin belongs to reversible DTI and among all agents used for HIT therapy presents most favorable pharmacokinetic profile. It has short half-life (25 min) and is primarily metabolized by plasma enzymatic degradation. It makes it drug of choice in patients with kidney and/or liver dysfunction (i.e. ICU patients). On the other hand due to plasma enzymatic degradation of bivalirudin any blood anticoagulated with this agent, which in stagnation will eventually clot. This property requires alternative approaches during CPB: the pump suckers must be replaced with cell saver and cardioplegia pump must be continuously flushed. Additionally, presence of clots in pericardium (stagnated blood) does not indicate that patient is not adequately anticoagulated. Therapy with Bivalirudin should be monitored with Ecarin Clotting Time (ECT), which is not available in many institutions. As an alternative one can use direct DTI assay or aPTT or plasma modified ACT if Bivalirudin is to be used for CPB purposes. Properties of Bivalirudin make it agent of choice for cardiac surgical procedures in HIT-positive patients who cannot be re-scheduled beyond time when HIT antibodies disappear.

5. HIT patient for CPB

One of the most challenging situations facing cardiac anaesthesiologists is intra-operative management of the patient who requires a cardiac surgical procedure who is HIT positive. Whenever possible it is recommended to delay surgery until the HIT antibodies have cleared (on average 100 days). Unfortunately, in some clinical situations it is not possible; for example: left main stenoses with symptoms of unstable angina, rapidly progressing endocarditis or heart transplantation are among the most common clinical scenarios. Among all of the presented agents (see **Table 3**), none of them is approved for anticoagulation during cardiopulmonary bypass (CPB). Therefore therapy with DTIs or indirect anti Xa inhibitors during cardiac surgery with use of CPB should be considered as an "off-label" application for these drugs. All of them have been used in different doses with varying protocols and outcomes were not always favorable. Their recommended doses and protocols for clinical use are presented in **Table 4.** When comparing all of these agents, Bivalirudin appears to offer that most favorable outcome with respect to control of anticoagulation during extracorporeal circulation. The features of Bivalirudin, which makes it a favorable agent for use with CPB are: a short half-life and metabolism that is independent from kidney and liver function. A protocol based on data from the literature and our own experience is presented in the **Appendix 1.**

Anticoagulant	Dosages for CPB
Danaparoid	Bolus 125 units kg^{-1} iv, post thoracotomy CPB prime 3 units ml^{-1} Infusion 7 units kg^{-1} h^{-1} iv on CPB If clotting noted additional bolus 1250 units Stop infusion 45 minutes before end of CPB
Ancrod	Infusion 8.4 units h^{-1} x 12hrs preoperatively check fibrinogen levels q 4hrs Stop infusion preoperatively once the target fibrinogen level of 0.4-0.8 gm L^{-1} is reached If fibrinogen > 0.8 gm L^{-1} restart the infusion at 2.1 units h^{-1}
Hirudin	Bolus 0.25 mg kg^{-1}, pre cannulation CPB prime 0.25 mg kg^{-1} Infusion 0.5 mg min^{-1} iv, maintain ECT > 400s Additional bolus to maintain ECT Stop infusion before end of CPB
Argatroban	Bolus 0.1 mg kg^{-1} iv, 20 minutes pre cannulation Infusion 5-10 ug kg^{-1} min^{-1} iv, maintain ACT > 400s CPB prime 0.05 mg kg^{-1} Additional 2 mg iv boluses to maintain ACT Stop infusion before end of CPB
Bivalirudin	Bolus 1.5 mg kg^{-1} iv, pre cannulation CPB prime 50mg Infusion 2.5 mg kg^{-1} h^{-1} iv, maintain ECT > 400s Stop infusion before end of CPB

Table 4. Dosages of alternative anticoagulants used for patients who are HIT positive and require cardiac surgery with the use of cardiopulmonary bypass

It should be mentioned that there are some reports in the literature recommending the use of strategies other than using a DTI or indirect Xa inhibitor for anticoagulation during CPB. The most encouraging of those are: use of plasmapheresis prior to CPB to clear all HIT antibodies followed by use of regular doses of heparin or to use a prostacyclin infusion combined with antiplatelet therapy with GPIIb/GPIIIa inhibitors.

Appendix 1 Scheme of CPB approach with bivalirudin anticoagulation for HIT positive patients

Requirements	For Anesthesiologist	For Surgeon	For Perfusionists
Staffing	2 anesthesiologist required, one responsible for anticoagulation, one for anesthesia	Regular setup	2 perfusionists required
Anticoagulation	Separate line for bivalirudin Bolus 1-1.5 mg/kg Followed by infusion 2.5mg/kg/h Discontinue infusion 15 min. prior to decannulation	Stagnant blood will clot (pericardium, pleura)-do not panic Suction-only from cell saver Consider continuous cardioplegia Consider flushing grafts with bivalirudin solution (0.1 mg/ml)	50 mg of bivalirudin into pump prime Monitor anticoagulation with Ecarin Clotting time (>400 sec) or ACT> 370 sec Additional bolus of 0.25mg/kg if ECT/ACT values below recommended, consider increasing infusion after bolus Cannot use suction units of CPB machine- only cell saver Have second circuit as a back-up solution
Hemostasis	Maintain normothermia after CPB Maximum dose of antifibrinolitic Be prepared for massive transfusion protocol No antidote for bivalirudin	Meticulous haemostasis Bleeding might continue for up to 45 min. after commencing CPB	Cell saver use to continue after CPB Be prepared to perform ultrafiltration after CPB to speed up elimination of bivalirudin. Extra pump blood must be stored in citrated bags
Other important points	Reduce doses in patients with kidney dysfunction	Flush you mammary every 10 min	Divede duties between 2 perfusionists prior to procedure
Equipment	Everything heparin free (lines, line flushed, PA catheters)	Lots of additional equipment in the room	Cell saver, additional pump as backup, ECT machine if available in your institution

Appendix 1.

6. Summary

HIT represents a rare but potentially life threatening complication of heparin therapy. Its pathogenesis is based on an immunological reaction specifically the formation of antibodies directed against a complex of heparin and PF-4. Secondary exposure to heparin triggers a reaction leading to activation of platelets, their aggregation and adhesion to endothelium leading to formation of clots (80% in the venous system and 20% in arteries) and subsequent thrombotic events.

The definitive diagnosis of HIT requires sophisticated laboratory tests that may take a while to get results from. Therefore treatment should be initiated before final results are obtained based on high clinical suspicion. The most important principles of therapy include: discontinuation of any form of heparin therapy, treatment with indirect inhibitors of factor Xa or direct thrombin inhibitors and reversal of vitamin K antagonists if they were used previously. Additionally, transfusion of platelets should be avoided since it will only precipitate their activation and aggravate the clinical symptoms.

7. Key points

- Heparin -induced thrombocytopenia (HIT) is a rare highly under-diagnosed but life threatening complication of heparin therapy.
- HIT is a clinico-pathological syndrome requiring multiple laboratory tests to make the final diagnosis. Most often treatment must be initiated before final diagnosis is established
- The most important principles of therapy include: discontinuation of any form of heparin, avoidance of platelet transfusion, treatment with indirect inhibitors of factor Xa or direct thrombin inhibitors and reversal of vitamin K antagonists if they were used previously.
- Management of a HIT-positive patient undergoing cardiac surgery with the use of CPB presents a challenge for the anesthesiologist.

8. References

[1] Warkentin TE. Agents for the treatment of Heparin-Induced Thrombocytopenia. Hematol Oncol Clin N Am 2010; 24: 755-75

[2] Ortel TL. Heparin Induced Thrombocytopenia: when low -platelet count is a mandate for anticoagulation. Hematology Am Soc Hematol Educ Program. 2009; 225-32.

[3] Levy JH, Winkler AM. Haparin-Induced Thrombocytopenia and cardiac surgery. Curr Opin Anaesthesiol 2010; 23: 74-79

[4] Wąsowicz M, Vegas A, Borger MA, Harwood S. Bivalirudin anticoagulation for cardiopulmonary bypass in a patient with Heparin-Induced Thrombocytopenia. Can J Anesth 2005; 52: 1093-98

[5] Sniecinski R, Hursting MJ, Paidas MJ, Levy JH. Etiology and assessment of hypercoagulability with lessons from Heparin-Induced Thrombocytopenia. Anesth Anal 2011; 112: 46-58.

13

Antiplatelet Drugs in Coronary Artery Disease

Susanne Maria Picker
Transfusion Medicine, University Hospital of Cologne
Germany

1. Introduction

Overview of diverse functional aspects

Human platelets (PLTs) are anucleate, discoid small cells (2 - 4 μm by 0.5 μm) that normally circulate at concentrations of 150 - 400 x 10^9/L for a maximum of 10 days. They are primed to undergo explosive activation following damage from the vessel wall and play a central role in both primary hemostasis and arterial thrombosis, including adhesion, aggregation, and coagulation but also chemotaxis, inflammation, and proliferation.

The normal vascular endothelium produces potent PLT inhibitors such as nitric oxide, prostacyclin and natural ADPase (CD39). However, once sub-endothelial components like collagen, fibronectin, laminin, or von Willebrand factor (vWF) become exposed, PLTs undergo a highly regulated set of functional responses including adhesion, followed by spreading, release reactions (degranulation), induction of pro-coagulant activity, microparticle formation, and clot retraction. These activities result in rapid formation of a vascular (white) plug, which then is stabilized by the activation of soluble plasma components resulting in the formation of fibrin and the inclusion of erythrocytes and leukocytes. This red plug initiates the healing process during which a part of fibrin is degraded again by fibrinolysis. Under physiological conditions thrombus formation is strongly limited to the region of the damaged vessel wall by inhibitory mechanisms of intact endothelial cells and the coagulation cascade.

PLTs are enriched in surface glycoprotein (GP) receptors that mediate interactions among PLTs themselves, with the sub-endothelium and with white blood cells. PLTs also contain specific granules for the storage of calcium (Ca^{++}), adenine/guanine nucleotides, and serotonin (dense bodies) and the storage of coagulation factors (e.g. vWF, FV), multimerin, thrombospondin-1, fibrinogen, IgE, growth factors (e.g. PDGF, TGF-β, ECGF, EGF, VEGF, bFGF, IGF-I), and cytokines (e.g. PF4, RANTES) (α granules). Serotonin (5-hydroxytryptamine) acts predominantly as a local vasoconstrictor but has also pro-inflammatory properties by stimulation of monocytes and attraction of T lymphocytes (IL-16). Contents of α granules mediate e.g. host defense, recruitment and activation of leukocytes as well as regulation of tissue repair by mitogenic effects on smooth muscle cells, macrophages, monocytes, and fibroblasts. Other important pro-inflammatory mediators are present in the cytosol (IL-1β, CD40L) and are generated from mRNA (relict from megacaryocytes) and are released upon PLT activation. CD40L stabilizes aggregation by interference with GP IIb-IIIa and stimulates endothelial cells to express ICAM-1, VCAM-1,

E-selectin, and the vitronectin receptor, thus modulates leukocyte-endothelium and PLT-endothelium interactions.

Due to specific binding between sub-endothelial agents and specific GP receptors, PLTs begin to slow down and transiently adhere or roll along the damaged area of the vessel wall. Under conditions of high shear, as found in the arterial circulation, the initial PLT-sub-endothelium interactions are exclusively mediated by vWF present in bridges between sub-endothelial collagen and GP Ib (V-IX) of the adhering PLTs. The following steps of activation via various signal transduction pathways (outside-in signaling) and the elevation of cytoplasmatic Ca^{++} levels are then mediated by other receptor-ligand interactions. When the cytoplasmatic Ca^{++} concentration exceeds a certain threshold, cytoskeletal changes occur, which mediate shape change from discoid to sphere, pseudopod formation, and conformational change of the fibrinogen receptor GP IIb-IIIa (receptor activation). Only the activated GP IIb-IIIa complex is able to bind soluble plasma fibrinogen (and vWF under high shear conditions) leading to further spreading of the stimulated PLTs along the site of injury and ultimate aggregation characterized by fibrinogen bridges between the activated GP IIb-IIIa complexes on adjacent PLTs. Simultaneous release and surface exposure of granule components (e.g. ADP and serotonin from dense bodies, vWF and p selectin from α-granules) and cyclooxygenase (COX)-related thromboxane A_2 (TxA_2) formation/expression result in further recruitment, activation and aggregation of other PLTs near to the growing plug. At least, internal, anionic, negatively charged phospholipids are exposed by transbilayer flip flop of the inner membrane leaflet and pro-coagulant microvesicles are generated. The exposure of anionic phospholipids, mainly phosphatidylserine, provides a surface upon which PLTs can support thrombin generation by accelerating the tenase and prothrombinase reactions of the plasmatic coagulation pathway. Thrombin, the key enzyme of the coagulation cascade and the most potent PLT agonist, interacts with two binding sites on PLTs, a) the region of GP Ib (high affinity) and b) a specific epitope of the thrombin receptor (moderate affinity). Binding of thrombin leads to cleavage of the extracellular domain (protease-activated receptor PAR), whereby the generated free polypeptide (SFLLRN-x) can directly activate further thrombin receptors (thrombin-receptor activating peptide TRAP). Human PLTs express two kinds of PARs activated either by lower (PAR-1) or higher concentrations of thrombin (PAR-4). Receptor activation by thrombin results in further activation of GP IIb-IIIa, TxA_2 formation, and secretion of granular components such as ADP that promotes recruitment and activation of adjacent PLTs into the vicinity of the growing plug and the inclusion of leukocytes. Thrombin also converts soluble fibrinogen into insoluble fibrin, which is cross-linked by the thrombin-activated FXIII to confer stability of the otherwise fragile plug/thrombus. At last, the activated PLTs rearrange their intracellular actin/myosin cytoskeleton, which leads to clot retraction. The latter is inhibited by blockade of GP IIb-IIIa receptors representing central links between the contractile elements.

Adhesion

As described, adhesion is mediated by GPs of the PLT surface that recognize specific structural components of the extracellular matrix such as collagen and elastic fibrils embedded in a gel of proteoglycans and water. This first contact *(contact phase)* between PLTs and the sub-endothelium is mediated by interaction between GP Ib-V-IX (vWF receptor belonging to the leucine-rich GPs) with collagen-bound vWF. Thus, the main task of GP Ib-V-IX is the adhesion of circulating PLTs to immobilized vWF despite high shear

forces. GP Ib-V-IX consists of four subunits: the central part is GP V surrounded by GP Ib_{α} and GP Ib_{β}, which are covalently linked to each other by disulfide bridges and non-covalently bound to GP IX. GP Ib_{α} possesses binding sites for vWF and thrombin. In contrast to GP IIb-IIIa, whose surface expression increases after thrombin activation, the surface density of GP Ib-V-IX is reduced by receptor internalization after PLT activation. Recent evidence suggests that, apart from GP Ib-V-IX, another PLT membrane receptor for collagen, GP VI, is strictly required for the initial PLT tethering following vascular injury. Both receptors appear to act in concert to recruit PLTs to the sub-endothelium in-vivo. GP VI mediates the activation (opening) of other adhesive receptors (GP IIb-IIIa, GP Ia-IIa) by shifting them from a low to a high affinity binding state required for stable PLT arrest. GP VI belongs to the immunoglobulin superfamily and forms complexes with the FcR γ-chain at the cell surface. In the absence of GP VI, PLTs completely failed to adhere and aggregate on the damaged vessel wall. Further immunoglobulin adhesion receptors, PECAM (PLT-endothelial cell adhesion molecule)-1 and ICAM (intracellular adhesion molecule)-2 probably mediate adhesion to leukocytes and PLT related inflammation, but their global role for PLT function is mostly unknown.
The contact phase is stabilized via further adhesion to collagen, fibronectin, laminin, and thrombospondin *(stabilization phase)*. Binding of collagen leads to the formation of pseudopods (shape change) and peptide as well as GP IIb-IIIa activation via tyrosine phosphorylation *(activation phase)*. Starting from released arachidonic acid (AA) the adhering PLTs form TxA_2, which slows down the blood flow due to its vasoconstricting activity. Additionally TxA_2 induces the release of soluble granule components like ADP *(secretion phase)* leading to the recruitment of still resting PLTs that then become activated and aggregate with already adhering PLTs through activated GP IIb-IIIa. By spreading of the PLT aggregate over the complete sub-endothelium, the vessel wall lesion is separated from blood flow, and blood loss is kept as low as possible.

Aggregation

Aggregation depends on three conditions: shear force, Ca^{++}, and fibrinogen. The latter are stored in PLT granules and are released in high concentrations during PLT activation. While the *primary aggregation phase* is reversible and characterized by "loose links" via fibrinogen bridges, the *secondary aggregation phase* is irreversible and induced by the degranulation process. GP IIb-IIIa, a β_3 integrin, plays a central role in aggregation. 60,000 to 100,000 GP IIb-IIIa receptors can be detected per PLT. 70% are bound to the surface, and 30% are only released from intracellular stores (open canalicular system, α-granules) upon PLT activation. Circulating PLTs carry resting, not activated GP IIb-IIIa complexes (low affinity functional state) that only can bind immobilized fibrinogen. The binding sites for soluble fibrinogen become accessible after conformational change during activation, which strongly depends on Ca^{++} (high affinity functional state). The binding of fibrinogen to the activated receptor induces a further conformational change (ligand-occupied functional state) with exposure of cryptic epitopes (LIBS = ligand-induced binding site) and transmembrane signal transduction (post-occupancy) events.

Activation

Upon changes in biochemical pathways several soluble PLT agonists (e.g. ADP, thrombin, TxA_2) are formed, which bind to specific G protein-linked receptors. Via signal transduction pathways, each agonist amplifies the activation step through the formation of *second*

messengers. One of these messengers, phospholipase C, forms inositol 1,4,5 triphosphate (IP_3) and diacylglycerol (DAG), whereby IP_3 enhances the intracellular Ca^{++} concentration and DAG activates proteinkinase C, which in turn phosphorylates a series of further signal proteins that control the degranulation process and the activation of GP IIb-IIIa. Cytoplasmatic Ca^{++} activates phospholipase A_2, which leads to the liberation of AA from phospholipids of the cell membrane. Aspirin-sensitive COX-1 and thromboxane synthetase then form TxA_2, which has vasoconstricting activity and stimulates the secretion of granule components after interaction with specific TxA_2 receptors. Two TxA_2 receptors can be distinguished on the PLTs surface (TPα and TPβ), of which TPα is most important. COX-1-inhibition results in reduced secretion and inhibition of secondary aggregation. Receptors that directly inhibit PLTs stimulate adenylate cyclase (increased formation of cAMT) via G_S proteins and are activated by PLT antagonists like adenosine, β-adrenergic substances, prostacyclin, prostaglandin E_1, and theophylline.
PLTs are presently the only cells that express ADP specific receptors (P_2Y_1, P_2Y_{12}, P_2X_1). Like other activation receptors, ADP receptors are linked to G-proteins. Due to their key role in the pathogenesis of arterial thrombosis, they are of particular pharmacological interest. The P_2Y_1 receptor is linked to the initiation of shape change, mediation of Ca^{++} mobilization and activation of phospholipase C. Activation of P_2Y_{12} inhibits cAMP formation via inhibitory G-proteins and is predominantly responsible for TxA_2 formation, p selectin surface expression and conformational changes of GP IIb-IIIa (receptor activation), thus sustained PLT aggregation. All of these mechanisms are affected by thienopyridines. Like P_2Y_1, P_2X_1 mediates Ca^{++} influx and shape change but seems not to be influenced by thienopyridines.

Secretion

During adhesion, PLTs begin to release stored components from the granules in the order dense bodies, α-granules, and lysosomes. Dependent on ATP and Ca^{++} the degranulation process initiates the secondary, irreversible phase of aggregation and reinforces the activation/recruitment of further circulating PLTs as well as fibrin formation resulting in thrombus consolidation. As described above, the interaction of released ADP (from PLTs, damaged vessel wall cells, endothelial cells, red blood cells) with its specific purinergic receptors plays a central role in this process. Released serotonin reinforces vasoconstriction and thus slows down the blood flow. Released α-granule contents attract leukocytes and fibroblasts (β-TG, PF4), promote mitogenic and proliferative effects in fibroblasts and smooth muscle cells (growth factors like PDGF), or exhibit pro-inflammatory activity (IL-1). P selectin is found in both PLTs (α-granules) and endothelial cells (Weibel-Palade bodies) and is expressed on cell surface only after cellular activation. P selectin is the decisive receptor for PLT adhesion to leukocytes and triggers inflammatory reactions but also plays a central part in vascular repair processes. Interestingly, p selectin is significantly increased in all states of coronary artery disease: stable angina (showing also increased TxA_2 formation and fibrinogen binding due to increased GP Ib and GP IIb-IIIa expression [1-3]), unstable angina (showing also increased LIBS expression [4]), and acute myocardial infarction (AMI). Here, increased p selectin levels are indicative for an increased thrombotic re-occlusion risk [5]. When coronary stenting is combined with dual antiplatelet therapy, p selectin expression and GP IIb-IIIa activation are as low as after conventional coronary angioplasty [6-8]. Besides p selectin, thrombin promotes chemotaxis of monocytes and mitogenesis in lymphocytes and mesenchymal cells (smooth muscle cells, fibroblasts). In addition, released coagulation factors (vWF, fibrinogen, FV, PAI-1) fulfill pro-coagulant or anti-fibrinolytic tasks. The pro-coagulant activity can be reinforced by microparticle formation, small membrane vesicles extruded from activated PLTs that exhibit a high binding affinity for FVa and FVIIIa, thus facilitating the formation of the tenase and prothrombinase complexes. Lysosomal enzymes like collagenease or elastase degradate surrounding fibrils and induce changes in atherosclerotic plaques.

2. The role of platelets in atherogenesis

Role of the arterial plaque

In contrast to stable angina pectoris, which is generally caused by a reduced oxygen supply to the myocardium due to coronary vasoconstriction, acute coronary syndromes (ACS) arise from an acute plaque rupture within an epicardial coronary artery with subsequent PLT aggregation and thrombus formation. Reperfusion strategies aim to dissolve the thrombotic plaque either through administration of fibrinolytic agents or direct coronary interventions. Paradoxically, despite a sufficiently reestablished blood flow, reperfusion injury occurs and myocardial dysfunction can progress. This is mainly triggered by activated PLTs released from the plaque area or the circulation itself (cardiovascular risk factors are per se associated with an increased basal activity of circulating PLTs [9,10]). Activated PLTs in turn promote inflammatory reactions within the ischemic myocardium, thus plug growing. Consequently, up to 50% of all patients with successful revascularization and normal epicardial blood flow following interventional therapy do not have adequate tissue reperfusion [11,12].
Following a modern concept of atherogenesis, apart from endothelial dysfunction (characterized by decreased vasodilatation upon stimulation with acetylcholine and increased pro-coagulant inflammatory activities) lipid deposition on the intima is one of the first pathological events in the genesis of an arterial plaque. The lipid-rich nucleus is separated from blood flow by a fibrous cap and rich in free cholesterol crystals, cholesteryl esters, oxidized LDL and monocytes/macrophages. The latter undergo phagocytosis of fatty acids and oxidized LDL and differ to foam cells. Additionally, there are particularly heavy PLT deposits and high amounts of tissue factor, which favors thrombin formation. Thrombin, in turn, activates additional PLTs and supports their aggregation to already adhering PLTs (recruitment), which, in parallel, stimulate the migration of smooth muscle cells and fibroblasts by a PDGF-dependent mechanism. After intima proliferation and monocyte migration increased shear forces (high blood flow or tension) and the liberation of proteolytic enzymes (plasminogen activator, metalloproteinases) can promote plaque rupture with all known sequelae. PLTs are not just involved in thrombotic complications by formation of vascular occlusions but also trigger plaque progression and promote myocardial malperfusion by participation in recurrent vasoconstrictions and local/systemic inflammatory reactions.

PLT-mediated microembolization

The regeneration of the afflicted myocardial area largely depends on the integrity and recovery of the microcirculation distal to the stenosis. Importantly, there is an increased embolization of thrombotic material from the arterial plaque lesion during plaque growing and particularly in the reperfusion phase after coronary interventions. This may promote intermittent coronary vasospasms distal to the stenosis through the release of serotonin and TxA_2 resulting in inadequate perfusion, myocardial ischemia, tissue damage, unstable angina or non-ST-segment elevation myocardial infarction. On the other hand, the contact of intact endothelial cells with activated PLTs has the potential to modify chemotactic, proteolytic and adhesive properties inducing increased surface expression of endothelial adhesion receptors (VCAM-1, ICAM-1, vitronectin receptor), which participate in the recruitment of PLTs to the inflamed endothelium. Additionally, the elevated release of endothelial pro-inflammatory substances (MIP-1, IL-6, IL-8) supports chemotaxis, adhesion, and transmigration of monocytes.

PLT-mediated inflammation

The exposure of sub-endothelial compounds is not required for PLT adhesion in acute inflammatory processes such as ischemia/reperfusion. E.g., p selectin expression of inflamed endothelial cells has been demonstrated to mediate PLT rolling through GP Ib indicating that the vWF receptor mediates both PLT adhesion to the sub-endothelial matrix and to "intact" endothelial cells. Additionally, endothelial adhesion receptors that bridge PLTs via fibrinogen are up-regulated in response to endothelial inflammation (e.g. by IL-1β or CD40L of activated PLTs or thrombin). In this manner, PLTs (if activated or resting) adhere to the vessel wall and promote the recruitment of neutrophils and monocytes by the release of a variety of pro-inflammatory mediators and growth hormones. Furthermore, adhering PLTs can induce up-regulation of NF-κB in endothelial cells leading to further inflammatory changes in the vessel wall. High doses of ASA (≥ 900 mg/d) can influence the NF-κB activation, thus promote the stillstand of atherosclerotic plaque progression [13]. Consequently, cardiac patients with elevated systemic CRP levels benefit especially from antiplatelet therapy with ASA [14]. Another strategy to limit reperfusion injury uses monoclonal antibodies to adhesion receptors such as p selectin (present on endothelial cells and PLTs), CD11/CD18 (present on leukocytes), and the vitronectin receptor (present on endothelial cells). Abciximab not only blocks GP IIb-IIIa on PLTs, but also the vitronectin receptor on endothelial cells explaining its favorable effect on myocardial perfusion, microcirculation, and recovery of left ventricular function [14-17].

3. Antiplatelet substances

Acetylic salicylic acid (ASA)

Of the five main groups of antiplatelet substances **(Tab.1.)**, ASA is probably the most important drug. Its use is considered as the gold standard in primary and secondary prophylaxis of coronary syndromes [18]. However, from the results of collagen and AA-induced aggregation, up to 30% of all patients respond insufficiently to ASA and may profit from a combined (dual) antiplatelet therapy to effectively reduce arterothrombotic events.

ASA selectively and irreversibly inhibits COX, an ubiquitous enzyme existing in two isoforms: COX-1 (forms short living prostaglandins (PgG_2, PgH_2) from which thromboxane synthetase forms TxA_2) and COX-2 (forms prostaglandins mainly in leukocytes that are involved in inflammatory and pain processes). After oral administration ASA is rapidly (5-16 min) and completely absorbed. Due to the hepatic first pass effect the bioavailability drops to about 50% **(Tab.2.)**. Thereafter, COX-1 of all bypassing PLTs is irreversibly acetylated at Ser_{529}. ASA thereby inhibits the production of the potent PLT activator TxA_2. However, with stronger agonists than TxA_2, especially thrombin, PLT aggregation is not markedly inhibited by ASA. ASA also inhibits synthesis of prostaglandins in endothelial cells (prostacyclin, a potent PLT inhibitor and powerful vasodilatator) and stomach mucosa cells (cytoprotective prostaglandins). Of note, in the absence of protein biosynthesis, COX-1

Mode of action	Substances
Increase of cyclic nucleotides	
• Activation of adenylat cyclase	PGE_1 (Alprostadil) PGI_2 (Epoprostenol) prostaglandin (Iloprost)
• Inhibition of phosphodiesterase	theophylline, dipyridamole
• Activation of guanylyl cyclase	NO, nitrate derivates, molsidomine
Interaction with arachidonic acid metabolism	
• Inhibition of cyclooxygenase	acetylsalicylic acid (ASA), sulphinpyrazone, indomethazine, ω3-fatty acids
• Inhibition of thromboxyne synthetase	dazoxibene, ozagrel
• Antagonism of TxA_2 receptor	ridogrel, nidrogrel
Interaction with aggregation receptors	
• Inhibition of ADP receptor	ticlopidine, clopidogrel
• Inhibition of thrombin receptor	peptide antagonists
• Inhibition of serotonin receptor	ketanserine
Inhibition of aggregation	
• Inhibition of fibrinogen receptor (GP IIb-IIIa)	i.v. moAB: abciximab (ReoPro) i.v. cyclic peptide: eptifibatide (Integrillin) i.v. peptide mimetics: tirofiban, lamifiban oral peptide mimetics: xemilofiban, orbofibane, gantofibane, roxifiban
Inhibition of adhesion	
• Inhibition of vWF receptor (GP Ib-V-IX)	recombinant vWF fragment
• Inhibition of collagen receptor (GP Ia-IIa)	antibodies, peptides

i.v. intravenous; moAB monoclonal antibody;

Table 1. Classification of antiplatelet substances [8]

	ASA	ticlopidine	clopidogrel	prasugrel
Bioavailability (%)	90	80-90	> 50	> 50
Protein binding (%)	50-80	98	94-98	98
Half life (h)	0,5	12,6	7-8	> 12
Metabolism	hepatic	hepatic	hepatic	hepatic
Active metabolites	no	no	yes	yes
Inhibited aggregation (onset)	minutes	< 4days	2 hours	< 30 minutes
Inhibited aggregation (steady state)	hours	8-11 days	3-7 days	2 days
Inhibited aggregation (duration)	7 days	5 days	2-3 days	7 days
Recommended daily dose (mg)	75 - 325	500 (2 x 250)	75	10

Impairment of hepatic function can diminish the antiplatelet effect. The onset of action of thienopyridines can be accelerated by higher initial doses. Compared to clopidogrel, prasugrel treatment is associated with more rapid, potent and prolonged PLT inhibition. Preliminary evidence suggests a similar safety profile compared to clopidogrel.

Table 2. Pharmacologic properties of oral antiplatelet drugs [8,23]

inhibition in anucleated PLTs persists for a cellular lifetime compared with nucleated vascular endothelial and stomach mucosa cells, which recover COX-1 activity shortly after exposure to ASA. Daily doses of 30-70 mg ASA are sufficient for complete inhibition of TxA_2 synthesis, whereas increasing doses can promote gastrointestinal side effects. The recommended daily dose ranges therefore from 75 to 325 mg. Other side effects include intracerebral hemorrhage (≤ 0.5%), hypersensitivity, respiratory alkalosis, and renal and liver dysfunction (cave Reye's syndrome in children characterized by encephalopathy with liver damage). Higher doses of ASA inhibit the nuclear factor κB (NF-κB) that regulates transcription of many inflammatory cytokines (e.g. MCP-1) and of immunoglobulin adhesion receptors (VCAM-1). Additionally, in ACE-inhibitor-treated patients, ASA should be replaced with thienopyridines, since much of the hemodynamic benefits of ACE inhibitors would be lost by the addition of ASA [19].

Thienopyridines (TPs)

TPs including drugs under late state development (cangrelor, elinogrel) inhibit PLT adhesion by inhibition of the ADP receptor P_2Y_{12} mediating recruitment and aggregation of further PLTs into the vicinity of a growing plug. After oral administration the antiplatelet effect is exerted by active metabolites formed by cytochrom (CYP) P450 activity upon hepatic metabolism **(Tab.2.)**. Since statins are also metabolized by CPY-P450 (mainly CYP3A4), co-administration is associated with decreased antiplatelet efficacy [20]. While ticlopidine (oral, approved), clopidogrel (oral, approved) and parasugrel (oral, approved) act irreversibly, ticagrelor (oral, approved), cangrelor (intravenous), and elinogrel (oral or intravenous) lead to reversible P_2Y_{12} receptor blockade.

In contrast to ASA, TPs do not influence the COX pathway in endothelial cells (no effect on prostacyclin production) but hinder the rapid degradation of extracellular ADP by impairment of ectoADPse released from the damaged vessel wall. Considerably more than ASA, TPs reduce key factors of arterial thrombosis: shear force-induced PLT activation, PLT-leukocyte formation, and inflammation [21]. Consequently, *ticlopidine,* the first developed TP, was found to be superior to ASA in reducing thrombotic risks (mainly stroke) during different pathological conditions including percutaneous coronary intervention (PCI) [22]. However, due to its unfavorable safety profile (20% diarrhea, 10% skin eruptions, 2.5% neutropenia and thrombotic-thrombocytopenic purpura) and its delayed onset of action (4-7 days), ticlopidine has been replaced by clopidogrel in routine clinical use.

Clopidogrel, a second generation TP, is equally effective as ticlopidine but has a markedly better tolerability profile. Additionally, clopidogrel achieves a significant antiplatelet effect even on the first day of treatment. Bleeding problems are as frequent as under ASA [23]. Clopidogrel, together with ASA, constitutes the current standard of care for high risk patients with cardiovascular diseases and has considerably improved the antithrombotic therapy after coronary stenting. Despite this, a considerable number of patients with recurrent ischemic cardiovascular events remains, which may only in part be attributed to suboptimal PLT inhibition. Less than 60% inhibition of ADP induced PLT aggregation following 75 mg/d clopidogrel in healthy volunteers [24] or 300 mg clopidogrel loading in PCI patients [25] indicates an incomplete P_2Y_{12} receptor blockade. In addition, inhibited ADP induced PLT aggregation < 10% is observed in 10-30% of treated patients [26-31], probably due to poor compliance, drug-drug interactions, genetic receptor polymorphisms, or variability in CYP P450 activity or intestinal absorption. Poor responsiveness to

clopidogrel was shown to be associated with recurrent cardiovascular events including stent thrombosis [32] and may be overcome by increased clopidogrel doses. This was demonstrated in the CLEAR PLATELETS study, where higher loading doses of clopidogrel prior to PCI acted more rapidly and increased the inhibitory effect on PLTs [25]. During maintenance, however, there was no significant difference in the composite end point (AMI, stroke, vascular death) between the double and the standard dose of clopidogrel [33]. Thus, the search for TPs (third generation) with less response variability is an ongoing feature.
Compared to clopidogrel, *cangrelor* exhibits more consistent and greater PLT inhibition as well as short onset and offset of action. The CHAMPION trials, however, were stopped early because of lack of efficiency [34,35]. Cangrelor is still being studied as a bridge for clopidogrel prior to surgery [36]. *Prasugrel* also combines a rapid onset of action (< 30min) with less response variability (0.3%) and a prolonged duration of action (> 3 days). While ticlopidine and clopidogrel require two CYP P450-dependent steps to form active metabolites (mainly CYP 3A4), prasugrel requires only one step (CYP3A4 or CYP2B6). This leads to less CYP P450 dependency and higher amounts of active metabolites [37] translating into a 10-fold (clopidogrel) to 100-fold (ticlopidine) greater potency [38]. As shown in the recent PRINCIPLE-TIMI 44 and TRITON-TIMI 38 studies [39,40], prasugrel increased the efficiency of PCI and improved cardiovascular outcomes (by 20%) but was associated with a significant increase in major bleedings [41]. This was reinforced by the recent CHARISMA trial testing prolonged dual antiplatelet therapy with ASA + prasugrel vs. ASA + clopidogrel [42], although the JUMBO-TIMI 26 trial demonstrated a similar bleeding risk compared to standard clopidogrel [43]. Prasugrel should not be used in adults > 75 years of age or < 60 kg of body weight and in those who have had a recent TIA/stroke or an increased bleeding risk. Like prasugrel, *ticagrelor* acts more potent and rapid but does not significantly increase major bleeding events. Drawbacks, however, are increased incidences of dyspnea and ventricular pauses [36]. The PLATO study demonstrated significantly increased reduction rates of cardiovascular syndromes and mortality vs. clopidogrel (- 16%), while bleeding events were as frequent as under prasugrel [44]. In addition to cangrelor, prasugrel, and ticagrelor *elinogrel* rapidly achieves nearly complete PLT inhibition even in subjects with low responsiveness to clopidogrel [45]. Patients undergoing PCI had greater PLT inhibition under elinogrel (100/150 mg twice daily) than under standard clopidogrel without exhibiting more bleeding events [46]. These results gave promise for further Phase III trials.

Fibrinogen receptor antagonists (FRAs)

FRAs currently prescribed only during PCI reversibly block one of the final steps of PLT activation irrespective of the stimulus. This is the binding of fibrinogen to GP IIb-IIIa mediating adhesion to the injured vessel wall or interactions with PLTs and other blood cells. Blockade of GP IIb-IIIa further leads to an attenuated formation of pro-coagulant microparticles and inhibits PLT-dependent formation of thrombin. Thus, in addition to inhibition of aggregation, an anticoagulant activity can also be achieved by the administration of FRAs. Side effects include hypotension, vertigo, vomiting, headache, and thrombocytopenia. Bleeding complications must be considered under ongoing therapy (especially in thrombocytopenic, female and elderly patients).
Chimeric monoclonal antibodies directed against the vicinity of the fibrinogen recognition (RGD) region (abciximab) can be distinguished from small low molecular mass antagonists (SMAs) including cyclic peptides (eptifibatide) or non-peptide molecules (tirofiban) with a

tyrosine like structure **(Tab.3)**. In contrast to SMAs that bind specifically to the RGD region (competitive inhibition) abciximab binds to a different site, even when the binding pocket is occupied by fibrinogen or vWF (steric inhibirion).

	abciximab	eptifibatide	tirofiban	lamifiban
Molecular mass (Dalton)	45.000	800	495	468
Receptor specificity	CR	no CR	no CR	no CR
Onset of action (after i.v. bolus)	minutes	minutes	minutes	minutes
Reversibility	slow (> 12 h)	rapid (< 6 h)	rapid (< 6 h)	rapid (< 6 h)
Half life **plasma (normally a few hours)** **receptor (normally a few hours)**	short long	DD DD	DD DD	DD DD
Intrinsic activity (LIBS expression)	+	+	+	+
Recommended dose **Initial bolus (μg/kg) prior to PCI** **MD (μg/kg/min) for 12-48 (72) h**	 250 0.125	 90.0 - 180.0 0.5 - 2.0	 0.4 - 10.0 0.10 - 0.15	 - 0.01 - 0.07

PCI percutaneous coronary intervention; CR cross reaction with the vitronectin (endothelium cells) and the MAC-1 receptor (leukocytes); DD dose dependency; MD maintenance dose
GP IIb-IIIa blockers administered intravenously (i.v.), have proven efficacious in mitigating arterial thrombosis in acute coronary syndromes and coronary interventions such as balloon dilatation and stent implantation but are associated with an increased bleeding risk. Currently, i.v. GP IIb-IIIa blockers are prescribed in high risk patients with acute coronary syndromes immediately before and after coronary intervention (for 24-72 h). Oral GP IIb-IIIa blockers have failed to demonstrate any benefit.

Table 3. Pharmacologic properties of intravenous (i.v.) GP IIb-IIIa antagonists [8]

In order to achieve an effective antithrombotic protection, a receptor blockade of at least 80% should be achieved. A blockade > 90% increases the risk of bleeding. This makes the dosing difficult. The latter is controlled by ADP-induced aggregation that should be carried out in hirudine- or PPACK-anticoagulated blood due to the Ca^{++} dependency of receptor binding. Unlike abciximab, the function of SMAs depends on the achieved plasma concentration. Excretion modalities are linked directly to body weight and are inversely correlated with age. Unlike SMAs that rapidly dissociate from the receptor, 70% of all GP IIb-IIIa receptors are still inhibited for up to 12 hours after termination of abciximab (PLT bound abciximab even lasts for up to 2 weeks). Thus, receptor blockade with abciximab can be reduced in patients with a strongly elevated PLT count. Due to the fact that internal GP IIb-IIIa receptors cannot adequately be blocked, TRAP-induced aggregation is only very incompletely be inhibited by standard doses of FRAs (in contrast to ADP induced aggregation that must completely be inhibited). Consequently, patients with ACS experience a markedly lower inhibition of aggregation than do patients with stable coronary artery disease. This suggests that higher doses of FRAs are required under conditions of increased PLT activation, especially with thrombin (occurring e.g. during fibrinolysis therapy). Additionally, the release of internal GP IIb-IIIa receptors can lead to a significant residual aggregation and thrombus formation despite the administration of FRAs.

Novel antiplatelet strategies

Currently, two groups of PLT inhibitors are approved for clinical use in ACS patients: ASA and oral TPs. These agents have shown improved short- and long-term clinical outcomes

but are associated with increased bleeding events. Thus, there is a need for new antiplatelet agents with higher PLT inhibition capacity and less bleeding risk.
A new TxA_2 receptor antagonist was tested in animals and has demonstrated fast and potent antiplatelet efficacy [47] comparable to that of ASA plus clopidogrel [48]. Additional desired effects were an improved endothelial function [49], an inhibited TxA_2-induced vasoconstriction [50], and a favorable bleeding risk profile [48]. *Picotamide,* already marketed in Italy, combines both TxA_2 receptor and thromboxane synthetase blockade and, unlike ASA, preserves prostacyclin formation in endothelial cells. Picotamide was shown to reduce atherosclerotic plaque progression, cardiovascular events and mortality without increased bleedings in ASA-refractory patients with peripheral artery disease without [51,52] or with diabetes [53]. Selective inhibition of the thrombin specific PAR-1 receptor *(vorapaxar, atopaxar)* represents a further strategy to reduce ischemic events and was tested in two Phase-II trials (TRA-PCI and LANCELOT-ACS) as secondary prophylaxis of ACS or on the top of standard antithrombotic therapy including ASA, clopidogrel and the heparin of choice. Despite significant dose-dependent increases in abnormal liver function parameters and QT elongation, there was a trend towards lower adverse cardiac events without increased bleeding events in the verum- vs. the placebo treated groups [54,55]. The first developed phosphodiesterase (PDE) inhibitor with an antiplatelet effect was *dipyridamole.* Together with ASA, dipyridamole demonstrated efficacy in the prevention of stroke [56]. However, ASA plus dipyridamole was not superior to clopidogrel in the prevention of recurrent stroke as seen in PRoFESS [57]. *Cilostazol,* a selective PDE III inhibitor, increases cAMP levels in PLTs, endothelial and smooth muscle cells leading to vasodilatatory and antiplatelet properties. Recent studies have shown that the addition of cilostazol to ASA and clopidogrel (triple antiplatelet therapy), particularly in diabetic patients, reduced risk of stent thrombosis (even of drug eluting stents) and increased cardiac outcomes after PCI without increased bleeding complications. However, due to headache, palpitations, and diarrhea, withdrawal of cilostazol approximated 15% [58,59]. Further antiplatelet strategies including blockade of inflammatory substances such as p selectin [60] or collagen receptors [61] are currently under clinical development. An accurate evaluation of the balance between the anti-ischemic effect and the hemorrhagic risk of these new drugs is highly warranted.

Antiplatelet-therapy-inherited bleeding risk

Sufficient hemostasis requires normal PLT function in at least 20% of circulating PLTs [62]. As the effects of antiplatelet drugs are not reversible by other drugs, PLT transfusions are the only manner to rapidly restore normal hemostasis. Today, prevention of cardiac events, especially stent thrombosis, is considered as being highly dependent on antiplatelet therapy during the first year after coronary intervention. In this period, however, up to 5% of patients have to undergo surgery for non cardiac reasons, whereby elderly patients, women, patients with anemia, renal dysfunction, and hypertension are at especially increased risk for perioperative bleeding. Not only does bleeding constitute an immediate threat, but is also associated with increased re-infarction and cardiac morbidity (5-fold/year) both in the short as well as the long term [63]. For this reason, the inherited bleeding risk of all antiplatelet drugs has to be outweighed against the concomitant cardioprotective effect **(Tab.4.)**. Of note, antiplatelet replacement by heparin does not provide protection against the risk of coronary artery or stent thrombosis. Based on a retrospective evaluation, we recommended discontinuation of antiplatelet therapy for at least 2 days prior to elective

Pharmacological properties	Indication (RRR)	Bleeding risk
GP IIb-IIIa antagonists		
Fibrinogen receptor antagonists	IST (50%)	SP: 3 - 4% (mostly catheters)
Clopidogrel (300 mg LD, 75/d mg MD)		
ADP receptor antagonist	AMI in ACS (18%) IST, recurrent ST (30%)	SP: 1 – 2% (higher plus ASA) ICH: 0.35% GIT: 0.68% GIT ulcers: 0.68% IOBL: 50% (ASA + clopidogrel) *
Acetylic salicylic acid ASA (100 – 325 mg/d)		
COX-1 inhibitor	Prim. prevention (40%) Sec. prevention (20%)	SP: 1 ‰/year ICH: 0.49% GIT: 2.66% GIT ulcers: 1.15% IOBL: 20%*

PCI percutaneous coronary intervention; LD loading dose; MD maintenance dose; AMI acute myocardial infarction; ACS acute coronary syndrome; ST stent thrombosis; IST immediate stent thrombosis; SP spontaneous; ICH intracranial hemorrhage; GIT gastrointestinal; intraoperative blood loss; * without bleeding-related increase in mortality.
The risk of cardiac events is maximal (increased up to 5-10-fold) in malignancy, diabetes mellitus, the early postoperative state and during stent re-endothelialization, especially of high risk stents (proximal, multiple, or overlapping stents, small vessels, bifurcated lesions). In these settings, the risk for stent thrombosis averages 35%. The associated mortality reaches 20-40%

Table 4. Relative risk reduction (RRR) and bleeding risk of common antiplatelet substances [59]

surgery [64]. However, since antiplatelet agents are maximally helpful when the thrombotic risk is highest, long-term dual antiplatelet therapy should be pursued until surgery, especially during stent re-endothelialization (4 – 6 weeks after bare metal stents, 12 months after drug-eluting stents). Due to the rise in fibrinogen, CRP and PAI-1, the risk of plaque rupture and consecutive thrombosis is maximal (2-4-fold higher) in the early postoperative setting. Here, the mortality rate due to stent thrombosis is estimated to about 20-40% [65]. After withdrawal of ASA, the cardiac complication rate increases 3-fold, and ASA should never be stopped when prescribed for secondary prophylaxis of ACS or in patients with stents. When prescribed for primary prevention, there is no evidence that ASA withdrawal 7 days prior to surgery is harmful. Clopidogrel withdrawal during the first month after coronary intervention makes patients 10 times more likely to die. When necessary, ADP receptor blockers could be bridged with short acting GP IIb-IIIa antagonists like eptifibatide. After surgery, both drugs ASA and clopidogrel should be resumed within 12-24 hours.

4. Antiplatelet therapy and coronary heart disease

Primary and secondary prophylaxis of cardiac syndromes

Since > 50 years ASA reduces vascular death by 15% and non-fatal vascular events by 30% as evidenced by meta-analyses of over 100 randomized trials [66,67]. ASA may also be of benefit in the primary prevention of cardiovascular events but the effect is more modest and its recommendation in this setting is highly debated due to the probably offset of the cardioprotective effect by bleeding complications [68,69]. Additionally, total mortality remains unaffected. Based on these and further data [70-74] daily doses of 160-325 mg ASA are recommended for all subjects > 50 years of age, who are at increased risk of AMI. Higher doses are not more effective in the prevention of cardiovascular events and may be associated with more serious side effects (reduced patient compliance) [33]. Younger subjects should use ASA only, when manifestations of atherosclerotic diseases (e.g. TIA, unstable angina) are present [8].

The CAPRIE study [75] examined the prophylactic efficacy of clopidogrel in comparison to ASA in patients with a history of ischemic stroke, prior AMI or symptomatic peripheral artery disease (PAD). In comparison to ASA (325 mg/d), a significant 8.7% risk reduction of non-fatal and fatal vascular deaths was found for clopidogrel (75 mg/d), which thereby occupies a firm place in secondary prophylaxis of cardiovascular events but is only marginally superior over ASA. Although not significant, ASA showed a trend towards better efficacy after prior AMI, whereas patients with PAD appeared to more profit from clopidogrel than from ASA. Despite this, a large portion of patients remains for whom no satisfactory therapeutic success can be obtained with ASA or clopidogrel monotherapy. Since both antiplatelet drugs have different target receptors and mechanisms of action (COX-1 inhibitor vs. P_2Y_{12} ADP receptor blockade), their combination as dual antiplatelet therapy offers additive effects and provides greater inhibition of PLT aggregation than therapy with either agent alone. As a consequence, the CURE study [76] demonstrated a risk reduction of 20% in patients with unstable angina, when ASA was combined with clopidogrel. The subsequent CREDO trial [77] showed that dual antiplatelet therapy reduced the risk of major adverse cardiovascular events after angioplasty compared with ASA alone. The tolerability profile was good, and major bleedings increased by only 1% as demonstrated in CLARITY-TIMI 28 [78] and COMMIT [79]. In the CHARISMA trial, however, patients with established vascular disease demonstrated a markedly increased bleeding risk, and no additional benefits were achieved with dual antiplatelet therapy over ASA therapy alone (probably due to clopidogrel resistance) [42]. Long-term dual antiplatelet therapy was beneficial only for high-risk patients with clinically evident atherothrombosis, especially for the prevention of stroke in cases with atrial fibrillation [80].

Fibrinolysis

Thrombin liberation in the region of the lysed thrombus may promote increased activation of circulating PLTs [81]. Moreover, due to high amounts of PAI-1, the PLT-rich core (white) thrombus is practically resistant to fibrinolytic agents. For these reasons, a successful reperfusion upon fibrinolysis can be achieved in only 50% of AMI and a TIMI-3 flow, which is a decisive survival parameter, is only insufficiently restored. For these reasons, antiplatelet drugs have been administered together with fibrinolytics: full dose fibrinolytics plus partial dose FRAs [82] or reduced-dose fibrinolytics plus full dose FRAs [83]. Pooled results from these studies and equivalent data suggest that FRAs together with ASA significantly increase the efficacy of fibrinolytics, reduce fatal and non fatal re-infarctions and the need for urgent revascularization [84-86]. Drawbacks, however, were increased intracranial bleeding and unaffected re-infarction rates after 30 days asking for safety and long-term efficacy of this combination [87].

Percutaneous transluminal coronary angioplasty (PTCA)

Pretreatment with ASA as well as with TPs significantly lower (up to 70%) the incidence of early acute thrombotic occlusions after PTCA [8]. Since the additional administration of FRAs to ASA and/or clopidogrel as well as to standard therapy including anticoagulants, nitrates, and beta-blockers, further reduce (40%) early cardiac incidents (partly, however, at cost of increased bleeding events [88-105]), the ACC/AHA guidelines recommend the addition of a FRA to ASA and heparin to patients in whom catheterization and coronary intervention are planned [106]. Furthermore, eptifibatide or tirofiban together with ASA and heparin should be given to patients with continuing ischemia or elevated troponin levels, in whom invasive management is not planned. Clopidogrel administered before cardiac catheterization enhances perioperative bleeding, if angiography reveals that bypass grafting is required rather than percutaneous coronary intervention. Thus, the American College of Chest Physicians (ACCP) guidelines recommend withholding clopidogrel until the coronary anatomy is determined [107]. Despite the efficacy of antiplatelet therapy concerning early thrombotic occlusions after PTCA, studies on the prevention of later re-stenosis (> 6 month) were disappointing [108,109]. Due to an excessive fibroproliferative response, up to 30% of PTCA patients developed recurrent ischemia and re-stenosis [110]. Only the results of the TACTICS study [104] showed that in patients with ACS early invasive strategy combined with immediate administration of FRAs was significantly better concerning late vascular deaths than the "wait and see" approach. Patients with elevated troponin levels had the greatest benefit from this strategy [8].

Coronary stenting

2 million patients of Western Countries undergo coronary dilatation each year [77], and coronary stents are placed in over 90% of these patients [111]. One of the greatest fears is subacute stent thrombosis triggered within minutes to hours after coronary intervention by activated PLTs. Predictors for increased risk of re-thrombosis are elevated GP IIb-IIIa expression or PLT degranulation markers prior to PCI as well as high post-interventional PLT reactivity to ADP [112]. Thus, long-term antiplatelet therapy is mandatory for the success of coronary stenting.

One of the first trials on stent thrombosis showed that ticlopidine (vs. anticoagulants) reduced the risk [113]. Thereafter, numerous clinical trials have demonstrated the superiority of dual antiplatelet therapy [114-116]. Based on these data, the American Heart Association/American College of Cardiology guidelines recommend ASA plus a 300 mg or 600 mg (better PLT inhibition) clopidogrel loading, followed by a 75 mg clopidogrel maintenance for 12 months for all patients undergoing PCI and/or stenting [117]. Recently, prasugrel demonstrated even higher efficiency than clopidogrel (plus 52%) irrespective of the clopidogrel loading dose: 300 mg [40] or 600 mg [39], however at cost of increased bleeding (2.4% vs. 1.8%, $p=0.03$) [40]. Moreover, the additional application of FRAs prior to PCI has significantly increased clinical outcomes as seen by improvements in early and late TIMI 3 flow rate, global left ventricular function, early re-stenosis, and recurrent ischemia [89,91,92,105,118,119] in spite of bleeding complications [92]. Abciximab could promote the re-establishment of the microcirculation, thus the functional recovery of the infarcted heart region. From the STOP-AMI trial [120] stenting + abciximab + dual antiplatelet therapy was superior over fibrinolysis with respect to myocardial salvage and the accumulation of death and thromboembolic complications for up to 6 months ($p=0.02$) and resulted in superior inhibition of inflammation [28]. In the ERASER study [121], however, the rate of late re-infarction (> 6 month) remained unaffected.

5. Conclusion

Despite its efficacy, ASA is a relatively weak antiplatelet drug, and ADP receptor antagonists like clopidogrel are only marginally superior to ASA in the reduction of AMI and stroke. Furthermore, adverse ischemic events probably due to drug resistance remain a serious clinical problem. The combination of different antiplatelet substances may implicate additive properties and is proven to be beneficial for patients, in whom monotherapy is not sufficient (non-responders) or who implicate a high thrombotic risk after coronary interventions. Given the predominate role of PLTs in the mechanism of stent thrombosis, dual antiplatelet therapy has reduced its incidence to less than 1.5% in most recent studies. Meanwhile, the combination of several (even three) antiplatelet drugs has become the standard of care in these situations. A future challenge, however, is to depict patients at especially high risk for post-interventional thrombotic complications, who may have additional benefit from the optimal antiplatelet therapy, probably with new antiplatelet regimens.

6. References

[1] Gawaz M, Reininger A, Neumann FJ. Platelet function and platelet-leukocyte adhesion in symptomatic coronary heart disease. Effects of intravenous magnesium. Thromb Res 1996; 83:341-349

[2] Trip MD, Cats VM, van Capelle FJ, Vreeken J. Platelet hyperreactivity and prognosis in survivors of myocardial infarction. N Engl J Med. 1990;322:1549-1554.

[3] Tschoepe D, Roesen P, Esser J, Schwippert B, Nieuwenhuis HK, Kehrel B, Gries FA. Large platelets circulate in an activated state in diabetes mellitus. Semin Thromb Hemost 1991;17:433-438

[4] Bihour C, Durrieu-Jaïs C, Macchi L, Poujol C, Coste P, Besse P, Nurden P, Nurden AT. Expression of markers of platelet activation and the interpatient variation in response to abciximab. Arterioscler Thromb Vasc Biol 1999;19:212-219

[5] Gawaz M, Neumann FJ, Ott I, Schiessler A, Schömig A. Platelet function in acute myocardial infarction treated with direct angioplasty. Circulation 1996;93:229-237

[6] Gawaz M, Neumann FJ, Ott I, May A, Rüdiger S, Schömig A. Role of activation-dependent platelet membrane glycoproteins in development of subacute occlusive coronary stent thrombosis. Coron Artery Dis 1997;8:121-128

[7] Gawaz M, Neumann FJ, Ott I, May A, Rüdiger S, Schömig A. Changes in membrane glycoproteins of circulating platelets after coronary stent implantation. Heart 1996;76:166-172

[8] Gawaz M. Blood platelets. Physiology, pathophysiology, membrane receptors, antiplatelet principles, and therapy for atherothrombotic diseases. Georg Thieme Verlag (eds.) Stuttgart, New York 2001

[9] Fitzgerald DJ, Roy L, Catella F, FitzGerald GA. Platelet activation in unstable coronary disease. N Engl J Med 1986;315:983-989

[10] Willerson JT, Golino P, Eidt J, Campbell WB, Buja LM. Specific platelet mediators and unstable coronary artery lesions. Experimental evidence and potential clinical implications. Circulation 1989;80:198-205

[11] Gawaz M. Role of platelets in coronary thrombosis and reperfusion of ischemic myocardium. Cardiovasc Res 2004;61:498-511

[12] Ito H. No reflow phenomenon in coronary heart disease. J Cardiol 2001;37:39-42

[13] Reininger AJ, Agneskirchner J, Bode PA, Spannagl M, Wurzinger LJ. c7E3 Fab inhibits low shear flow modulated platelet adhesion to endothelium and surface-absorbed fibrinogen by blocking platelet GP IIb/IIIa as well as endothelial vitronectin receptor--results from patients with acute myocardial infarction and healthy controls. Thromb Haemost 2000;83:217-223

[14] Neumann FJ, Blasini R, Schmitt C. Effect of glycoprotein IIb/IIIa receptor blockade on recovery of coronary flow and left ventriculkar function after the placement of coronary-artery stents in acute myocardial infarction. Circulation 1998;98:2695-2701

[15] Neumann FJ, Kastrati A, Schmitt C, Blasini R, Hadamitzky M, Mehilli J, Gawaz M, Schleef M, Seyfarth M, Dirschinger J, Schömig A. Effect of glycoprotein IIb/IIIa receptor blockade with abciximab on clinical and angiographic restenosis rate after the placement of coronary stents following acute myocardial infarction. J Am Coll Cardiol 2000;35:915-921

[16] Gawaz M, Neumann FJ, Ott I, May A, Rüdiger S, Schömig A. Role of activation-dependent platelet membrane glycoproteins in development of subacute occlusive coronary stent thrombosis. Coron Artery Dis 1997;8:121-128

[17] Neumann FJ, Gawaz M, Ott I, May A, Mössmer G, Schömig A. Prospective evaluation of hemostatic predictors of subacute stent thrombosis after coronary Palmaz-Schatz stenting. J Am Coll Cardiol 1996;27:15-21

[18] Schrör K. Aspirin and platelets: the antiplatelet action of aspirin and its role in thrombosis treatment and prophylaxis. Semin Thromb Hemost 1997;23:349-356

[19] Hall D. The aspirin-angiotensin-converting enzyme inhibitor tradeoff: to halve and halve not. J Am Coll Cardiol 2000;35:1808-1812

[20] Bates ER, Lau WC. Controversies in antiplatelet therapy for patients with cardiovascular disease. Circulation 2005;111:267-271

[21] Dorsam RT, Kunapuli SP. Central role of the P2Y12 receptor in platelet activation. J Clin Invest 2004;113:340-345

[22] Patrono C, Coller B, FitzGerald GA, Hirsh J, Roth G. Platelet-active drugs: the relationships among dose, effectiveness, and side effects: the Seventh ACCP Conference on Antithrombotic and Thrombolytic Therapy. Chest 2004;126:234S-264S

[23] Tantry US, Bliden KP, Gurbel PA. Prasugrel. Expert Opin Investig Drugs 2006;15:1627-1633

[24] Savcic M, Hauert J, Bachmann F, Wyld PJ, Geudelin B, Cariou R. Clopidogrel loading dose regimens: kinetic profile of pharmacodynamic response in healthy subjects. Semin Thromb Hemost 1999;25:15-19

[25] The CLEAR PLATELETS Investigators. Gurbel PA, Bliden KP, Zaman KA, Yoho JA, Hayes KM, Tantry US. Clopidogrel loading with eptifibatide to arrest the reactivity of platelets: results of the Clopidogrel Loading With Eptifibatide to Arrest the Reactivity of Platelets (CLEAR PLATELETS) study. Circulation 2005;111:1153-1159

[26] Matetzky S, Shenkman B, Guetta V, Shechter M, Bienart R, Goldenberg I, Novikov I, Pres H, Savion N, Varon D, Hod H. Clopidogrel resistance is associated with increased risk of recurrent atherothrombotic events in patients with acute myocardial infarction. Circulation 2004;109:3171-3175

[27] Cuisset T, Frere C, Quilici J, Morange PE, Nait-Saidi L, Mielot C, Bali L, Lambert M, Alessi MC, Bonnet JL. High post-treatment platelet reactivity is associated with a high incidence of myonecrosis after stenting for non-ST elevation acute coronary syndromes. Thromb Haemost;97:282-287

[28] The CLEAR PLATELETS 1b Investigators. Gurbel PA, Bliden KP, Tantry US. Effect of clopidogrel with and without eptifibatide on tumor necrosis factor-alpha and C-reactive protein release after elective stenting: results from the CLEAR PLATELETS 1b study. J Am Coll Cardiol 2006;48:2186-2191

[29] Gurbel PA, Tantry US. Clopidogrel resistance? Thromb Res 2007;120:311-321

[30] Hochholzer W, Trenk D, Bestehorn HP, Fischer B, Valina CM, Ferenc M, Gick M, Caputo A, Büttner HJ, Neumann FJ. Impact of the degree of peri-interventional platelet inhibition after loading with clopidogrel on early clinical outcome of elective coronary stent placement. J Am Coll Cardiol 2006;48:1742-1750

[31] Sweeny JM, Gorog DA, Fuster V. Antiplatelet drug 'resistance'. Part 1: mechanisms and clinical measurements. Nat Rev Cardiol 2009;6:273-282

[32] The RESPONSE Investigators. Gurbel PA, Bliden KP, Butler K, Antonino MJ, Wei C, Teng R, Rasmussen L, Storey RF, Nielsen T, Eikelboom JW, Sabe-Affaki G, Husted S, Kereiakes DJ, Henderson D, Patel DV, Tantry US. Response to ticagrelor in clopidogrel nonresponders and responders and effect of switching therapies: the RESPOND study. Circulation 2010;121:1188-1199

[33] The CURRENT-OASIS 7 Investigators. Mehta SR, Tanguay JF, Eikelboom JW, Jolly SS, Joyner CD, Granger CB, Faxon DP, Rupprecht HJ, Budaj A, Avezum A, Widimsky P, Steg PG, Bassand JP, Montalescot G, Macaya C, Di Pasquale G, Niemela K, Ajani AE, White HD, Chrolavicius S, Gao P, Fox KA, Yusuf S; CURRENT-OASIS 7 trial investigators. Double-dose versus standard-dose clopidogrel and high-dose versus low-dose aspirin in individuals undergoing percutaneous coronary intervention for acute coronary syndromes (CURRENT-OASIS 7): a randomised factorial trial. Lancet 2010;376:1233-1243

[34] The CHAMPION Investigators. Harrington RA, Stone GW, McNulty S, White HD, Lincoff AM, Gibson CM, Pollack CV Jr, Montalescot G, Mahaffey KW, Kleiman NS, Goodman SG, Amine M, Angiolillo DJ, Becker RC, Chew DP, French WJ, Leisch F, Parikh KH, Skerjanec S, Bhatt DL. Platelet inhibition with cangrelor in patients undergoing PCI. N Engl J Med 2009;361:2318-2329

[35] The CHAMPION-PLATFORM Investigators. Bhatt DL, Lincoff AM, Gibson CM, Stone GW, McNulty S, Montalescot G, Kleiman NS, Goodman SG, White HD, Mahaffey KW, Pollack CV Jr, Manoukian SV, Widimsky P, Chew DP, Cura F, Manukov I, Tousek F, Jafar MZ, Arneja J, Skerjanec S, Harrington RA. Intravenous platelet blockade with cangrelor during PCI. N Engl J Med 2009;361:2330-2341

[36] Ueno M, Kodali M, Tello-Montoliu A, Angiolillo DJ. Role of Platelets and Antiplatelet Therapy in Cardiovascular Disease. J Atheroscler Thromb 2011 [Epub ahead of print]

[37] Farid NA, Kurihara A, Wrighton SA. Metabolism and disposition of the thienopyridine antiplatelet drugs ticlopidine, clopidogrel, and prasugrel in humans. J Clin Pharmacol 2010;50:126-142. Erratum in J Clin Pharmacol 2010;50:483

[38] Jakubowski JA, Payne CD, Brandt JT, Weerakkody GJ, Farid NA, Small DS, Naganuma H, Li GY, Winters KJ. The platelet inhibitory effects and pharmacokinetics of prasugrel after administration of loading and maintenance doses in healthy subjects. J Cardiovasc Pharmacol 2006;47:377-384

[39] The PRINCIPLE-TIMI 44 Investigators. Wiviott SD, Trenk D, Frelinger AL, O'Donoghue M, Neumann FJ, Michelson AD, Angiolillo DJ, Hod H, Montalescot G, Miller DL, Jakubowski JA, Cairns R, Murphy SA, McCabe CH, Antman EM, Braunwald E; PRINCIPLE-TIMI 44 Investigators. Prasugrel compared with high loading- and maintenance-dose clopidogrel in patients with planned percutaneous coronary intervention: the Prasugrel in Comparison to Clopidogrel for Inhibition of Platelet Activation and Aggregation-Thrombolysis in Myocardial Infarction 44 trial. Circulation 2007;116:2923-2932

[40] The TRITON-TIMI 38 Investigators. Montalescot G, Wiviott SD, Braunwald E, Murphy SA, Gibson CM, McCabe CH, Antman EM. Prasugrel compared with clopidogrel in patients undergoing percutaneous coronary intervention for ST-elevation myocardial infarction (TRITON-TIMI 38): double-blind, randomised controlled trial. Lancet 2009;373:723-731

[41] Freeman MK. Thienopyridine antiplatelet agents: focus on prasugrel. Consult Pharm 2010;25:241-257

[42] The CHARISMA Investigators. Berger PB, Bhatt DL, Fuster V, Steg PG, Fox KA, Shao M, Brennan DM, Hacke W, Montalescot G, Steinhubl SR, Topol EJ; CHARISMA Investigators. Bleeding complications with dual antiplatelet therapy among patients with stable vascular disease or risk factors for vascular disease: results from the Clopidogrel for High Atherothrombotic Risk and Ischemic Stabilization, Management, and Avoidance (CHARISMA) trial. Circulation 2010;121:2575-2583

[43] The JUMBO-TIMI 26 Investigators. Wiviott SD, Antman EM, Winters KJ, Weerakkody G, Murphy SA, Behounek BD, Carney RJ, Lazzam C, McKay RG, McCabe CH, Braunwald E. Randomized comparison of prasugrel (CS-747, LY640315), a novel thienopyridine P2Y12 antagonist, with clopidogrel in percutaneous coronary intervention: results of the Joint Utilization of Medications to Block Platelets Optimally (JUMBO)-TIMI 26 trial. Circulation 2005;111:3366-3373

[44] The PLATO Investigators. Held C, Asenblad N, Bassand JP, Becker RC, Cannon CP, Claeys MJ, Harrington RA, Horrow J, Husted S, James SK, Mahaffey KW, Nicolau JC, Scirica BM, Storey RF, Vintila M, Ycas J, Wallentin L. Ticagrelor versus clopidogrel in patients with acute coronary syndromes undergoing coronary artery bypass surgery: results from the PLATO (Platelet Inhibition and Patient Outcomes) trial. J Am Coll Cardiol 2011;57:672-684

[45] Gurbel PA, Bliden KP, Antonino MJ, Stephens G, Gretler DD, Jurek MM, Pakyz RE, Shuldiner AR, Conley PB, Tantry US. The effect of elinogrel on high platelet reactivity during dual antiplatelet therapy and the relation to CYP2C19*2 genotype: first experience in patients. J Thromb Haemost 2010;8:43-53

[46] The INNOVATE-PCI Investigatos. Leonardi S, Rao SV, Harrington RA, Bhatt DL, Gibson CM, Roe MT, Kochman J, Huber K, Zeymer U, Madan M, Gretler DD,

McClure MW, Paynter GE, Thompson V, Welsh RC. Rationale and design of the randomized, double-blind trial testing INtraveNous and Oral administration of elinogrel, a selective and reversible P2Y(12)-receptor inhibitor, versus clopidogrel to eVAluate Tolerability and Efficacy in nonurgent Percutaneous Coronary Interventions patients (INNOVATE-PCI). Am Heart J 2010;160:65-72

[47] Maalej N, Osman HE, Shanmuganayagam D, Shebuski RJ, Folts JD. Antithrombotic properties of the thromboxane A2/prostaglandin H2 receptor antagonist S18886 on prevention of platelet-dependent cyclic flow reductions in dogs. J Cardiovasc Pharmacol 2005;45:389-395

[48] Vilahur G, Casaní L, Badimon L. A thromboxane A2/prostaglandin H2 receptor antagonist (S18886) shows high antithrombotic efficacy in an experimental model of stent-induced thrombosis. Thromb Haemost 2007;98:662-669

[49] Belhassen L, Pelle G, Dubois-Rande JL, Adnot S. Improved endothelial function by the thromboxane A2 receptor antagonist S 18886 in patients with coronary artery disease treated with aspirin. J Am Coll Cardiol 2003;41:1198-1204

[50] Verbeuren TJ, Vallez MO, Lavielle G, Bouskela E. Activation of thromboxane receptors and the induction of vasomotion in the hamster cheek pouch microcirculation. Br J Pharmacol 1997;122:859-866

[51] Balsano F, Violi F. Effect of picotamide on the clinical progression of peripheral vascular disease. A double-blind placebo-controlled study. The ADEP Group. Circulation 1993;87:1563-1569

[52] Milani M, Longoni A, Maderna M. Effects of picotamide, an antiplatelet agent, on cardiovascular, events in 438 claudicant patients with diabetes: a retrospective analysis of the ADEP study. Br J Clin Pharmacol 1996;42:782-785

[53] The DAVID Investigators. Neri Serneri GG, Coccheri S, Marubini E, Violi F; Drug Evaluation in Atherosclerotic Vascular Disease in Diabetics (DAVID). Picotamide, a combined inhibitor of thromboxane A2 synthase and receptor, reduces 2-year mortality in diabetics with peripheral arterial disease: the DAVID study. Eur Heart J 2004;25:1845-1852

[54] The TRA-PCI Investigators. Becker RC, Moliterno DJ, Jennings LK, Pieper KS, Pei J, Niederman A, Ziada KM, Berman G, Strony J, Joseph D, Mahaffey KW, Van de Werf F, Veltri E, Harrington RA. Safety and tolerability of SCH 530348 in patients undergoing non-urgent percutaneous coronary intervention: a randomised, double-blind, placebo-controlled phase II study. Lancet 2009;373:919-928

[55] The LANCELOT-ACS Investigators. O'Donoghue ML, Bhatt DL, Wiviott SD, Goodman SG, Fitzgerald DJ, Angiolillo DJ, Goto S, Montalescot G, Zeymer U, Aylward PE, Guetta V, Dudek D, Ziecina R, Contant CF, Flather MD. Safety and tolerability of atopaxar in the treatment of patients with acute coronary syndromes: the lessons from antagonizing the cellular effects of Thrombin–Acute Coronary Syndromes Trial. Circulation 2011;123:1843-1853

[56] The ESPS 2 Investigators. Diener HC, Cunha L, Forbes C, Sivenius J, Smets P, Lowenthal A. European Stroke Prevention Study. 2. Dipyridamole and acetylsalicylic acid in the secondary prevention of stroke. J Neurol Sci 1996;143:1-13

[57] The PRoFESS Investigators. Diener HC, Sacco RL, Yusuf S, Cotton D, Ounpuu S, Lawton WA, Palesch Y, Martin RH, Albers GW, Bath P, Bornstein N, Chan BP, Chen ST, Cunha L, Dahlöf B, De Keyser J, Donnan GA, Estol C, Gorelick P, Gu V,

Hermansson K, Hilbrich L, Kaste M, Lu C, Machnig T, Pais P, Roberts R, Skvortsova V, Teal P, Toni D, VanderMaelen C, Voigt T, Weber M, Yoon BW; Prevention Regimen for Effectively Avoiding Second Strokes (PRoFESS) study group. Effects of aspirin plus extended-release dipyridamole versus clopidogrel and telmisartan on disability and cognitive function after recurrent stroke in patients with ischaemic stroke in the Prevention Regimen for Effectively Avoiding Second Strokes (PRoFESS) trial: a double-blind, active and placebo-controlled study. Lancet Neurol 2008;7:875-84, Erratum in Lancet Neurol 2008;7:985

[58] The ACCEL-AMI Investigators. Jeong YH, Hwang JY, Kim IS, Park Y, Hwang SJ, Lee SW, Kwak CH, Park SW. Adding cilostazol to dual antiplatelet therapy achieves greater platelet inhibition than high maintenance dose clopidogrel in patients with acute myocardial infarction: Results of the adjunctive cilostazol versus high maintenance dose clopidogrel in patients with AMI (ACCEL-AMI) study. Circ Cardiovasc Interv 2010;3:17-26

[59] The DECREASE Investigators. Lee SW, Park SW, Yun SC, Kim YH, Park DW, Kim WJ, Lee JY, Lee CW, Hong MK, Kim JJ, Park SJ. Triple antiplatelet therapy reduces ischemic events after drug-eluting stent implantation: Drug-Eluting stenting followed by Cilostazol treatment REduces Adverse Serious cadiac Events (DECREASE registry). Am Heart J 2010;159:284-291

[60] Kozlowski EO, Pavao MS, Borsig L. Ascidian dermatan sulfates attenuate metastasis, inflammation and thrombosis by inhibition of P-selectin. J Thromb Haemost 2011;1111:1538-7836

[61] Surin WR, Barthwal MK, Dikshit M. Platelet collagen receptors, signaling and antagonism: emerging approaches for the prevention of intravascular thrombosis. Thromb Res 2008;122:786-803

[62] Di Minno MN, Prisco D, Ruocco AL, Mastronardi P, Massa S, Di Minno G. Perioperative handling of patients on antiplatelet therapy with need for surgery. Intern Emerg Med 2009;4:279-288

[63] Segev A, Strauss BH, Tan M, Constance C, Langer A, Goodman SG; Canadian Acute Coronary Syndromes Registries Investigators. Predictors and 1-year outcome of major bleeding in patients with non-ST-elevation acute coronary syndromes: insights from the Canadian Acute Coronary Syndrome Registries. Am Heart J 2005;150:690-694

[64] Picker SM, Kaleta T, Hekmat K, Kampe S, Gathof BS. Antiplatelet therapy preceding coronary artery surgery: implications for bleeding, transfusion requirements and outcome. Eur J Anaesthesiol 2007;24:332-329

[65] Iakovou I, Schmidt T, Bonizzoni E, Ge L, Sangiorgi GM, Stankovic G, Airoldi F, Chieffo A, Montorfano M, Carlino M, Michev I, Corvaja N, Briguori C, Gerckens U, Grube E, Colombo A. Incidence, predictors, and outcome of thrombosis after successful implantation of drug-eluting stents. JAMA 2005;293:2126-2130

[66] Antithrombotic Trialists' (ATT) Collaboration, Baigent C, Blackwell L, Collins R, Emberson J, Godwin J, Peto R, Buring J, Hennekens C, Kearney P, Meade T, Patrono C, Roncaglioni MC, Zanchetti A. Aspirin in the primary and secondary prevention of vascular disease: collaborative meta-analysis of individual participant data from randomised trials. Lancet 2009;373:1849-1860

[67] Lièvre M, Cucherat M. Aspirin in the secondary prevention of cardiovascular disease: an update of the APTC meta-analysis. Fundam Clin Pharmacol 2010;24:385-391
[68] Antiplatelet trialists collaboration. Collaborative overview of randomized trials of antiplatelet therapy-I: Prevention of death, myocardial infarction and stroke by prolonged antiplatelet therapy in various categories of patients. BMJ 1994;308:81-106
[69] Peto R, Gray R, Collins R, Wheatley K, Hennekens C, Jamrozik K, Warlow C, Hafner B, Thompson E, Norton S. Randomised trial of prophylactic daily aspirin in British male doctors. Br Med J (Clin Res Ed) 1988;296:313-316
[70] Lewis HD Jr, Davis JW, Archibald DG, Steinke WE, Smitherman TC, Doherty JE 3rd, Schnaper HW, LeWinter MM, Linares E, Pouget JM, Sabharwal SC, Chesler E, DeMots H. Protective effects of aspirin against acute myocardial infarction and death in men with unstable angina. Results of a Veterans Administration Cooperative Study. N Engl J Med 1983;309:396-403
[71] Cairns JA, Gent M, Singer J, Finnie KJ, Froggatt GM, Holder DA, Jablonsky G, Kostuk WJ, Melendez LJ, Myers MG. Aspirin, sulfinpyrazone, or both in unstable angina. Results of a Canadian multicenter trial. N Engl J Med 1985;313:1369-1375
[72] The RISK Group. Risk of myocardial infarction and death during treatment with low dose aspirin and intravenous heparin in men with unstable coronary artery disease. Lancet 1990;336:827-830
[73] Juul-Möller S, Edvardsson N, Jahnmatz B, Rosén A, Sørensen S, Omblus R. Double-blind trial of aspirin in primary prevention of myocardial infarction in patients with stable chronic angina pectoris. The Swedish Angina Pectoris Aspirin Trial (SAPAT) Group. Lancet 1992;340:1421-1425
[74] Théroux P, Ouimet H, McCans J, Latour JG, Joly P, Lévy G, Pelletier E, Juneau M, Stasiak J, deGuise P. Aspirin, heparin, or both to treat acute unstable angina. N Engl J Med 1988;319:1105-1111
[75] The CAPRIE Steering Committee. A randomised, blinded, trial of clopidogrel versus aspirin in patients at risk of ischaemic events (CAPRIE). Lancet 1996;348:1329-1339
[76] The CURE committee. The Clopidogrel in Unstable angina to prevent Recurrent Events (CURE) trial programme. Rationale, design and baseline characteristics including a meta-analysis of the effects of thienopyridines in vascular disease. Eur Heart J 2000;21:2033-2041
[77] The CREDO Investigators. Steinhubl SR, Berger PB, Mann JT 3rd, Fry ET, DeLago A, Wilmer C, Topol EJ. Clopidogrel for the Reduction of Events During Observation. Early and sustained dual oral antiplatelet therapy following percutaneous coronary intervention: a randomized controlled trial. JAMA 2002;288:2411-2420, Erratum in JAMA 2003;289:987
[78] The CLARITY-TIMI 28 Investigators. Sabatine MS, Cannon CP, Gibson CM, López-Sendón JL, Montalescot G, Theroux P, Lewis BS, Murphy SA, McCabe CH, Braunwald E; Clopidogrel as Adjunctive Reperfusion Therapy (CLARITY)-Thrombolysis in Myocardial Infarction (TIMI) 28. Effect of clopidogrel pretreatment before percutaneous coronary intervention in patients with ST-elevation myocardial infarction treated with fibrinolytics: the PCI-CLARITY study. JAMA 2005;294:1224-1232

[79] The COMMIT Investigators. Chen ZM, Jiang LX, Chen YP, Xie JX, Pan HC, Peto R, Collins R, Liu LS; COMMIT (ClOpidogrel and Metoprolol in Myocardial Infarction Trial) collaborative group. Addition of clopidogrel to aspirin in 45,852 patients with acute myocardial infarction: randomised placebo-controlled trial. Lancet 2005;366:1607-1621

[80] Hart RG, Bhatt DL, Hacke W, Fox KA, Hankey GJ, Berger PB, Hu T, Topol EJ. Clopidogrel and aspirin versus aspirin alone for the prevention of stroke in patients with a history of atrial fibrillation: subgroup analysis of the CHARISMA randomized trial. Cerebrovasc Dis 2008;25:344-347

[81] Gurbel PA, Serebruany VL, Shustov AR, Bahr RD, Carpo C, Ohman EM, Topol EJ. Effects of reteplase and alteplase on platelet aggregation and major receptor expression during the first 24 hours of acute myocardial infarction treatment. GUSTO-III Investigators. Global Use of Strategies to Open Occluded Coronary Arteries. J Am Coll Cardiol 1998;31:1466-1473

[82] The TAMI 8 Investigators. Kleiman NS, Ohman EM, Califf RM, George BS, Kereiakes D, Aguirre FV, Weisman H, Schaible T, Topol EJ. Profound inhibition of platelet aggregation with monoclonal antibody 7E3 Fab after thrombolytic therapy. Results of the Thrombolysis and Angioplasty in Myocardial Infarction (TAMI) 8 Pilot Study. J Am Coll Cardiol 1993;22:381-289

[83] The TIMI 14 Investigators. Antman EM, Gibson CM, de Lemos JA, Giugliano RP, McCabe CH, Coussement P, Menown I, Nienaber CA, Rehders TC, Frey MJ, Van der Wieken R, Andresen D, Scherer J, Anderson K, Van de Werf F, Braunwald E. Combination reperfusion therapy with abciximab and reduced dose reteplase: results the Thrombolysis in Myocardial Infarction (TIMI) 14 study. Eur Heart J 2000;21:1944-1953

[84] The IMPACT-AMI Investigators. Ohman EM, Kleiman NS, Gacioch G, Worley SJ, Navetta FI, Talley JD, Anderson HV, Ellis SG, Cohen MD, Spriggs D, Miller M, Kereiakes D, Yakubov S, Kitt MM, Sigmon KN, Califf RM, Krucoff MW, Topol EJ. Combined accelerated tissue-plasminogen activator and platelet glycoprotein IIb/IIIa integrin receptor blockade with Integrilin in acute myocardial infarction. Results of a randomized, placebo-controlled, dose-ranging trial. Circulation 1997;95:846-854

[85] The PARADIGM Investigators. Combining thrombolysis with the platelet glycoprotein IIb/IIIa inhibitor lamifiban: results of the Platelet Aggregation Receptor Antagonist Dose Investigation and Reperfusion Gain in Myocardial Infarction (PARADIGM) trial. J Am Coll Cardiol 1998;32:2003-2010

[86] The GUSTO V Investigators. Topol EJ. Reperfusion therapy for acute myocardial infarction with fibrinolytic therapy or combination reduced fibrinolytic therapy and platelet glycoprotein IIb/IIIa inhibition: the GUSTO V randomised trial. Lancet 2001;357:1905-1914

[87] Fernandez JS, Sadaniantz BT, Sadaniantz A. Review of antithrombotic agents used for acute coronary syndromes in renal patients. Am J Kidney Dis 2003;42:446-455

[88] The CAPTURE investigators. Randomized placebo-controlled trial of abciximab before and during coronary intervention in refractory unstable angina: the CUPTURE study. Lancet 1997;349:1429-1435

[89] The EPIC Investigators. Topol EJ, Califf RM, Weisman HF, Ellis SG, Tcheng JE, Worley S, Ivanhoe R, George BS, Fintel D, Weston M. Randomised trial of coronary intervention with antibody against platelet IIb/IIIa integrin for reduction of clinical restenosis: results at six months. Lancet 1994;343:881-886

[90] The EPILOG Investigators. Platelet glycoprotein IIb/IIIa receptor blockade and low-dose heparin during percutaneous coronary revascularization. N Engl J Med 1997;336:1689-1696

[91] The CADILLAC Investigators. Stone GW, Grines CL, Cox DA, Garcia E, Tcheng JE, Griffin JJ, Guagliumi G, Stuckey T, Turco M, Carroll JD, Rutherford BD, Lansky AJ; Controlled Abciximab and Device Investigation to Lower Late Angioplasty Complications (CADILLAC). Comparison of angioplasty with stenting, with or without abciximab, in acute myocardial infarction. N Engl J Med 2002;346:957-966

[92] The ESPRIT Investigators. Enhanced Suppression of the Platelet IIb/IIIa Receptor with Integrilin Therapy. Lancet 2000;356:2037-44. Erratum in Lancet 2001;357:1370

[93] The EPISTENT Investigators. Topol EJ, Mark DB, Lincoff AM, Cohen E, Burton J, Kleiman N, Talley D, Sapp S, Booth J, Cabot CF, Anderson KM, Califf RM. Outcomes at 1 year and economic implications of platelet glycoprotein IIb/IIIa blockade in patients undergoing coronary stenting: results from a multicentre randomised trial. EPISTENT Investigators. Evaluation of Platelet IIb/IIIa Inhibitor for Stenting. Lancet 1999;354:2019-2024, Erratum in Lancet 2000;355:1104

[94] The STENT Investigators. Lincoff AM, LeNarz LA, Despotis GJ, Smith PK, Booth JE, Raymond RE, Sapp SK, Cabot CF, Tcheng JE, Califf RM, Effron MB, Topol EJ. Abciximab and bleeding during coronary surgery: results from the EPILOG and EPISTENT trials. Improve Long-term Outcome with abciximab GP IIb/IIIa blockade. Evaluation of Platelet IIb/IIIa Inhibition in STENTing. Ann Thorac Surg 2000;70:516-526

[95] The PARAGON Investigators. International, randomized, controlled trial of lamifiban (a platelet glycoprotein IIb/IIIa inhibitor), heparin, or both in unstable angina. Platelet IIb/IIIa Antagonism for the Reduction of Acute coronary syndrome events in a Global Organization Network. Circulation 1998;97:2386-2395

[96] The PRISM-PLUS Investigators. Inhibition of the platelet glycoprotein IIb/IIIa receptor with tirofiban in unstable angina and non-Q-wave myocardial infarction. Platelet Receptor Inhibition in Ischemic Syndrome Management in Patients Limited by Unstable Signs and Symptoms (PRISM-PLUS). N Engl J Med 1998;338:1488-1497 Erratum in N Engl J Med 1998;339:415

[97] The PRISM Investigators. A comparison of aspirin plus tirofiban with aspirin plus heparin for unstable angina. Platelet Receptor Inhibition in Ischemic Syndrome Management (PRISM). N Engl J Med 1998;338:1498-1505

[98] The PURSUIT Investigators. Inhibition of platelet glycoprotein IIb/IIIa with eptifibatide in patients with acute coronary syndromes. N Eng J Med 1998;339:436-443

[99] Dyke CM, Bhatia D, Lorenz TJ, Marso SP, Tardiff BE, Hogeboom C, Harrington RA. Immediate coronary artery bypass surgery after platelet inhibition with eptifibatide: results from PURSUIT. Platelet Glycoprotein IIb/IIIa in Unstable Angina: Receptor Suppression Using Integrelin Therapy. Ann Thorac Surg 2000;70:866-871

[100] The GUSTO IV-ACS Investigators. Simoons ML. Effect of glycoprotein IIb/IIIa receptor blocker abciximab on outcome in patients with acute coronary syndromes without early coronary revascularisation: the GUSTO IV-ACS randomised trial. Lancet 2001;357:1915-1924

[101] The RAPPORT Investigators. Brener SJ, Barr LA, Burchenal JE, Katz S, George BS, Jones AA, Cohen ED, Gainey PC, White HJ, Cheek HB, Moses JW, Moliterno DJ, Effron MB, Topol EJ. Randomized, placebo-controlled trial of platelet glycoprotein IIb/IIIa blockade with primary angioplasty for acute myocardial infarction. ReoPro and Primary PTCA Organization and Randomized Trial (RAPPORT). Circulation 1998;98:734-741

[102] The RESTORE Investigators. Effects of platelet glycoprotein IIb/IIIa blockade with tirofiban on adverse cardiac events in patients with unstable angina or acute myocardial infarction undergoing coronary angioplasty. Randomized Efficacy Study of Tirofiban for Outcomes and REstenosis. Circulation 1997;96:1445-1453

[103] The IMPACT-II Investigators. Blankenship JC, Sigmon KN, Pieper KS, O'Shea C, Tardiff BE, Tcheng JE. Effect of eptifibatide on angiographic complications during percutaneous coronary intervention in the IMPACT-II Trial-(Integrilin to Minimize Platelet Aggregation and Coronary Thrombosis II Trial). Am J Cardiol 2001;88:969-973

[104] The TACTICS Investigators. Cannon CP, Weintraub WS, Demopoulos LA, Vicari R, Frey MJ, Lakkis N, Neumann FJ, Robertson DH, DeLucca PT, DiBattiste PM, Gibson CM, Braunwald E; TACTICS (Treat Angina with Aggrastat and Determine Cost of Therapy with an Invasive or Conservative Strategy)--Thrombolysis in Myocardial Infarction 18. Comparison of early invasive and conservative strategies in patients with unstable coronary syndromes treated with the glycoprotein IIb/IIIa inhibitor tirofiban. N Engl J Med 2001;344:1879-1887

[105] The TARGET Investigators. Topol EJ, Moliterno DJ, Herrmann HC, Powers ER, Grines CL, Cohen DJ, Cohen EA, Bertrand M, Neumann FJ, Stone GW, DiBattiste PM, Demopoulos L. Do Tirofiban and ReoPro Give Similar Efficacy Trial. Comparison of two platelet glycoprotein IIb/IIIa inhibitors, tirofiban and abciximab, for the prevention of ischemic events with percutaneous coronary revascularization. N Engl J Med 2001;344:1888-1894

[106] Braunwald E, Antman EM, Beasley JW, Califf RM, Cheitlin MD, Hochman JS, Jones RH, Kereiakes D, Kupersmith J, Levin TN, Pepine CJ, Schaeffer JW, Smith EE 3rd, Steward DE, Theroux P, Gibbons RJ, Alpert JS, Faxon DP, Fuster V, Gregoratos G, Hiratzka LF, Jacobs AK, Smith SC Jr; American College of Cardiology; American Heart Association. Committee on the Management of Patients With Unstable Angina.ACC/AHA 2002 guideline update for the management of patients with unstable angina and non-ST-segment elevation myocardial infarction--summary article: a report of the American College of Cardiology/American Heart Association task force on practice guidelines (Committee on the Management of Patients With Unstable Angina). J Am Coll Cardiol 2002;40:1366-1374

[107] Harrington RA, Becker RC, Ezekowitz M, Meade TW, O'Connor CM, Vorchheimer DA, Guyatt GH. Antithrombotic therapy for coronary artery disease: the Seventh ACCP Conference on Antithrombotic and Thrombolytic Therapy. Chest 2004;126:513S-548S

[108] White HD, Frensh JK, Elllis CJ. New antiplatelet agents. Auts N Z J Med 1998;28:558-564

[109] Bourassa MG, Alderman EL, Bertrand M, de la Fuente L, Gratsianski A, Kaltenbach M, King SB, Nobuyoshi M, Romaniuk P, Ryan TJ. Report of the joint meeting of the International Society and Federation of Cardiology and the World Health Organization Task Force on Coronary Angioplasty. Arch Mal Coeur Vaiss 1989;82:2053-2063

[110] Popma JJ, Topol EJ. Factors influencing restenosis after coronary angioplasty. Am J Med 1990;88:16N-24N

[111] Chassot PG, Delabays A, Spahn DR. Perioperative antiplatelet therapy: the case for continuing therapy in patients at risk of myocardial infarction. Br J Anaesth 2007;99:316-328

[112] The CLEAR PLATELETS 2 Investigators. Gurbel PA, Bliden KP, Saucedo JF, Suarez TA, DiChiara J, Antonino MJ, Mahla E, Singla A, Herzog WR, Bassi AK, Hennebry TA, Gesheff TB, Tantry US. Bivalirudin and clopidogrel with and without eptifibatide for elective stenting: effects on platelet function, thrombelastographic indexes, and their relation to periprocedural infarction results of the CLEAR PLATELETS-2 (Clopidogrel with Eptifibatide to Arrest the Reactivity of Platelets) study. J Am Coll Cardiol 2009;53:648-657

[113] Schömig A, Neumann FJ, Kastrati A, Schühlen H, Blasini R, Hadamitzky M, Walter H, Zitzmann-Roth EM, Richardt G, Alt E, Schmitt C, Ulm K. A randomized comparison of antiplatelet and anticoagulant therapy after the placement of coronary-artery stents. N Engl J Med 1996;334:1084-1089

[114] The MATTIS Investigator. Urban P, Macaya C, Rupprecht HJ, Kiemeneij F, Emanuelsson H, Fontanelli A, Pieper M, Wesseling T, Sagnard L. Randomized evaluation of anticoagulation versus antiplatelet therapy after coronary stent implantation in high-risk patients: the multicenter aspirin and ticlopidine trial after intracoronary stenting (MATTIS). Circulation 1998;98:2126-2132

[115] The FANTASTIC Investigators. Bertrand ME, Legrand V, Boland J, Fleck E, Bonnier J, Emmanuelson H, Vrolix M, Missault L, Chierchia S, Casaccia M, Niccoli L, Oto A, White C, Webb-Peploe M, Van Belle E, McFadden EP. Randomized multicenter comparison of conventional anticoagulation versus antiplatelet therapy in unplanned and elective coronary stenting. The full anticoagulation versus aspirin and ticlopidine (FANTASTIC) study. Circulation 1998;98:1597-1603

[116] The STARS Investigators. Leon MB, Baim DS, Popma JJ, Gordon PC, Cutlip DE, Ho KK, Giambartolomei A, Diver DJ, Lasorda DM, Williams DO, Pocock SJ, Kuntz RE. A clinical trial comparing three antithrombotic-drug regimens after coronary-artery stenting. Stent Anticoagulation Restenosis Study. N Engl J Med 1998;339:1665-1671

[117] King SB 3rd, Smith SC Jr, Hirshfeld JW Jr, Jacobs AK, Morrison DA, Williams DO, Feldman TE, Kern MJ, O'Neill WW, Schaff HV, Whitlow PL; ACC/AHA/SCAI, Adams CD, Anderson JL, Buller CE, Creager MA, Ettinger SM, Halperin JL, Hunt SA, Krumholz HM, Kushner FG, Lytle BW, Nishimura R, Page RL, Riegel B, Tarkington LG, Yancy CW. 2007 focused update of the ACC/AHA/SCAI 2005 guideline update for percutaneous coronary intervention: a report of the American College of Cardiology/American Heart Association Task Force on Practice guidelines. J Am Coll Cardiol 2008;51:172-209

[118] The ADMIRAL Investigators. Montalescot G, Barragan P, Wittenberg O, Ecollan P, Elhadad S, Villain P, Boulenc JM, Morice MC, Maillard L, Pansiéri M, Choussat R, Pinton P;. Abciximab before Direct Angioplasty and Stenting in Myocardial Infarction Regarding Acute and Long-Term Follow-up. Platelet glycoprotein IIb/IIIa inhibition with coronary stenting for acute myocardial infarction. N Engl J Med 2001;344:1895-1903
[119] The ISAR-II Investigators. Schömig A, Kastrati A, Dirschinger J, Mehilli J, Schricke U, Pache J, Martinoff S, Neumann FJ, Schwaiger M. Coronary stenting plus platelet glycoprotein IIb/IIIa blockade compared with tissue plasminogen activator in acute myocardial infarction. N Engl J Med 2000;343:385-391
[120] The STOP-AMI Investigators. Schömig A, Kastrati A, Dirschinger J, Mehilli J, Schricke U, Pache J, Martinoff S, Neumann FJ, Schwaiger M. Coronary stenting plus platelet glycoprotein IIb/IIIa blockade compared with tissue plasminogen activator in acute myocardial infarction. Stent versus Thrombolysis for Occluded Coronary Arteries in Patients with Acute Myocardial Infarction. N Engl J Med 2000;343:385-391
[121] The ERASER Investigators. Acute platelet inhibition with abciximab does not reduce in-stent restenosis (ERASER study). Circulation 1999;100:799-806

14

Thyroid Hormone Therapy for the Cardiac Surgical Patient

Aaron M. Ranasinghe[1,2] and Robert S. Bonser[1,2]
[1]*University of Birmingham, Cardiovascular Medicine, School of Clinical and Experimental Medicine, Birmingham*
[2]*UHB NHS FT, Department of Cardiothoracic Surgery, Edgbaston, Birmingham*
UK

1. Introduction

Thyroid hormones (THs) are key regulators of metabolism. The thyroid gland produces both thyroxine (T4) and triiodothyronine (T3). T4 is the main product and is converted in the periphery via deiodination to T3 which is the main biologically active TH. The production of THs is regulated by thyrotrophin (TSH) in response to TSH releasing hormone (TRH). This, in turn, is regulated by a negative feedback mechanism related to serum levels of free T3 and T4 (fT3 and fT4). Binding of T3 to TH receptors (TR) followed by binding of T3-TR complex to thyroid response elements within TH responsive genes leads to changes in gene transcription. These effects of TH are present through a wide number of tissues and organ systems including the cardiovascular system.

2. Thyroid hormone and its actions on the cardiovascular system

The effects of TH on both the heart and peripheral vascular system have been well documented[1-9]. In states of TH excess (hyperthyroidism) a high cardiac output state secondary to increased heart rate and contractility with a reduction in systemic vascular resistance (SVR) is seen. In hypothyroidism, the reciprocal effects are observed. The reduction that is seen in SVR is an early response to TH administration[10, 11]. This may be partly due to the release of local vasodilators liberated as a result of increasing metabolic activity and oxygen consumption. The effects of TH on vascular tone may also be attributable to its direct effects on arteriolar smooth muscle. Intracoronary administration of TH in Langendorff preparations has been demonstrated to lead to coronary vasodilatation within 15 seconds[12] and in normal human subjects reductions in SVR are seen within minutes of administration[11], with this effect lasting for several hours when administered intra-operatively[13].

TH is able to manifest its effects on the cardiovascular system at both a genomic and non-genomic level; this means that with administration of TH there are immediate non-genomic cardiovascular consequences[6, 11, 14], followed by later genomic alterations which include alterations in the expression of the beta one adrenergic receptor (ADRB1). However, despite increasing receptor expression, there is a paucity of evidence that T3 administration increases sensitivity to catecholamines[15, 16]. TH also acts upon the expression of calcium handling proteins within the myocyte including the sarcoplasmic reticulum calcium ATPase (SERCA) and its negative regulator phospholamban (PLB). Administration of T3 increases the level of SERCA mRNA and protein and also lowers phospholamban levels and increases its phosphorylation state, which enhances the activity of SERCA[17-22]. The combined effect of these changes is an increase in the force of contraction and speed of diastolic relaxation.

3. The consequences of the hypo-and hyperthyroid states

Hypothyroid patients may have symptoms or signs associated with heart failure including dyspnoea, oedema, cardiomegaly and effusions. Low cardiac output in these patients is due to decreased heart rate, reduced ventricular filling and decreased myocardial contractility. Hypothyroidism is a risk factor for coronary artery disease[23], the incidence of angina and myocardial infarction is however lower and this may relate to a reduction in metabolic requirements of the myocardium. Hypothyroidism is associated with hypertension, secondary to alterations in peripheral vascular resistance. Prolongation of the cardiac action potential and QT interval are also noted [24] and this leads to an increased risk of ventricular arrhythmias in this group. Supplementation with TH can lead to a reversal of some of these cardiovascular manifestations[25]. However, in the setting of cardiac surgery post-operative reductions in circulating THs have been demonstrated to be associated with an increase in the occurrence of atrial fibrillation[26, 27]. The vast majority of patients who are hypothyroid are receiving hormone replacement therapy and are therefore euthyroid at the time of surgery. However, in theory, in the untreated hypothyroid patient acute TH replacement could worsen myocardial ischaemia if myocardial oxygen consumption were increased in the face of fixed oxygen delivery[28]. Surgery in the hypothyroid patient may be performed without increased risk. In patients with untreated mild to moderate hypothyroidism undergoing cardiac surgery, Drucker reported no adverse effects[29] and Syed et al. reported no increase in complications in patients with known hypothyroidism on treatment who were biochemically hypothyroid over those that were biochemically euthyroid without utilising additional TH replacement therapy[30]. O'Connor et al[31] in undiagnosed patients with hypothyroidism have reported the occurrence of severe myxoedema post cardiac surgery leading to significant haemodynamic compromise which recovered with replacement TH therapy.

Hyperthyroid patients commonly have a resting tachycardia. The most common rhythm disturbances are supraventricular arrhythmias including atrial fibrillation which predispose to thromboembolic diseases. Cardiac output may be supranormal (between 50-300% higher than in normal subjects). This is secondary to increases in heart rate, left ventricular contractility, blood volume and a reduction in SVR[8]. Improvements in LV systolic and diastolic function are believed to be modulated by changes in the expression of contractile and calcium regulating proteins (SERCA and PLB). Even though cardiac output is high it may be suboptimal at times of exertion[32], due to an inability to further augment heart rate or lower systemic vascular resistance. Long-term follow-up of patients with hyperthyroidism reveals an increased cardiovascular and cerebrovascular mortality. This may partially be related to the increased rate of supraventricular dysrhythmias[33,34]. In the setting of overt clinical and biochemical hyperthyroidism surgery should be deferred if possible, until the patient can be rendered euthyroid in order to avoid thyroid storm.

4. The non-thyroidal illness syndrome

In response to severe physiological stress including cardiac surgery, changes in circulating concentrations of T3, T4 and TSH occur. The term non-thyroidal illness syndrome (NTIS) has been used to describe this phenomenon as it makes no presumption regarding the metabolic state of the patient. Whether hormone supplementation to correct these abnormalities is beneficial or not is unproven and much debated[35]. There are a variety of mechanisms that could potentially explain the biochemical profile observed in the NTIS including modifications of the hypothalamic-pituitary-thyroid axis, altered binding of TH to circulating proteins, modified entry of TH into tissues, changes in TH metabolism due to modification of the iodothyronines deiodinases as well as changes in TH receptor expression or function[36]. Circulating levels of T3 decrease within two hours of severe physiological stress and this is thought to reflect a reduction in the peripheral conversion of T4 to T3[37, 38]. The most common abnormality observed in severely ill hospitalised patients is a low T3 syndrome, which occurs in up to 70% of patients[39]. Reduction in concentrations of free T3 (fT3) in hospitalised patients have been demonstrated to be predictive of mortality[40]. Deficiencies in TH metabolism have also been demonstrated to occur at a tissue level with a positive correlation between circulating and tissue TH levels[41]. As T3 levels fall reverse T3 (rT3, an inactive metabolite) increases. With increasing severity of illness, T4 levels also begin to fall (low T3-low T4 syndrome). Whether these observed responses are energy conserving to reduce metabolic rate or pathological requiring TH supplementation still remains a matter of debate.

5. The effects of cardiopulmonary bypass on circulating levels of thyroid hormone

With the stress response associated with surgery, concentrations of fT3 are noted with a more precipitous decline following institution of cardiopulmonary bypass (CPB). These further reductions may relate either to a secondary increase in the stress response or to haemodilution[42]. Occurrence of the NTIS has been well documented in the context of both adult and paediatric cardiac surgery[13, 43, 44]. Supplementation with both oral and intravenous T3 has been demonstrated to raise circulating T3 levels to normal or supra-normal levels[13, 45].

It was believed that occurrence of NTIS may be related to the stress response and haemodilution associated with CPB. However, data from patients undergoing cardiac surgery without CPB have demonstrated that the reductions in T3 that have previously been observed in trials of patients undergoing cardiac surgery utilising CPB also occur in the off-pump group to a similar magnitude. This implies that the NTIS during cardiac surgery is a non-specific stress response and CPB is not the only contributing factor to its occurrence[46, 47].

6. The rationale for treatment of the NTIS in patients undergoing cardiac surgery

If the NTIS is truly a maladaptive phenomenon, therapy with TH supplementation may have potentially beneficial effects by rectifying the observed abnormalities and increasing myocardial performance via both genomic and non-genomic mechanisms, thereby having the potential to improve patient outcomes.

In addition to the beneficial haemodynamic effects seen with T3 administration, there is a mounting body of both animal and clinical data suggesting that T3 may have a positive influence on protecting the myocyte following ischaemia. Two weeks administration of T4, followed by ischaemia and reperfusion in an isolated rodent heart model has been demonstrated to improve post-ischaemic function in T4 treated hearts with attenuation of activation of the p38 mitogen activated protein kinase (MAPK)[48]. In a murine coronary artery ligation model of acute myocardial ischaemia, animals administered T3 demonstrated improved haemodynamic function as well as reducing ischaemia induced apoptosis with an associated increase in Akt signalling compared with placebo[49]. In addition, following a period of global ischaemia in a rodent isolated heart model, T3 administered at reperfusion led to a reduction in apoptotic damage with reduced caspase-3 activity and activated p38 MAPK after one hour of reperfusion. These effects were associated with improved recovery of post-ischaemic function when compared to control hearts[50]. In patients undergoing isolated coronary artery bypass graft surgery (CABG) administration of T3 at reperfusion and for six hours after has been demonstrated to improve haemodynamic function in the immediate post-operative period with an associated reduction in the release of troponin I compared with placebo therapy[51].

7. Development of the use of thyroid hormone as an inotropic agent during cardiac surgery

The salutary effects of acute T3 supplementation have previously been demonstrated in a number of animal models that aimed to recreate the post-ischaemic dysfunction observed after cardiac surgery.

Novitzky demonstrated in both a porcine and canine models of ischaemia-reperfusion that T3 administration was able to attenuate the post-ischaemic left ventricular dysfunction compared with control[52, 53]. In isolated canine hearts subjected to hyperkalaemic arrest, Klemperer demonstrated that T3 supplementation following reperfusion led to an increase in preload recruitable stroke work area. This occurred without an increase in myocardial oxygen consumption, suggesting that administration of T3 in patients with a myocardial oxygen debt does not exacerbate this debt[54].

8. Thyroid hormone supplementation in paediatric cardiac surgery

There are a number of randomised controlled trials of T3 supplementation in paediatric cardiac surgery. These studies have been mainly performed in heterogeneous groups of patients with a variety of CPB and temperature management strategies, age ranges and diagnoses.

During paediatric cardiac surgery, Murzi et al. noted a significant reduction in fT3 with a nadir at 48 hours post-operatively and levels still below baseline values up to six days post-operatively. Levels of fT4 were reduced at six hours with a nadir at 72 hours, however, the magnitude of the decline was not as great as that seen with fT3[43]. Saatvedt et al. demonstrated in a population of paediatric cardiac surgical patients a reduction in fT3 and TSH with an increase in fT4 in the first 48 hours following surgery[55]. They attributed the increase in fT4 to the competition with free fatty acids (which are liberated by systemic heparinisation) in binding to plasma proteins, thus increasing fT4 levels. Marks et al demonstrated a reduction in TSH to lower limits of normal and reduced fT4 total T3 and fT3 index to below normal ranges and correlations between increased intensive care unit stay and mechanical ventilation to the degree of NTIS was observed[44].

Bettendorf et al conducted a randomised double-blind placebo controlled trial of 40 paediatric patients randomised to receive either T3 ($2\mu g.kg^{-1}$ on the first post-operative day, followed by 1μg.kg^{-1} on subsequent days) or placebo for up to 12 days following surgery. T3 therapy led to significantly higher serum circulating TH levels and the mean change in cardiac index was significantly higher in those that received T3 (20.4% vs. 10.0%, $p=0.004$). A sub group of patients with increased operative and CPB times were demonstrated to have improvements in systolic function measured by transthoracic echocardiography for T3 treated patients. The level of post-operative inotropic support was not different between groups[56].

In 28 children under seven years of age, Chowdhury et al randomised patients to receive either T3 at an infusion rate of 0.05-0.15μg.kg^{-1}.h^{-1} to maintain serum T3 levels within a normal range or placebo for a maximum of seven days[57].Sub-group analysis of the nine neonatal patients (less than one month) demonstrated a reduction in inotrope and therapeutic intervention scores. No significant difference was noted in the main trial group.

Mackie et al reported on the effects of T3 supplementation (0.05μg.kg^{-1}.h^{-1}) following termination of CPB and continued for a maximum of 48 hours in a randomised double-blind placebo controlled trial (n= 42) on neonates undergoing Norwood repair or repair of interrupted aortic arch with ventricular septal defect. Administration of T3 was noted to be safe but did not improve haemodynamic function. T3 treated patients had a shorter time to negative fluid balance compared with controls[58].

The largest randomised controlled trial to date of T3 supplementation in the paediatric surgical population is the triiodothyronine supplementation in infants and children undergoing cardiopulmonary bypass (TRICC) trial [59]. Portman and colleagues randomised 198 (analysed 193) children less than two years of age. They stratified to account for the heterogeneity of pathologies seen. T3 was administered as boluses of 0.4μg.kg^{-1} prior to CPB, a further 0.4μg.kg^{-1} at reperfusion, followed by three equally timed doses of 0.2μg.kg^{-1} up to nine hours post reperfusion. The safety of T3 administration in this group of patients with complex congenital cardiac defects was noted. In the entire study group, no difference in haemodynamic, inotropic or post-operative outcomes were detected. However, on planned sub-group analysis a reduction in time to extubation, improvements in cardiac function and reduced inotrope requirements were noted for children less than five months of age.

9. Thyroid hormone supplementation in adult cardiac surgery

Novitzky performed two small randomised blinded trials assessing the administration of T3 in patients undergoing CABG. In the first of these, 24 patients with a left ventricular ejection fraction (LVEF) < 30% were administered either placebo or T3 (n= 12) at aortic cross clamp (AXC) removal and at pre-defined intervals post-operatively. Patients treated with T3, demonstrated a reduction in, inotrope and diuretic requirements. In the following study (n= 24) of this series T3 was administered to those patients with an LVEF > 40%. Those patients treated with T3 (n=13) demonstrated a significant increase in cardiac output with an associated reduction in systemic vascular resistance in the first 24 hours following removal of the AXC[60]. Following the encouraging results of these trials and the preceding animal work, a number of larger trials have been performed.

Klemperer et al randomised 142 patients undergoing first time CABG with LVEF < 40% to receive either placebo or T3 therapy[13]. T3 was administered as a bolus of 0.8μg.kg^{-1} at AXC removal followed by an infusion of 0.113μg.kg^{-1}.h^{-1} for six hours post AXC removal. Treatment with T3 led to supra-physiological levels of T3 (and remained significantly higher during T3 treatment compared to placebo) and were associated with haemodynamic improvements manifest by an increase in cardiac index and reduction in SVR. No statistically significant difference was noted in the requirement of inotropic or vasoconstrictor support during the six hours of T3 therapy following surgery. The incidence of post-operative atrial fibrillation was significantly reduced in the T3 group[61].

Bennett-Guerro et al randomised 211 patients undergoing CABG surgery[62] believed to be at higher risk of requiring post-operative inotropic support (LVEF < 40%, age > 65 years or cardiac re-operation) to receive either T3, dopamine (as a positive control) or placebo. T3 treatment dose was again a $0.8\mu g\ kg^{-1}$ bolus at AXC removal followed by an infusion of $0.12\mu g\ kg^{-1}.h^{-1}$ for six hours, weaned over the next five hours. The dopamine group received $5\mu g.kg^{-1}.min^{-1}$ for six hours, weaned over the next six hours. The post-operative low T3 state was prevented with T3 administration, however, this study failed to demonstrate any significant difference in post-operative haemodynamic performance or inotrope requirements for patients receiving T3 therapy.

In a third study of patients undergoing CABG, Mullis-Jansson et al randomised 170 patients to receive either T3 $1\mu g\ kg^{-1}$ at AXC removal followed by an infusion of $1\mu g.kg^{-1}$ for six hours. In this trial, T3 therapy was demonstrated to have a significant haemodynamic benefit with an increase in cardiac index in the 12 hours following removal of the AXC but with no significant reduction in the SVR. The requirement for post-operative inotropic and post-operative mechanical circulatory support was also reduced in patients receiving T3 therapy. Post-operative myocardial injury as measured by biochemical markers and electrocardiographic criteria (assessed by an independent blinded cardiologist) was also reduced for patients receiving T3 therapy[63].

In a randomised trial of metabolic and hormonal therapy in patients undergoing first-time isolated CABG patients receiving T3 were demonstrated to have improved haemodynamic performance, reduced inotrope requirements and release of troponin I was significantly reduced for those patients administered T3 [51]. T3 therapy was administered as per the protocol originally set out in the trial by Klemperer et al[13].

In addition to the studies investigating peri-operative intravenous supplementation, the potential benefits of pre-operative oral administration of T3 have been investigated. Sirlak et al[64] attempted to optimise TH levels in patients undergoing CABG with reduced LVEF (<30%). In this study, patients (n= 80) were randomised to receive either oral T3 therapy 125µg per day for seven days prior to surgery and from the first post-operative day until time of discharge or placebo therapy. At anaesthetic induction patients in the T3 treatment group were demonstrated to have significantly higher levels of serum fT3 and significantly reduced serum levels of TSH and T4. Although both groups had reductions in serum fT3 associated with surgery and institution of CPB, the magnitude of the effect was reduced in patients receiving oral T3 and with post-operative re-institution of T3 a more rapid return to baseline levels was noted. Although no benefit was seen in terms of improvement in haemodynamic performance at baseline between the groups, T3 treated patients had a significant increase in both cardiac index and mixed venous oxygen saturations in the first 24 hours when compared with the placebo group. In addition, inotrope requirements, requirement for mechanical circulatory support and intensive care unit length of stay were reduced for the T3 group[64].

Kaptein and colleagues performed a meta-analysis to investigate the effects of TH therapy on post-operative NTIS in adults, They analysed 14 randomised controlled trials (13 of which were in patients undergoing cardiac surgery)[45]. Patients were divided into low and high dose intravenous T3 groups and oral T3 groups. Patients in the high dose group tended towards supra-physiological concentrations of T3, whereas those in the low dose group were more physiological. For those patients undergoing CABG, both the low (0.0275-0.0333μg.kg^{-1}.h^{-1} for 14 to 24 hours) and high (0.175-0.333μg.kg^{-1}.h^{-1} for six to nine hours) dose treatment groups demonstrated significantly increased cardiac index at four to six hours in pooled analyses. In the low and high dose treatment groups, serum T3 levels were 90-108% and 241-571% of baseline values respectively. No correlation was noted between cardiac index (percentage of basal) and total T3 dose, implying that there may be no additional benefit on cardiac index with increasing T3 dose. No difference in mortality was noted and there was insufficient data to comment on hospital and intensive care unit stay. The overall conclusions of the meta-analysis were that although cardiac index was increased, further information is required to investigate potential deleterious effects such as an increase in myocardial oxygen consumption[45], although this has not been demonstrated in animal studies[54].

10. Summary

The NTIS is a common occurrence following cardiac surgery in both paediatric and adult populations. Supplementation with T3 leads to supra-normal T3 levels and has been shown in a number of studies to

1. Improve haemodynamic performance
2. Reduce inotrope requirements
3. Reduce the need for mechanical circulatory support
4. Attenuate myocardial injury.

As yet none of these trials has demonstrated a major benefit in terms of a significant reduction in post-operative morbidities and mortality and further work is required to ascertain the optimal dose and timing of administration to maximise the potential benefits of T3 therapy in the post-operative cardiac surgical patient.

11. References

[1] Ojamaa K, Balkman C, Klein IL. Acute effects of triiodothyronine on arterial smooth muscle cells. *Ann.Thorac.Surg.* 1993;56(1 Suppl):S61-S66.

[2] Park KW, Dai HB, Ojamaa K, Lowenstein E, Klein I, Sellke FW. The direct vasomotor effect of thyroid hormones on rat skeletal muscle resistance arteries. *Anesth.Analg.* 1997;85(4):734-738.

[3] Klein I, Ojamaa K. Thyroid hormone: targeting the vascular smooth muscle cell. *Circ.Res.* 2001;88(3):260-261.

[4] Klein I, Ojamaa K. Thyroid hormone and the cardiovascular system. [Review] [82 refs]. *New England Journal of Medicine.* 2001;344(7):501-509.

[5] Klein I, Ojamaa K. Thyroid hormone-targeting the heart.[comment]. [Review] [30 refs]. *Endocrinology.* 2001;142(1):11-12.

[6] Danzi S, Klein I. Thyroid hormone-regulated cardiac gene expression and cardiovascular disease. [Review] [57 refs]. *Thyroid.* 2002;12(6):467-472.

[7] Klein I. Thyroid and the heart. *Thyroid.* 2002;12(6):439.

[8] Klein I, Danzi S. Thyroid disease and the heart. *Circulation.* 2007;116(15):1725-1735.

[9] Klein I, Danzi S. Thyroid hormone treatment to mend a broken heart. *Journal of Clinical Endocrinology Metabolism.* 2008;93(4):1172-1174.

[10] Klein I. Thyroid hormone and the cardiovascular system. [Review] [64 refs]. *American Journal of Medicine.* 1990;88(6):631-637.

[11] Schmidt BMW, Martin N, Georgens AC, Tillmann HC, Feuring M, Christ M, Wehling M. Nongenomic Cardiovascular Effects of Triiodothyronine in Euthyroid Male Volunteers. *Journal of Clinical Endocrinology Metabolism.* 2002; 87(4): 1681-1686.

[12] Yoneda K, Takasu N, Higa S, Oshiro C, Oshiro Y, Shimabukuro M, Asahi T. Direct effects of thyroid hormones on rat coronary artery: nongenomic effects of triiodothyronine and thyroxine. *Thyroid.* 1998;8(7):609-613.

[13] Klemperer JD, Klein I, Gomez M, Helm RE, Ojamaa K, Thomas SJ, Isom OW, Krieger K. Thyroid hormone treatment after coronary-artery bypass surgery. *N.Engl.J.Med.* 1995;333(23):1522-1527.

[14] Davis PJ, Davis FB. Nongenomic actions of thyroid hormone on the heart. [Review] [62 refs]. *Thyroid.* 2002;12(6):459-466.

[15] Bahouth SW. Thyroid hormones transcriptionally regulate the beta 1-adrenergic receptor gene in cultured ventricular myocytes. *Journal of Biological Chemistry.* 1991;266(24):15863-15869.

[16] Hoit BD, Khoury SF, Shao Y, Gabel M, Liggett SB, Walsh RA. Effects of Thyroid Hormone on Cardiac {beta}-Adrenergic Responsiveness in Conscious Baboons. *Circulation.* 1997;96(2):592-598.

[17] Khoury SF, Hoit BD, Dave V, Pawloski-Dahm CM, Shao Y, Gabel M, Periasamy M, Walsh RA. Effects of Thyroid Hormone on Left Ventricular Performance and Regulation of Contractile and Ca2+-Cycling Proteins in the Baboon: Implications for the Force-Frequency and Relaxation-Frequency Relationships. *Circulation Research.* 1996;79(4):727-735.

[18] Simmerman HK, Jones LR. Phospholamban: Protein Structure, Mechanism of Action, and Role in Cardiac Function. *Physiological Reviews.* 1998;78(4):921-947.

[19] Kiss E, Brittsan AG, Edes I, Grupp IL, Grupp G, Kranias EG. Thyroid Hormone–Induced Alterations in Phospholamban-Deficient Mouse Hearts. *Circulation Research.* 1998;83(6):608-613.

[20] Yen PM. Physiological and Molecular Basis of Thyroid Hormone Action. *Physiological Reviews.* 2001;81(3):1097-1142.

[21] Bluhm WF, Meyer M, Sayen MR, Swanson EA, Dillmann WH. Overexpression of sarcoplasmic reticulum Ca2+-ATPase improves cardiac contractile function in hypothyroid mice. *Cardiovascular Research.* 1999;43(2):382-388.

[22] Ojamaa K, Kenessey A, Klein I. Thyroid hormone regulation of phospholamban phosphorylation in the rat heart. *Endocrinology.* 2000;141(6):2139-2144.

[23] Auer J, Weber T, Eber B. Low triiodothyronine and cardiovascular disease. *Circulation.* 2003;108(4):e29-e30.

[24] Ojamaa K, Sabet A, Kenessey A, Shenoy R, Klein I. Regulation of rat cardiac Kv1.5 gene expression by thyroid hormone is rapid and chamber specific. *Endocrinology.* 1999;140(7):3170-3176.

[25] Faber J, Petersen L, Wiinberg N, Schifter S, Mehlsen J. Hemodynamic changes after levothyroxine treatment in subclinical hypothyroidism. *Thyroid.* 2002;12(4):319-324.

[26] Cerillo AG, Bevilacqua S, Storti S, Mariani M, Kallushi E, Ripoli A, Clerico A, Glauber M. Free triiodothyronine: a novel predictor of postoperative atrial fibrillation. *European Journal of Cardio-Thoracic Surgery.* 2003;24(4):487-492.

[27] Park YJ, Yoon JW, Kim KI, Lee YJ, Kim KW, Choi SH, Lim S, Choi DJ, Park K-H, Choh JH, Jang HC, Kim SY, Cho BY, Lim C. Subclinical Hypothyroidism Might Increase the Risk of Transient Atrial Fibrillation After Coronary Artery Bypass Grafting. *Ann Thorac Surg.* 2009;87(6):1846-1852.

[28] Bennett-Guerrero E, Kramer DC, Schwinn DA. Effect of chronic and acute thyroid hormone reduction on perioperative outcome. [see comments.]. [Review] [68 refs]. *Anesthesia & Analgesia.* 1997;85(1):30-36.

[29] Drucker DJ, Burrow GN. Cardiovascular surgery in the hypothyroid patient. *Arch Intern Med.* 1985;145(9):1585-1587.

[30] Syed AU, El Watidy AF, Akhlaque NB, Wahba A, El Oakley RM, Imran K, Al Bukhari EA, Al Fagih MR. Coronary Bypass Surgery in Patients on Thyroxin Replacement Therapy. *Asian Cardiovascular Thoracic Annals.* 2002;10(2):107-110.

[31] O'Connor CJ, March R, Tuman KJ. Severe myxedema after cardiopulmonary bypass. *Anesth Analg.* 2003;96(1):62-64, table of contents.

[32] Forfar JC, Muir AL, Toft AD. Left ventricular function in hypothyroidism. Responses to exercise and beta adrenoceptor blockade. *Br.Heart J.* 1982;48(3):278-284.

[33] Osman F, Gammage MD, Franklyn JA. Hyperthyroidism and cardiovascular morbidity and mortality. *Thyroid.* 2002;12(6):483-487.

[34] Parle JV, Maisonneuve P, Sheppard MC, Boyle P, Franklyn JA. Prediction of all-cause and cardiovascular mortality in elderly people from one low serum thyrotropin result: a 10-year cohort study. *The Lancet.* 2001;358(9285):861-865.

[35] De Groot LJ. Dangerous Dogmas in Medicine: The Nonthyroidal Illness Syndrome. *Journal of Clinical Endocrinology Metabolism.* 1999;84(1):151-164.

[36] Warner MH, Beckett GJ. Mechanisms behind the non-thyroidal illness syndrome: an update. *J Endocrinol.* 2010;205(1):1-13.

[37] Chopra IJ, Huang TS, Beredo A, Solomon DH, Chua Teco GN, Mead JF. Evidence for an inhibitor of extrathyroidal conversion of thyroxine to 3,5,3'-triiodothyronine in sera of patients with nonthyroidal illnesses. *Journal of Clinical Endocrinology Metabolism.* 1985;60(4):666-672.

[38] Van den BG. The neuroendocrine response to stress is a dynamic process. *Best.Pract.Res.Clin Endocrinol Metab.* 2001;15(4):405-419.

[39] Chopra IJ. Euthyroid Sick Syndrome: Is It a Misnomer? *Journal of Clinical Endocrinology Metabolism.* 1997;82(2):329-334.

[40] Iglesias P, Munoz A, Prado F, Guerrero MT, Macias MC, Ridruejo E, Tajada P, Diez JJ. Alterations in thyroid function tests in aged hospitalized patients: prevalence, aetiology and clinical outcome. *Clin.Endocrinol.(Oxf).* 2009;70(6):961-967.

[41] Peeters RP, van der GS, Wouters PJ, Darras VM, van Toor H, Kaptein E, Visser TJ, Van den BG. Tissue thyroid hormone levels in critical illness. *J Clin Endocrinol Metab.* 2005;90(12):6498-6507.

[42] Bremner WF, Taylor KM, Baird S, Thomson JE, Thomson JA, Ratcliffe JG, Lawrie TD, Bain WH. Hypothalamo-pituitary-thyroid axis function during cardiopulmonary bypass. *J Thorac Cardiovasc Surg.* 1978;75(3):392-399.

[43] Murzi B, Iervasi G, Masini S, Moschetti R, Vanini V, Zucchelli G, Biagini A. Thyroid Hormones Homeostasis in Pediatric Patients During and After Cardiopulmonary Bypass. *The Annals of Thoracic Surgery.* 1995;59(2):481-485.

[44] Marks SD, Haines C, Rebeyka IM, Couch RM. Hypothalamic-Pituitary-Thyroid Axis Changes in Children after Cardiac Surgery. *J Clin Endocrinol Metab.* 2009;94(8):2781-2786.

[45] Kaptein EM, Sanchez A, Beale E, Chan LS. Thyroid Hormone Therapy for Postoperative Nonthyroidal Illnesses: A Systematic Review and Synthesis. *J Clin Endocrinol Metab.* 2010:jc.2010-1052.

[46] Cerillo AG, Sabatino L, Bevilacqua S, Farneti PA, Scarlattini M, Forini F, Glauber M. Nonthyroidal illness syndrome in off-pump coronary artery bypass grafting. *The Annals of Thoracic Surgery.* 2003;75(1):82-87.

[47] Velissaris T, Tang ATM, Wood PJ, Hett DA, Ohri SK. Thyroid function during coronary surgery with and without cardiopulmonary bypass. *Eur J Cardiothorac Surg.* 2009;36(1):148-154.

[48] Pantos C, Malliopoulou V, Paizis I, Moraitis P, Mourouzis I, Tzeis S, Karamanoli E, Cokkinos DD, Carageorgiou H, Varonos D, Cokkinos DV. Thyroid hormone and cardioprotection: study of p38 MAPK and JNKs during ischaemia and at reperfusion in isolated rat heart. *Molecular & Cellular Biochemistry.* 2003;242(1-2):173-180.

[49] Chen YF, Kobayashi S, Chen J, Redetzke RA, Said S, Liang Q, Gerdes AM. Short term triiodo-L-thyronine treatment inhibits cardiac myocyte apoptosis in border area after myocardial infarction in rats. *J Mol.Cell Cardiol.* 2008;44(1):180-187.

[50] Pantos C, Mourouzis I, Saranteas T, Clave G, Ligeret H, Noack-Fraissignes P, Renard PY, Massonneau M, Perimenis P, Spanou D, Kostopanagiotou G, Cokkinos DV. Thyroid hormone improves postischaemic recovery of function while limiting apoptosis: a new therapeutic approach to support hemodynamics in the setting of ischaemia-reperfusion? *Basic Res Cardiol.* 2009;104(1):69-77.

[51] Ranasinghe AM, Quinn DW, Pagano D, Edwards N, Faroqui M, Graham TR, Keogh BE, Mascaro J, Riddington DW, Rooney SJ, Townend JN, Wilson IC, Bonser RS. Glucose-Insulin-Potassium and Tri-Iodothyronine Individually Improve Hemodynamic Performance and Are Associated With Reduced Troponin I Release After On-Pump Coronary Artery Bypass Grafting. *Circulation.* 2006;114(1_suppl):I-245.

[52] Novitzky D, Human PA, Cooper DK. Inotropic effect of triiodothyronine following myocardial ischemia and cardiopulmonary bypass: an experimental study in pigs. *The Annals of Thoracic Surgery.* 1988;45(1):50-55.

[53] Novitzky D, Matthews N, Shawley D, Cooper DK, Zuhdi N. Triiodothyronine in the recovery of stunned myocardium in dogs. *The Annals of Thoracic Surgery.* 1991;51(1):10-16.

[54] Klemperer JD, Zelano J, Helm RE, Berman K, Ojamaa K, Klein I, Isom OW, Krieger K. Triiodothyronine improves left ventricular function without oxygen wasting effects after global hypothermic ischemia. *Journal of Thoracic & Cardiovascular Surgery.* 1995;109(3):457-465.

[55] Saatvedt K, Lindberg H, Geiran OR, Fiane A, Seem E, Michelsen S, Pedersen T, Hagve TA. Thyroid function during and after cardiopulmonary bypass in children. *Acta Anaesthesiologica Scandinavica.* 1998;42(9):1100-1103.

[56] Bettendorf M, Schmidt KG, Grulich-Henn J, Ulmer HE, Heinrich UE. Tri-iodothyronine treatment in children after cardiac surgery: a double-blind, randomised, placebo-controlled study. *Lancet.* 2000;356(9229):529-534.

[57] Chowdhury D, Ojamaa K, Parnell VA, McMahon C, Sison CP, Klein I. A prospective randomized clinical study of thyroid hormone treatment after operations for complex congenital heart disease. *The Journal of Thoracic and Cardiovascular Surgery.* 2001;122(5):1023-1025.

[58] Mackie AS, Booth KL, Newburger JW, Gauvreau K, Huang SA, Laussen PC, DiNardo JA, del Nido PJ, Mayer JE, Jr., Jonas RA, McGrath E, Elder J, Roth SJ. A randomized, double-blind, placebo-controlled pilot trial of triiodothyronine in neonatal heart surgery. *The Journal of Thoracic and Cardiovascular Surgery.* 2005;130(3):810-816.

[59] Portman MA, Slee A, Olson AK, Cohen G, Karl T, Tong E, Hastings L, Patel H, Reinhartz O, Mott AR, Mainwaring R, Linam J, Danzi S, for the TRICC Investigators. Triiodothyronine Supplementation in Infants and Children Undergoing Cardiopulmonary Bypass (TRICC): A Multicenter Placebo-Controlled Randomized Trial: Age Analysis. *Circulation.* 2010;122(11_suppl_1): S224-233.

[60] Novitzky D, Cooper DK, Barton CI, Greer A, Chaffin J, Grim J, Zuhdi N. Triiodothyronine as an inotropic agent after open heart surgery. *The Journal of Thoracic and Cardiovascular Surgery.* 1989;98(5):972-977.

[61] Klemperer JD, Klein IL, Ojamaa K, Helm RE, Gomez M, Isom OW, Krieger KH. Triiodothyronine therapy lowers the incidence of atrial fibrillation after cardiac operations. *Ann.Thorac.Surg.* 1996;61(5):1323-1327.

[62] Bennett-Guerrero E, Jimenez JL, White WD, D'Amico EB, Baldwin BI, Schwinn DA. Cardiovascular effects of intravenous triiodothyronine in patients undergoing coronary artery bypass graft surgery. A randomized, double-blind, placebo-controlled trial. Duke T3 study group. *JAMA: The Journal of the American Medical Association.* 1996;275(9):687-692.

[63] Mullis-Jansson SL, Argenziano M, Corwin S, Homma S, Weinberg AD, Williams M, Rose EA, Smith CR. A randomised double-blind study of the effect of triiodothyronine on cardiac function and morbidity after coronary bypass surgery. *The Journal of Thoracic and Cardiovascular Surgery.* 1999;117(6):1128-1135.

[64] Sirlak M, Yazicioglu L, Inan MB, Eryilmaz S, Tasoz R, Aral A, Ozyurda U. Oral thyroid hormone pretreatment in left ventricular dysfunction. *Eur J Cardiothorac Surg.* 2004;26(4):720-725.

15

A Pathophysiological Approach to Understanding Pulmonary Hypertension in Cardiac Surgery

Anne Q. N. Nguyen, Alain Deschamps,
France Varin, Louis P. Perrault
and André Y. Denault
Montreal Heart Institute and Université de Montréal
Canada

1. Introduction

Pulmonary hypertension (PH) is associated with increased morbidity and mortality and is an important prognostic factor in cardiac surgery. As the average age and associated co-morbidities of cardiac surgical patients increase, the prevalence of PH is likely to rise. In this chapter, we will define PH, classify it on the basis of pathophysiological etiology, and suggest treatment therapies according to this classification. The importance of PH in cardiac surgery, its relationship to right ventricular dysfunction and preventive therapies will also be discussed. When applicable, we will draw from our clinical experience with PH to suggest strategies for the prevention of possible complications.

2. Definition of pulmonary hypertension

2.1 Hemodynamic parameters used in clinical settings

There are several hemodynamic parameters used in defining PH (Table **1**) (Gomez & Palazzo, 1998). These definitions have been used in various studies.

2.2 Diagnosis in awake and anesthetized patients

Pulmonary hypertension is usually diagnosed prior to cardiac surgery in awake patients. The diagnosis is obtained either directly by cardiac catheterization or indirectly by using Doppler signals from transesophageal echocardiography (TEE) and using Bernoulli's equation. In the presence of tricuspid regurgitation, the simplified Bernoulli's equation gives an estimation of the pressure gradient across the tricuspid valve (Fig. **1**) (Denault et al., 2010a). This pressure gradient is equal to the difference in systolic pressure between the right ventricle (RV) and the right atrium. Therefore, with the measurement of right atrial pressure (Pra), the estimation of systolic right ventricular pressure (Prv) is possible. In the absence of right ventricular outflow tract obstruction (RVOTO) and pulmonic valve stenosis, systolic Prv represents a reliable estimation of the systolic pulmonary artery pressure (SPAP).

Hemodynamic parameter	Normal value	Abnormal value
Systolic pulmonary artery pressure (SPAP)	15-30 mmHg	> 30 or ≥ 40 mmHg
Mean pulmonary artery pressure (MPAP)	9-16 mmHg	Moderate > 18 mmHg Significant > 25 mmHg Exercise-induced > 30 mmHg
Pulmonary vascular resistance (PVR) = (MPAP – PAOP) X 80/CO	60-120 dyn·sec·cm^{-5}	Mild > 125 dyn·sec·cm^{-5} Moderate > 200-300 dyn·sec·cm^{-5} Severe > 600 dyn·sec·cm^{-5}
Indexed pulmonary vascular resistance (PVRI) = (MPAP – PAOP) X 80/CI	250-340 dyn·sec·cm^{-5}·m^{-2}	> 340 dyn·sec·cm^{-5}·m^{-2}
Pulmonary to systemic vascular resistance index (PVRI/SVRI) X 100%	≤ 10%	> 10%
Transpulmonary gradient (MPAP – PAOP)	≤ 14 mmHg	> 14 mmHg
Mean pulmonary to systemic pressure ratio (MPAP/MAP) X 100%	< 25%	Moderate 33-50% Severe > 50%
Mean systemic to pulmonary pressure ratio (MAP/MPAP) X 100%	≥ 4	< 4 (Robitaille et al., 2006)

CI: cardiac index; CO: cardiac output; MAP: mean arterial pressure; PAOP: pulmonary artery occlusion pressure; SVRI: indexed systemic vascular resistance. Adapted from Gomez (Gomez & Palazzo, 1998).

Table 1. Definitions of Pulmonary Hypertension Used in Clinical Settings

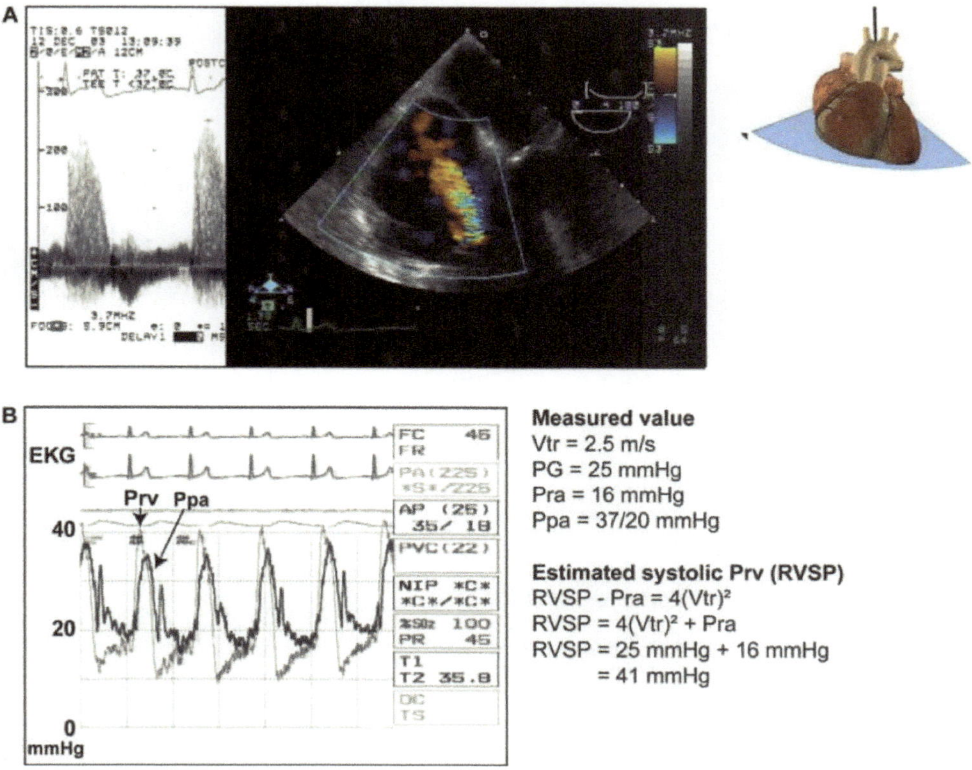

Fig. 1. (**A**) Estimation of right ventricular systolic pressure (systolic Prv or RVSP) using the pressure gradient (PG) obtained from tricuspid regurgitation (TR) and right atrial pressure (Pra). (**B**) Note that the RVSP is higher than the systolic pulmonary artery pressure (Ppa) due to a small gradient across the pulmonic valve. (EKG: electrocardiogram; V: velocity). With permission from Denault *et al.* (Denault et al., 2010a).

2.3 Comparison of absolute and relative values in the assessment of pulmonary hypertension

Following the induction of general anesthesia, a reduction in both the systemic and the pulmonary artery pressures is observed. Consequently, using absolute values of SPAP in defining PH would underestimate its severity. To address this issue, Robitaille *et al.* studied 1557 patients undergoing cardiac surgery (Robitaille et al., 2006). In the 32 patients with preoperative PH, induction of general anesthesia resulted in a significant reduction in mean arterial pressure (MAP) and mean pulmonary artery pressure (MPAP) but the ratio of MAP/MPAP remained stable (Fig. **2**). The normal value for this ratio is > 4, and lower values can be used to quantify the severity of PH.

The relevance of the MAP/MPAP ratio was demonstrated after comparing its ability to estimate the probability of postoperative complications with the ability of other normally used hemodynamic parameters for this purpose (listed in Table **1**). Values of the ratio obtained after induction of general anesthesia but before cardiopulmonary bypass (CPB) in 1439 patients undergoing cardiac surgery showed similar trend when compared to other

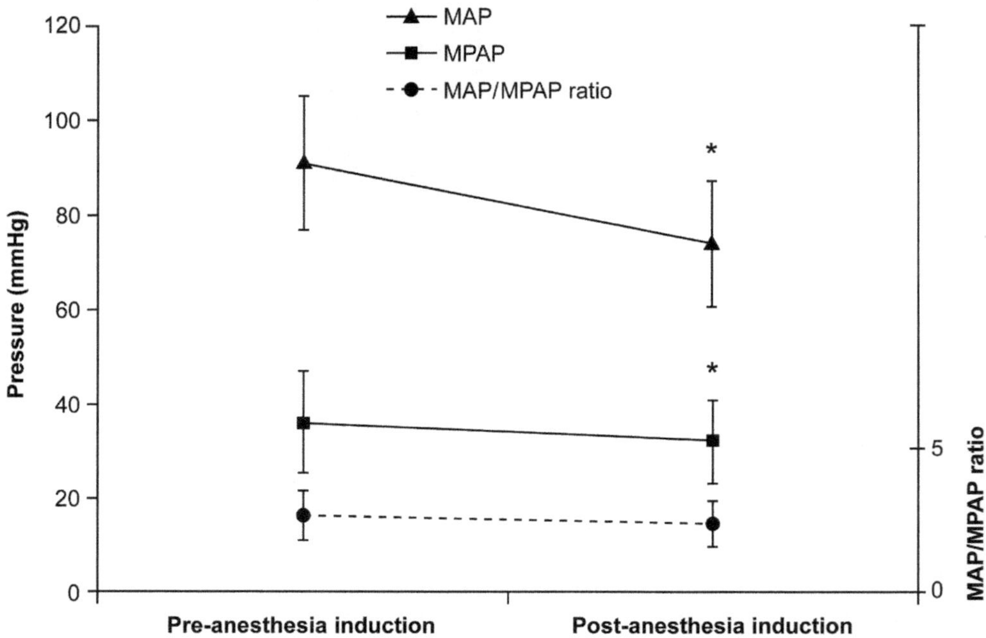

Fig. 2. Changes in mean arterial pressure (MAP), mean pulmonary artery pressure (MPAP), and the MAP/MPAP ratio after the induction of anesthesia in 32 patients with preoperative pulmonary hypertension. No significant change in the MAP/MPAP ratio was observed (*p < 0.05). (Robitaille et al., 2006)

hemodynamic parameters (Fig. **3**). Furthermore, the ratio turned out to be the best predictor of perioperative complications, defined as death, need for intra-aortic balloon pump, cardiac arrest, or use of vasoactive support for more than 24 hours.

An abnormal MAP/MPAP ratio was also recognized to be significantly correlated with abnormal systolic and/or diastolic cardiac function (Fig. **4**) (Robitaille et al., 2006). The use of relative instead of absolute values to estimate PH is currently used in congenital cardiology (Therrien et al., 2001a; Therrien et al., 2001b).

In summary, the evaluation and diagnostic of PH in cardiac surgical patients must be done using specific criteria. In awake patients, the absolute values can be used since they correlate well with outcomes. However, in patients under general anesthesia, the ratio of MAP/MPAP allows to screen for PH when systolic blood pressures are lower due to the anesthetic agents.

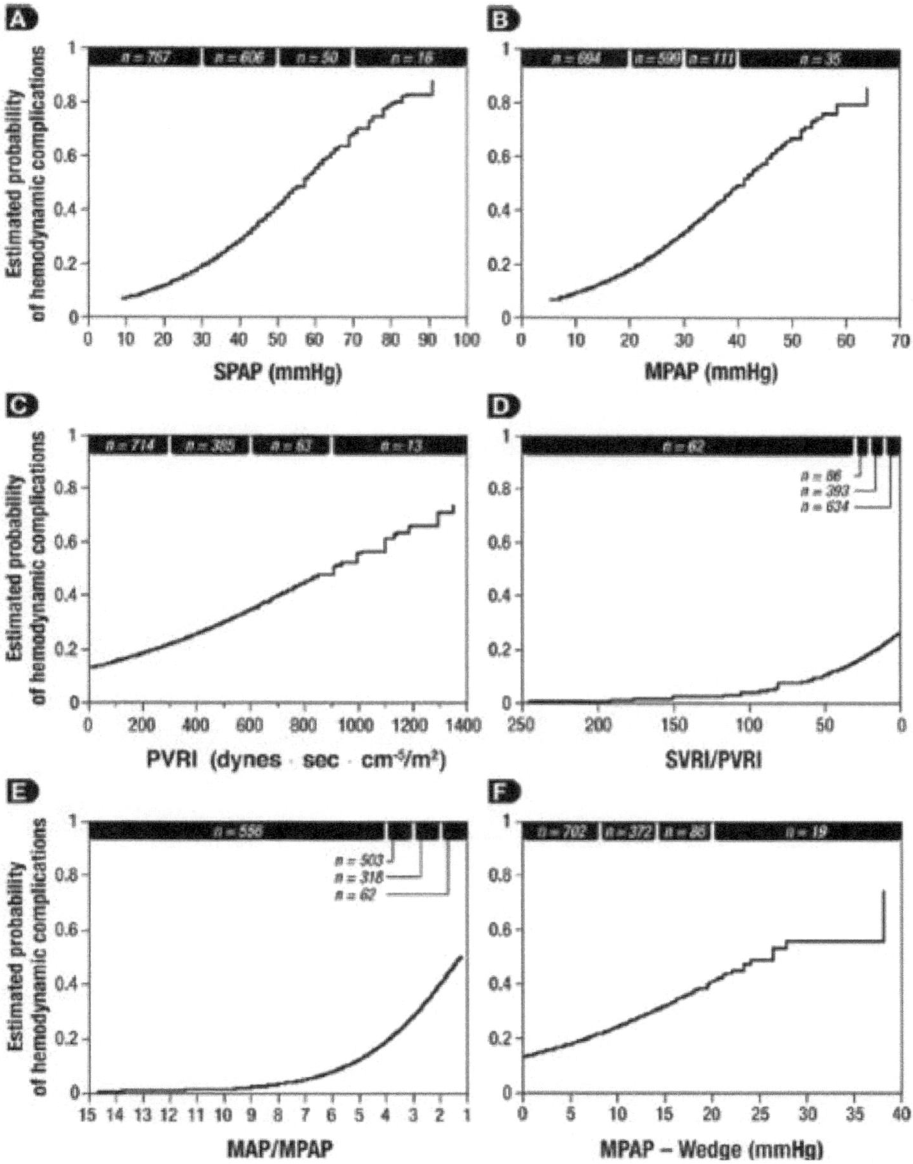

Fig. 3. Relationship between the estimated probability of hemodynamic complications and variables used in the evaluation of pulmonary hypertension: (**A**) systolic pulmonary artery pressure (SPAP), (**B**) mean pulmonary artery pressure (MPAP), (**C**) indexed pulmonary vascular resistance (PVRI), (**D**) systemic to pulmonary vascular resistance index ratio (SVRI/PVRI), (**E**) mean systemic to pulmonary pressure ratio (MAP/MPAP), and (**F**) transpulmonary gradient defined as MPAP - Wedge or pulmonary artery occlusion pressure (PAOP). For easier comparison, the scale of the x axis of the SVRI/PVRI and the MAP/MPAP are inverted. (n = number of patients). (Robitaille et al., 2006)

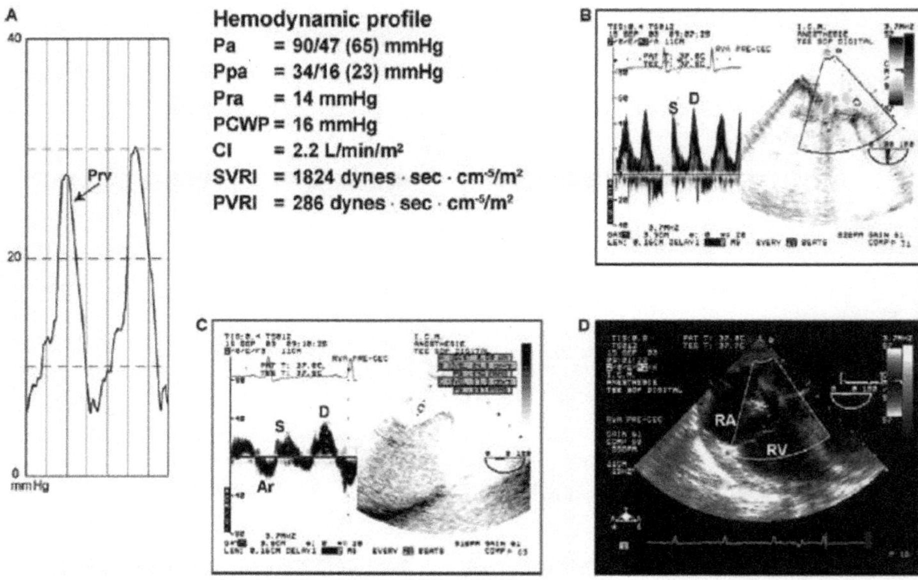

Fig. 4. Hemodynamic and transesophageal echocardiographic evaluation of a 46-year-old woman scheduled for aortic valve surgery. Despite a normal pulmonary artery pressure (Ppa) of 34/16 mmHg and pulmonary vascular resistance index (PVRI) at 286 dyn $\cdot s \cdot cm^{-5} \cdot m^{-2}$, this patient had an abnormal right ventricular diastolic filling pressure waveform characterized by a rapid upstroke (**A**) and reduced systolic (S) to diastolic (D) pulmonary (**B**) and hepatic (**C**) venous flows consistent with left and right ventricular diastolic dysfunction. In addition, a dilated right atrium and ventricle were present without significant tricuspid regurgitation in a mid-esophageal right ventricular view (**D**). The mean systemic to pulmonary pressure ratio (MAP/MPAP) was 65/23 or 2.8. (CI: cardiac index; Pa: arterial pressure; PCWP: pulmonary capillary wedge pressure; Pra: right atrial pressure; Prv: right ventricular pressure; RA: right atrium; RV: right ventricle; SVRI: systemic vascular resistance index). (Robitaille et al., 2006)

3. Classification of pulmonary hypertension based on pathophysiology and etiology

The 2008 World Symposium on PH endorsed by The World Health Organization (WHO) proposed a classification system divided into 5 groups: 1) Pulmonary arterial hypertension, 2) PH owing to left heart disease, 3) PH owing to lung diseases and/or hypoxia, 4) Chronic thromboembolic PH, and 5) PH with unclear or multifactorial etiologies (Simonneau et al., 2009).
In cardiac surgery, PH is more frequently classified as pre-capillary, capillary or post-capillary, depending on the site where the underlying cause of PH is found. In this context, PH during cardiac surgery is typically post-capillary since the cause is mainly of left ventricular (LV) origin, past the pulmonary capillary bed. To confirm this diagnosis, pulmonary artery catheterization can be used to demonstrate an equal value for diastolic pulmonary artery pressure (DPAP) and pulmonary artery occlusion pressure (PAOP). When the cause for PH is at the pre-capillary or capillary level, in absence of tachycardia, DPAP is significantly higher than PAOP (Gomez & Palazzo, 1998).
The causes underlying PH in cardiac surgery can be complex and may result from several mechanisms acting alone or in combination (Fig. **5**). These mechanisms may exist before the operation or appear during or after the procedure. Exacerbation of PH may happen at any time during cardiac surgery, before, during or after CPB. Indeed, patients are at risk of LV failure at all times, especially after CPB when the reperfusion of the ischemic lungs can cause pulmonary reperfusion syndrome. Finally, PH can persist postoperatively secondary to a patient-prosthesis-mismatch (PPM) after mitral or aortic valve replacement. The treatment of PH is based on the identification of its etiology, whence the importance of distinguishing between the different pathophysiologies.

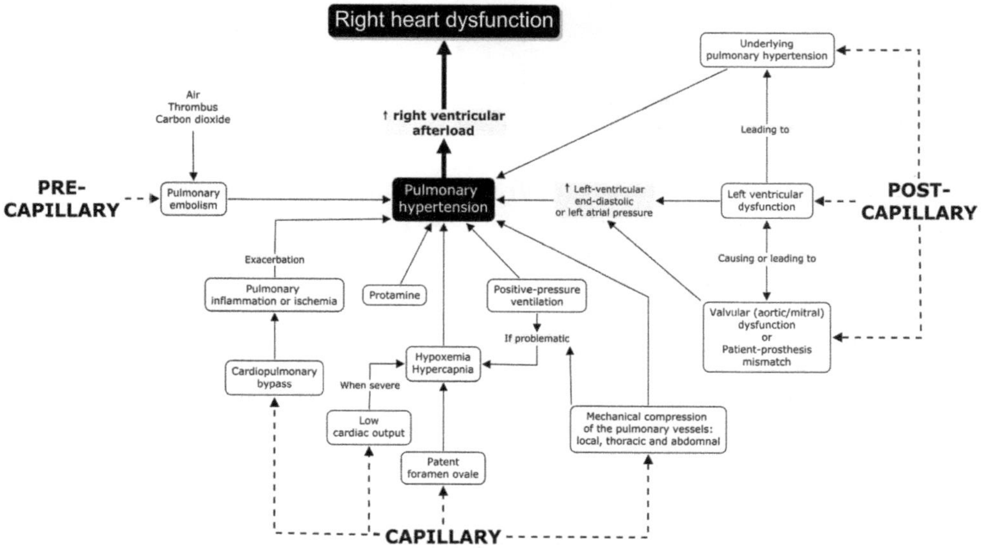

Fig. 5. Major mechanisms of pulmonary hypertension in cardiac surgery. Other mechanisms may be operating at several levels: for instance, hypoxia (capillary) may lead to pulmonary hypertension, right ventricular systolic failure and, through interventricular interaction, left ventricular diastolic function (post-capillary).

3.1 Review of the factors involved

The most important causes of PH in cardiac surgery, illustrated in Fig. 5, are classified according to their originating anatomical site: pre-capillary, capillary and post-capillary.

3.1.1 Pre-capillary

Pulmonary embolism

Pulmonary embolism is an example of a pre-capillary PH. It may occur before, during or after CPB leading to the development or the exacerbation of PH. Thrombus, air and even carbon dioxide (Martineau et al., 2003) can cause pulmonary embolism. Pulmonary embolisms are rare in the immediate cardiac postoperative period. However, patients at risk include patients with predisposing factors to PH and patients with chronic thromboembolic pulmonary hypertension (CTEPH) (Fig. 6). The incidence of CTEPH is uncertain, but it represents a frequent cause of PH occurring in up to 4% of patients after an acute pulmonary embolism (Pengo et al., 2004; Tapson & Humbert, 2006).

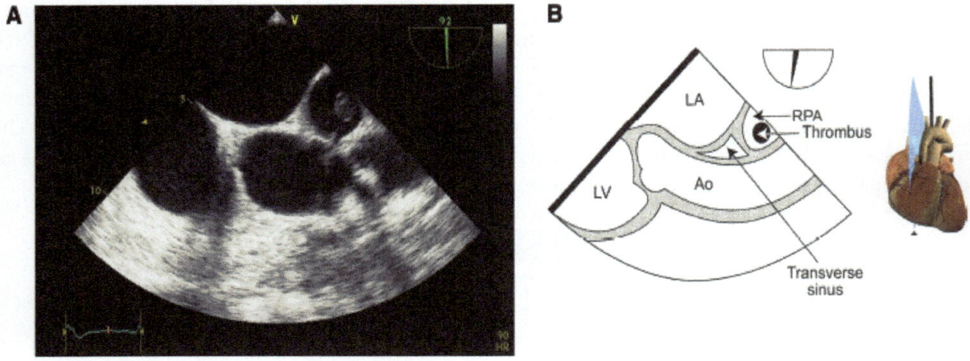

Fig. 6. Chronic pulmonary embolism. (**A, B**) Mid-esophageal ascending aorta (Ao) long-axis view in a 65-year-old woman with chronic pulmonary embolism shows the mobile clot adherent to the right pulmonary artery (RPA) wall. (LA: left atrium; LV: left ventricle). With permission from Denault *et al.* (Denault et al., 2010a).

3.1.2 Capillary

Cardiopulmonary bypass

Pulmonary damage during cardiopulmonary bypass (CPB) is one of the important etiologies of PH in cardiac surgery. This is mainly due to the fact that the lungs are ischemic during CPB. The underlying mechanisms include 1) release of cytokines through endotoxin production (Downing & Edmunds, Jr., 1992), 2) complement activation and 3) ischemia reperfusion injury (Wan et al., 1997; Asimakopoulos et al., 1999) which leads to the production of free radicals, endothelin and prostacyclin derivatives with nitric oxide inhibition (Wan et al., 1997). The resulting systemic inflammatory response, pulmonary reperfusion syndrome as well as the transfusion of blood products may all exacerbate PH (Fig. 7) (Lesage et al., 1966; Kaul & Fields, 2000).

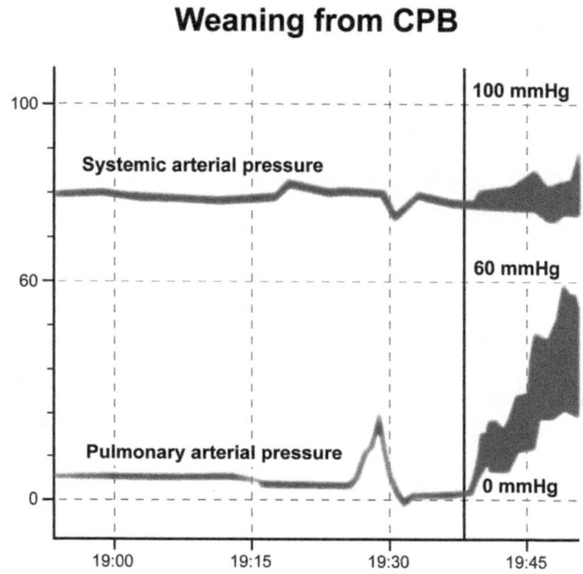

Fig. 7. Unexpected pulmonary hypertension upon weaning from cardiopulmonary bypass (CPB) in a 76-year-old woman after aortic valve replacement (AVR). The CPB duration was 71 minutes. A significant increase in pulmonary arterial pressure in relation to the systemic arterial pressure was observed as the patient was weaned from CPB. No mechanical causes were found.

During CPB, blood is exposed to an artificial surface for oxygenation before it is sent back into the systemic circulation. This is associated with an inflammatory reaction secondary to endothelial activation, activation of the complement cascade, neutrophils, thrombin and platelets. Since the heart and lungs do not receive blood during CPB, cardioplegia solutions are used to preserve heart function, however, no specific protection is undertaken for the pulmonary circulation. In some patients, this may result in pulmonary reperfusion syndrome associated with postoperative endothelial dysfunction and PH or in post-CPB respiratory distress syndrome. The latter phenomenon, similar to the respiratory distress syndrome in adults, is characterized by an increased capillary permeability leading to a reduction in oxygenation, increased alveolar-arterial gradient, decreased lung compliance, increased pulmonary vascular resistance (PVR), and exacerbation of preoperative PH. Activation of the endothelin system during CPB increases endothelin ET-1 concentrations and correlates with CPB duration, severity of PH and post-CPB myocardial dysfunction. For this reason, CPB duration plays a major role in the incidence of mortality in cardiac surgery. Post-CPB PH can lead to RV dysfunction which, when severe, is fraught with a 44 to 86% mortality rate.

Protamine

The administration of protamine can induce catastrophic pulmonary vasoconstriction in up to 1.8% of patients (Ocal et al., 2005). Protamine is administered in CPB to neutralize the anti-clotting effects of heparin and has the capacity to activate the complement cascade. Thus, when given at the end of CPB, it can induce PH associated with adverse hemodynamic responses that range from minor perturbations to cardiovascular collapse, and may occur in three forms: systemic hypotension, anaphylactoid reaction and catastrophic PH (Viaro et al., 2002). The mechanism of protamine-induced PH is thought to be caused by an imbalance of vasoconstrictors and vasodilators leading to a reduction in nitric oxide release from the pulmonary vasculature (Viaro et al., 2002).

Lung diseases and/or hypoxia

In this category, the predominant cause of PH is alveolar hypoxia as a result of impaired control of breathing or lung disease.

Lung volumes exert a differential effect on the resistance of intra- and extra-alveolar vessels, which accounts for the unique U-shaped relationship between lung volume and pulmonary vascular resistance (PVR) (Fig. **8**). At functional residual capacity (FRC), PVR is minimal but increases at large or total lung capacity (TLC) and small lung volumes. Clinically, this may be observed when hyperinflation of the lungs greatly increases PVR (Fischer et al., 2003).

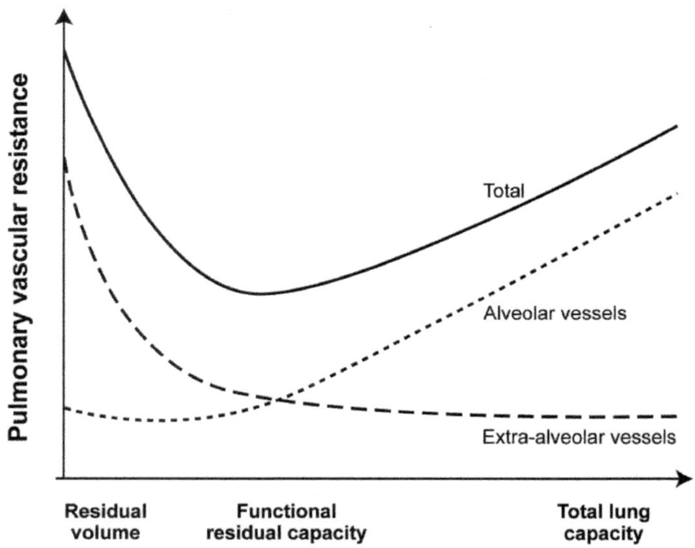

Fig. 8. Relationship between lung volume and pulmonary vascular resistance (PVR). At functional residual capacity (FRC) PVR is minimal and increases at large or total lung capacity (TLC) and residual volume decreases at small lung volumes. The differential effect on intra- and extra-alveolar vessels accounts for the U-shaped relationship of PVR and lung volume. Adapted from Fischer *et al.* (Fischer et al., 2003).

Changes in cardiac output (CO), airway pressure, and gravity may affect the pulmonary circulation. Therefore, patients with PH already have a restricted pulmonary circulation and increases in oxygen demand may further worsen PH and lead to right heart failure.

Application of high levels of positive end-expiratory pressure (PEEP) may narrow capillaries in well-ventilated lung areas (intra-alveolar) and divert blood flow to less well-ventilated or non-ventilated areas (extra-alveolar). Thus, intrapulmonary shunts may result in desaturation of mixed venous blood, potentially leading to hypoxia.

Hypoxia may also be caused by right-to-left intracardiac shunting through a patent foramen ovale (PFO) or a congenital heart defect. Pulmonary hypertension can lead to RV dysfunction causing increased pressure in the right atrium. In turn, the increase in Pra may result in opening of a PFO, present in 20-30% of the general population (Sukernik et al., 2001), increasing the severity of hypoxia. In contrast to systemic arteries, pulmonary vessels constrict with hypoxia (Euler-Liljestrand reflex) and dilate in the presence of hyperoxia (Fischer et al., 2003), which explains the exacerbation of PH with hypoxia.
Hypercapnia can occur especially in the case of acute lung injury during or after the procedure. The increase in partial pressure of carbon dioxide (PCO_2) will cause vasoconstriction and therefore worsen PH.
Increases in CO distend open vessels and recruit previously closed vessels so that when the cross-sectional area of pulmonary circulation increases, PVR decreases.
Mechanical compression of pulmonary vessels is transmitted to the surrounding cardiac pressure and contributes to increase PAP. Hemothorax or tension pneumothorax may be responsible for an elevation in intrathoracic pressure.
In addition, gravity influences blood flow in the pulmonary circulation. Both regional blood flow and ventilation are greater in the dependent areas of the lung (intra-alveolar). Hence, the relationship between alveolar and hydrostatic pressure bears important clinical consequences.
Multiple molecular pathways are involved in the regulation of PVR, namely nitric oxide, prostacyclin, endothelin-1 and serotonin pathways (Humbert et al., 2004). Nitric oxide and prostacyclin are endogenous vasodilators produced in the pulmonary vascular endothelium. Endothelin-1 is an endogenous vasoconstrictor peptide secreted by the vascular endothelium and plays a role in pulmonary vasoconstriction and vascular smooth muscle proliferation (McLaughlin & McGoon, 2006). The neurotransmitter serotonin and the serotonin receptor transporter are also involved in the regulation of pulmonary vascular tone. Therefore, an imbalance in these pathways may result in vasoconstriction and vascular remodelling, potentially leading to progressive pulmonary vascular disease.

3.1.3 Post-capillary

Left heart disease

Left ventricular disease represents the most frequent cause of PH in cardiac surgery (Oudiz, 2007). Left-sided dysfunction includes three distinct etiologies: systolic dysfunction, diastolic dysfunction, and valvular heart disease (mitral and/or aortic). Pre- or postoperative left-sided ventricular or valvular diseases may produce an increase in left atrial pressure, with passive backward transmission of the pressure leading to increased PAP. The elevation of PAP and PVR is due to either the increase of pulmonary artery vasomotor tone and/or pulmonary vascular remodeling (Delgado et al., 2005; Moraes et al., 2000).

Patient-prosthesis mismatch

Aortic patient-protheis mismatch (PPM) through a reduction in coronary reserve would also contribute to postoperative PH (Bakhtiary et al., 2007) and persistent postoperative valvular gradients (Fig. 9). There is general agreement that the postoperative indexed effective orifice area (EOA) of the prosthesis being implanted should not be < 0.85 to 0.90 cm^2/m^2. Mitral PPM was recently described as another cause of residual postoperative PH. Magne *et al.*

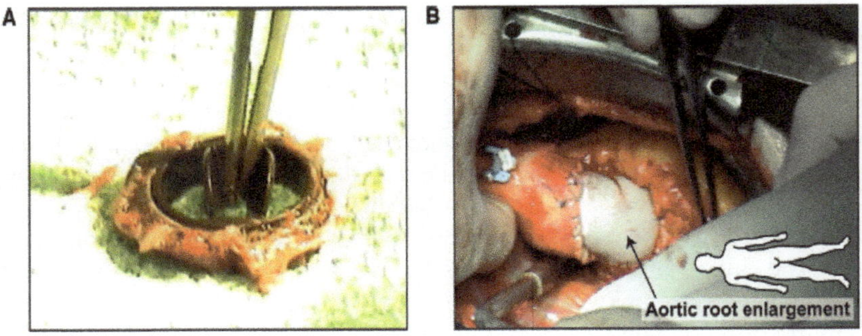

Fig. 9. Patient-prosthesis aortic valve mismatch. A 71-year-old man with a body surface area of 1.89 m^2 was re-operated for symptoms of severe aortic valve stenosis. He had an aortic vavle replacement (AVR) 4 years before with a Carbomedics 19 mm mechanical bileaflet prosthesis (non-indexed effective orifice area = 1.06 cm^2). (**A**) The preoperative mean gradient was 41 mmHg although the intraoperative inspection of the prosthetic valve was completely normal. (**B**) Intraoperative view of an aortic root enlargement procedure in a 69-year-old patient with a reduced aortic diameter requiring AVR. Courtesy of Dr. Michel Carrier. With permission from Denault *et al.* (Denault et al., 2010a).

(Magne et al., 2007) studied 929 patients who underwent mitral valve replacement (MVR), following them up to 15 years. Mitral valve PPM was defined according to the indexed valve EOA as not clinically significant (EOA > 1.2 cm^2/m^2), moderate (1.2 $cm^2/m^2 \geq$ EOA > 0.9 cm^2/m^2), and severe (EOA $\leq$ 0.9 cm^2/m^2). Prevalence of moderate and severe PPM was 69% and 9%, respectively. In addition, severe PPM was found to be associated with residual PH and a 3-fold increase in postoperative mortality after adjustment for other risk factors. This relevant new finding is currently absent from the majority of studies involving predictors of survival in mitral valve surgery.

4. Treatment of pulmonary hypertension in cardiac surgery based on pathophysiology and etiology

The approach to pharmacological and non-pharmacological treatment of PH will be directed towards the cause or the consequence of PH, as illustrated in Fig. **5**. Most often, treatment of the underlying mechanism causing PH requires non-pharmacological approaches, while pharmacological approaches will usually be the solution for the treatment of persisting PH and its consequence, RV failure.

4.1 Pharmacological and non-pharmacological approaches

Therapeutic management of PH has dramatically improved in the last years, offering both relief from symptoms and prolonged survival. However, there is still no cure for this disease. Moreover, in presence of PH, the choice of the appropriate therapy should rely on evidence-based medicine. By performing a Medline search using the keywords 'randomized controlled trial', 'humans', 'adults', 'pulmonary hypertension' and 'English', a total of 14 articles in cardiac surgery were retrieved. These publications were then classified according to their levels of evidence (Sackett, 1989; Moher et al., 2001) and summarized in Table **2**. Most of the studies reviewed were based on a small number of patients and had

Author	Country	Date	Agents used	Design	N	Inclusion criteria	Primary end-point	Efficacy	Level of evidence
Fernandes *et al.*	Brazil	2011	iNO *vs* oxygen	Single-center	29	MVR + PH after surgery	Hemodynamic	Yes	A1b
Kim *et al.*	Korea	2010	oral sildenafil + beraprost *vs* placebo	Single-center	50	PH before surgery	Hemodynamic	No	A1b
Khan *et al.*	USA	2009	$iPGI_2$ *vs* iNO	Crossover Single-center	25	PH, refractory hypoxemia, or RV dysfunction	Hemodynamic and oxynegation	Idem	A1b
Wang *et al.*	China	2009	Inhaled milrinone *vs* intravenous milrinone	Single-center	48	MVR + PH after surgery	Hemodynamic	Yes	A1b
Fattouch *et al.*	Italy	2006	$iPGI_2$ *vs* iNO vs intravenous vasodilators	Single-center	58	MVR + PH before the end of CPB	Hemodynamic	Yes	A1b
Ocal *et al.*	Turkey	2005	$iPGI_2$ *vs* NTG	Multicenter	68	CABG with protamine reaction after CPB	Hemodynamic	Yes	A1b
Stafford *et al.*	USA	2005	Heparinase *vs* protamine	Multicenter	167	CABG on + off pump after CPB	Bleeding	No	A1b
Fattouch *et al.*	Italy	2005	$iPGI_2$ *vs* iNO *vs* intravenous vasodilators	Single-center	58	MVR + PH in the intensive care unit	Hemodynamic	Yes	A1b
Hache *et al.*	Canada	2003	$iPGI_2$ *vs* placebo	Single-center	20	PH before CPB	Hemodynamic	Yes	A1b
Solina *et al.*	USA	2001	iNO *vs* milrinone	Single-center	62	PH after surgery	Hemodynamic	Yes	B
Feneck *et al.*	UK	2001	Milrinone *vs* dobutamine	Multicenter	120	CO < 2 $L/min/m^2$ et PAOP > 10 mmHg after cardiac surgery	Hemodynamic	Idem	A1b
Solina *et al.*	USA	2000	iNO *vs* milrinone	Single-center	45	PH after surgery	Hemodynamic	Yes	A1b
Schmid *et al.*	Switzerland	1999	iNO *vs* NTG *vs* PGE_1	Crossover Single-center	14	PH after surgery	Hemodynamic	Idem	B
Hachenberg *et al.*	Germany	1997	Enoximone *vs* dobutamine+NTG	Single-center	20	PH in MVR before and after surgery	Hemodynamic	Idem	A1b

CABG: coronary artery bypass graft; CO: cardiac output; CPB: cardiopulmonary bypass; iNO: inhaled nitric oxide; iPGI2: inhaled prostacyclin; MVR: mitral valve replacement; NO: nitric oxide; NTG: nitroglycerin; PAOP: pulmonary artery occlusion pressure; PGE_1: prostaglandin E1; PGI_2: prostacyclin; PH: pulmonary hypertension; RCT: randomized controlled trial; UK: United Kingdom; USA: United States of America.

Table 2. Randomized Controlled Trial in the Treatment of Pulmonary Hypertension in Adult Cardiac Surgery

hemodynamic changes as their primary end-points. Various pharmacological agents were studied: inhaled prostacyclin I_2 ($iPGI_2$), inhaled nitric oxide (iNO), heparinase, protamine and intravenous vasodilators including prostaglandin E1 (PGE_1), nitroglycerin (NTG), nitroprusside, milrinone, enoximone, dobutamine, oral sildenafil, beraprost and oxygen. Findings on pharmacological and non-pharmacological approaches for the treatment of PH in cardiac surgery will be discussed together in this section.

4.1.1 Pre-capillary

Pulmonary embolism

Acute pulmonary embolism during cardiac surgery can lead to PH and, in some cases, evolve into CTEPH. Pulmonary thromboembolectomy, when surgically indicated, can help control PH and is currently the only curative treatment in patients with CTEPH (Jamieson & Nomura, 2000; Jamieson et al., 2003) (Fig. **6**). In case of CTEPH, evaluation of the feasibility of surgery mainly depends on the location of the obstruction (central vs. more distal pulmonary arteries) (Dartevelle et al., 2004). Patients who are not candidates for surgery may also benefit from PH-specific medical therapy, however, the use of these medications in CTEPH requires further evaluation in randomized controlled trials (Jais et al., 2008; Rubin et al., 2006; Suntharalingam et al., 2008).

The rationale for systemic anticoagulant therapy for chronic lung embolism in patients with PH may be justified by well-recognized risk factors for venous thromboembolism, such as heart failure, a sedentary lifestyle, and a thrombophilic predisposition (Bjornsson & Edwards, 1985). However, no data actually support anticoagulant therapy specifically in patients with PH. Warfarin has been evaluated in only two nonrandomized studies, one retrospective and the other prospective, involving a small number of patients (Fuster et al., 1984; Rich et al., 1992).

4.1.2 Capillary

Cardiopulmonary bypass

As discussed, CPB causes pulmonary damage during surgery through different mechanisms, potentially leading to PH but, more frequently, it contributes to the exacerbation of PH caused by other factors during the surgical procedure. In this context, patients can benefit from PH-specific medical therapy (Table **2**) and prophylactic treatments for PH use in cardiac surgery, which will be discussed later in this chapter.

In 62 patients with preoperative PH (PVR > 125 dyn·sec·cm^{-5} immediately before induction of anesthesia) Solina *et al.* (Solina et al., 2001) explored the dose-responsiveness of 10, 20, 30 and 40 ppm of iNO administered upon termination of CPB in comparison to an intravenous bolus of 50 mg/kg of milrinone given 15 minutes before separation from CPB followed by a 0.5 mg/kg/min regimen administered in the operating room thereafter. Treatment with iNO was associated with significant reductions in PVR at all doses but no improved benefit was observed for doses higher than 10 ppm. No significant difference was observed between iNO and milrinone in terms of reduction in PVR and inotropic requirement.

The same team compared 20 and 40 ppm of iNO to the same dose of intravenous milrinone in 45 patients after cardiac surgery (Solina et al., 2000). Study drugs were administered upon termination of CPB for a 24h-period in the intensive care unit (ICU). The group receiving 20 ppm iNO had a significantly higher MAP while the group receiving 40 ppm had higher right ventricular ejection fraction (RVEF) on arrival in the ICU. The milrinone group required significantly more phenylephrine in the ICU with a trend towards higher heart rates.

In a crossover study, Schmid *et al.* (Schmid et al., 1999) compared iNO, PGE_1 and NTG in 14 adult patients with severe PH (MPAP > 30 mmHg; PVR > 300 dyn·sec·cm^{-5}) after cardiac surgery. The investigation was performed in the ICU within the first 24 h after the procedure. The generalization of results obtained from this study was limited, since it only included patients in stable postoperative circulatory conditions. However, in contrast to PGE_1 and NTG, iNO decreased PVR without exerting concomitant systemic vasodilatory effects. In addition, iNO did not affect the right coronary perfusion pressure and increased oxygen transport.

Protamine

The administration of protamine can be associated with severe PH followed by RV failure. This condition requires immediate treatment. In coronary artery bypass graft (CABG) patients (*n*=3800), Ocal *et al.* (Ocal et al., 2005), two therapeutic approaches were compared for the treatment of the protamine reaction observed in 68 of them (1.8%). One group received $iPGI_2$ and the other intravenous NTG in addition to standard vasoactive agents. The $iPGI_2$ group showed improved hemodynamics and only 14 patients (39%) had to return to CPB compared with all 30 patients (100%) in the NTG group. A trend towards a shorter length of stay in the ICU and reduced mortality was observed in the $iPGI_2$ group, but the numbers were too small to achieve statistical significance.

In order to avoid protamine reaction, heparinase I, a heparin degrading enzyme, was compared to protamine in a multicenter randomized controlled trial (Stafford-Smith et al., 2005). The prevention of protamine-induced PH was also explored as a secondary end-point. Heparinase I was not associated with a reduction in bleeding or reduction in the need for intervention in the treatment of PH.

Lung diseases and/or hypoxia

Low CO during cardiac surgery may affect the pulmonary circulation, potentially leading to hypoxia and worsen PH and RV failure. Thus, an acute perioperative low-output state should be reversed whenever possible before clinical manifestation of chronic hypoperfusion and organ dysfunction.

Khan *et al.* (Khan et al., 2009) compared iNO to $iPGI_2$ in 25 heart and lung transplant recipients with PH, refractory hypoxia, or RV dysfunction. Patients were randomized to iNO (20 ppm) or $iPGI_2$ (20,000 ng/ml) as initial treatment in the operating room, followed by a crossover to the other agent after 6 hours. Both iNO and $iPGI_2$ reduced PAP and central venous pressure (CVP), and improved cardiac index (CI) and mixed venous oxygen saturation on initiation of therapy. At the 6-hour crossover trial, there were no significant differences between groups in the reduction of PAP and CVP, and the improvement of CI and mixed venous oxygen saturation on initiation of therapy. Neither iNO nor $iPGI_2$ affected the oxygenation index or systemic blood pressure.

In the case of chronic hypoxia, supplemental oxygen may be indicated to maintain arterial oxygen saturation at a level above 90 percent (Rubin & Rich, 1997).

In the presence of lung disease, improvement of symptoms of PH may be obtained using basic therapy for PH, for instance, therapy for chronic obstructive pulmonary disease COPD and corticosteroids for interstitial lung disease. Antibiotic therapy for pneumonia as well as elimination of ventilation/perfusion mismatch from and atelectasis can also help control PH.

Chest drainage is required in patients with elevated intrathoracic pressure resulting from accumulated air or blood. However, chest closure may be associated with hemodynamic instability in patients requiring long procedures associated with prolonged CPB due to myocardial edema. The solution to this "thoracic compartment syndrome" consists in leaving the chest temporarily opened in order to reduce surrounding pressures until edema recedes.

4.1.3 Post-capillary

Left heart disease

Left and right ventricular functions are interdependent. All LV function abnormalities induced by coronary artery disease, congestive heart failure, valvular heart disease, or systemic hypertension will influence RV function through ventricular interdependence mainly through an effect on the interventricular septum. Hence, a dilated LV and left atrium can shift the interatrial and interventricular septum and compress the right atrium and ventricule and reduce RV end-diastolic volume.

Fernandes *et al.* (Fernandes et al., 2011) compared iNO to oxygen in 29 patients with PH after MVR. Treatments were initiated for 48 hours immediately after surgery. After 24 and 48 hours, patients receiving iNO had a significantly greater increase in CI compared to patients receiving oxygen ($p < 0.0001$). Pulmonary vascular resistance was also more significantly reduced in patients receiving iNO versus oxygen ($p = 0.005$) at 48 hours. Patients in the iNO group required less systemic vasoactive drugs and had a shorter ICU stay ($p = 0.02$).

Kim *et al.* (Kim et al., 2010) compared the pulmonary vasodilation effect of combined preoperative oral sildenafil (50 mg) and beraprost (40 μg) (pulmonary vasodilators) to placebo in 50 patients scheduled for valvular heart surgery with PH (MPAP > 30 mmHg). Medication was initiated 15 min before the induction of anesthesia. The treatment group had a significantly lower systemic vascular resistance index (SVRI) at 60 min after medication. No other significant intergroup differences in hemodynamic variables were observed. In addition, significantly more patients in the treatment group required vasopressor therapy. In both groups, the PAP was significantly reduced by general anesthesia, and almost normalized after valvular heart surgery. The combination of preoperative oral sildenafil and beraprost treatment resulted in a loss of pulmonary selectivity, and did not provide any additional pulmonary vasodilation or benefits perioperatively.

Wang *et al.* (Wang et al., 2009) investigated the postoperative effects of inhaled milrinone in 48 patients with PH undergoing MVR. Patients were randomly assigned to receive inhaled milrinone (nebulized for 4 hours) or intravenous milrinone (control group bolus of 50 microg/kg i.v. milrinone and then received a continuous milrinone infusion, 0.5 microg/kg/min, for 4 hours) After milrinone administration, MPAP and PVR showed a comparable decrease in both groups. However, both mean MPAP and SVR in the inhaled group were significantly higher than in the control group. MPAP and PVR returned to baseline values 60 minutes after termination of milrinone inhalation. In addition, in the inhaled group, there was a reduction in intrapulmonary shunt fraction (Qs/Qt), with an improvement in arterial oxygen tension/fraction of inspired oxygen (PaO_2/FiO_2).

A study by Fattouch *et al.* (Fattouch et al., 2005) evaluated the effects of inhaled prostacyclin $iPGI_2$ and iNO and compared them with those of conventional intravenous vasodilators (i.e. NTG and nitroprusside) in 58 patients with PH (PVR > 250 dyn·sec·cm^{-5} and MPAP > 25 mmHg) suffering from severe mitral valve stenosis. Both drugs were administered by inhalation 5 min before weaning from CPB and continued in the ICU for up to 2 hours. Significant decreases in MPAP and PVR, as well as increases in CO and RVEF, were noted in both inhaled groups, which was not the case in the conventional group. Furthermore, patients in the inhaled groups showed easier separation from CPB, lower requirements for vasoactive drugs and shorter ICU and hospital lengths of stay.
The same investigators also compared the same three strategies in 58 patients with mitral valve stenosis and elevated PVR (>200 dyn·sec·cm^{-5} and/or a transpulmonary gradient (MPAP-PAOP)>10 mmHg) after MVR (Fattouch et al., 2006). Intravenous nitroprusside (5–15 g/min), $iPGI_2$ (10 g/min) or iNO (20 ppm) were started immediately after patient admission to the ICU. Reduction in MPAP, PVR, and transpulmonary gradient were observed in all groups. Only $iPGI_2$ was associated with a significant increase in stroke volume and CO. Administration of nitroprusside was associated with a reduction in SVR and occurrence of systemic hypotension.
Feneck *et al.* (Feneck et al., 2001) compared milrinone to dobutamine in 120 patients with PAOP > 10 mmHg and low output syndrome after CBP (CO < 2 L/min/m^2). In a subset of patients with PH (PVR > 200 dyn·sec·cm^{-5}; MPAP > 25 mmHg), milrinone and dobutamine had similar effects in reducing PVR and increasing CI. However, milrinone was more effective in reducing PAOP and systemic vascular resistance (SVR).
Finally, in 20 patients scheduled for mitral valve surgery with PH (MPAP > 25 mmHg), Hachenberg *et al.* (Hachenberg et al., 1997) explored the role of enoximone compared to a combination of NTG and dobutamine, given after induction of anesthesia and then restarted before the end of CPB. Only enoximone was associated with a decrease in MPAP and PVR.
In the presence of PH secondary to LV failure, intra-aortic balloon counterpulsation may facilitate LV recovery.

Patient-prosthesis mismatch (PPM)

In the presence of prosthetic valve dysfunction after CPB, returning under CPB to correct the problem is considered the treatment of choice (Fig. **9**).

4.2 Experience at the Montreal Heart Institute

At the Montreal Heart Institute, $iPGI_2$ (Hache et al., 2001; Hache et al., 2003) and inhaled milrinone (Lamarche et al., 2005; Lamarche et al., 2007) are commonly administered to patients when PH and RV dysfunction occur before or after cardiac surgery. Oral sildenafil and iNO are also used in refractory cases in the ICU. Administration by inhalation has the advantage of selectively reaching well-ventilated regions of the lung and thus avoiding undesired decreases of systemic pressures. Future strategies may include the combination of currently available drugs and improvement of methods of administration for current drugs.

5. Importance and impact of pulmonary hypertension in cardiac surgery

Preoperative PH is associated with increased morbidity and mortality in cardiac surgery (Tuman et al., 1992; Tremblay et al., 1993; Reich et al., 1999; Bernstein & Parsonnet, 2000; Malouf et al., 2002). Therefore, awareness of PH is very important and its presence in any form should be routinely reported to the surgeon and be evaluated in risk stratification models. Yet, this is not always the case, since only 4/19 risk stratification models in cardiac surgery include preoperative PH as a risk factor (Nilsson et al., 2006). Interestingly, PH is included in the EuroSCORE model which had the greatest discriminatory power over all other models. In a Swedish study including 4351 CABG patients, the receiver operating characteristics (ROC) of the EuroSCORE model was found to be 0.86 and 0.75 for the 30-day and one year mortality rates, respectively.

Analysis performed using the Montreal Heart Institute anesthesia database in 1999 on a total of 1439 patients revealed a mean preoperative SPAP of 31±10 mmHg. PH was defined as SPAP > 30 mmHg and was observed in 605 patients (42%). The type of procedures performed in this subpopulation were mainly MVR (*n*=80, 40±14 mmHg), followed by combined CABG and valve procedures (*n*=126, 36±13 mmHg), multiple valve procedures (*n*=60, 36±16 mmHg) and heart transplantations (*n*=6, 36±14 mmHg). Severe PH defined as MAP/MPAP ratio < 2 was observed in 16 patients, who all experienced difficult separation from CPB, half of them required postoperative vasoactive support for more than 24 hours while 3 of them died (18.7%).

Thus, PH present before, during or after the operation has an impact on survival mostly through its deleterious effect on right-sided heart function. The most dreaded consequence of PH is the increase in RV afterload and RV dysfunction which will be addressed herein.

5.1 Right ventricular dysfunction

Regardless of the underlying cause, uncontrolled PH leads to RV dysfunction. There is growing evidence showing that morbidity and mortality associated with PH depends on RV adaptation to the disease rather than on the absolute values of PAP (D'Alonzo et al., 1991; Yeo et al., 1998; Ramakrishna et al., 2005; Voelkel et al., 2006; Haddad et al., 2009). Furthermore, studies addressing hemodynamic variables and survival in idiopathic pulmonary arterial hypertension show that high mean Pra and low CO are consistently associated with poorer survival while PAP values are only moderately related to outcome (D'Alonzo et al., 1991; Chin et al., 2005).

Many studies, in a variety of clinical settings, have demonstrated the importance of RV function in cardiac surgery (Table **3**) (Haddad et al., 2009). Typical pathologies and treatments in these studies included high risk coronary or valvular heart disease, congenital heart disease, heart transplantation, patients requiring mechanical assist devices, and unstable patients postoperatively. However, most of the evidence supporting the importance of RV function pertains to retrospective and small prospective studies. Moreover, parameters of RV function have not yet been included in large scale models of risk stratification and thus, their incremental value to the Parsonnet Score and the EuroSCORE has not been well established (Bernstein & Parsonnet, 2000; Nashef et al., 2002; Shroyer et al., 2003; Ambler et al., 2005). A panel in 2006 from the National Institute of Health (NIH) has emphasized the importance of conducting research to better understand RV failure (Voelkel et al., 2006).

5.1.1 Before the procedure

In patients with severe aortic stenosis, Boldt *et al.* (Boldt et al., 1992) demonstrated that preoperative RV dysfunction was associated with increased requirements for postoperative inotropic support.

Study	Population	Study Design	RV dysfunction	Results
Reitchert *et al.*	Unstable post-operative patients	Prospective *n*=60	RVFAC < 35%	RV dysfunction associated with high mortality rates
Pinzani *et al.*	Mitral and combined mitro-aortic surgery	Retrospective *n*=382	Clinical definition	Postoperative RV failure is the strongest predictor of postoperative mortality
Cullen *et al.*	Tetralogy of Fallot	Prospective *n*=35	Restrictive RV physiology	Restrictive physiology predicts longer intensive care unit stay post repair and lower cardiac output
Gatzoulis *et al.*	Tetralogy of Fallot	Prospective *n*=41	Restrictive RV physiology	Restrictive physiology predicts smaller RV and better exercise tolerance
Kromos *et al.*	LVAD and RV failure	Retrospective *n*=31	Clinical mean RVEF = 11.8%	Preoperative clinical factors such as fever, pulmonary edema, and intraoperative blood transfusions were associated with RVAD need
Hosenpud *et al.*	Heart Transplantation	Retrospective (International Society for Heart & Lung transplantation) *n*=69,205	RV failure associated with circulatory failure	RV failure accounts for up to 20% of early deaths
Oehiai *et al.*	LVAD	Retrospective *n*=245	RV failure requiring RVAD	23 patients (9%) required RVAD. The need for circulatory support, female gender, and non-ischemic etiology were predictors of RVAD need
Maslow *et al.*	CAD undergoing coronary bypass surgery with LVEF < 25%	Retrospective *n*=41	RVFAC < 35%	RV dysfunction is associated with decreased long term survival
Therrien *et al.*	Tetralogy of Fallot	Prospective *n*=17	RV remodeling	Severe RV dilatation (RVEDV ≥ 170 ml/m^2 or RVESV > 85 ml/m^2) associated with incomplete RV remodeling
Webb *et al.*	Atrial septal defect	Retrospective series	RV remodeling	Older age at repair and abnormal RV myocardial relaxation were associated with incomplete RV remodeling
Denault *et al.*	Patients undergoing bypass surgery	Retrospective and prospective *n*=800	Dynamic RVOTO (Gradient> 25 mmHg)	Incidence: 4%, dynamic obstruction of RVOTO was associated with a higher incidence of difficult weaning from bypass
Haddad *et al.*	High risk valvular surgery	Prospective *n*=50	RVFAC < 32% or RVMPI > 0.50	Preoperative RV dysfunction was associated with a higher incidence of post-operative circulatory failure

CAD: coronary artery disease; LVEF: left ventricular ejection fraction; LVAD: left ventricular assist device; RV: right ventricular; RVAD: right ventricular assist device; RVESV: right ventricular end-systolic volume; RVEDV: right ventricular end-diastolic volume; RVEF: right ventricular ejection fraction; RVFAC: right ventricular fractional area change; RVMPI: right ventricular myocardial performance index; RVOTO: right ventricular outflow tract obstruction. (Haddad et al., 2009)

Table 3. Prognostic Value of Right Ventricular Function in Cardiac Surgery (selected studies)

In a retrospective study involving patients undergoing mitral and mitral-aortic valvular surgery, Pinzani *et al.* (Pinzani et al., 1993) showed that preoperative RV failure was associated with increased perioperative mortality. Furthermore, in that study, postoperative RV failure was the most important independent predictor of late survival.
In a small prospective study of 14 patients with severe non-ischemic mitral regurgitation presenting high risk descriptors (LV ejection fraction (LVEF) ≤45% or RVEF ≤ 20%), Wencker *et al.* (Wencker et al., 2000) found that preoperative RVEF ≤ 20% predicted late postoperative death.
In a retrospective study of 41 patients undergoing non-emergent coronary artery bypass surgery, Maslow *et al.* (Maslow et al., 2002) have shown than RV dysfunction (right ventricular fractional area change (RVFAC)< 35%) in presence of severe LV dysfunction (LVEF ≤ 25%) was associated with an increased risk of postoperative morbidity and mortality. Furthermore, patients with RV dysfunction presented a higher prevalence of diabetes mellitus and renal disease, a higher incidence of postoperative support (inotropic or mechanical), longer ICU and hospital stays, as well as a decrease in short and long term survival.

Experience at the Montreal Heart Institute

Haddad *et al.* (Haddad et al., 2007) further assessed the value of RV function relative to other validated risk factors in open valvular heart surgery on 50 patients undergoing valvular surgery. Patients with RV myocardial performance index (RVMPI) < 50% (n=20) presented a significantly higher occurrence of circulatory failure (16/20 (80%) *vs* 6/30 (20%), p<0.0001) as well as a higher postoperative heart failure mortality (14/20 (74%) *vs* 3/30 (10%), p<0.0001). In addition, multivariate analysis revealed RVMPI as the only independent predictor of heart failure and mortality among all other demographic, hemodynamic and echocardiographic variables (p<0.0001).

5.1.2 After the procedure

Right ventricular failure after CPB is associated with a mortality rate ranging from 44% to 86% (Davila-Roman et al., 1995). The incidence of acute refractory RV failure ranges from 0.04 to 0.1% after cardiac surgery. Acute refractory RV failure has also been reported in 2-3% patients after heart trasplantationand in 20-30% patients receiving support from a LV assist device with a reported initial salvage rate as low as 25-30% (Kaul & Fields, 2000).

5.2 Treatment of right ventricular failure

A proposed algorithm for the treatment of RV failure used at the Montreal Heart Instituteis summarised in Fig. **10**. Assessment of RV function is performed visually when the chest is opened, by analysing RV pressure waveforms and using transesophageal echocardiography. Once RVOTO is ruled out, the etiology of RV systolic dysfunction is divided in two categories, either ischemic or not and with or without LV failure. If ischemia is suspected of causing either RV failure or bi-ventricular failure, treatments (medical and surgical) will be oriented towards the promotion of RV perfusion by means of thrombolysis, percutaneous transluminal coronary angioplasty, or CABG. Finally, pulmonary artery balloon pump, RV assist device or cavopulmonary diversion have also been described as potential treatments for severe RV dysfunction (Kaul & Fields, 2000). Otherwise, if a non-ischemic etiology is more likely or if no LV failure is present, treatments will rather be oriented towards an increase in contractility (inotropes) and a reduction in RV afterload (iNO, $iPGI_2$, inhaled milrinone, oral sildenafil).

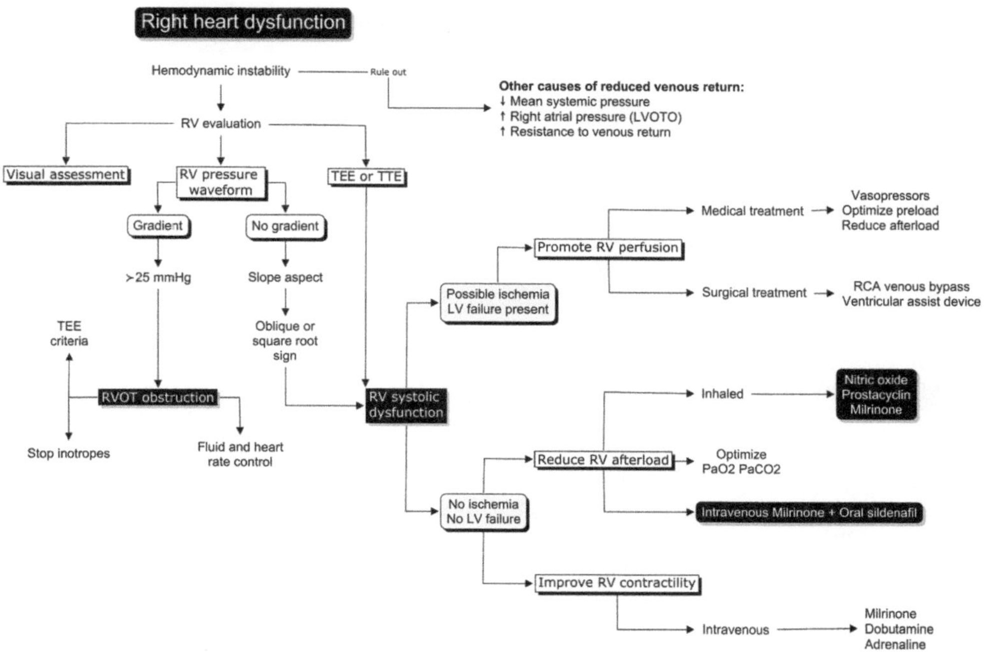

Fig. 10. Proposed approach in the treatment of right ventricular (RV) dysfunction. (LVOTO: left ventricular outflow tract obstruction; RCA: right coronary artery; RVOTO: right ventricular outflow tract obstruction; TEE: transesophageal echocardiography; TTE: transthoracic echocardiography). Presented at the 2011 Canadian Anesthesiologist Society Annual Meeting in Toronto, ON, Canada.

Optimizing oxygenation and ventilation and ruling out other reversible causes of reduction in venous return such as reduction in MAP, increase in Pra and increase in resistance to venous return will also be important in managing these patients.

6. Prevention of pulmonary hypertension in cardiac surgery

6.1 Pharmacological

Prevention of PH represents a promising strategy to prevent RV failure, its most important consequence after cardiac surgery. To date, very few studies have addressed this issue and one of the potential avenues constitutes the prevention of the pulmonary reperfusion syndrome. In this regard, both $iPGI_2$ (Fortier et al., 2004) and inhaled milrinone (Lamarche et al., 2005) have been demonstrated to prevent CPB-induced endothelial dysfunction, in an animal model. A pilot randomized controlled trial (RCT) conducted by Hache *et al.* (Hache et al., 2003) in patients with preoperative PH concluded that $iPGI_2$ was superior to placebo in reducing PH and was also associated with lower requirements for vasoactive support.

A pilot RCT was conducted on the administration of inhaled milrinone before CPB in 21 patients, all undergoing valvular surgeries (Denault et al., 2010b). Procedures consisted of 14 complex surgeries and 5 reoperations. The study included a total of 8 males and 13 females with a mean age of 70±6.3 years old and a mean Parsonnet Score of 32±9. Inhaled milrinone (n=10) significantly reduced mean SPAP, which decreased from 66±20 mmHg (pre-CPB) to

46±20 mmHg (after CPB) (p<0.001). In contrast, SPAP remained unchanged in the control group (*n*=11) and no significant differences between groups were observed in decreased systemic arterial pressures.
A retrospective study reporting the preliminary experience on the use of inhaled milrinone at the Montreal Heart Institute was conducted in 70 high risk patients with a mean Parsonnet Score of 27±14 (Bernstein & Parsonnet, 2000; Lamarche et al., 2007). Results were compared to those of a control group with similar baseline characteristics. In conclusion, the administration of inhaled milrinone prior to CPB (*n*=30) was associated with a lower chance of CPB re-initiation (9 *vs* 1; p=0.021) and lower postoperative PAP. Further studies (# NCT00819377) are underway to determine the efficacy of this approach.

6.2 Non-pharmacological

In addition to therapeutic approaches to the prevention of PH, the choice of type and size of aortic prosthetic valve may be a very important factor. As previously discussed, it has been shown that, if the EOA of the aortic valve is too small relative to body size, the so-called PPM, the intraoperative and long-term mortality will increase (Milano et al., 2001; Rao et al., 2000; Pibarot & Dumesnil, 2000; Blais et al., 2003; Ruel et al., 2004; Pibarot & Dumesnil, 2006; Tasca et al., 2006; Kulik et al., 2006). Hence, prevention of PPM may contribute to reducing PH after cardiac surgery and facilitate separation from CPB. This includes strategies such as the implantation of a prosthesis with better performance (stentless bioprosthesis, new generation bileaflet mechanical valve, new generation supra-annular stented bioprosthetic valve) or enlargement of the aortic root (Fig. **9**) in order to accommodate a larger prosthesis. On the other hand, some strategies used to prevent PPM are complex and may even increase the risk of difficult weaning from CPB extending the duration of the surgical procedure and consequently, CPB duration. Unfortunately, in some cases, the drawbacks of using alternative procedures may supercede the benefits of avoiding PPM. Therefore, the establishment of accurate criteria for a better assessment of the benefit-risk ratio with respect to the prevention of PPM is essential. In the case of mitral valve PPM, the best option would be to favor mitral valve repair rather than replacement. However, mitral valve repair may not be possible in a significant number of patients, which limits the options when compared to aortic valve replacement (Magne et al., 2007).

7. Conclusion

Pulmonary hypertension and its most dreaded consequence, RV dysfunction, are important mortality risk factors in cardiac surgery. Accordingly, all cardiac patients may benefit from early diagnosis and/or treatment prior to the surgical procedure. In patients with PH, further evaluation of potential alterations in the RV function would be relevant. Thus, future trials should prioritize in-depth exploration of preventive approaches in order to address the role of preemptive reduction of PH severity before cardiac surgery and to determine its impact on postoperative outcomes and survival improvement.

8. Acknowledgements

The authors sincerely thank Antoinette Paolitto and Denis Babin for their_help with the chapter submission and Sybil Skinner Robertson and Paul Gavra for their help with the chapter review.

9. Abbreviations

Ao	aorta
AVR	aortic valve replacement
CABG	coronary artery bypass graft
CAD	coronary artery disease
CI	cardiac index
CO	cardiac output
COPD	chronic obstructive pulmonary disease
CPB	cardiopulmonary bypass
CTEPH	chronic thromboembolic pulmonary hypertension
CVP	central venous pressure
D	diastolic
DPAP	diastolic pulmonary arterial pressure
EKG	electrocardiogram
EOA	effective orifice area
FRC	functional residual capacity
ICU	intensive care unit
iNO	inhaled nitric oxide
$iPGI_2$	inhaled prostacyclin
LA	left atrium
LV	left ventricle or left ventricular
LVAD	left ventricular assist device
LVEF	left ventricular ejection fraction
LVOTO	left ventricular outflow tract obstruction
MAP	mean arterial pressure
MPAP	mean pulmonary artery pressure
MVR	mitral valve replacement
NIH	National Institutes of Health
NO	nitric oxide
NTG	nitroglycerin
PaO_2/FiO_2	arterial oxygen tension/fraction of inspired oxygen
PAOP	pulmonary artery occlusion pressure
PAP	pulmonary artery pressure
PCWP	pulmonary capillary wedge pressure
PEEP	positive end-expiratory pressure
PFO	patent foramen ovale
PG	pressure gradient
PGE_1	prostaglandin E_1
PGI_2	prostacyclin
PH	pulmonary hypertension
Pa	arterial pressure
PCO_2	partial pressure of carbon dioxide
Ppa	pulmonary artery pressure
PPM	patient-prosthesis mismatch
Pra	right atrial pressure
Prv	right ventricular pressure

PVR	pulmonary vascular resistance
PVRI	indexed pulmonary vascular resistance
Qs/Qt	intrapulmonary shunt fraction
RA	right atrium
RCA	right coronary artery
RCT	randomized controlled trial
ROC	receiver operating characteristics
RPA	right pulmonary artery
RV	right ventricle or right ventricular
RVAD	right ventricular assist device
RVEDV	right ventricular end-diastolic volume
RVEF	right ventricular ejection fraction
RVESV	right ventricular end-systolic volume
RVFAC	right ventricular fractional area change
RVMPI	right ventricular myocardial performance index
RVOTO	right ventricular outflow tract obstruction
RVSP	right ventricular systolic pressure
S	systolic
SAP	systemic arterial pressure
SPAP	systolic pulmonary artery pressure
SVR	systemic vascular resistance
SVRI	indexed systemic vascular resistance
TEE	transesophageal echocardiography
TLC	total lung capacity
Tr	tricuspid regurgitation
TTE	transthoracic echocardiography
UK	United Kingdom
USA	United States of America
V	velocity

10. References

Ambler, G., Omar, R. Z., Royston, P., Kinsman, R., Keogh, B. E., & Taylor, K. M. (2005). Generic, simple risk stratification model for heart valve surgery. *Circulation*. 112, 2, 224-231, ISSN 1524-4539

Asimakopoulos, G., Smith, P. L., Ratnatunga, C. P., & Taylor, K. M. (1999). Lung injury and acute respiratory distress syndrome after cardiopulmonary bypass. *Ann Thorac Surg*. 68, 3, 1107-1115, ISSN 0003-4975

Bakhtiary, F., Schiemann, M., Dzemali, O., Dogan, S., Schachinger, V., Ackermann, H., Moritz, A., & Kleine, P. (2007). Impact of patient-prosthesis mismatch and aortic valve design on coronary flow reserve after aortic valve replacement. *J Am Coll Cardiol*. 49, 7, 790-796, ISSN 1558-3597

Bernstein, A. D. & Parsonnet, V. (2000). Bedside estimation of risk as an aid for decision-making in cardiac surgery. *Ann Thorac Surg*. 69, 3, 823-828, ISSN 0003-4975

Bjornsson, J. & Edwards, W. D. (1985). Primary pulmonary hypertension: a histopathologic study of 80 cases. *Mayo Clin Proc*. 60, 1, 16-25, ISSN 0025-6196

Blais, C., Dumesnil, J. G., Baillot, R., Simard, S., Doyle, D., & Pibarot, P. (2003). Impact of valve prosthesis-patient mismatch on short-term mortality after aortic valve replacement. *Circulation*. 108, 8, 983-988, ISSN 1524-4539

Boldt, J., Zickmann, B., Ballesteros, M., Dapper, F., & Hempelmann, G. (1992). Right ventricular function in patients with aortic stenosis undergoing aortic valve replacement. *J Cardiothorac Vasc Anesth*. 6, 3, 287-291, ISSN 1053-0770

Chin, K. M., Kim, N. H., & Rubin, L. J. (2005). The right ventricle in pulmonary hypertension. *Coron Artery Dis*. 16, 1, 13-18, ISSN 0954-6928

D'Alonzo, G. E., Barst, R. J., Ayres, S. M., Bergofsky, E. H., Brundage, B. H., Detre, K. M., Fishman, A. P., Goldring, R. M., Groves, B. M., & Kernis, J. T. (1991). Survival in patients with primary pulmonary hypertension. Results from a national prospective registry. *Ann Intern Med*. 115, 5, 343-349, ISSN 0003-4819

Dartevelle, P., Fadel, E., Mussot, S., Chapelier, A., Herve, P., de Perrot, M., Cerrina, J., Ladurie, F. L., Lehouerou, D., Humbert, M., Sitbon, O., & Simonneau, G. (2004). Chronic thromboembolic pulmonary hypertension. *Eur Respir J*. 23, 4, 637-648, ISSN 0903-1936

Davila-Roman, V. G., Waggoner, A. D., Hopkins, W. E., & Barzilai, B. (1995). Right ventricular dysfunction in low output syndrome after cardiac operations: assessment by transesophageal echocardiography. *Ann Thorac Surg*. 60, 4, 1081-1086, ISSN 0003-4975

Delgado, J. F., Conde, E., Sanchez, V., Lopez-Rios, F., Gomez-Sanchez, M. A., Escribano, P., Sotelo, T., Gomez, d. l. C., Cortina, J., & de la Calzada, C. S. (2005). Pulmonary vascular remodeling in pulmonary hypertension due to chronic heart failure. *Eur J Heart Fail*. 7, 6, 1011-1016, ISSN 1388-9842

Denault, A. Y., Couture, P., Vegas, A., Buithieu, J., & Tardif, J. C. (2010a). *Transesophageal Echocardiography Multimedia Manual: A Perioperative Transdisciplinary Approach,* (Second Edition), Informa Healthcare, ISBN 9781-420-08070-4, New York

Denault, A. Y., Haddad, F., Lamarche, Y., Nguyen, A. Q. N., Varin, F., Levesque, S., Shi, Y., Perrault, L. P., Tardif, J. C., and Lambert, J. (2010b). Inhaled Milrinone in Cardiac Surgery, *Procedings of Canadian Anesthesiologists' Society*, Montreal, QC, Canada, June 2010b

Downing, S. W. & Edmunds, L. H., Jr. (1992). Release of vasoactive substances during cardiopulmonary bypass. *Ann Thorac Surg*. 54, 6, 1236-1243, ISSN 0003-4975

Fattouch, K., Sbraga, F., Bianco, G., Speziale, G., Gucciardo, M., Sampognaro, R., & Ruvolo, G. (2005). Inhaled prostacyclin, nitric oxide, and nitroprusside in pulmonary hypertension after mitral valve replacement. *J Card Surg*. 20, 2, 171-176, ISSN 0886-0440

Fattouch, K., Sbraga, F., Sampognaro, R., Bianco, G., Gucciardo, M., Lavalle, C., Vizza, C. D., Fedele, F., & Ruvolo, G. (2006). Treatment of pulmonary hypertension in patients undergoing cardiac surgery with cardiopulmonary bypass: a randomized, prospective, double-blind study. *J Cardiovasc Med (Hagerstown)*. 7, 2, 119-123, ISSN 1558-2027

Feneck, R. O., Sherry, K. M., Withington, P. S., & Oduro-Dominah, A. (2001). Comparison of the hemodynamic effects of milrinone with dobutamine in patients after cardiac surgery. *J Cardiothorac Vasc Anesth*. 15, 3, 306-315, ISSN 1053-0770

Fernandes, J. L., Sampaio, R. O., Brandao, C. M., Accorsi, T. A., Cardoso, L. F., Spina, G. S., Tarasoutchi, F., Pomerantzeff, P., Auler, J. O., Jr., & Grinberg, M. (2011). Comparison of inhaled nitric oxide versus oxygen on hemodynamics in patients with mitral stenosis and severe pulmonary hypertension after mitral valve surgery. *Am J Cardiol*. 107, 7, 1040-1045

Fischer, L. G., Van, A. H., & Burkle, H. (2003). Management of pulmonary hypertension: physiological and pharmacological considerations for anesthesiologists. *Anesth Analg*. 96, 6, 1603-1616, ISSN 0003-2999

Fortier, S., DeMaria, R. G., Lamarche, Y., Malo, O., Denault, A. Y., Desjardins, F., Carrier, M., & Perrault, L. P. (2004). Inhaled prostacyclin reduces cardiopulmonary bypass-induced pulmonary endothelial dysfunction via increased cyclic adenosine monophosphate levels. *J Thorac Cardiovasc Surg*. 128, 1, 109-116, ISSN 0022-5223

Fuster, V., Steele, P. M., Edwards, W. D., Gersh, B. J., McGoon, M. D., & Frye, R. L. (1984). Primary pulmonary hypertension: natural history and the importance of thrombosis. *Circulation*. 70, 4, 580-587, ISSN 0009-7322

Gomez, C. M. & Palazzo, M. G. (1998). Pulmonary artery catheterization in anaesthesia and intensive care. *Br J Anaesth*. 81, 6, 945-956, ISSN 0007-0912

Hache, M., Denault, A. Y., Belisle, S., Couture, P., Babin, D., Tetrault, F., & Guimond, J. G. (2001). Inhaled prostacyclin (PGI2) is an effective addition to the treatment of pulmonary hypertension and hypoxia in the operating room and intensive care unit. *Can J Anaesth*. 48, 9, 924-929, ISSN 0832-610X

Hache, M., Denault, A. Y., Belisle, S., Robitaille, D., Couture, P., Sheridan, P., Pellerin, M., Babin, D., Noel, N., Guertin, M. C., Martineau, R., & Dupuis, J. (2003). Inhaled epoprostenol (prostacyclin) and pulmonary hypertension before cardiac surgery. *J Thorac Cardiovasc Surg*. 125, 3, 642-649, ISSN 0022-5223

Hachenberg, T., Mollhoff, T., Holst, D., Hammel, D., & Brussel, T. (1997). Cardiopulmonary effects of enoximone or dobutamine and nitroglycerin on mitral valve regurgitation and pulmonary venous hypertension. *J Cardiothorac Vasc Anesth*. 11, 4, 453-457, ISSN 1053-0770

Haddad, F., Couture, P., Tousignant, C., & Denault, A. Y. (2009). The right ventricle in cardiac surgery, a perioperative perspective: II. Pathophysiology, clinical importance, and management. *Anesth Analg*. 108, 2, 422-433

Haddad, F., Denault, A. Y., Couture, P., Cartier, R., Pellerin, M., Levesque, S., Lambert, J., & Tardif, J. C. (2007). Right ventricular myocardial performance index predicts perioperative mortality or circulatory failure in high-risk valvular surgery. *J Am Soc Echocardiogr*. 20, 9, 1065-1072

Humbert, M., Sitbon, O., & Simonneau, G. (2004). Treatment of pulmonary arterial hypertension. *N Engl J Med*. 351, 14, 1425-1436

Jais, X., D'Armini, A. M., Jansa, P., Torbicki, A., Delcroix, M., Ghofrani, H. A., Hoeper, M. M., Lang, I. M., Mayer, E., Pepke-Zaba, J., Perchenet, L., Morganti, A., Simonneau, G., & Rubin, L. J. (2008). Bosentan for treatment of inoperable chronic thromboembolic pulmonary hypertension: BENEFiT (Bosentan Effects in iNopErable Forms of chronIc Thromboembolic pulmonary hypertension), a randomized, placebo-controlled trial. *J Am Coll Cardiol*. 52, 25, 2127-2134, ISSN 1558-3597

Jamieson, S. W., Kapelanski, D. P., Sakakibara, N., Manecke, G. R., Thistlethwaite, P. A., Kerr, K. M., Channick, R. N., Fedullo, P. F., & Auger, W. R. (2003). Pulmonary endarterectomy: experience and lessons learned in 1,500 cases. *Ann Thorac Surg*. 76, 5, 1457-1462

Jamieson, S. W. & Nomura, K. (2000). Indications for and the results of pulmonary thromboendarterectomy for thromboembolic pulmonary hypertension. *Semin Vasc Surg*. 13, 3, 236-244

Kaul, T. K. & Fields, B. L. (2000). Postoperative acute refractory right ventricular failure: incidence, pathogenesis, management and prognosis. *Cardiovasc Surg*. 8, 1, 1-9

Khan, T. A., Schnickel, G., Ross, D., Bastani, S., Laks, H., Esmailian, F., Marelli, D., Beygui, R., Shemin, R., Watson, L., Vartapetian, I., & Ardehali, A. (2009). A prospective, randomized, crossover pilot study of inhaled nitric oxide versus inhaled prostacyclin in heart transplant and lung transplant recipients. *J Thorac Cardiovasc Surg*. 138, 6, 1417-1424

Kim, S. Y., Shim, J. K., Shim, Y. H., Hong, S. W., Choi, K. H., & Kwak, Y. L. (2010). Sildenafil and beraprost combination therapy in patients with pulmonary hypertension undergoing valvular heart surgery. *J Heart Valve Dis*. 19, 3, 333-340

Kulik, A., Burwash, I. G., Kapila, V., Mesana, T. G., & Ruel, M. (2006). Long-term outcomes after valve replacement for low-gradient aortic stenosis: impact of prosthesis-patient mismatch. *Circulation*. 114, 1 Suppl, I553-I558

Lamarche, Y., Malo, O., Thorin, E., Denault, A. Y., Carrier, M., Roy, J., & Perrault, L. P. (2005). Inhaled but not intravenous milrinone prevents pulmonary endothelial dysfunction after cardiopulmonary bypass. *J Thorac Cardiovasc Surg*. 130, 1, 83-92

Lamarche, Y., Perrault, L. P., Maltais, S., Tetreault, K., Lambert, J., & Denault, A. Y. (2007). Preliminary experience with inhaled milrinone in cardiac surgery. *Eur J Cardiothorac Surg*. 31, 6, 1081-1087

Lesage, A. M., Tsuchioka, H., Young, W. G., Jr., & Sealy, W. C. (1966). Pathogenesis of pulmonary damage during extracorporeal perfusion. *Arch Surg*. 93, 6, 1002-1008

Magne, J., Mathieu, P., Dumesnil, J. G., Tanne, D., Dagenais, F., Doyle, D., & Pibarot, P. (2007). Impact of Prosthesis-Patient Mismatch on Survival After Mitral Valve Replacement. *Circulation*. 115, 11, 1417-1425

Malouf, J. F., Enriquez-Sarano, M., Pellikka, P. A., Oh, J. K., Bailey, K. R., Chandrasekaran, K., Mullany, C. J., & Tajik, A. J. (2002). Severe pulmonary hypertension in patients with severe aortic valve stenosis: clinical profile and prognostic implications. *J Am Coll Cardiol*. 40, 4, 789-795

Martineau, A., Arcand, G., Couture, P., Babin, D., Perreault, L. P., & Denault, A. Y. (2003). Transesophageal echocardiographic diagnosis of carbon dioxide embolism during minimally invasive saphenous vein harvesting and treatment with inhaled epoprostenol. *Anesth Analg*. 96, 4, 962-964

Maslow, A. D., Regan, M. M., Panzica, P., Heindel, S., Mashikian, J., & Comunale, M. E. (2002). Precardiopulmonary bypass right ventricular function is associated with poor outcome after coronary artery bypass grafting in patients with severe left ventricular systolic dysfunction. *Anesth Analg*. 95, 6, 1507-1518

McLaughlin, V. V. & McGoon, M. D. (2006). Pulmonary arterial hypertension. *Circulation*. 114, 13, 1417-1431

Milano, A. D., Blanzola, C., Mecozzi, G., D'Alfonso, A., De Carlo, M., Nardi, C., & Bortolotti, U. (2001). Hemodynamic performance of stented and stentless aortic bioprostheses. *Ann Thorac Surg*. 72, 1, 33-38

Moher, D., Schulz, K. F., & Altman, D. G. (2001). The CONSORT statement: revised recommendations for improving the quality of reports of parallel-group randomised trials. *Lancet*. 357, 9263, 1191-1194

Moraes, D. L., Colucci, W. S., & Givertz, M. M. (2000). Secondary pulmonary hypertension in chronic heart failure: the role of the endothelium in pathophysiology and management. *Circulation*. 102, 14, 1718-1723, ISSN 1524-4539

Nashef, S. A., Roques, F., Hammill, B. G., Peterson, E. D., Michel, P., Grover, F. L., Wyse, R. K., & Ferguson, T. B. (2002). Validation of European System for Cardiac Operative Risk Evaluation (EuroSCORE) in North American cardiac surgery. *Eur J Cardiothorac Surg*. 22, 1, 101-105

Nilsson, J., Algotsson, L., Hoglund, P., Luhrs, C., & Brandt, J. (2006). Comparison of 19 pre-operative risk stratification models in open-heart surgery. *Eur Heart J*. 27, 7, 867-874

Ocal, A., Kiris, I., Erdinc, M., Peker, O., Yavuz, T., & Ibrisim, E. (2005). Efficiency of prostacyclin in the treatment of protamine-mediated right ventricular failure and acute pulmonary hypertension. *Tohoku J Exp Med*. 207, 1, 51-58

Oudiz, R. J. (2007). Pulmonary hypertension associated with left-sided heart disease. *Clin Chest Med*. 28, 1, 233-41, x, ISSN 0272-5231

Pengo, V., Lensing, A. W., Prins, M. H., Marchiori, A., Davidson, B. L., Tiozzo, F., Albanese, P., Biasiolo, A., Pegoraro, C., Iliceto, S., & Prandoni, P. (2004). Incidence of chronic thromboembolic pulmonary hypertension after pulmonary embolism. *N Engl J Med*. 350, 22, 2257-2264, ISSN 1533-4406

Pibarot, P. & Dumesnil, J. G. (2000). Hemodynamic and clinical impact of prosthesis-patient mismatch in the aortic valve position and its prevention. *J Am Coll Cardiol*. 36, 4, 1131-1141

Pibarot, P. & Dumesnil, J. G. (2006). Prosthesis-patient mismatch: definition, clinical impact, and prevention. *Heart*. 92, 8, 1022-1029

Pinzani, A., de Gevigney, G., Pinzani, V., Ninet, J., Milon, H., & Delahaye, J. P. (1993). [Pre- and postoperative right cardiac insufficiency in patients with mitral or mitral-aortic valve diseases]. *Arch Mal Coeur Vaiss*. 86, 1, 27-34

Ramakrishna, G., Sprung, J., Ravi, B. S., Chandrasekaran, K., & McGoon, M. D. (2005). Impact of pulmonary hypertension on the outcomes of noncardiac surgery: predictors of perioperative morbidity and mortality. *J Am Coll Cardiol*. 45, 10, 1691-1699

Rao, V., Jamieson, W. R., Ivanov, J., Armstrong, S., & David, T. E. (2000). Prosthesis-patient mismatch affects survival after aortic valve replacement. *Circulation*. 102, 19 Suppl 3, III5-III9

Reich, D. L., Bodian, C. A., Krol, M., Kuroda, M., Osinski, T., & Thys, D. M. (1999). Intraoperative hemodynamic predictors of mortality, stroke, and myocardial infarction after coronary artery bypass surgery. *Anesth Analg*. 89, 4, 814-822

Rich, S., Kaufmann, E., & Levy, P. S. (1992). The effect of high doses of calcium-channel blockers on survival in primary pulmonary hypertension. *N Engl J Med*. 327, 2, 76-81, ISSN 0028-4793

Robitaille, A., Denault, A. Y., Couture, P., Belisle, S., Fortier, A., Guertin, M. C., Carrier, M., & Martineau, R. (2006). Importance of relative pulmonary hypertension in cardiac surgery: the mean systemic-to-pulmonary artery pressure ratio. *J Cardiothorac Vasc Anesth*. 20, 3, 331-339

Rubin, L. J., Hoeper, M. M., Klepetko, W., Galie, N., Lang, I. M., & Simonneau, G. (2006). Current and future management of chronic thromboembolic pulmonary hypertension: from diagnosis to treatment responses. *Proc Am Thorac Soc*. 3, 7, 601-607, ISSN 1546-3222

Rubin, L. J. & Rich, S. (1997). *Primary pulmonary hypertension*, M. Dekker, ISBN 0824795059, New York

Ruel, M., Rubens, F. D., Masters, R. G., Pipe, A. L., Bedard, P., Hendry, P. J., Lam, B. K., Burwash, I. G., Goldstein, W. G., Brais, M. P., Keon, W. J., & Mesana, T. G. (2004). Late incidence and predictors of persistent or recurrent heart failure in patients with aortic prosthetic valves. *J Thorac Cardiovasc Surg*. 127, 1, 149-159

Sackett, D. L. (1989). Rules of evidence and clinical recommendations on the use of antithrombotic agents. *Chest*. 95, 2 Suppl, 2S-4S

Schmid, E. R., Burki, C., Engel, M. H., Schmidlin, D., Tornic, M., & Seifert, B. (1999). Inhaled nitric oxide versus intravenous vasodilators in severe pulmonary hypertension after cardiac surgery. *Anesth Analg*. 89, 5, 1108-1115

Shroyer, A. L., Coombs, L. P., Peterson, E. D., Eiken, M. C., DeLong, E. R., Chen, A., Ferguson, T. B., Jr., Grover, F. L., & Edwards, F. H. (2003). The Society of Thoracic Surgeons: 30-day operative mortality and morbidity risk models. *Ann Thorac Surg*. 75, 6, 1856-1864

Simonneau, G., Robbins, I. M., Beghetti, M., Channick, R. N., Delcroix, M., Denton, C. P., Elliott, C. G., Gaine, S. P., Gladwin, M. T., Jing, Z. C., Krowka, M. J., Langleben, D., Nakanishi, N., & Souza, R. (2009). Updated clinical classification of pulmonary hypertension. *J Am Coll Cardiol*. 54, 1 Suppl, S43-S54, ISSN 1558-3597

Solina, A., Papp, D., Ginsberg, S., Krause, T., Grubb, W., Scholz, P., Pena, L. L., & Cody, R. (2000). A comparison of inhaled nitric oxide and milrinone for the treatment of pulmonary hypertension in adult cardiac surgery patients. *J Cardiothorac Vasc Anesth*. 14, 1, 12-17

Solina, A. R., Ginsberg, S. H., Papp, D., Grubb, W. R., Scholz, P. M., Pantin, E. J., Cody, R. P., & Krause, T. J. (2001). Dose response to nitric oxide in adult cardiac surgery patients. *J Clin Anesth*. 13, 4, 281-286

Stafford-Smith, M., Lefrak, E. A., Qazi, A. G., Welsby, I. J., Barber, L., Hoeft, A., Dorenbaum, A., Mathias, J., Rochon, J. J., & Newman, M. F. (2005). Efficacy and safety of heparinase I versus protamine in patients undergoing coronary artery bypass grafting with and without cardiopulmonary bypass. *Anesthesiology*. 103, 2, 229-240

Sukernik, M. R., Mets, B., & Bennett-Guerrero, E. (2001). Patent foramen ovale and its significance in the perioperative period. *Anesth Analg*. 93, 5, 1137-1146

Suntharalingam, J., Treacy, C. M., Doughty, N. J., Goldsmith, K., Soon, E., Toshner, M. R., Sheares, K. K., Hughes, R., Morrell, N. W., & Pepke-Zaba, J. (2008). Long-term use of sildenafil in inoperable chronic thromboembolic pulmonary hypertension. *Chest*. 134, 2, 229-236, ISSN 0012-3692

Tapson, V. F. & Humbert, M. (2006). Incidence and prevalence of chronic thromboembolic pulmonary hypertension: from acute to chronic pulmonary embolism. *Proc Am Thorac Soc.* 3, 7, 564-567, ISSN 1546-3222

Tasca, G., Mhagna, Z., Perotti, S., Centurini, P. B., Sabatini, T., Amaducci, A., Brunelli, F., Cirillo, M., DallaTomba, M., Quaini, E., Troise, G., & Pibarot, P. (2006). Impact of prosthesis-patient mismatch on cardiac events and midterm mortality after aortic valve replacement in patients with pure aortic stenosis. *Circulation.* 113, 4, 570-576

Therrien, J., Dore, A., Gersony, W., Iserin, L., Liberthson, R., Meijboom, F., Colman, J. M., Oechslin, E., Taylor, D., Perloff, J., Somerville, J., & Webb, G. D. (2001a). CCS Consensus Conference 2001 update: recommendations for the management of adults with congenital heart disease. Part I. *Can J Cardiol.* 17, 9, 940-959

Therrien, J., Gatzoulis, M., Graham, T., Bink-Boelkens, M., Connelly, M., Niwa, K., Mulder, B., Pyeritz, R., Perloff, J., Somerville, J., & Webb, G. D. (2001b). Canadian Cardiovascular Society Consensus Conference 2001 update: Recommendations for the Management of Adults with Congenital Heart Disease--Part II. *Can J Cardiol.* 17, 10, 1029-1050

Tremblay, N. A., Hardy, J. F., Perrault, J., & Carrier, M. (1993). A simple classification of the risk in cardiac surgery: the first decade. *Can J Anaesth.* 40, 2, 103-111

Tuman, K. J., McCarthy, R. J., March, R. J., Najafi, H., & Ivankovich, A. D. (1992). Morbidity and duration of ICU stay after cardiac surgery. A model for preoperative risk assessment. *Chest.* 102, 1, 36-44

Viaro, F., Dalio, M. B., & Evora, P. R. (2002). Catastrophic cardiovascular adverse reactions to protamine are nitric oxide/cyclic guanosine monophosphate dependent and endothelium mediated: should methylene blue be the treatment of choice? *Chest.* 122, 3, 1061-1066

Voelkel, N. F., Quaife, R. A., Leinwand, L. A., Barst, R. J., McGoon, M. D., Meldrum, D. R., Dupuis, J., Long, C. S., Rubin, L. J., Smart, F. W., Suzuki, Y. J., Gladwin, M., Denholm, E. M., & Gail, D. B. (2006). Right ventricular function and failure: report of a National Heart, Lung, and Blood Institute working group on cellular and molecular mechanisms of right heart failure. *Circulation.* 114, 17, 1883-1891

Wan, S., LeClerc, J. L., & Vincent, J. L. (1997). Inflammatory response to cardiopulmonary bypass: mechanisms involved and possible therapeutic strategies. *Chest.* 112, 3, 676-692

Wang, H., Gong, M., Zhou, B., & Dai, A. (2009). Comparison of inhaled and intravenous milrinone in patients with pulmonary hypertension undergoing mitral valve surgery. *Adv Ther.* 26, 4, 462-468

Wencker, D., Borer, J. S., Hochreiter, C., Devereux, R. B., Roman, M. J., Kligfield, P., Supino, P., Krieger, K., & Isom, O. W. (2000). Preoperative predictors of late postoperative outcome among patients with nonischemic mitral regurgitation with 'high risk' descriptors and comparison with unoperated patients. *Cardiology.* 93, 1-2, 37-42

Yeo, T. C., Dujardin, K. S., Tei, C., Mahoney, D. W., McGoon, M. D., & Seward, J. B. (1998). Value of a Doppler-derived index combining systolic and diastolic time intervals in predicting outcome in primary pulmonary hypertension. *Am J Cardiol.* 81, 9, 1157-1161

16

The Physiology and the Clinical Significance of Postoperative Hyperlactatemia After Pediatric Cardiac Surgery

Vered Molina-Hazan and Gideon Paret
Department of Pediatric Critical Care,
Safra Children's Hospital,
Chaim Sheba Medical Center, Tel Hashomer,
Affiliated to The Sackler School of Medicine,
Tel Aviv University, Tel Aviv
Israel

1. Introduction

Lactate was first described by Berzelius in 1807 when he discovered it in its modified form in meat juices. It has been used as a marker of cellular hypoxia and tissue malperfusion, and hyperlactatemia has been associated with postoperative complications and mortality. Notably, high blood lactate concentrations have been associated with increased mortality and morbidity in children after cardiac operations (Siegel et al., 1996). Hyperlactatemia associated with metabolic acidosis is a major predictor of mortality of patients with sepsis or after cardiovascular shock, and the evolution of lactate concentration after therapeutic management can more accurately predict the outcome (Bakker et al., 1996; Weil & Afifi, 1970). Blood lactate concentrations are more easily obtained and measured than other monitoring variables, even before any invasive monitoring, such as mean arterial blood pressure, is available. This use of lactate as a clinical endpoint is based on a substantial body of literature, including multiple prospective studies on trauma, surgery or sepsis, patients and in mixed populations of critically ill patients.

2. The physiology of lactate production

Lactate is a glycolytic product that is either used within the cells or transported through the interstitium and vasculature to adjacent and anatomically distributed cells for utilization. As such, lactate is a quantitatively important oxidizable substrate and gluconeogenetic precursor, as well as a means by which metabolism in diverse tissues is coordinated (Brooks, 2002; Stacpoole et al., 1994). Furthermore, lactate measurement in critically ill animals is practical and can provide information on illness severity and prognosis, because a high lactate level is most frequently, but not always, interpreted as resulting from anaerobic metabolism, particularly when associated with metabolic acidosis (Handy, 2006).
Lactic acid is derived from the metabolism of pyruvic acid, a reaction that is catalyzed by lactate dehydrogenase and one that involves the conversion of NADH into NAD+ (reduced

and oxidized nicotine adenine dinucleotide, respectively) (Phypers, 2006). Under aerobic conditions, pyruvate is converted to acetyl CoA to enter the Kreb's cycle. Under anaerobic conditions, pyruvate is converted by lactate dehydrogenase (LDH) to lactic acid. In aqueous solutions, lactic acid dissociates almost completely to lactate and H^{+}þ (Phypers, 2006). Once having been believed to be the consequence of oxygen lack in contracting skeletal muscle, it is now known that lactate is also formed and utilized continuously under fully aerobic conditions (Brooks, 2002).

Normal plasma lactate concentration is 0.3–1.3 mmol/liter (3-12 mg/dL), and normal basal lactate production is 0.8 mmol/kg/hour (1300 mmol/day) (Phypers, 2006). Normal subjects produce between 15 to 20 mmol/kg of lactic acid/day, most of which is generated either from glucose via the glycolytic pathway or from the deamination of alanine (Huckabee, 1961). Its concentration can rise to over 20 mmol/L (180 mg/dL) during intense exertion or severe illness (Mizock & Falk, 1992).

Lactate has two chemical isomers in nature. The first, D-lactate, is produced from non-absorbed carbohydrates by colonic bacteria (which may also proliferate in the ileum). The D isomer is mostly exogenous from Ringer's lactate solution infusion, and its non-iatrogenic presence in humans is uncommon. In the blood, it is a reflection of bacterial overgrowth in the gastrointestinal tract. Its clearance is much slower than the other chemical isomer, L-lactate, with the clearance mainly depending on liver function (Uribarri et al., 1998). L-lactate is the product of anaerobic glycolysis in humans and has been used as a marker of cellular hypoxia and tissue malperfusion. It can only be produced or consumed from pyruvate via the enzyme LDH in the cytosol, by means of a process of fermentation during normal metabolism and exercise (Mizock, 1989). It does not increase in concentration until the rate of lactate production exceeds the rate of lactate removal, a process which is governed by a number of factors, including monocarboxylate transporters, concentration and isoform of LDH, and oxidative capacity of the tissues.

Both the production and the removal of lactate are active functions of every tissue of the body. Tissue sources of lactate production include erythrocytes, perivenous hepatocytes, skeletal myocytes and skin. The liver is the major organ of lactate utilization, followed by the kidneys (Huckabee, 1961; Mizock, 1989). The liver removes 70% of lactate and less than 5% of lactate is renally excreted. Liver uptake involves both a monocarboxylate transporter and the less efficient process of diffusion, while renal fraction may increase and become more clinically significant during hyperlactatemia. Following the liver, skeletal muscle, brain, erythrocytes, and the renal medulla are considered to be the most important sources of lactate in the body (Phypers, 2006).

3. Causes for hyperlactatemia

Hyperlactatemia is usually defined as more than >4 mmol/liter or 40 mg/dL, a result of conditions in which production exceeds utilization. Hyperlactatemia can be associated with acidosis, alkalosis and normal blood pH, and can also be found in conditions of normoxia, hypoxia and anoxia (Handy, 2006).

Since lactate is a byproduct of anaerobic metabolism, it becomes elevated in hypoperfusion states when pyruvate cannot enter the Krebs cycle due to insufficient oxygen supply and is converted to lactate. Lactate-producing tissues include the skin, erythrocytes, brain, skeletal muscles, leukocytes and the renal medulla. Lactate-consuming tissues include the liver, renal cortex and heart. Overproduction and under-consumption result in hyperlactatemia, which can be *physiologic* or *pathologic*. Specifically, increased lactate production can be physiologic as a result of postprandial rest, postabsorptive rest, sustained submaximal exercise or catecholamine-stimulated glycolysis (Mizock, 1989). The primary role of lactate overproduction is clear in certain disorders: for example, plasma lactate levels may transiently be as high as 15 mmol/L during a grand mal seizure, and 20-25 mmol/L during maximally intense exercise, with the systemic pH falling to as low as 6.80. Studies on these subjects have demonstrated rapid recovery of acid-base balance with a maximum rate of lactate utilization that can reach as high as 320 mmol/h.

Impairment of oxidative pathways during lactate production results in a net gain of H^+ whereupon acidosis occurs. The pathologic causes of hyperlactatemia were historically divided between those with evidence of one or another of the well-known causes of hypoxia; and those with no detectable disturbance in oxygen transport in the usual sense (Huckabee, 1961). As a result, hyperlactatemia may occur without (primary) or with (secondary) tissue hypoperfusion, a distinction proposed by Cohen and Woods in 1976 (as cited in Mizock, 1989). However, many critically ill patients can have hyperlactatemia as a result from both of those mechanisms (Phypers, 2006).

3.1 Primary (type B)

The more clinically prevalent hyperlactatemia is not associated with poor tissue perfusion (i.e., alkalosis or increased metabolic activity). In such cases, body-buffering mechanisms can compensate for the decreasing pH (Smith et al., 2001). Among the mechanisms that may be involved are a toxin-induced impairment of cellular metabolism or regional areas of ischemia. Primary hyperlactatemia is usually associated with an underlying disease (e.g., diabetes mellitus, liver disease, malignancy, sepsis, pheochromocytoma, and thiamine deficiency), with drugs or toxins (e.g., ethanol, methanol, ethylene glycol, fructose, sorbitol, xylitol, salicylates, acetaminophen, epinephrine, terbutaline, cyanide, nitroprusside, isoniazid and propylene glycol), and with inborn errors of metabolism (e.g., glucose + phosphatase deficiency [van Gierke's disease], fructose-l + diphosphatase deficiency, pyruvate carboxylase deficiency, pyruvate dehydrogenase deficiency, and oxidative phosphorylation defects), or following hypoglycemia (Mizock, 1989). D-lactic acidosis is a unique form of acidosis that occurs in patients with short bowel syndrome or other forms of malabsorption.

3.2 Secondary (type A)

Secondary hyperlactatemia is due to poor tissue perfusion and the body-buffering mechanisms are not able to compensate for the decreasing pH (Smith et al., 2001). This is the common post-cardiac surgery type of hyperlactatemia. The most frequent cause for secondary hyperlactatemia is the hypoperfusion and tissue hypoxia that are associated with significant cardiopulmonary compromise. Either systemic or regional hypoperfusion may result in hyperlactatemia (Mizock & Falk, 1992). The major causes of secondary hyperlactatemia are shock (cardiogenic, septic, hypovolemic), regional hypoperfusion (limb, mesenteric ischemia), severe hypoxemia, severe anemia, carbon monoxide poisoning, and severe respiratory acidosis (asthma) (Juneja et al., 2011; Mizock, 1989).

The relationship between regional oxyhemoglobin saturation ($rS0_2$) and lactate is exponential in nature, as demonstrated in a study which aimed to determine whether there is a relationship between $rS0_2$ measured at various body locations by near-infrared spectroscopy and blood lactate level in children after cardiac surgery (Chakravarti et al., 2009).

3.3 Summary

Hyperlactatemia may be physiologic or pathologic. It can be caused by increased lactate production (i.e., an increase in the rate of glycolysis or unregulated substrate entry into glycolysis) as well as a decrease in its clearance (i.e., liver or renal insufficiency).
Common causes for type A hyperlactatemia include intense exercise or hypoxemia, anemia, systemic or regional hypoperfusion, shock, CO poisoning and impaired liver blood flow below 25%. This type is more common in postoperative patients.

4. The prevalence and incidence of postoperative hyperlactatemia

The prevalence and incidence of postoperative hyperlactatemia after pediatric cardiac surgery

An increase in serum lactate reflects anaerobic metabolism, and this yardstick has been used in many studies of postoperative management in congenital heart defects (CHD) as a predictor of adverse outcome, given that an elevated serum lactate is common at the time of ICU admission after surgical correction of CHD.
Postoperative hyperlactatemia was seen in 38% of a cohort of 68 patients who underwent isolated atrial septal defect repair at Arkansas Children's Hospital between January 2001 and March 2006 (Abraham et al., 2010).
Our previous studies and validated data of a clinical database encompassing all the consecutive children who underwent surgery for CHD between 1999 and 2001 at the Sheba Medical Center, revealed a prevalence of 41% (89 out of 215 patients) of hyperlactatemia on pediatric cardiac critical-care unit (PCCU) admission, and of 49% in the last blood lactate level taken at the operating room post-CHD repair (our unpublished data). The prevalence declined to 27% and 17% at 6 and 12 hours, respectively, post-PCCU admission after CHD repair. Moreover the mean initial postoperative lactate level was significantly lower for survivors (42.2 ±32.0 mg/dL) than for nonsurvivors (85.4 ± 54.1 mg/dL) ($p<0.01$) (Molina Hazan et al., 2010).
In another study in which 23 pediatric non-cyanotic patients were included, lactate was measured at 0, 2, 4, 6, and 24 hours after admission to the pediatric intensive care unit (PICU), and more often if clinically indicated (Chakravarti et al., 2009). A total of 163 lactate measurements were recorded, of which 18% had a value greater than 3 mmol/L (27 mg/dL).

The prevalence and incidence of postoperative hyperlactatemia in adults

Maillet et al. (2003) found immediate postoperative hyperlactatemia in 20.6% patients, and early postoperative hyperlactatemia in 17.2% patients among 325 patients following coronary heart disease repair. Hyperlactatemia was observed in a substantial proportion of patients who had been operated on under extracorporeal circulation in a Russian study which included 270 patients after cardiac surgery (Bakanov et al., 2009).
Ranucci et al. (2006) reported the rate of patients with hyperlactatemia during cardiopulmonary bypass (CPB) as being relatively low (5.7%) when they measured

progressive hyperlactatemia during the procedure (excluding 30 patients who had pre-existing hyperlactatemia). The overall incidence of hyperlactatemia was 11.4%. Non-pre-existing hyperlactatemia during CPB for cardiac operations in adults occurred in approximately 6% of the patients.
O'Connor and Fraser's (2010) single-center review of prospectively collated data from 529 post-cardiac surgical patients in a tertiary Australian cardiac surgical ICU showed 25% late hyperlactatemia (above 2.5 mmol/L [23 mg / dL]).
Demers et al. (2000) reported higher rates: they recorded peak blood lactate levels of 4.0 mmol/L (36 mg/dL) or higher during CPB in 18.0% of their patients

The prevalence and incidence of hyperlactatemia upon general admission to the ICU

Hyperlactatemia was present in 199 of 653 (30.47%) patients, admitted over 15 months to an 8-bed general ICU of a tertiary care hospital in India (Juneja et al., 2011). Khosravani et al. (2009) documented the incidence of hyperlactatemia in critically ill patients and found a significantly variation according to the major admitting diagnostic category. Specifically, the incidence of hyperlactatemia was highest among neuro/trauma patients (1053/2328, 45%), followed by medical (2047/4935, 41%), other surgical (900/2274, 40%), and cardiac surgical (1578/4395, 36%).

5. Predictive factors for hyperlactatemia

Hyperlactatemia appears in association with peripheral circulatory failure (reduced arterial blood pressure, tachycardia, sweating and mental confusion), with low arterial blood 0_2 saturation, and with acid base disturbance. Significant hyperlactatemia and dangerous hypoperfusion can exist despite the lack of acidosis. Patients with hyperlactatemia may have variable blood pyruvate concentrations because renal dysfunction, electrolyte abnormalities serum lactate and base deficits may not always be linked due to alterations in the body's buffer base. Also relevant is whether the patients did or did not undergo treatment.
While they may present clinically with normal vital signs and are hemodynamically stable, many surgical patients have increased blood lactate levels ('occult hypoperfusion' or 'compensated shock') (Jansen et al., 2008; Meregalli et al., 2004).

5.1 Nonoperative factors

Hyperlactatemia could be present in a critically ill patient due to multiple factors that are either secondary to increased production (shock, sepsis, or respiratory failure) or because of reduced lactate clearance (liver or renal failure). Shock was the most common cause for non-surgical hyperlactatemia, followed by respiratory and renal failures in one study (Juneja et al., 2011). Patients with or without shock who had higher blood lactate levels on admission to the ICU were also found to have higher APACHE II scores, and a greater need for vasopressors or renal replacement therapy and mechanical ventilation, (Juneja et al., 2011).

5.2 Operative factors

Lactic acidosis is often observed as being related to cardiac surgery with CPB, low output syndrome and hypoxemia, which usually show clinical evidence of poor tissue oxygen delivery. Early postoperative hyperlactatemia is seen in some children after surgical repair of CHD despite evidence of good cardiac output. Cardiac arrest or severe hypovolemia triggers anaerobic metabolism and hyperlactatemia, all of which can appear pre-, peri- or postoperatively due to the many cardiac or resuscitation problems found in pediatric patients with CHD.

Changes in lactate levels in post-cardiac surgery patients are not homogenous in nature, due to the fact that early hyperlactatemia and late hyperlactatemia differ in both risk profile and physiological rationale (O'Connor & Fraser, 2010).

5.2.1 Preoperative

The Risk-Adjusted Classification for Congenital Heart Surgery (RACHS-1) system for mortality risk adjustment has recently been proposed as a universal objective score for adjusting differences in case mix when examining in-hospital death rates after congenital heart surgery, and for predicting the risk involved in specific types of cardiac surgery (Jenkins & Gauvreau, 2002; Jenkins et al., 2002). RACHS-1 assigns congenital heart surgical cases to one of six risk categories based on the presence or absence of specific diagnosis and procedure codes, where category 1 has the lowest risk of death and category 6 has the highest. When the mean lactate level was measured at four time points for each RACHS-1 subgroup, blood lactate levels absolutely correlated with the RACHS-1 subgroups at each of the time points ($r^2 > 0.89$ for all) (Molina Hazan et al., 2010). In addition, the progression of lactate levels over time differs significantly between patients with different RACHS-1 scores ($P = 0.029$).

The patient's age affects the risk for postoperative hyperlactatemia. Children younger than 1 year of age would be primed with banked red blood cells and have comparatively more banked blood peri-operatively and higher risk for developing postoperative hyperlactatemia and lactic acidosis (Zhou & Liu, 2011). The adult patient's age is not a predictor for hyperlactatemia.

The electivity/urgency of the surgery are also influential: the more elective the surgery, the lower the postoperative blood lactate levels are expected (Maillet et al., 2003). Urgent or emergency surgery is usually performed for patients who are hemodynamically unstable, and so the preoperative lactate values might have already been abnormal in some of them.

Non-pre-existing hyperlactatemia during CPB for cardiac operations in *adults* is favored by the preoperative risk profile (high serum creatinine values and active endocarditis) and by prolonged (> 96 minutes) CPB times, in addition to being associated with hyperglycemia (Ranucci et al., 2006). Patients with a blood lactate level of 4.0 mmol/L (36 mg/dL) or higher were older and were more often females. The prevalence of congestive heart failure, left ventricular ejection fraction less than 30%, and arteriosclerosis was significantly higher among the patients with hyperlactatemia (Demers et al., 2000).

5.2.2 Peri-operative

Hyperlactatemia occurring early after CPB may represent intra-operative or early postoperative tissue oxygen debt, impaired lactate clearance, or both. It may, however, follow CPB despite well-maintained oxygen delivery and a normal perioperative course. The duration of CPB and, especially, the occurrence of hypotension at the start of the bypass period appears to be related to the development of lactic acidosis. Non-pulsatile, hypothermic CPB itself has a potential for impairment of peripheral perfusion and thus of metabolic balance, since it is associated with collapse and sludging in capillary vessels according to duration of the CPB and to lactate concentration fluctuations (increase after the start of CPB, remaining elevated during CPB, decreasing after CPB, and increasing again after surgery).

Patients with lactate levels of 4.0 mmol/L (36 mg/dL) or higher had significantly longer CPB time and aortic cross-clamping time, and the lowest hemoglobin value recorded during CPB tended to be lower in patients with lactate levels of 4.0 mmol/L (36 mg/dL) or higher (Demers et al., 2000).

Postoperative hyperlactatemia following cardiac surgery was associated with the longest CPB duration and the more frequent intraoperative administration of vasopressors (Maillet et al., 2003). A significant association was found between either duration of CPB or arterial pH and lactate in a retrospective study (Duke et al., 1997). Type A lactic acidosis during CPB appears to be multifactorial.

In a retrospective study where hyperlactatemia was defined as 5 mmol/L (45 mg/dL) or more, CPB duration in the hyperlactatemia group was significantly longer than for the normal lactatemia group in adults undergoing cardiac surgery. Moreover, significant elevations of serum lactate were observed after the start of CPB in the hyperlactatemia group, while other intraoperative variables, including the degree of induced hypothermia, were similar between the two groups (Inoue et al., 2001). In that study, significant correlations between maximal lactate concentration and duration of CPB and aortic cross-clamping were observed as well.

Abraham et al. (2010) compared perioperative factors in 26 patients with postoperative hyperlactatemia (lactate greater than 3 mmol/L (27 mg/dL))) to 42 patients with low-normal lactatemia, including bypass time, crossclamp time, mixed venous oxygen levels, peripheral oxygen saturation, pump flow, intraoperative mean arterial blood pressure, lowest intraoperative core temperature, rewarming time, duration of surgery, duration of anesthesia, average intraoperative hemoglobin, intraoperative oxygen content, and intraoperative oxygen delivery. Of all these intra-operative measurements, the authors found the two groups to differ significantly only in pump flow and intra-operative oxygen delivery. The weight-indexed CPB flow rate was an independent predictor of postoperative high lactate ($P<.007$), and the odds ratio was 7.67 for postoperative hyperlactatemia when it was less than 100 mL/kg/min. Higher mean arterial blood pressure was associated with a reduced risk of high lactate blood levels. An increase of 1 mm Hg, with a fixed CPB flow, resulted with odds ratio for postoperative hyperlactatemia of 0.8343 ($P<.009$) (Abraham et al., 2010). The nadir temperature, duration of cooling and rewarming, hematocrit during and after CPB, and systemic inflammatory response to CPB were also proposed as being likely predictors for postoperative hyperlactatemia (Abraham et al., 2010; Cheung et al., 2005; Munoz et al., 2000).

An association was found between the duration of extracorporeal circulation and the magnitude of hyperlactatemia developing in the early post-pediatric cardiac operation period in Bakanov et al.'s (2009) work as well.

Finally, massive exogenous D-lactate Ringer's solution infusion during surgery can also cause iatrogenic hyperlactatemia in infants with immature liver function (Zhou & Liu, 2011).

5.2.3 Postoperative

Metabolic disturbances, such as changes in blood acid-base balance and electrolytic composition, hyperglycemia and hyperlactatemia, are factors that frequently complicate the early postoperative period in patients after cardiac surgery under extracorporeal circulation. Post-cardiac surgery hyperlactatemia is mostly the consequence of excess lactate production, although a reduction of hepatic lactate clearance may contribute to the condition. Early postoperative measurable adverse effects, such as base deficit, maximal anion gap and bicarbonate levels, were significantly different between patients with postoperative hyperlactatemia and patients with low-normal lactatemia in the early postoperative period (i.e., less than 12 hours after admission to the ICU), while postoperative lactate and glucose levels were significantly correlated (Abraham et al., 2010; Chiolero et al., 2000).

Inadequate tissue oxygen delivery because of impaired cardiac output after pediatric cardiac surgery is a relatively common problem which can be expressed in early stages by hyperlactatemia, and one that has been associated with significant morbidity and mortality (Chakravarti et al., 2009).

Elevated lactate concentrations were associated with metabolic acidosis following cardiac surgery. Moreover, postoperative episodes of hypotension, hyperglycemia, and epinephrine, norepinephrine or dobutamine consumption were more frequent in patients with hyperlactatemia following cardiac surgery compared to patients with non-elevated blood lactate levels (Maillet et al., 2003).

Clinical indicators used for diagnosing decreased cardiac output other than hyperlactatemia include a low peripheral temperature/core temperature gradient, long capillary refill time, high pulse and low blood pressure, decreased urine output and base deficit (Bohn, 2011). Most of these indicators do not reflect cardiovascular performance very well (Tibby et al., 1997).

Averaged cerebral and renal $rS0_2$ levels of less than 65% as measured by near-infrared spectroscopy (NIRS) predict hyperlactatemia (>3 mmol/L, 27 mg/dL) in acyanotic children after congenital heart surgery (Chakravarti et al., 2009). The averaged cerebral and renal $rS0_2$ was a good predictor of the lactate status, with a value less than or equal to 65%, predicting a lactate level of greater than or equal to 3.0 mmol/L (27 mg per dL), with a sensitivity of 95% and a specificity of 83% in the studied patients. Consequently, monitoring of $rS0_2$ could aid in the prompt identification of patients at risk for hyperlactatemia and low-cardiac-output syndrome (Chakravarti et al., 2009). A combination of cerebral and renal $rS0_2$ with an average value less than 65% using the intravenous NIRS device could, therefore, predict hyperlactatemia (>3 mmol/L (>27 mg/dL)) in acyanotic children after congenital heart surgery.

Patients with higher blood lactate levels during CPB were also more likely to have myocardial infarction and postoperative neurologic, hemodynamic, pulmonary, digestive, or renal complications (Demers et al., 2000).

Moreover, sepsis as postoperative complication, can be the cause for late postoperative hyperlactatemia.

5.3 Summary

Patients without signs of clinical shock can still be hypoperfused and are at high risk for pre- peri- and postoperative complications. They tend to develop postoperative hyperlactatemia. Patients undergoing surgery with a RACHS-1 score of IV and higher are not expected to maintain good cardiac output in the postoperative period, emphasizing the importance of combining pre- peri- and postoperative prognosis predictors, especially for the so called "preoperative good prognosis" groups.

6. Blood lactate levels as a biomarker

6.1 General

Biomarkers that are sensitive and rapidly measurable could allow early intervention and improve patient outcomes. Efforts are aimed at developing novel biomarkers and surrogates for disease severity to indicate conditions associated with organ dysfunction early on and by early intervention lead to improved outcome. Lactate levels are commonly used to stratify risk and to assess adequacy of resuscitation among high risk patients in the ICU (Smith et al., 2001). Lactate may have prognostic value in critically ill patients with either observed or occult tissue hypoperfusion.

Lactate levels higher than 2 mmol/L (18 mg/dL) after 48 hours predicted mortality with a specificity of 86% and poor neurologic outcome with a specificity of 87%. Sensitivity for both end points was 31%. Lactate at 48 hours after cardiac arrest is an independent predictor of mortality and unfavorable neurologic outcome. Persisting hyperlactatemia over 48 hours. predicts a poor prognosis (Kliegel et al., 2004). Sensitivity and specificity of lactate >2 mmol/L (18 mg/dL) to predict ICU mortality was 74.8% and 77.8%, respectively. The odds ratio for dying in patients with hyperlactatemia was 10.39 (95% CI, 6.378-16.925), with a relative risk of 1.538 (95% CI, 1.374-1.721) (Juneja et al., 2011). In one multicenter, open-label randomized controlled study on patients who had hyperlactatemia on general ICU admission, lactate monitoring followed by hyperlactatemia-targeted treatment significantly reduced length of stay in the ICU. In addition, ICU and hospital mortality were reduced when adjusting for predefined risk factors (Jansen et al., 2010). In that study, the time of the first available lactate level immediately after ICU admission was taken as the baseline and patients were randomly allocated to either treatment aimed to decrease lactate levels by at least 20%/2 hours or to standard therapy for the following 8 hours.

Elevated blood lactate levels in the presence of normal vital signs (occult hypoperfusion) are good markers of mortality in surgical patients. It is therefore important to identify the high-risk surgical patients who have had a stable hemodynamic course during surgery and immediately after admission to the ICU. Blood lactate levels are superior to several clinical markers of shock or organ failure, including the heart rate, diuresis and the mean arterial pressure, or indices of metabolic acidosis.

In adults following cardiac surgery, blood lactate levels at admission to the ICU were the best predictors of ICU mortality (AUC, 0.84; 95% CI, 0.73 to 0.95), compared to lactatemia measured during the ICU stay (Maillet et al., 2003). Early postoperative hyperlactatemia is associated with adverse outcome of surgery. When they were compared with patients with a normal lactate profile, patients with late hyperlactatemia showed no increase in hospital mortality (OR 0.57, 95%CI 0.07 to 5.05) (O'Connor & Fraser 2010). However, Nichol et al. (2010) reported that early (at admission) and late (post-admission) hyperlactatemia were both strongly associated with mortality in cardiac/vascular surgical patients of whom a significant number were postoperative cardiac patients).

Boyd et al. (1993) demonstrated a 75% reduction in postoperative mortality in adults when targeted therapy was guided by blood lactate levels as predictors for poor prognosis.

Moreover, Kliegel et al. (2004) claimed that sequential measurements during therapy may be more useful than a single measurement since the rapidity at which lactate is cleared from the blood during resuscitation correlates better with outcome – including mortality or organ failure – than a single measure. They showed that survivors' blood lactate levels decreased significantly with time, while those levels remained stable in the non-survivor group.

Among a cohort of 9107 first admissions with an ICU stay of at least one day, both hyperlactatemia at presentation and its later development were associated with significantly increased fatality rates compared with patients without elevated lactate (20% vs. 5%; $P < 0.001$ and 27% vs. 4%; $P < 0.001$, respectively). After controlling for confounding effects in multivariable logistic regression analyses, hyperlactatemia was an independent risk factor for death (Khosravani et al., 2009). When broadly implemented in routine practice, measurement of lactate in patients with infection and possible sepsis can affect assessment of mortality risk. Specifically, an initial lactate level equal to or greater than 4.0 mmol/l (36 mg/dL) substantially increases the probability of acute phase death (Trzeciak et al., 2007).

Blood lactate concentrations greater than 5 mmol/L in patients with severe acidosis (pH less than 7.35 or base deficit greater than 6) carries a mortality of 80% (Stacpoole et al., 1994).

It is well established that hyperlactatemia is also a postoperative prognostic factor. Historically, a rise in blood lactate levels was associated with a decrease in survival rates (Weil & Afifi 1970). These results were recently repeated by a number of investigators. The severity of hyperlactatemia was shown to correlate with oxygen debt and poor survival (Mizock & Falk, 1992), and sustained presence of hyperlactatemia was confirmed as being an important risk factor for poor outcome of critically ill patients (Abubacker et al., 2003; Bakker et al., 1996; Gogos et al., 2003; Kobayashi et al., 2001).

Patients with lactic acidosis were shown to have a higher mortality rate and are at a greater risk of developing multiple organ failure (Bakker et al. 1996). ICU mortality was significantly increased in patients with hyperlactatemia who did not have hypotension ($P = .009$) (Juneja et al., 2011). Similarly to other changes in blood acid-base balance and electrolytic composition, this metabolic disturbance is a factor that frequently complicates the early postoperative period in patients after cardiac surgery under extracorporeal circulation.

6.2 Post-pediatric congenital heart disease repair

An elevated lactate level has been associated with an increased risk for morbidity and mortality after pediatric cardiac surgery (Basaran et al., 2006; Charpie et al., 2000; Cheifetz et al., 1997; Duke et al., 1997). Elevated blood lactate levels were associated with a higher mortality rate and postoperative complications in hemodynamically stable surgical patients, and failure of serum lactate levels to reach normal values within a specific time during critical illness could be even more closely related to survival than the initial level (Meregalli et al., 2004). Hyperlactatemia during and after CPB has been linked to increased morbidity and mortality in children undergoing surgical repair of complex CHD (Cheung et al., 2005; Munoz et al., 2000). Several factors contribute to lactic acidosis because of global ischemia occurring during circulatory arrest and the hypocirculatory state during cardiopulmonary resuscitation. Oxygen deficiency leads to anaerobic metabolism and therefore to overproduction of lactate. At the same time, the profound ischemic state may impair liver function, leading to reduced lactate elimination. Basaran et al. (2006) reported that mean lactate levels correlated significantly with inotrope score, intubation time, and duration of intensive care unit stay.

In their prospective cohort study of 90 children post-congenital heart surgery, Duke et al.'s (1997) multivariable logistic regression analysis showed that lactate levels were an independent predictor of major adverse events. These adverse events included death, cardiac arrest, emergency chest reopening, and an increased risk of failure of 3 or more organ systems. The only measurement that those authors found to consistently predict major adverse events was an elevated serum lactate concentration at the time of ICU admission and at 4, 8, 12, and 24 hours postoperatively (Duke et al., 1997). Of the all variables tested by Seear et al. by stepwise discriminant analysis, serum lactate and $Scv0_2$ emerged as the only ones with significant predictive power for major adverse events. This predictive effect was present at all measurement time points (3, 6, 9, 12, and 24 hours, postoperatively) (Seear et al., 2008). Initial postoperative lactate levels above 4.2 mmol/L (38 mg/dL), above 4.5 mmol/L (40.5 mg/dL), and above 6 mmol/L (54 mg/dL) were associated with a positive predictive value for mortality of 16.7%, 32% and 100% respectively (Hatherill et al., 2000; Siegel et al., 1996).

Hyperlactatemia during CPB is relatively frequent and is associated with an increased postoperative morbidity. Hyperlactatemia has an independently predictive value for major adverse events post-CHD surgical repair, when measured at ICU admission and at 4 and 8 hours, with an odds ratio of 5.1, 8.3 and 9.3 respectively, and with a specificity of 91%, 94% and 95%, respectively (Duke et al., 1997). Death was predicted at ICU admission only by the patient's blood lactate value ($p = 0.03$) and not by any of the other physiologic measures. The odds ratio for death was 29.3 (with a confidence interval of 2.7 to 315) when the admission blood lactate level was greater than 4.5 mmol/L (40.5 mg/dL). However, it should be emphasized that the finding of a normal lactate level did not preclude the possibility of a major adverse event. A lactate level greater than 3 mmol/L (27 mg/dL) at the time of admission to the ICU identified only 50% of those who subsequently had a major complication, thus the sensitivity was relatively low but the specificity was very high (Duke et al., 1997).

As noted earlier, hyperlactatemia post-CHD repair is usually due to decreased cardiac output and hypoperfusion (secondary, type A). Basaran et al. (2006) prospectively studied 60 infants undergoing surgery for CHD and showed that mortality was higher in the group with a mean lactate of greater than 4.8 in the early postoperative period. In another group of 46 infants, the mean initial lactate level was significantly higher in patients who had a poor outcome (as defined as death or the need for extracorporeal membrane oxygenation in the first 72 Hours) than in patients with a good outcome (Charpie et al., 2000).

Studies have shown that blood lactate levels are even superior to mixed venous oxygen saturation in predicting outcome (Duke et al., 1997). Our previous work has validated the measurement of lactate levels as a reliable tool for predicting the postoperative survival of children undergoing cardiac surgery (Molina Hazan et al., 2010). The progression of lactate levels with time was significantly different between the patients in different RACHS-1 subgroups ($p = 0.029$), and the lower the RACHS-1 score at each time point, the lower were the mean lactate levels for each time point ($p < 0.001$). Moreover, postoperative blood lactate levels differed significantly between survivors and non-survivors within the same RACHS-1 subgroup. The lactate level at admission to the PCCU compared with the postoperative lactate level was the most significant parameter for predicting non-survival (odds ratio = 1.038, AUC =0.881, $p < 0.001$). Lactate levels above 53 mg/dL had the sensitivity for non-survival of 88.9% and specificity of 23.4%: accordingly, a patient admitted to the PCCU with lactate levels higher than 53 mg/dL would have an almost 90% risk of dying. Patients who died or survived with complications had higher admission lactate levels compared with survivors without complications (8.5 vs. 4.6 vs. 2.0 mmol/L) (Munoz et al., 2000).

Serum lactate best predicted major adverse events for values greater than 8 mmol/L (>72 mg/dL) with a low sensitivity (73.7%), a high specificity (96.3%) and a low positive predictive value (63.6%) in high risk cases (Seear et al., 2008). The ratio of central venous oxygen sampling (Scv02, measured in %) per lactate (measured in mmol/L) had a better predictive value for major adverse events than each individual value measured alone (if the value of the ratio fell below 5 at any time after surgery, the positive predictive value for major adverse events was above 90%).

The length of time it took for serum lactate levels to reach normal values was a useful predictor of mortality in children undergoing repair or palliation of CHD under CPB, while initial and peak lactate levels had a poor positive predictive value for mortality in that retrospective study (Kalyanaraman et al., 2008). Hyperlactatemia was described as the only predictor of persistent renal impairment at 48 hours at the time of admission to the intensive care unit was the admission blood lactate level (p = 0.018) (Duke et al., 1997). The odds ratio for renal impairment was 3.2 (with a confidence interval of 1.1 to 9.5) for patients whose admission lactate level was greater than 4 mmol/L (36 mg/dL) (Duke et al., 1997). According to the results of a retrospective review of children aged 0-21 years who had been admitted to a cardiac ICU, the length of time during which the lactate level remained greater than 2 mmol/L (18 mg/dL) was associated with the number of ventilator days and hospital days for the survivors. They all had surgery for CHD and required CPB (DeCampli & Burke, 2009; Kalyanaraman et al., 2008).

The lactate level was also considered as being a risk factor for cerebral damage, which was defined as the development of seizures, movement disorders, developmental disorders, cerebral hemorrhage, infarction, hydrocephalus, or marked cerebral atrophy in children after they had undergone cardiac surgery (Trittenwein et al., 2003).

6.3 Summary

Measurements of blood lactate reflect oxygen delivery to tissues and, therefore, are useful in guiding clinical management. Levels of serum lactate are indirect markers of tissue hypoxia secondary to insufficient peripheral oxygen delivery. They have been used to monitor progress after pediatric heart surgery and to report positive predictive values (Duke et al., 1997; Hatherill et al., 2000; Munoz et al., 2000).

Lactate levels differed significantly between survivors and non-survivors even within the same preoperative prognosis subgroup. As such, a combination of preoperative scores and postoperative serial lactate measurements is needed in order to serve as a useful marker for the postoperative course of cardiac patients, allowing the targeting of appropriately intensive interventions and therapies for the sickest among them, especially for the apparently low risk groups whose poorer perioperative course and worse outcome may not have been predictable from the preoperative scores alone. A cutoff threshold of 3 mmol/L (27 mg/dL) at ICU admission will identify a subpopulation of patients at higher postoperative risk.

7. Treatment of postoperative hyperlactatemia after pediatric cardiac surgery

Poor outcome was associated with multi-organ involvement, as reflected by high blood lactate values, and the need for ventilatory or inotropic support. The therapy for type A hyperlactatemia is optimal hemodynamic resuscitation combined with supportive treatment, such as alkalinization, thiamine, dialysis, and dichloroacetate (Mizock 1989).

Resuscitation of surgical patients has traditionally been guided by the normalization of vital signs, e.g., blood pressure, urine output, and heart rate. A goal-oriented protocol targeting a normal blood lactate level can shorten the length of hospitalization among cardiac surgical patients (Polonen et al., 2000). Polonen et al. showed that therapy aimed at achieving an $Sv0_2$ level greater than 70% and a lactate concentration less than 2 mmol/L (18 mg/dL) immediately after cardiac surgery improves outcome. Specifically, early monitoring of lactate levels with the added target to reduce levels by 20%/2 hours on top of currently recommended resuscitation guidelines significantly reduced the length of ICU stay of patients with a lactate level at or above 3.0 mmol/L on admission (Jansen et al., 2010). The deliberate increasing of peri- and postoperative oxygen delivery ($D0_2I$) for the guided postoperative therapy which decreased mortality by 75%, was monitored by lactate levels, and that maneuver was maintained in the protocol group until blood lactate levels had fallen below 1.5 mmol/L (13.5 mg/dL) for 2 consecutive measurements (Boyd et al., 1993).
Early postoperative supply of oxygen improved the outcome during the early stages of surgery-related sepsis in cases of late postoperative hyperlactatemia. This was accomplished by the administration of D02I and by the use of intravenous dopexamine, a novel dopamine analogue with action at b2-adrenoceptors and DA1 receptors.
Dichloroacetate enhanced the activity of pyruvate dehydrogenase and lowered blood lactate concentrations in these septic patients but had no effect on hemodynamics or survival (Stacpoole et al., 1994).

8. Recommendations - The function of lactate as a warning signal

Serial lactate monitoring can be used to assess the severity of illness and response to therapy. Although conventional monitoring with blood gases during CPB may detect inadequate tissue oxygenation, blood lactate concentration monitoring during CPB might be more sensitive for detecting an imbalance between oxygen supply and demand. Monitoring alone, however, cannot improve outcome, and the therapeutic plan shares equal importance.
When high blood lactate levels are identified, consideration must be given to the ratio of lactate production to lactate metabolism, oxygen status and blood pH before those levels can be meaningfully interpreted. Normal levels do not exclude and high levels do not confirm the presence of critical illness.
We recommend the administration of additional fluids and the increased use of vasodilators in patients considered as having higher lactate levels. Another recommendation is the perioperative increase of oxygen delivery with dopexamine hydrochloride, in agreement with Boyd et al. (Boyd et al., 1993).
In summary, the combination of serial measurements of postoperative lactate levels after surgical repair for CHD in children assigned to a preoperative risk subgroup was predictive of prognosis after surgery. Lactate levels differed significantly between survivors and non-survivors in the same subgroup. This combination should serve as a useful marker for the child's postoperative course, allowing the targeting of appropriately intensive interventions and therapies for the sickest patients. It should be borne in mind, however, that although the measurement of blood lactate level is relatively a low invasive procedure, it is carried out intermittently, whereupon an acute deterioration may be missed. Finally, frequent blood sampling leads to increased blood loss and an increased risk of infection (Chakravarti, Mittnacht, Katz, Nguyen, Joashi and Srivastava 2009).

9. Conclusions

We recommend maintaining a high level of vigilance for the earliest signs of developing multiorgan involvement, as reflected by high lactate levels. We also recommend priority triage of these postoperative children to the PICU for the purpose of taking measures to prevent systemic complications and reduce mortality rates.

10. Acknowledgment

We thank Ms. Esther Eshkol for editorial assistance.

11. References

Abraham, B. P.; Prodhan, P., Jaquiss, R. D., Bhutta, A. T., Gossett, J. M., Imamura, M., Johnson C. E., Schmitz, M. L., Morrow, W. R. & Dyamenahalli, U. (2010). Cardiopulmonary Bypass Flow Rate: a Risk Factor for Hyperlactatemia after Surgical Repair of Secundum Atrial Aeptal Defect in Children. *Journal of Thoracic and Cardiovascular Surgery,* Vol.139, No.1, pp.170-173.

Abubacker, M., Yoxall, C. W. & Lamont, G. (2003). Peri-operative Blood Lactate Concentrations in Pre-Term Babies with Necrotising Enterocolitis. *European Journal of Pediatric Surgery,* Vol.13, No.1, pp. 35-39.

Bakanov, A., Naimushin, A. V., Mikhaĭlov, A. P., Khudonogova, S. V., Kadyshkina, E. B., Malaia, E. Ia., Bel'ianinova, I. V., Polianitsa, A. V., & Shatalkin, I. V. (2009). [Early Postoperative Hyperlactatemia in Patients After Surgery Under Extracorporeal Circulation]. *Anesteziologicai reanimatologia,* Vol.2, No.9-12, pp. 0201-7563.

Bakker, J., Gris, P., Coffernils, M., Kahn, R. J. & Vincent, J. L. (1996). Serial Blood Lactate Levels Can Predict The Development of Multiple Organ Failure Following Septic Shock. *American Journal of Surgery,* Vol.171, No.2, pp. 221-226.

Basaran, M., Sever, K., Kafali, E., Ugurlucan, M., Sayin, O. A., Tansel, T., Alpagut, U., Dayioglu, E. & Onursal, E. (2006). Serum Lactate Level Has Prognostic Significance After Pediatric Cardiac Surgery. *Journal of Cardiothoracic and Vascular Anesthesia,* Vol.20, No.1, pp. 43-47.

Bohn, D. (2011). Objective Assessment of Cardiac Output in Infants After Cardiac Surgery. *Seminars in Thoracic and Cardiovascular Surgery. Pediatric Cardiac Surgery Annual,* Vol.14, No.1, pp. 19-23.

Boyd, O., Grounds, R. M. & Bennett, E. D. (1993). A Randomized Clinical Trial of The Effect of Deliberate Perioperative Increase of Oxygen Delivery on Mortality in High-Risk Surgical Patients. *JAMA,* Vol.270, No.22, pp. 2699-2707.

Brooks, G. A. (2002). Lactate Shuttles in Nature. *Biochemical Society Transactions,* Vol.30, No.2, pp 258-264.

Chakravarti, S. B., Mittnacht, A. J., Katz, J. C., Nguyen, K., Joashi, U., & Srivastava S. (2009). Multisite Near-Infrared Spectroscopy Predicts Elevated Blood Lactate Level in Children After Cardiac Surgery. *Journal of Cardiothoracic and Vascular Anesthesia,* Vol.23, No.5, pp. 663-667.

Charpie, J. R., Dekeon M. K., Goldberg, C. S., Mosca, R. S., Bove, E. L. & Kulik, T. J. (2000). Serial Blood Lactate Measurements Predict Early Outcome After Neonatal Repair or Palliation for Complex Congenital Heart Disease. *Journal of Thoracic and Cardiovascular Surgery,* Vol.120, No.1, pp. 73-80

Cheifetz, I. M., Kern, F. H., Schulman, S. R., Greeley, W. J., Ungerleider, R. M. & Meliones, J. N. (1997). Serum Lactates Correlate With Mortality After Operations For Complex Congenital Heart Disease. *Annals of Thoracic Surgery,* Vol.64, No.3, pp. 735-738.

Cheung, P. Y., Chui, N., Joffe, A. R., Rebeyka, I. M. & Robertson, C. M.; Western Canadian Complex Pediatric Therapies Project, Follow-up Group. (2005). Postoperative Lactate Concentrations Predict The Outcome of Infants Aged 6 Weeks or Less After Intracardiac Surgery: A Cohort Follow-Up to 18 Months. *Journal of Thoracic and Cardiovascular Surgery,* Vol.130, No.3, pp. 837-843.

Chiolero, R. L., Revelly, J. P., Leverve, X., Gersbach, P., Cayeux, M. C., Berger, M. M. & Tappy, L. (2000). Effects of Cardiogenic Shock on Lactate And Glucose Metabolism After Heart Surgery. *Critical Care Medicine,* Vol.28, No.12, pp. 3784-3791.

DeCampli, W. M. & Burke, R. P. (2009). Interinstitutional Comparison of Risk-Adjusted Mortality And Length of Stay in Congenital Heart Surgery. *Annals of Thoracic Surgery,* Vol.88, No.1, pp. 151-156.

Demers, P., Elkouri, S., Martineau, R., Couturier, A. & Cartier, R. (2000). Outcome with High Blood Lactate Levels During Cardiopulmonary Bypass in Adult Cardiac Operation. *Annals of Thoracic Surgery,* Vol.70, No.6, pp. 2082-2086.

Duke, T., Butt, W., South, M. & Karl, T. R. (1997). Early Markers of Major Adverse Events in Children After Cardiac Operations. *Journal of Thoracic and Cardiovascular Surgery* Vol.114, No.6, pp. 1042-1052.

Gogos, C. A., Lekkou, A., Papageorgiou, O., Siagris, D., Skoutelis, A. & Bassaris, H. P. (2003). Clinical Prognostic Markers in Patients with Severe Sepsis: A Prospective Analysis of 139 Consecutive Cases. *Journal of Infection,* Vol.47, No.4, pp. 300-306.

Handy, J. (2006). Lactate—The Bad Boy of Metabolism, or Simply Misunderstood? *Current Anaesthesia & Critical Care,* Vol.17, No.17, pp. 71-76.

Hatherill, M., McIntyre, A. G., Wattie, M. & Murdoch, I. A. (2000). Early Hyperlactataemia in Critically Ill Children. *Intensive Care Medicine,* Vol.26, No.3, pp. 314-318.

Huckabee, W. E. (1961). Abnormal Resting Blood Lactate. I. The Significance of Hyperlactatemia in Hospitalized Patients. *American Journal of Medicine,* Vol.30, pp. 840-848.

Inoue, S., Kuro, M. & Furuya, H. (2001). What Factors Are Associated with Hyperlactatemia After Cardiac Surgery Characterized By Well-Maintained Oxygen Delivery And A Normal Postoperative Course? A Retrospective Study. *European Journal of Anaesthesiology,* Vol.18, No.9, pp. 576-584.

Jansen, T. C., van Bommel, J. Mulder, P. G., Rommes, J. H., Schieveld, S. J. & Bakker, J. (2008). The Prognostic Value of Blood Lactate Levels Relative to That of Vital Signs in The Pre-Hospital Setting: A Pilot Study. *Critical Care,* Vol.12, No.6, pp. R160.

Jansen, T. C., van Bommel, J., Schoonderbeek, F. J., Sleeswijk Visser, S. J., van der Klooster, J. M., Lima, A. P., Willemsen, S. P. & Bakker. J.; LACTATE Study Group. (2010). Early Lactate-Guided Therapy in Intensive Care Unit Patients: A Multicenter, Open-Label, Randomized Controlled Trial. *American Journal of Respiratory and Critical Care Medicine,* Vol.182, No.6, pp. 752-761.

Jenkins, K. J. & Gauvreau, K. (2002). Center-Specific Differences In Mortality: Preliminary Analyses Using The Risk Adjustment In Congenital Heart Surgery (RACHS-1) Method. *Journal of Thoracic and Cardiovascular* Surgery, Vol.124, No.1, pp. 97-104.

Jenkins, K. J., Gauvreau, K., Newburger, J. W., Spray, T. L., Moller, J. H. & Iezzoni, L. I. (2002). Consensus-Based Method for Risk Adjustment for Surgery for Congenital Heart Disease. *Journal of Thoracic and Cardiovascular Surgery,* Vol.123. No.1, pp. 110-118.

Juneja, D., Singh, O. & Dang, R. (2011). Admission Hyperlactatemia: Causes, Incidence, And Impact on Outcome of Patients Admitted in A General Medical Intensive Care Unit. *Journal of Critical Care,* Vol.26, No.3, pp. 316-320.

Kalyanaraman, M., DeCampli, W. M., Campbell, A. I., Bhalala, U., Harmon, T. G., Sandiford, P., McMahon, C. K., Shore, S. & Yeh, T. S. (2008). Serial Blood Lactate Levels As A Predictor of Mortality in Children After Cardiopulmonary Bypass Surgery. *Pediatric Critical Care Medicine,* Vol.9, No.3, pp. 285-288.

Khosravani, H., Shahpori, R., Stelfox, H. T., Kirkpatrick, A. W. & Laupland, K. B. (2009). Occurrence And Adverse Effect on Outcome of Hyperlactatemia in The Critically Ill. *Critical Care,* Vol.13, No.3, pp. R90.

Kliegel, A., Losert, H., Sterz, F., Holzer, M., Zeiner, A., Havel, C. & Laggner, A. N. (2004). Serial Lactate Determinations for Prediction of Outcome After Cardiac Arrest. *Medicine (Baltimore),* Vol.83, No.5, pp. 274-279.

Kobayashi, S., Gando, S., Morimoto, Y., Nanzaki, S. & Kemmotsu, O. (2001). Serial Measurement of Arterial Lactate Concentrations As A Prognostic Indicator in Relation To The Incidence of Disseminated Intravascular Coagulation in Patients with Systemic Inflammatory Response Syndrome. *Surgery Today,* Vol.31, No.10, pp. 853-859.

Maillet, J. M., Le Besnerais, P., Cantoni, M., Nataf, P., Ruffenach, A., Lessana, A. & Brodaty, D. (2003). Frequency, Risk Factors, And Outcome of Hyperlactatemia After Cardiac Surgery. *Chest,* Vol.123, No.5, pp. 1361-1366.

Meregalli, A., Oliveira, R. P. & Friedman, G. (2004). Occult Hypoperfusion Is Associated with Increased Mortality in Hemodynamically Stable, High-Risk, Surgical Patients. *Critical Care,* Vol.8, No.2, pp. R60-65.

Mizock, B. A. (1989). Lactic Acidosis. *Disease-A-Month,* Vol.35, No.4, pp. 233-300.

Mizock, B. A. & Falk, J. L. (1992). Lactic Acidosis in Critical Illness. *Critical Care Medicine* Vol.20, No.1, pp. 80-93.

Molina Hazan, V., Gonen, Y., Vardi, A., Keidan, I., Mishali, D., Rubinshtein, M., Yakov, Y. & Paret, G. (2010). Blood Lactate Levels Differ Significantly Between Surviving And Nonsurviving Patients Within The Same Risk-Adjusted Classification for Congenital Heart Surgery (RACHS-1) Group After Pediatric Cardiac Surgery. *Pediatric Cardiology,* Vol.31, No.7, pp. 952-960.

Munoz, R., Laussen, P. C., Palacio, G., Zienko, L., Piercey, G. & Wessel, D. L. (2000). Changes in Whole Blood Lactate Levels During Cardiopulmonary Bypass for Surgery for Congenital Cardiac Disease: An Early Indicator of Morbidity And Mortality. *Journal of Thoracic and Cardiovascular Surgery,* Vol.119, No.1, pp. 155-162.

Nichol, A. Egi, D. M., Pettila, V., Bellomo, R., French, C., Hart, G., Davies, A., Stachowski, E., Reade, M. C., Bailey, M., Cooper, D. J.. Pettila, V., Bellomo, R., French, C., Hart, G.,

Davies, A., Stachowski, E., Reade, M. C., Bailey, M. & Cooper, D. J. (2010). Relative Hyperlactatemia And Hospital Mortality in Critically Ill Patients: A Retrospective Multi-Centre Study. *Critical Care,* Vol.14, No.1, pp. R25.

O'Connor, E. D. & Fraser, J. F. (2010). Hyperlactatemia in Critical Illness And Cardiac Surgery. *Critical Care* Vol.14, No.3, pp. 421.

Phypers, B. (2006). Lactate Physiology in Health And Disease. *Continuing Education in Anaesthesia, Critical Care & Pain,* Vol. 6, No.3, pp. 128-132.

Polonen, P., Ruokonen, E, Hippeläinen, M., Pöyhönen, M., Takala, J., Hippeläinen, M., Pöyhönen, M. & Takala J. (2000). A Prospective, Randomized Study of Goal-Oriented Hemodynamic Therapy in Cardiac Surgical Patients. *Anesthesia and Analgesia,* Vol. 90, No.5, pp. 1052-1059.

Ranucci, M., De Toffol, B. Isgrò, G., Romitti, F., Conti, D. & Vicentini, M. (2006). Hyperlactatemia During Cardiopulmonary Bypass: Determinants And Impact on Postoperative Outcome. *Critical Care,* Vol.10, No.6, pp. R167.

Seear, M. D., Scarfe, J. C. & LeBlanc J. G. (2008). Predicting major adverse events after cardiac surgery in children. *Pediatric Critical Care Medicine,* Vol.9, No.6, pp. 606-611.

Siegel, L. B., Dalton, H. J., Hertzog, J. H., Hopkins, R. A., Hannan, R. L., Hauser, G. J.. Hertzog, J. H., Hopkins, R. A., Hannan, R. L.& Hauser, G. J. (1996). Initial Postoperative Serum Lactate Levels Predict Survival in Children After Open Heart Surgery. *Intensive Care Medicine,* Vol.22, No.12, pp. 1418-1423.

Smith, I., Kumar, P., Molloy, S., Rhodes, A., Newman, P. J., Grounds, R. M. & Bennett, E. D. (2001). Base Excess And Lactate As Prognostic Indicators for Patients Admitted to Intensive Care. *Intensive Care Medicine,* Vol.27, No.1, pp. 74-83.

Stacpoole, P. W., Wright, E. C., Baumgartner, T. G., Bersin, R. M., Buchalter, S., Curry, S.H., Duncan, C., Harman, E. M., Henderson, G,N., & Jenkinson, S, et al. (1994). Natural History And Course of Acquired Lactic Acidosis in Adults. DCA-Lactic Acidosis Study Group. *American Journal of Medicine,* Vol.97, No.1, pp. 47-54.

Tibby, S. M., Hatherill, M., Marsh, M. J. & Murdoch, I. A. (1997). Clinicians' Abilities to Estimate Cardiac Index in Ventilated Children And Infants. *Archives of Disease in Childhood,* Vol.77, No.6, pp. 516-518.

Trittenwein, G., Nardi, A., Pansi, H., Golej, J., Burda, G., Hermon, M., Boigner, H. & Wollenek, G; Verein zur Durchführung wissenschaftlichter Forschung auf dem Gebeit der Neonatologie und Pädiatrischen Intensivmedizin. (2003). Early Postoperative Prediction of Cerebral Damage After Pediatric Cardiac Surgery. *Annals of Thoracic Surgery,* Vol.76, No.2, pp. 576-580.

Trzeciak, S., Dellinger, R. P. (2007). Serum Lactate As A Predictor of Mortality in Patients with Infection. *Intensive Care Medicine,* Vol.33, No.6, pp. 970-977.

Uribarri, J., Oh, M. S. & Carroll, S. J. (1998). D-Lactic Acidosis. A Review of Clinical Presentation, Biochemical Features, And Pathophysiologic Mechanisms. *Medicine (Baltimore),* Vol.77, No.2, pp. 73-82.

Weil, M. H. & Afifi, A. A. (1970). Experimental And Clinical Studies on Lactate And Pyruvate As Indicators of The Severity of Acute Circulatory Failure (Shock). *Circulation,* Vol.41, No.6, pp. 989-1001.

Zhou, R. & Liu, J. (2011). A Risk Factor for Hyperlactatemia After Surgical Repair of Secundum Atrial Septal Defect in Children: What Is The Problem? *Journal of Thoracic and Cardiovascular Surgery*, Vol.141, No.2, pp. 598-599.

17

Sticking Up for the Immune System Integrity: Should the Thymus Be Preserved During Cardiac Surgery?

Sara Ferrando-Martínez[1,2],
M. Ángeles Muñoz-Fernández[2] and Manuel Leal[1]
[1]*Laboratory of Immunovirology, Infectious Diseases Service, HU Virgen del Rocío, Institute of Biomedicine of Seville (IBiS), Seville*
[2]*Laboratory of Molecular Immuno-Biology, HGU Gregorio Marañón, Madrid*
Spain

1. Introduction

Thymus is the site of maturation of T lymphocytes (TL) from bone marrow-derived precursors and, therefore, a major organ in the immune system generation and maintenance. Thymic function starts as early as during embryonic development and its activity is maximal after birth. However, maintain the high mitotic rate that the thymus shows during fetal life and first months of life is not cost-effective after childhood. A progressive atrophy, enhanced by adolescence, will lead to the thymic output exhaustion later on life. Accordingly, it has been long accepted that TL repertory is fixed during childhood and thymus activity is no longer necessary in either adulthood or elderly. Thymus anatomical situation, in the anterior mediastinum above the heart, situates it in the surgical field of important open heart procedures and is therefore routinely removed (partially or totally) in patients of any age. Thymic ablation impact during children's cardiac surgery is being studied to determine its potential influence in peripheral TL dynamics, despite only partial results are still available. Conversely, since adult and elderly thymic function is usually disregarded, thymic ablation during adult's cardiac surgery is accepted as appropriate and harmless. Recent results, however, indicate that thymus could have an active role in elderly immune system maintenance, increasing the importance of maximal preservation during any-age cardiac surgery. Thus, the aim of this chapter is to analyze the importance of thymic function during the different stages of life and to review current evidences of the potential clinical impact of both, early childhood and adulthood thymectomy.

2. Overview of the human thymic gland

2.1 Embryonic development, anatomy and histology

During embryonic development thymic epithelium and neighboring mesenchyme are derived from the cephalic region of the neural crest. Initially, thymus originates from the third pharyngeal pouch as two endodermic buds. Sprouts descend upon the superior mediastinum and will thereafter be fused as a V-shaped solid epithelial mass. Epithelium undergoes critical morphological changes and express the major histocompatibility class (MHC)-II complex at high levels as well as epidermal growth factor-like proteins that control several steps of tissue development and homeostasis, thus playing an important role in subsequent TL maturation processes. During the third gestation month thymus is colonized, via the bloodstream, by bone marrow-derived multipotential lymphoid stem cells (CFU-L), transforming the thymus in a lymphoepithelial organ. Under the inductive influence of modified thymic epithelial cells (TECs) lymphoid precursors mature in their passage through the thymus to be dumped back to peripheral blood as fully functional TL.

Developed thymus is a bilobed organ, surrounded by a connective-tissue capsule, located in the anterior mediastinum, just behind the sternum, above the heart and ahead the great vessels. Fibrous septa divide each thymic lobe into multiples smaller lobes. Thymocytes (lymphocytes undergoing maturation process in the thymus) locate heavily packed in the periphery of each lobe while the center is only sparsely populated. Therefore, a cortex and medulla region are usually identified despite there is no defined anatomical limitation. Cortex and medulla compose the true thymic epithelial space (TES), keratin-positive thymic epithelium that nourishes immature thymocytes, in which thymopoiesis actually occurs. In the human thymus a non-thymopoietic perivascular space (PVS), keratin-negative stroma, can also be found. In addition, non-lymphoid epithelial cells, bone marrow-derived macrophages and dendritic cells are spread over the thymus. Finally, Hassall's corpuscles, isolated tight whorls of epithelial cells located in the medullar region, are a thymic hallmark. Despite its function is still unclear, Interleukin (IL)-4 and IL-7 production could be its important contribution to thymocyte maturation and tuition. Vascular supply is rich in the thymus, and efferent lymphatic vessels drain into mediastinal lymph nodes. Young human thymus description and microphotography are showed in Figure 1A-B.

A fully functional thymus contains 10% of immature precursors and 15% of mature thymocytes waiting to reach the bloodstream as naive (antigen-inexperienced) TL. Remaining 75% of the thymocytes are in an intermediate maturation step (CD4+CD8+ double positive - DP - thymocytes) and undergoing selection processes. Approximately 99% of these immature thymocytes will not fulfilled the strict criteria to be safely poured to peripheral blood (extended information about the maturation process is provided in the next section) and endure programmed cell death in the cortical region, which is full of dying individual thymocytes. Phagocyted cells can also be found inside macrophages or cortical epithelial cells. Thus, the thymus has a dramatically high rate of both, mitosis and cell death. This situation of extensive proliferation and mass death cannot be cost-effectively maintained and thymus undergoes a chronically age-related atrophy as evolutionary energy-saving method. Atrophy starts from the first year of life (Steinmann et al., 1985) and is enhanced by hormonal changes during puberty (Chiodi, 1940). During the atrophy process the PVS (adipocytes, peripheral blood lymphocytes and stroma) increases, intensely diminishing the amount of TES. Loss of TES - it can be as low as 10% in elderly thymus - together with architecture damage that breaks up the cortex/medulla structure leads to a less efficient thymopoiesis. Immature DP thymocytes percentages diminish and *in situ* TCR rearrangement is impaired (Sempowski et al., 2000). In addition, lymphoid component within the remaining TES also decreases in around 3%/year during the first 35 to 45 years of life and 1%/year thereafter (reviewed in Lynch et al., 2009). As a consequence, elderly thymuses are mostly adipocyte-filled PVS with isolated lymphoepithelial islets. Figure 1 C-D show a schematic representation and microphotography of an atrophied thymus.

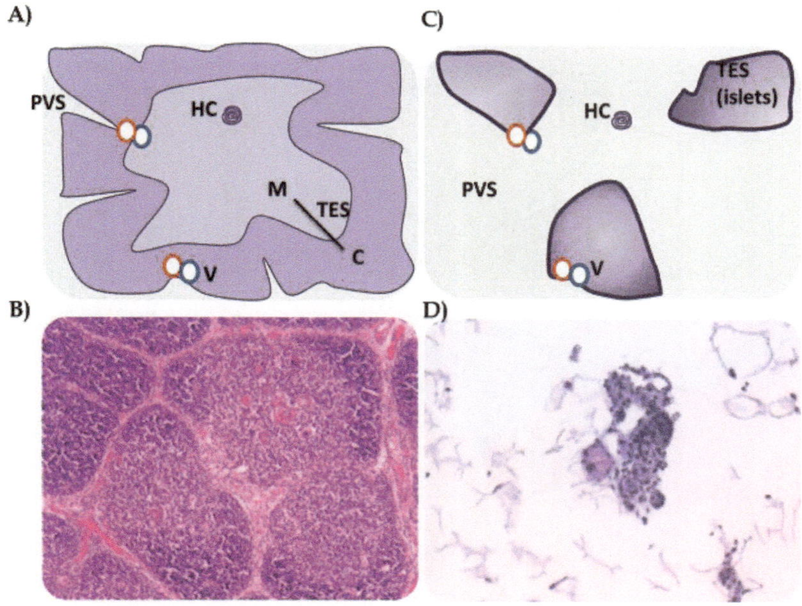

Fig. 1. Schematic representation and microphotography of young (A-B) and atrophied (C-D) thymus. C = Cortex; HC = Hassall's corpuscles; M = Medulla; PVS = Perivascular space; TES = Thymic epithelial space; V = blood vessels;

2.2 T Lymphocyte (TL) maturation

Thymus is the major site of maturation of TL. Bone marrow-derived lymphoid precursor entering the thymus commit to the T lineage. Maturation processes begin in the cortex and thymocytes move toward the medulla as they progress in the tuition program. Thymus is not only the provider of new mature naive TL to preserve the immune system integrity but also ensures that all departing cells are functional and non-self-reactive.

As shown in Figure 2 most immature cells of the T lineage enter the thymic cortex through the blood vessels. After a proliferation step Pro-T thymocytes, CD4-CD8- double negative (DN) irresponsive cells that still do not express the T cell receptor (TCR), start expressing the terminal deoxynucleotidyl transferase (TdT) enzyme, which adds random nucleotides to the TCR genomic sequence to increase lymphocyte diversity. Expression of the Rag-1 and Rag-2 proteins, necessary for the TCR rearrangement, marks the pre-T cell stage. Pre-T cells are still DN thymocytes. Beta chain of the TCR is rearranged at this stage. Β-chain rearrangement success is tested in the cellular membrane using a pre-T α-chain. Expression of a functional β-chain triggers another proliferation round and the entry into the CD4+CD8+ double positive (DP) stage. Thymus atrophy diminishes TES lymphoid components by impairing this proliferation step. As a consequence, DP numbers, or DN to DP proliferation rates, are the best indicative of thymic functionality. DP thymocytes rearrange then the α-chain of the TCR. Once a functional αβ TCR protein is expressed, DP thymocytes start a strict scrutiny program. TCR affinity and avidity is checked from every thymocyte. Positive selection ensures that only cells presenting a functional TCR reach the next step. Thymocytes that do not receive a positive signaling thru a successful TCR

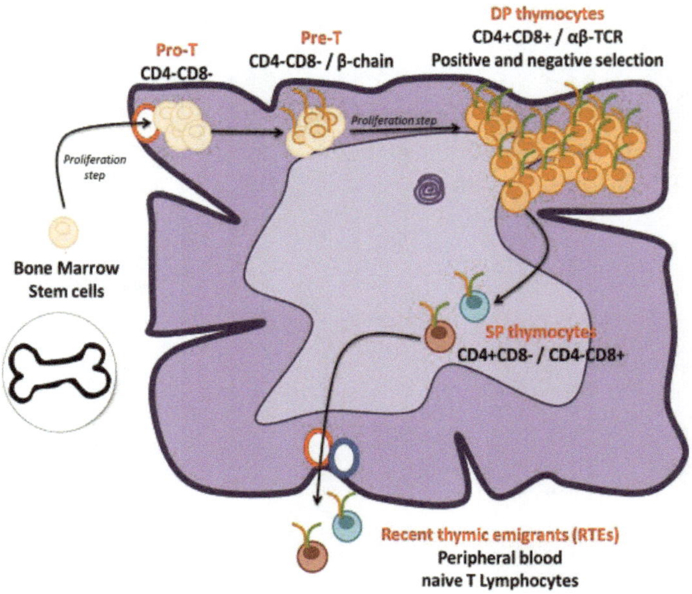

Fig. 2. Thymocyte maturation process.

recognition go to programmed cell death. Afterwards, a negative selection warrants that survivors do not have self-reactivity. Thymocytes with strong TCR signaling due to self-antigen recognition will be also directed to cell death. A small percentage of DP thymocytes, approximately 1%, qualify to further maturation. Thymocytes migrate to the medullar space expressing a fully functional non-self-reactive TCR. CD4 and CD8 co-receptor expression is modulated in this stage and mature thymocyte are CD4 or CD8 single positive (SP) cells.

Thymocyte maturation and selection need the stimuli provided by the thymic microenvironment. TECs, bone marrow-derived macrophages and dendritic cells locate in the pathways of thymocyte migration, allowing physical interactions necessary for the maturation process. MHC class I and class II molecules (expressed by epithelial and dendritic cells); cytokines and chemokines (secreted by thymic stromal cells) provide signaling for selection process, stimulate thymocyte proliferation and coordinate the cortical to medullary transit. Therefore, non-lymphoid thymic cells play a crucial role in the immune system generation.

2.3 Thymic function-related markers

Study of thymic function is of great interest either to determine immune system impairment in lymphopenia scenarios or to monitor immune reconstitution. However, despite the necessity, lack of accurate measurement tools has hampered thymic output assessment. Due to its anatomical situation (in the anterior mediastinum, above the heart and ahead the great vessels) thymic biopsies are formally contraindicated and indirect measurements are needed. Thymic volume determination by thoracic computed tomography (CT) or magnetic resonance imaging (MRI) is an accurate indirect approximation and has been very useful to determine the role of thymic function in HIV-infected patients' immune reconstitution

(Ruiz-Mateos et al. 2004). Nevertheless, both are expensive techniques where thymic inference needs specifically trained radiologists. Moreover, thoracic CT generates high levels of radiation. Thus, thymic function-related markers that could be determined from peripheral blood samples have usually been first choice for thymic output determination.

Naive TL quantification was the first proposed related-marker and is still being used. Controversy exist regarding the surface markers election that best discriminate the naive subset by flow cytometry. High expression of CD45RA, CCR7 and CD27 are commonly used to categorize this TL subset, and CD45RA+CD27+ or CD45RA+CCR7+ phenotypes seem to both be accurate enough to identify naive T cells (Ferrando-Martínez et al., 2010). However, naive TL are defined as mature lymphocytes that still have not find their specific antigen (non-experienced lymphocytes), disregarding whether they are recent thymic emigrants (RTEs) or long-lived cells. As a consequence, surface markers that could truthfully identify RTEs have been long chased. CD31-positive naive TL have very short proliferative history and are a RTE-enriched population (Junge et al., 2007). Moreover, protein tyrosine kinase 7 (PTK7)-expressing lymphcytes are proposed as precursor cells for later differentiation into mature naive TL (Haines et al., 2009). However, a marker that specifically characterizes mature thymocytes leaving the thymus is still missing.

T cell receptor excision circles (TREC) description was a milestone in thymic function quantification. TRECs are circular episomal DNA discarded through TCR rearrangement processes that can only be thymically produced and lack of replication origin (they cannot be copied in periphery). Signal-joint (sj)-TREC quantification, discarded product of the α-chain rearrangement at DP stage, was described as a new thymic output-related marker (Douek et al., 1998). However, TREC counts are deeply affected by peripheral proliferation (Hazenberg et al., 2000), increasing the difficulty of interpretation (Harris et al., 2005). Moreover, subsequent mathematical models showed that, even in the steady state, the sj-TREC content is not a good measurement of thymic function (Ribeiro and Perelson, 2007). To overcome these limitations, Dion et al. (2004) proposed an elegant technique to quantify the ratio between sj-TREC and the β-TRECs, discarded during the β-chain rearrangement at a more immature stage (see Figure 2). A proliferation step, directly related to thymic function, occurs between the β- and the α-chain rearrangement. Thus, the sj/β-TREC ratio is an indirect measure of this intrathymic proliferation step and a thymic function-related marker. In addition, since the proportion between both TREC types is evaluated, rather than TREC numbers, the results are not affected by peripheral proliferation, even if absolute TREC numbers are. Recently, we have described a simplified version of this technique that allows an accurate and time- and cost-effective quantification of human thymic function from peripheral blood samples (Ferrando-Martínez et al., 2010b). Table 1 summarizes different techniques that have been used to determine thymic function together with their advantages and disadvantages.

3. Thymic function and age

Thymus functionality starts during fetal life and is maximal at birth. After the first year of life, thymus goes through a chronic atrophy that progressively diminishes its function, eventually leading to thymic function exhaustion in later life. During this process TES loses the cortical/medullar architecture, lymphoid components are greatly reduced and TCR rearrangement is somehow impaired. Besides, TES is progressively reduced and this space is filled with adipocyte-packed PVS. Clinical implications of the age-related loss of thymic function and the specific burden of thymic output during different life-stages are still controversial.

Quantification method	Type	Advantages	Disadvantages
Double positive (DP) thymocytes *ex-vivo* quantification	Thymic ***function***-related marker	Thymic function ***gold standard***	Needs thymic biopsy
Thymic volume	Thymic ***function***-related marker	Accurate indirect approximation	Irradiation (CT) Specifically trained radiologist Coarser quantification
Naive T lymphocytes	Thymic ***output***-related marker	Peripheral blood sample	Cannot discriminate long-lived naive TL Controversy regarding markers
CD31-expressing naive T Lymphocytes	Thymic ***output***-related marker	Peripheral blood sample Short proliferative history	Quantifies a recent thymic emigrant (RTE)-enriched subset rather than RTEs
PTK7-expressing T lymphocytes	Thymic ***output***-related marker	Peripheral blood sample Immature naive TL	Quantifies a recent thymic emigrant (RTE)-enriched subset rather than RTEs
sjTREC quantification	Thymic ***output***-related marker	Peripheral blood sample Intrathymic generation	Deeply affected by peripheral proliferation
sj/β-TREC ratio	Thymic ***function***-related marker	Peripheral blood samples Intrathymic generation Not affected by peripheral proliferation	Technically difficult

Table 1. Advantages and disadvantages of the different thymic function quantification methods

3.1 Thymic failure during childhood

Thymus is the major site of TL maturation and, therefore, essential for the adaptive immune system formation. Few clinical situations involve lack of thymus, but all they lead to serious consequences.

3.1.1 DiGeorge syndrome: Defective thymic development

DiGeorge syndrome is a congenital malformation involving defective development of the structures derived from the third and fourth pharyngeal pouch during fetal life, as thymus and parathyroid glands, among others. Depending on the severity of the syndrome, thymus can be completely absent or just reduced or misplaced. When thymus is present, thymic structure and functionality, despite reduced, is normal. Approximately 90% of all DiGeorge syndromes present a specific deletion on the region q11.2 of chromosome 22, while the remaining 10% show other chromosomic defects due to gestational diabetes, fetal alcoholism syndrome or prenatal exposure to Accutane® (cystic acne treatment). A similar defect in thymic development has been reported when mutation in gene T box 1 (TBX1) occurs. Principal characteristics of the DiGeorge syndrome are shown in Table 2.

Immune system alterations	Aplasia or hypoplasia of thymus
	Lymphocyte counts under 1500 cells / μL
	T lymphocytes absent or greatly reduced
	T lymphocyte irresponsiveness to polyclonal T cell activators and mixed lymphocyte reactions (MLRs)
	Immunoglobulin levels and antibody function about normal (may be reduced in severely affected patients)
Infectious diseases	Susceptible to mycobacterial, viral and fungal infections
Cardiac affectations	Frequent congenic cardiac illness
Aesthetic affectations	Characteristic facial abnormalities
Others	Aplasia or hypoplasia of the parathyroid glands
	Hypocalcemia

Table 2. Clinical features of DiGeorge syndrome.

Most urgent treatment for children with DiGeorge syndrome is *Pneumocistiis jirovenci* prophylaxis. General care includes treating hypocalcemia and correcting cardiac abnormalities. When TL immunity is severely compromised, thymus and bone marrow transplant can partially restore the adaptive immune system. Severe syndromes usually lead to sudden or cardiac-derived death. Surprisingly, less severe syndromes, where TL are reduced but not absent, natural improvement due to regrowth of remaining thymic tissue, extra-thymic TL maturation or ectopic thymus development can be observed.

3.1.2 Infectious ablation of the thymus

Human immunodeficiency virus (HIV)-infected children usually show faster AIDS progression than their adult counterparts. Newborns infected during fetal development (intra-uterine infection versus infection in the birth canal) show important immune alterations from the first day of life. Due to lack of thymic function measurements, thymus ablation was defined thru peripheral observations as T lymphopenia involving both CD4 and CD8 T cell subsets. More severe thymic deficiency was associated with worse clinical prognosis. Some of these vertically-infected children present an immunophenotypic profile even comparable with DiGeorge syndrome. Infectious thymus ablation is strongly correlated with earlier and faster AIDS progression (Kourtis et al., 1996) and increased mortality rates (Nahmias et al., 1998) when compared with children with preserved thymic function (usually infected at the birth canal).

3.2 Thymic failure during adulthood and elderly

Atrophy implies thymic function reduction and it has been long time assumed that TL repertory was fixed during childhood and the thymus was no longer needed during adult life. However, different studies showed that adult thymus not only is functional but it can even booster its function to expedite immune reconstitution in different scenarios as chemotherapy (Mackall et al., 1995) or HIV-infected patients under highly active antiretroviral therapy (HAART) (de la Rosa and Leal, 2003).
During elderly, thymus shows even more reduced functionality. However, despite TES reduction and architectural changes, elderly thymus is able to maintain a certain degree of thymopoiesis (Jamieson et al., 1999). Thymopoietic degree is widely heterogeneous among individuals (Figure 3). In addition, thymic function in elderly people has an active role in the peripheral immune system rejuvenation (Ferrando-Martínez et al., 2009). Higher thymic function in elderly human is associated with a better preservation of the immune system. To add "insult to injury", thymic failure in healthy elderly leads to a discrete lymphopenia and naive T cell drop that eventually allows non-antigen driven homeostatic proliferation (Ferrando-Martinez et al., 2011). Homeostatic proliferation correlates with naive TL gathering age-related defects leading to irresponsiveness. Despite causality still needs to be assessed, altogether these results strongly suggest that elderly thymic function preservation or rejuvenation could be of great importance to ameliorate the age-related immune system deterioration. In fact, recent results show that thymic function, accurately measured with the sj/β-TREC ratio quantification method, in healthy elderly subjects (aged over 65) is independently associated with two-years all-cause mortality (Ferrando-Martínez et al., 2011b).Thus, elderly thymic function still has an active role in the maintenance of the immune system and this information should be taken into account to design innovative therapies capable of improve elderly quality of life through the immune system rejuvenation.

4. Surgical thymic ablation

Thymus anatomically locates in the anterior mediastinum, just behind the sternum, facing the heart and the great vessels. This location places the thymus in the surgical field of critical open heart surgery. Since short-time consequences of either children or adult thymectomy have not been reported, thymus is partially or completely removed during this surgical procedure. However, recent studies suggest that individuals thymectomized during early childhood could have an immunological misbalance later on adulthood. Despite still a controversial topic, a continuously increasing body of knowledge supports the choice of preserving, as far as possible, thymus integrity.

4.1 Neonatal thymectomy during congenital heart disease correction

Congenital heart disease (CHD) comprises aberrant embryonic development or failure to progress beyond some early stage during fetal development of any cardiac structure. Septal or cyanotic defects, defects causing obstruction in either the heart or blood vessels and complex abnormalities are encompassed into CHD. Complex multifactorial genetic and environmental causes, rather chromosomal aberrations or single gene mutation (less than

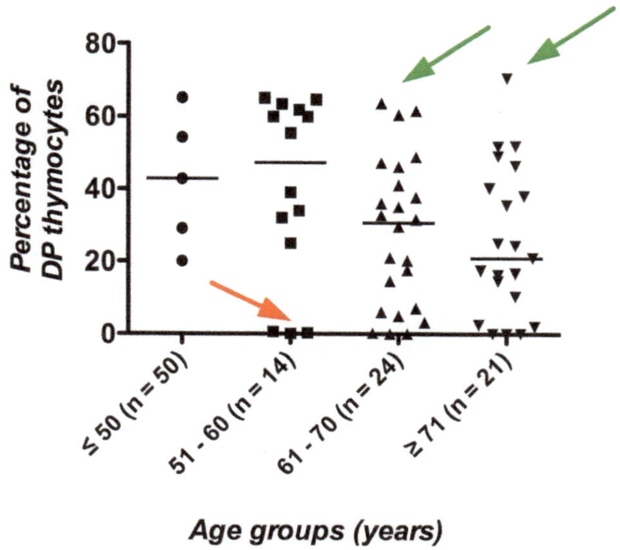

Fig. 3. Heterogeneity of the thymic function. Functionality was measured by ex-vivo quantification of DP thymocytes. Green arrows show high thymic function among elderly individuals (older than 65) while the red arrow show lack of functionality in adult individuals (50 to 60 years old). Modified from Ferrando-Martinez et al., 2009.

10% of diagnosed CHD), are the origin this disease. Prevalence in general population is estimated in 1% of all live deliveries. However, frequency rises up to 4% for childbirths of women which have been diagnosed with CHD during childhood. Disorders showing mild seriousness usually need little or no medical treatment lifetime. However, CHD can be a life-threatening condition. Since CHD is a progressive disease from prenatal to adulthood, severe conditions can be lethal immediately after birth and also during child/adulthood. Deathly forms of CHD usually need invasive surgery to guarantee the patient's survival. All forms together, more than 85% of diagnosed newborns reach adulthood thanks to positive adaptation to their condition (non-severe forms) or to successful medical and surgical interventions (lethal forms). Over the last 30 years, neonatal surgery to correct serious CHD has become usual and, since surgical access is obstructed by the thymus, thymectomy is a common practice.

Several studies, with case-control designs, assessed the potential immune failure of thymectomyzed children. Despite data are scarce and methodology heterogeneous, some conclusion can be already extracted. When short-term consequences are analyzed (less than one year after surgery) low peripheral lymphocyte counts are already reported (Wells et al., 1998; Turan et al., 2004). From the lymphocyte populations, T cells are preferentially decreased. Normal responsiveness to mitogens and none clinical consequence have been reported despite the described lymphopenia. Other studies focused in children that underwent surgery one to five years before, in order to analyze medium-term consequences of thymectomy. The fast drop of the lymphocyte populations was still observed, suggesting that peripheral homeostasis is not enough to maintain normal lymphocyte numbers during childhood (Halnon et al., 2005; Mancebo et al., 2006). In addition, low sj-TREC levels are also associated with thymectomy. Low levels of sj-TREC per million of cells in the thymectomyzed group has been associated with insufficient thymic function. Therefore, despite thymectomy is only partial in some individuals and thymic regeneration could be observed in some reoperated children, the general appreciation is that remaining thymopoietic degree will never reach normal levels in early thymectomyzed individuals. However it should be noted that sj-TREC counts are not a good measure of thymic function, especially when high peripheral proliferation is involved. On account of thymectomyzed individuals evidence low lymphocyte counts early after the surgical procedure, it can be assumed that homeostatic-driven proliferation will try to adjust lymphopenia to normal levels. High proliferation rates will dilute the sj-TREC content, disregarding changes of thymic function. Consequently, even if inefficient thymic function is indisputable due to persistently low lymphocyte counts, thymic function dynamics need to be further analyzed. It is noteworthy that medium-time costs of thymectomy still do not involve any clinical consequence.

In addition, long-term consequences should be evaluated. Interestingly, long-term studies also report persistent lymphopenia (preferentially T lymphocyte drops, as expected) and maintained low sj-TREC levels. However, when 20 to 30 years old individuals are analyzed, a trend to normalization in naive TL is observed, despite not in all studies. On the other hand Eysteinsdottir et al., 2004 reported new immune defects, as impaired Th2 T cell response despite normal Th1 response. In this study, thymectomyzed subjects also present higher numbers of neutrophils and low platelet counts but normal B lymphocyte and natural killer (NK) cell numbers. Low naive T cell counts, high proliferation rates among the naive subset and increased IL-7 bioavailability have been also observed (Prelog et al., 2009). This later result is especially interesting, since this naive T lymphocytes alteration is also a hallmark feature of immune senescence on healthy aging (Ferrando-Martínez et al., 2011). Whether this non-antigen driven proliferation is also leading to a naive T cell pool exhaustion (described in age-related changes of naive TL) needs to be explored.

Accordingly, more recent works specifically focused on premature aging. Immune senescence, or *immunosenescence*, comprises the age-related changes of the immune system that gather phenotypic and functional defects in both, the innate and adaptive immune response. It is generally accepted that thymic atrophy, as the first age-related change, triggers the accumulation of lymphocyte frailty. Despite causality needs to be established, the prevalence and severity of infectious diseases, probable direct immunosenescence consequence, discloses de outstanding importance of the age-related immune exhaustion. Immune senescence has also been linked to lack of vaccination response, autoimmunity and increase in oncological pathology in elderly subjects. Other clinical situations involving immune weakness (as HIV-infection or immune reconstitution after extensive chemotherapy) have been analyzed under this point of view, interestingly finding that TL which are forced to replenish a strongly damaged immune space usually show premature immunosenescence-related defects. Thymic function defects in early childhood can be an added model of premature immunosenescence. In this regard, thymectomyzed children show several features usually reported in chronological immunosenescence. Naive TL have increased proliferation rates, strong oligoclonal CMV-specific responses (that probably can accumulate because thymus is not able to replenish the immune space with naive TL), CD57-expressing exhausted cells or systemic inflammation biomarkers (Sauce et al., 2009). Lack of vaccine response, as elderly individuals, seems to focus on new antigens, despite normal memory responses (Zlamy et al., 2010). As a difference, thymectomyzed children have delayed vaccine response, rather that complete lack of immunization.

Finally, some studies report about normal TL counts after 20 - 30 years post-thymectomy, suggesting a reestablishment of thymic function later on life. Van Gent et al. (2011) report normal naive T cell numbers, adjusted proliferation rates and sj-TRECs numbers, concluding that thymectomization has an early impact on the LT compartment that will be restored later on life. Thymic regeneration (as measure by image techniques and inferred by sj-TREC dynamics) is proposed as major restoration mechanism. The reason why some cohorts can observe thymic and LT renewal (van Gen et al., 2011) while other do not (Prelog et al., 2009), remains a matter of debate. Partial results and animal models point to the possibility that younger thymus (months after birth) could have higher epithelial precursor content and, then, higher regeneration potential. However, further studies are needed to better clarify whether thymus actually have an age-related drop of regeneration capability. The lack of clinical consequences reported by all studies could be explained by thymic renewal and immune system restoration during adulthood. Despite all these results are very reassuring, it should be note that thymectomyzed individuals grow up with a frail immune system the first five to ten years of life and premature immunosenescence features have been reported in young adulthood (20 - 30 years old), suggesting that early thymectomy have immune consequences that, despite not being overwhelming, could have clinical consequences once premature immunosenescence joins the age-related exhaustion of the immune system.

4.2 Adult thymectomy: Open heart surgery

Valve replacement and ischemic cardiopathy are common open heart surgical procedures in adulthood / elderly subjects. Despite neonatal thymus size is larger than the atrophied adult thymus is; thymectomy to gain unrestricted view of the operation site is performed at any age. Moreover, the widespread belief that thymus from adult individuals completely lacks of functionality makes it usually despised. Anyhow, several factors should be pondered. First of all, despite the atrophy, elderly thymus still impacts on the peripheral T cell pool rejuvenation (Ferrando-Martínez et al., 2009). The more important, thymic function failure, in subjects over 65, predicts two-year all-cause mortality (Figure 4) (Ferrando-Martínez et al., 2011b). Moreover, myasthenia gravis patients (neuromuscular autoimmune disease where thymectomy is associated with better prognosis by unknown mechanisms) benefit of complete thymectomy even if thymus is already atrophied (Chen et al., 2011). All results together strongly suggest that atrophied thymus is active in different ways rather than an inactive surplus.

In addition, immune system of adult and elderly subjects undergoing open heart surgery already present exhaustion and senescence features. Thus, short- and medium-time defects induced by thymectomy (clearly present in children up to five to ten years old) will be acting on a previously damaged system. Clinical consequences of this damage have not been studied yet. Associated comorbidities of an elderly cohort with major cardiac illness is not easy, but further studies are needed to evaluate the potential effect of thymus removal on survival rates.

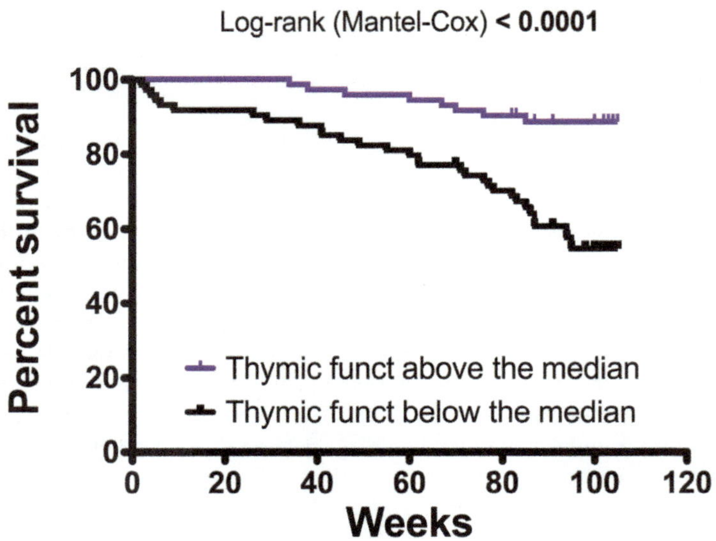

Fig. 4. Relationship between thymic function and two-year all-cause mortality in healthy elderly. Modified from Ferrando-Martínez et al., 2011b.

5. Conclusions and recommendations

Neonatal thymectomy have immunological consequences in short- and medium-time, despite these defects are not associated with clinical outcomes. T lymphocytes show a trend to normalization and stabilization in long-term analysis. Normalization could be due to thymic tissue regeneration. However, several features of exhaustion and senescence are detected in young adults 20 years old that underwent thymectomy in the first year of life. Premature immunosenescence is not found in age-matched non-thymectomized controls. In a reassuring way, despite the immune response to newly encountered antigens is delayed, clinical consequences (increased infection rates or other clinical signs of immune weakness) are not observed at any age. Subsequent studies are needed to determine the consequences, if any, of the thymectomy-induced premature senescence once chronological immunosenescence starts exhausting the immune system. On the other hand, elderly thymectomy data is still missing, but information showing that thymus still has relevance in seniors strongly suggest the need of caution before performing complete thymectomy: thymus removal in elderly individuals aggravates a previously frail immune system.

The topic remains controversial, and strong data are still scarce. Moreover, open heart surgery is an important procedure with priority over an immunosenescent scenario. However, our recommendation in children's surgery, where the great size of the thymus forces the surgeon to resect to gain unrestricted view of the operation site, is to proactively preserve the maximum possible tissue. During interventions of adult or elderly patients, which atrophied thymus is no longer a critical problem to reach the surgical field; our recommendation is to preserve the complete organ to guarantee the maximal integrity of the immune system.

6. Acknowledgements

Authors want to thank the cardiac surgery team of the Virgen del Rocío University Hospital. Their support and interest in Immunology research have been critical for us. Similarly, we are thankful to Dr. Felipe Borderas and the Service of Anatomical Pathology of the HUVR as key help with H&E slides preparation and interpretation. This work has been supported by Red de Investigación en SIDA (ISCIII RETIC RD06/0006/0021 and RD06/0006/0035).

7. References

Chen, Z.; Luo, H.; Peng, Y.; Cai, L.; Zhang, J.; Su, C. and Zou, J. (2011). Comparative clinical features and immune responses after extended thymectomy for myasthenia gravis in patients with atrophic versus hyperplastic thymus. *The Annals of Thoracic Surgery*, Vol.91 No.1, pp.212-218

Chiodi, H. (1940). The relationship between the thymus and the sexual organs. *Endocrinology*, Vol.26, No.1, pp.107-116

De la Rosa, R. & Leal, M. (2003). Thymic involvement in immune recovery among chronic-HIV-infected adults under highly active antiretroviral therapy. *Journal of Antimicrobial therapy*, Vol.52, No.2, pp.155-158

Dion, M.L.; Poulin, J.F.; Bordi, R.; Sylvestre, M.; Corsini, R.; Kettaf, N.; Dalloul, A.; Boulassel, M.R.; Debré, P.; Routy, J.P.; Grossman, Z.; Sekaly, R.P. & Cheynier, R. (2004). HIV infection rapidly induces and maintains a substantial suppression of thymocyte proliferation. *Immunity*, Vol.21, No.6, pp.757-768

Douek, D.C.; McFarland, R.D.; Keiser, P.H.; Gage, E.A.; Massey, J.M.; Haynes, B.F.; Polis, M.A.; Haase, A.T.; Feinberg, M.B.; Sullivan, J.L.; Jamieson B.D.; Zack, J.A.; Picker, L.J. & Koup, R.A. (1998). Changes in thymic function with age and during the treatment of HIV infection. *Nature*, Vol.396, No.6712, pp.690-695

Eysteinsdottir, J.H.; Freysdottir, J.; Haraldsson, A.; Stefansdottir, J.; Skaftadottir, I.; Helgason, H. & Ogmudsdottir, H.M. (2004). The influence of partial or total thymectomy during open heart surgery in infants on the immune function later on life. *Clinical and Experimental Immunology*, Vol. 136, No.2, pp.349-355

Ferrando-Martínez, S.; Franco, J.M.; Hernández, A.; Ordóñez, A.; Gutiérrez, E.; Abad, A. & Leal, M. (2009). Thymopoiesis in elderly human is associated with systemic inflammatory status. *Age (Dodr)*, Vol.31, No.2, pp.87-97

Ferrando-Martínez, S.; Ruiz-Mateos, E. & Leal, M. (2010) CD27 and CCR7 expression on naive T cells: are both necessary? *Immunology Letters*, Vol.127, No.2, pp.157-158

Ferrando-Martínez, S.; Franco, J.M.; Ruiz-Mateos, E.; Hernández, A.; Ordoñez, A.; Gutiérrez, E. & Leal, M. (2010b). A reliable and simplified sj/β-TREC ratio quantification method for human thymic output measurement. *Journal of Immunological Methods*, Vol.352, No.1-2, pp.111-117

Ferrando-Martínez, S.; Ruiz-Mateos, E.; Hernández, A.; Gutiérrez, E.; Rodríguez-Méndez, M.M.; Ordoñez, A. & Leal M. (2011). Age-related deregulation of naive T cell homeostasis in elderly humans. *Age (Dodr)*, Vol.33, No.2, pp.197-207

Ferrando-Martínez, S.; Romero-Sánchez, M.C.; Delgado, J.; de la Rosa, R.; Solana, R.; Ruiz-Mateos, E. & Leal, M. (2011b). Thymic function and inflammation markers are independently associated with elderly human survival rates. *VII IAGG European congress, "Healthy and active ageing for all Europeans – II"*, Bologna, April 2011 (oral communication)

Haines, C.J.; Giffon, T.D.; Li-Sheng, L.; Lu, X.; Tessier-Lavigne, M.; Ross, D.T. & Lewis, D.B. (2009). Human CD4+ T cell recent thymic emigrants are identified by protein tyrosine kinase 7 and have reduced immune function. *Journal of Experimental Medicine*, Vol.206, No.2, pp.275-285

Halnon, N.J.; Jamieson, B.; Plunkett, M.; Kitchen, C.M.; Pham, T. and Krogstad, P. (2005). Thymic function and impaired maintenance of peripheral T cell populations in children with congenital heart disease and surgical thymectomy. *Pediatric Research*, Vol.57, No.1, pp.42-48

Harris, J.M.; Hazenberg, M.D.; Poulin, J.F.; Higuera-Alhino, D.; Schmidt, D.; Gotway, M. & McCune, J.M. (2005). Multiparameter evaluation of human thymic function: interpretation and caveats. *Clinical Immunology*, Vol.115, No.2, pp.138-146

Hazenberg, M.D.; Otto, S.A.; Cohen Stuart, J.W.; Verschuren, M.C.; Borleffs, J.C.; Boucher, C.A.; Coutinho,R.A.; Lange, J.M.; Rinke de Wit, T.F.; Tsegaye, A.; von Dengen, J.J.; Harmann, D.; de Boer, R.J. & Miedema, F. (2000). Increased cell division but not thymic dysfunction rapidly affects the T cell receptor excision circle content of the naive T cell population in HIV-1 infection. *Nature Medicine*, Vol.6, No9, pp.1036-1042

Jamieson, B.D.; Douek, D.C.; Killian, S.; Hultin, L.E.; Scripture-Adams, D.D.; Giorgi, J.V.; Marellin D.; Koup R.A. & Zack, J.A. (1999). Generation of functional thymocytes in the human adult. *Immunity*, Vol.10, No.5, pp.569-575

Junge, S.; Kloeckener-Gruissem, B.; Zufferey, R.; Keisker, A.; Salgo, B.; Fauchere, J.C.; Scherer, F.; Shalaby, T.; Grotzer, M.; Seger, R. & Güngör, T. (2007). Correlation between recent thymic emigrants and CD31+ (PECAM-1) CD4+ T cells in normal individuals during aging and in lymphopenic children. *European Journal of Immunology*, Vol.37, No.11, pp.3270-3280

Kourtis, A.P.; Ibegbu, C.; Nahmias, A.J.; Lee, F.K.; Clark, W.S.; Sawyer, M.K & Nesheim, S. (1996). Early progression of disease in HIV-infected infants with thymus dysfunction. *New England Journal of Medicine*, vol.335, No.19, pp.1431-1436

Lynch, H.E.; Goldberg, G.L.; Chidgey, A.; Van den Brink, M.R.M.; Boyd, R. & Sempowski, G.D. (2009). Thymic involution and immune reconstitution. *TRENDS in Immunology*, Vol. 30, No.7, pp.366-373

Mackall, C.L.; Fleisher, T.A.; Brown, M.R.; Andrich, M.P.; Chen, C.C.; Feuerstein, I.M.; Horowitz, M.E.; Magrath, I.T.; Shed, A.T.; Steinberg, S.M.; Wexler, L.H. & Gress, R.E. (1995). Age, thymopoiesis and CD4+ T-lymphocyte regeneration after intensive chemotherapy. *New England Journal of Medicine*, Vol.332, No.3, pp.143-149

Mancebo, E.; Clemente, J.; Sanchez, J.; Ruiz-Contreras, J.; De Pablos, P.; Cortezon, S.; Romo, E.; Paz-Artal, E. and Allende, L.M. (2008). Longitudinal analysis of immune function in the first 3 years of life in thymectomyzed neonates during cardiac surgery. *Clinical and Experimental Immunology*, Vol.154, No.3, pp.375-383

Nahmias, A.J.; Clark, W.S.; Kourtis, A.K.; Lee, F.K.; Cotsonis, G.; Ibegbu, C.; Thea, D.; Palumbo, P.; Vink, P.; Simonds, R.J.; Nesheim, S.R. & the CDC Perinatal AIDS Collaborative Transmission Study Group. (1998). Thymic dysfunction and time of infection predict mortality in human immunodeficiency virus-infected infants. *The Journal of Infectious Diseases*, Vol.178, No.3, pp.680-685

Prelog, M.; Keller, M.; Geiger, R.; Brandstätter, A.; Würzner R.; Schweigmann, U.; Zlamy, M.; Zimmerhackl, L.B. & Grubeck-Loebenstein, B. (2009). Thymectomy in early childhood: significant alterations of the CD4(+)CD45RA(+)CD62L(+) T cell compartment in later life. *Clinical Immunology*, Vol.130, No.2, pp.123-132

Ribeiro, R.M. & Perelson, A.S. (2007). Determining thymic output quantitatively: using models to interpret experimental T-cell receptor excision circle (TREC) data. *Immunological Reviews*, Vol.216, pp.21-34

Ruiz-Mateos, E.; Rubio, A.; Vallejo, A.; de la Rosa, R.; Sánchez-Quijano, A.; Lissen, E. & Leal, M. (2004). Thymic volume is associated independently with the magnitud of short- and long-term repopulation of CD4+ T cells in HIV-infected adults after highly active antiretroviral therapy (HAART). *Clinical and Experimental Immunology*, Vol.136, No.3, pp.501-506

Sauce, D.; Larsen, M.; Fastenackels, S.; Duperrier, A.; Keller, M.; Grubeck-Loebestein, B.; Ferrand, C.; Debré, P.; Sidi, D. & Appay, V. (2009). Evidence of premature immune aging in patients thymectomyzed during early childhood. *Journal of Clinical Investigation*, Vol.119, No.10, pp.3070-3078

Sempowski, G.D.; Hale, L.P.; Sundy, J.S.; Massey, J.M.; Koup, R.A.; Douek, D.C.; Patel, D.D. & Haynes, B.F. (2000). Leukemia inhibitory factor, oncostatin M, IL-6 and stem cell factor mRNA expression in human thymus increases with age and is associated with thymic atrophy. *Journal of Immunology*, Vol.164, No.4, pp.2180-2187

Steinmann, G.G.; Klaus, B. & Müller-Hermelink, H.K. (1985). The involution of the ageing human thymic epithelium is independent of puberty. A morphometric study. *Scandinavian Journal of Immunology*, Vol.22, No.5, pp.563-575

Turan, T.; Turan, M.; Arslan, C.; Kinoglu, B. and Sarioglu, T. (2004). How does neonatal thymectomy affect the immune system? *Acta Cardiologica*, Vol.59, No.5, pp.511-513

Van Gent, R.; Schadenberg, A.W.L.; Otto, S.A.; Nievelstein, R.A.J.; Sieswerda, G.T.; Haas, F.; Miedema, F.; Tesselaar, K.; Jansen, N.J.G. & Borghans, J.A.M. (2011). Long-term restoration of the human T-cell compartment after thymectomy during infancy: a role for thymic regeneration? *Blood*, in press (DOI: 101182/blood-2011-03-341396)

Wells, W.J.; Parkman, R.; Smogorzewska, E. & Barr, M. (1998). Neonatal thymectomy: does it affect immune function? *The Journal of Thoracic and Cardiovascular Surgery*, Vol.115, No.5, pp.1041-1046

Zlamy, M.; Würzner, R.; Holzmann, H.; Brandstätter, A.; Jeller, V.; Zimmerhackl, L.B. & Prelog, M. (2010). Antibody dynamics after tick-born encephalitis and measles-mumps-rubella vaccination in children post early thymectomy. *Vaccine*, Vol.28, No.51, pp.8053-8060

18

Relationship Between Natriuretic Peptides and Hemodynamic Parameters Following Heart Surgery in Infancy

Andrea Székely, Tamás Breuer and Béla Merkely
Department of Anesthesiology and Intensive Care,
Department of Cardiology, Semmelweis University
and Department of Cardiology Gottsegen György
Hungarian Institute of Cardiology, Budapest
Hungary

1. Introduction

Critically ill states, perioperative period of major surgery, particularly cardiac operations are often encountered with large hemodynamic alterations and fluid shifts. Cardiac failure in patients with congenital heart defect has heterogeneous origin therefore diagnosis related treatment is difficult to apply. During the postoperative period, hemodynamic instability has multifactorial origin and cardiorespiratory dysfunction has several manifestation e.g. myocardial dysfunction, pulmonary hypertension etc (Laussen & Roth, 2003).
Biochemical markers play an important role in the risk stratification of patients with cardiovascular disease. Elevated brain natriuretic peptide level has been shown to reveal congestive heart failure among adult patients admitted to emergency department with dyspnoe (Maisel et al, 2002; de Lemos et al, 2001), and to predict adverse events in acute coronary syndromes (de Lemos et al, 2001). Cardiac troponin, creatine kinase-MB, brain natriuretic peptide and C-reactive protein have been shown to predict mortality and morbidity in unstable coronary artery disease (Lindahl et al, 2000). In patients with pulmonary embolism, brain natriuretic peptide and other cardiac markers, such as troponin predict adverse outcomes much more accurately than any other clinical signs (Kucher et al, 2003). In the last decade, several papers investigating the prognostic, diagnostic and therapeutic relevance of natriuretic peptides in the pediatric population have been published (in rev. Cantinotti et al, 2011; Cantinotti et al, 2011).

2. Physiology of the natriuretic peptides

The natriuretic peptides are a family of peptides produced by the myocardium, vascular endothelium and the kidneys (Clerico et al, 2006). The "hormone" of the heart is involved in the regulation of intravascular homeostasis, myocardial function. On the other hand, natriuretic peptides counteract with the renin-angiotensin-aldosterone system, symphathetic nervous system, vasopressin release. Receptors of natriuretic peptides are mainly presented in the myocardium, kidneys, lungs and vascular endothelium. The action is mediated by c-

GMP, the cytoplasmatic calcium availability will be decreased in the smooth muscles and it will result in vasodilatation.(Silberbach & Roberts, 2001).

Atrial stretching triggers release of the preformed prohormone of atrial natriuretic peptide (NT-proANP) in the atrial wall. During secretion, the prohormone of atrial natriuretic peptide (ANP) is cleaved to atrial natriuretic peptide and N-terminal pro-atrial natriuretic peptide (Kangawa et al, 1984). Although brain natriuretic peptide chemically resembles atrial natriuretic peptide to some extent, it is synthetized both in the atrial and ventricular myocardium due to volume and pressure overload. The production of BNP requires time (6-12 hours), since RNA transcription of the prohormone precedes the secretion. Then, the prohormone of brain natriuretic peptide is cleaved to brain natriuretic peptide (BNP) and N-terminal pro-brain natriuretic peptide (NT-proBNP). N-terminal peptides have several times higher concentrations and longer half life time in blood circulation than atrial natriuretic peptide and brain natriuretic peptide, making them reliable markers (Ham et al, 1995).

3. Diagnostic application of the natriuretic peptides

3.1 Adult population

In adults, diastolic dysfunction or asymptomatic aortic stenosis confirmed by echocardiography or angiography show marked correlations with brain natriuretic peptide (Gerber et al, 2003). Right-sided heart failure or complications after pulmonary embolism can accurately be detected by measuring natriuretic peptides, though the cut-off levels were only half of those for left ventricular dysfunction (Kucher et al, 2003). There are two widely accepted area for BNP testing; exclusion of non-cardiac origin of dyspnoe in emergency settings and prognostic information of various states of heart failure. NT-proBNP above 1065 pmol/l had a very high specificity and sensitivity for cardiac failure in our population, similar levels were found in decompensated heart failure, septic shock and acute pulmonary embolism with New York Heart Association III and IV symptoms (Seino et al, 2004). Additionally, lower postoperative cut-off value (513 pmol/l) bore high negative predictive power, indicating a level below which the occurrence of heart failure is unlikely. In these cases, NT-proBNP or BNP measurements are used. Levels above the cut-off level were independently associated with increased risk for mortality and cardiovascular morbidity including cardiac fibrillation. In adults, it has been shown that hyperthyroidism increases the NT-pro BNP level and could reflect cardiac dysfunction secondary to thyreotoxicosis [Kato 2008, Welisch 2011].

ANP or NT-proANP reflect acute changes in atrial wall stress (Ruskoaho, 2003). Therefore, it is not suitable for long-term follow-up of congestive heart failure. Recently, a new immunoassay has been developed for a hybrid peptide (referred to as NT-proXNP) containing peptide sequences from both NT-proANP and NT-proBNP (Ala-Kopsala et al, 2005). This novel assay mimics the physiological signaling pathway since the actions of the different active natriuretic fragments on the target cells are mediated by a single natriuretic peptide receptor. The NT-proXNP assay measures the concentration of the new virtual natriuretic peptide, and thus provides combined information about the plasma levels of NT-proANP and NT-proBNP. In cardiac diseases, the neurohormonal system of the heart is activated. The diagnostic performances of NT-proXNP in adults for coronary artery disease and valvular heart disease are greater than or equal to those of NT-proANP or NT-proBNP, individually. NT-proXNP seems to combine the characteristics of the two natriuretic peptides. Therefore, NT-proXNP will increase earlier during myocardial wall stress than the NT-proBNP alone.

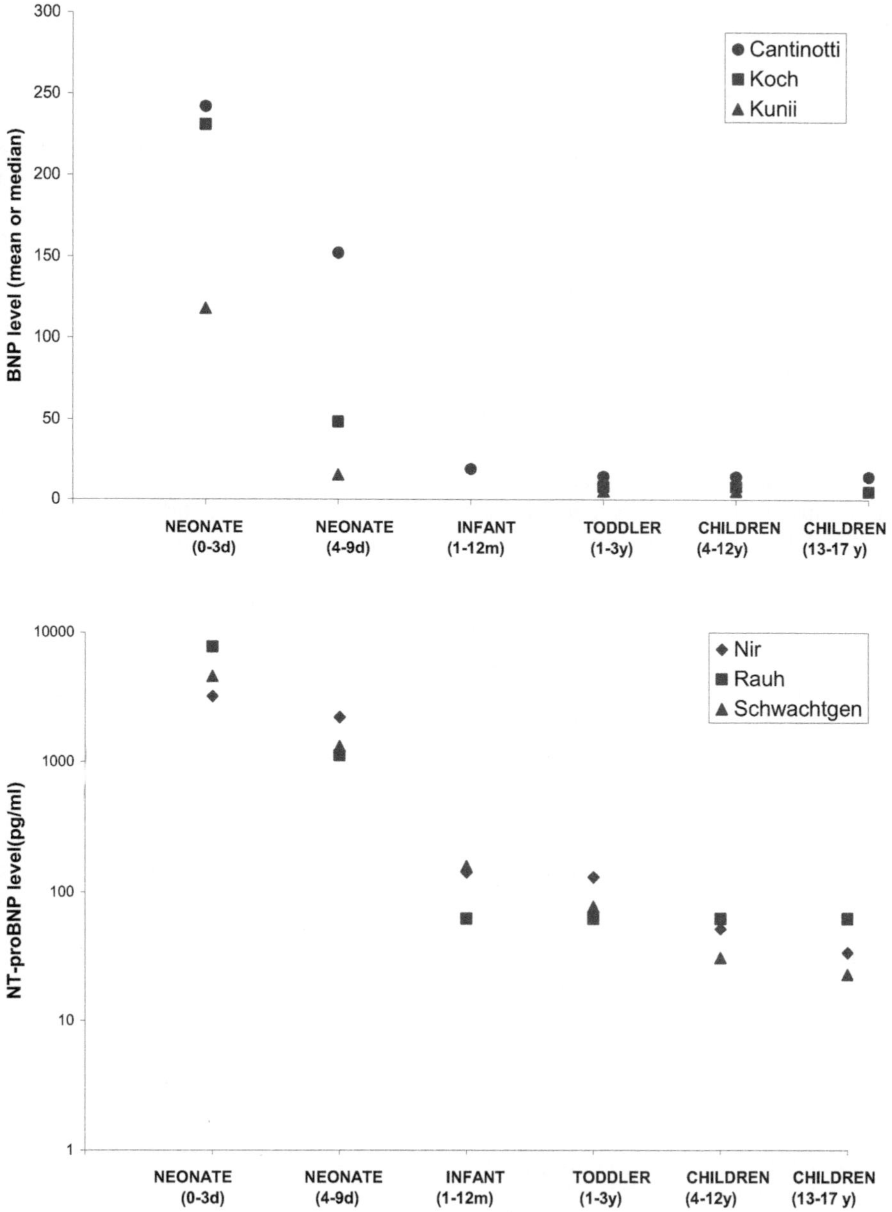

Fig. 1. Refence mean and median values of healthy subjects

3.2 Pediatric population

Based on physiological considerations, BNP and NT-proBNP levels are age dependent in the first two weeks after birth (Albers et al, 2006-Schwachtgen et al, 2005). The perinatal transition from fetal to neonatal circulation is accompanied by an increase in the pulmonary blood flow and an increase in the systemic vascular resistance. These hemodynamic changes lead to pressure and volume load of the heart and it may stimulate the secretion and release of natriuretic peptides. From 31 days to 12 years of age, there is no significant change in healthy subjects (Cantinotti et al, 2010). From 14 years of age, gender related differences should be accounted and it is probably due to steroid sex hormones (Soldin et al, 2006). Age-corrected brain natriuretic peptide and NT-proBNP values should be used in the neonatal population (Cantinotti et al, 2010b), while gender should be considered in the adolescent population. Additionally, it is important to note that reference ranges, decision values are method dependent and it shows variations between the assays and consequently between the studies (Soldin et al, 2006, Cantinotti et al, 2010). These variations are seen in Figure 1. As in the adult population NT-proBNP is significantly higher in children with sepsis. In children with sepsis NT-proBNP levels are higher in some patients with leftventricular dysfunction (Fried 2006). In comparison to the adult population there are no paediatric studies in hyperthyroidism available at present (Welisch 2011).

3.3 Pediatric population – Congenital heart disease

Different requirements have been formulated for the natriuretic peptide assays in the pediatric population. One major area is the exclusion of cardiovascular disease particularly below one year of age. The clinical signs are poor or share the ones with other noncardiac diseases. The major symptoms are dyspnea, tachypnea, cold extremities, murmurs, tachycardia, hypotension, etc. The assay is easy to carry out and requires only 0.5 ml blood. The recent studies showed convincing results that the BNP test could be performed without difficulties from capillary stick and it had a high negative power both in neonates and infants (Law et al, 2009,Maher et al, 2008).

The anatomy of the congenital heart diseases is heterogenous. Additionally, the situation after different types of surgery complicates the hemodynamic state. An arbitrary classification is the following: ventricle volume overload, including left-right shunts, ventricular septal defects, patent ductus arteriosus, atrial septal defect, atrioventricular malformations, truncus arteriosus, etc; pressure overload, as a consequence of outflow tract obstruction or valvular stenosis, such as tetralogy of Fallot, pulmonary or aorta stenosis; univentricular physiology and non-clusterable complex malformations. Despite the age related BNP elevation in the neonatal period, the severity of heart failure can be determined and diagnosed (Cantinotti et al, 2010b, Law et al, 2009). Other studies have been described the linear relationship between BNP or NT-proBNP levels and the magnitude of left-right shunting (Kunii et al, 2003) and BNP levels were able to predict the need for ductus arteriosus closure (Paul et al, 2009). Echocardiographic studies have been confirmed the association between pressure gradient and natriuretic peptide levels (Cowley et al, 2004). In right sided pressure overload, the BNP levels were lower compared to left sided pressure overload (Cantinotti et al, 2009, Holmgren et al, 2005). In Table 1 and 2 pediatric studies measuring BNP and NT-proBNP levels are shown.

3.4 Pediatric cardiac population postoperative period

Monitoring of cardiac output is still a problematic issue, although early recognition of hemodynamic complications is essential in pediatric critical care. During the postoperative period, hemodynamically unstable patients are characterized by high volume intake, the need for considerable inotropic support, edema formation, hepatic congestion, lung

Author	Key words	n	result	Congenital HD	cut-off// lowest level
Lowenthal, A (Lowenthal 2010)	BNP, pediatric Carvedilol trial, heterogenous subject population, cut off values in subgroups	29	positive predictive of heart failure	single ventricle physiology	>30pg/ml
Hall, EK (Hall 2011)	orthotope heart transplantation, follow up, cardiac catheterization, acute cellular rejection	62	Corr betw BNP&right sided pressure measurements	OHT	mean 171pg/ml
Shah A (Shah 2009)	single ventricle, heart failure, BNP	29	Positive predictive of heart failure	single ventricle physiology	>30pg/ml
Cowley C (Cowley 2004)	catherization, BNP correlation pressures espec left ventr outflow obstruction	107	BNP correlates with left ventricular outflow obstruction		median 19pg/ml
Muta H (Muta 2002)	catherization, ASD closure	14	natriuretic peptides may reflect hemodynamic changes	ASD	ANP 24ng/l, BNP23ng/l
Hsu J (Hsu 2007)	neonates, cardiac surgery	36	in neonates BNP predicts poor outcome after cardiac surgery	group 1: stage 1 Norwood,group 2: biventricular repair	
Hsu J (Hsu 2008)	bidirectional cavopulmonary anastomosis, total cavopulmonary connection	36	BNP predicts unplanned surgical/transcatheter interventions includ transplantation	functionally single ventricle	BNP>500pg /ml
Knirsch W (Knirsch 2011)	BNP, PulmHT, AqHD, CongHD	522	BNP useful as follow-up, e.g. BNP decrease after Fontan proc, e.g. BNP decrease after initialization of treatment for PulmHT	yes (heterogeneous group before med treatment,surgery or catherization)	no cut-off values
Berry J (Berry 2008)	single ventricle, prognostic BNP	25	early postoperative BNP levels correlate with ensuing duration of hospitalization and duration of inotropic support	single ventricle to undergo Norwood, Bidirectional cavopulmonary Anastomosis, Fontan	
Law Y (Law 2009)	BNP, rapid triage tool, identify CardVascDisease	100	BNP reliable test to diagnose significant structural or functional CVD in children		BNP: neonatal 170pg/ml, older age 41pg/ml, combined group 44pg/ml
Maher K (Maher 2008)	acute care setting, CongHD, AqHD	103	BNP in acute care settings valuable diagnostic tool	yes, (heterogenous group of 33 children)no	highest median in hypoplastic left heart syndr 4920pg/ml
El-Khuffash, A (El-Khuffash 2011)	PDA, neurodevelopmental outcome, cTNT,preterm	60	possibl assoc cTNT/BNP & hd significant PDA: no statistic significance foud	exclusion criteria	1664vs9209p mol/lNT-proNBNP

Table 1. Usefulness of Brain Natriuretic Peptide measurements. Prospective observational study PO, Brain natriuretic peptide BNP, Atrial natriuretic peptide ANP, cardiac Troponin cTNT, orthotope heart transplantation OHT, persistent Ductus arteriosus PDA, Atria septum defect ASD, pulmonary hypertension pulmHT, aquired heart disease AqHD, congenital heart disease congHD, cardiovascular disease CardVascDis.

Author	Key words	n	Result	Congenital HD	Cut-off// lowest level	Special remarks
Heise G (Heise 2008)	serial, natriuretic hormone system, pulsatile MCS (Berlin Heart EXCOR)	19	serial NP correlate with level of unloading of heart & potential recovery	15 DCM, 2 myocarditis, 1 CongHD, 1 Cardiac arrest in rejection after HTX	250pg/ml on MCS	none
Gessler P (Gessler 2006)	risk stratification for low-risk surgery in CongHD, RACHS-1 score, lactate, duration of CBP, cyanotic defect	40	high NT-proBNP preop predictive of postop prolonged need for inotropic therapy	obstructive lesions/ l-r-shunt/ cyanotic defects		risk stratificati on for surgery in CongHD
Pietrzak R (Pietrzak 2009)	Fallot correction, rigth ventricular failure, transannular patch, duration of QRS	20	high NT-proBNP may help identify patients at risk for arythmias, rigth ventr failure after Fallot correction	postop correction of Fallot tetralogy	18fmol/l	NT-proBNP higher after TOFl correction
Breuer T (Breuer 2010)	NT-proXNP, neonates/infants <1 year, complete biventriculair repair	26	NT-proXNP correlates with CI	biventriculair repair, <1year	NT-proXNP 3079pmol/l or NT-proBNP 2051pmol/l ~CI<3l/min/m2	none
Kaneko K (Kaneko 2011)	kawasaki syndrome,NT-proBNP, coronary arterial lesions	43	risk to develop coronary artery lesions 10x higher with NT-proBNP>1000pg/ml		NT-proBNP>1000pg /ml	none
Joseph L (Joseph 2010)	Bronchopulmonarydysplasia,natriureticpeptides,prematurity <34weeks gest	34	NT-proBNP signif higher with BPD, NT-signif higher with Resp Distress Syndr	Cong HD/ sepis/ current PDA exclusion criteria		none
Mazurek B (2009)	idiopathic ventricular arrhythmia, asymptomatic circulatory failure	36	NT-proBNPincreases with malignant ventricular arrhythmia	none,idiopathic ventricular arrhythmia	66pg/ml median in group malign arryhthmia	none
Rusconi P (Rusconi 2010)	dilated cardiomyopathy (idiopathic, anthracycline-related, uremic, muscular dystrophy), heart failure, changes in echocardiographic evalutaion of HF	36	serial NT-proBNP >1000pg/ml correlates with HF, echodardiographic measures correlate with NT-proBNP changes within patients	none	NT-proBNP>1000pg /ml; NT-proBNP <450pg/ml asymptomatic patients;	retrospect ive ;NT-proBNP <450pg/ ml
Nir A (Nir 2009)	reference values neonates/infants, log-normal distribution, high NT-proBNP in pubertal girls	690	reference values for pediatr population	no, no cardiac disease, no respiratory disease	see table 1	combined study data
Cohen S (Cohen 2005)	differenciate between cardiac or respiratory problem	48	BNP differentiates between heart failure and lung disease, BNP for monitoring treatment for heart failure	yes (heterogeneous group)	2940pg/ml	none

Author	Key words	n	Result	Congenital HD	Cut-off// lowest level	Special remarks
Mir T (Mir 2002)	establish normal age-related NT-proBNP levels in children form infant to adulthood, compare CongestiveHF with controlgrou	164	NT-proBNP is higher in children with CHF, correlates with severity of clinical signs and echocardiographic EF	yes, (heterogenous group of 31 children)	no	none
Wong D (Wong 2011)	mechanical circulatory support, transplantation, acute decompensated heart failure	24	signif diff MCS/no-MCS, but not predictive	4 CHD, 17 cardiomyopathy, 3 "other"	Median of max value 40pg/ml	none

Table 2. Usefulness of NT-proBrain Natriuretic Peptide measurements. Retrospective study r, n-terminal pro-brainnatriureticpeptide NT pro-BNP, brain natriuretic peptide BNP, dilated cardiomyopathy DCM, congestive heart failure congestiveHF, mechanical circulatory support MCS; cardiopulmonary bypass CPB, total corretion of Fallot TOF, persistent Ductus arteriosus PDA, Risk Adjustement for Congenital Heart Surgery RACHS-1 (Jenkins 2004)

dysfunction or the combination of them (Laussen & Roth, 2003). High lactate levels and low base excess on the first postoperative day have been reported to predict mortality and outcome in pediatric cardiac patients (Tibby et al, 1999, Carmona et al, 2008). Mir et al.found limited value of NT-proBNP levels in the perioperative period. In their study, dosage and duration of catecholamines and length of mechanical ventilation correlated with postoperative troponin T and arterial lactate levels, but not with NT-proBNP (Mir et al, 2006). Since catecholamine therapy is a consequence of hemodynamic instability and prolonged mechanical ventilation can be influenced by certain non-cardiac factors, the direct relationship might be concerned. Indeed, clinical signs and scores of congestive heart failure is difficult to apply as diaphoresis, respiratory rate, heart rate in the early postoperative period are strongly modified by inotropic, analgesic and sedative medication (Tibby et al, 1999). Preoperative NT-proBNP was associated with adverse postoperative outcome in children undergoing heart surgery, like duration of mechanical ventilation, dose of inotropic support, length of intensive care unit stay (33-Hsu et al, 2007). BNP and NT-proBNP levels usually exceed the peak maximum at 12 hours, and a second peak may occur about five days after surgery (Koch et al, 2007). Postoperative BNP and NT-proBNP levels have also been shown to have prognostic value after pediatric cardiac surgery. After cavopulmonary anastomosis a decrease in natriuretic peptides level compared to preoperative level were correlated with better outcomes (Hsu et al, 2008). Prognostic role of BNP was also reported after switch surgery in neonates (Lehot et al, 1992).

Our study investigated the prognostic role of NT-proXNP, a hybride analyte. NT-proXNP level correlated significantly with the simultaneously measured NT-proANP level ($r = 0.60$, $p < 0.001$), but more strongly with NT-proBNP level ($r = 0.89$, $p < 0.001$) and the arithmetic sum of both peptides throughout the perioperative period ($r = 0.88$, $p < 0.001$). Baseline NT-proXNP level correlated with the age ($r = -0.72$, $p < 0.001$) and the weight of the patients ($r = -0.47$, $p = 0.026$). Preoperative creatinine level (53.3 ± 13.1 μmol/l) correlated with baseline NT-proXNP ($r = 0.53$, $p = 0.013$). The duration of operation and the duration of CPB were associated with the preoperative NT-proXNP level ($r = 0.58$, $p = 0.005$ and $r = 0.62$ $p = 0.002$,

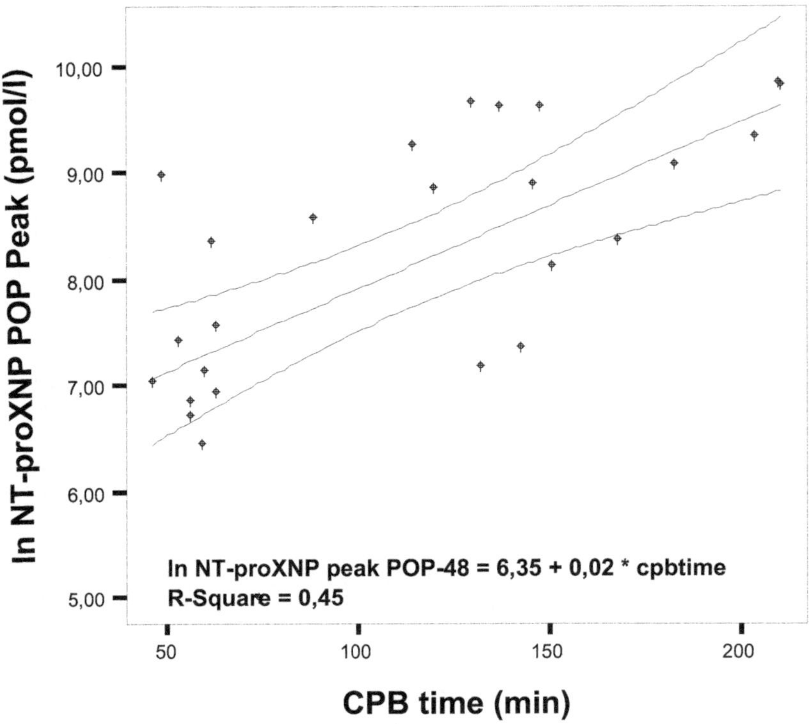

Fig. 2. Correlation between logarithmic transformed NT-proXNP levels and cardiopulmonary bypass time

respectively) and the peak postoperative NT-proXNP level (r = 0.64, p < 0.001 and r = 0.67, p < 0.001, respectively). NT-proBNP showed similar correlations with the duration of operation and CPB (Breuer et al, 2010). In the postoperative period, natriuretic peptide levels correlated significantly with the simultaneously assessed hemodynamic parameters. NT-proXNP correlated stronger with the hemodynamic parameters except for extravascular lung water index than the arithmetic sum of NT-proANP and NT-proBNP. The correlation between NT-proXNP and CI remained significant after adjusting for age (r = 0.60, p = 0.018) or weight (r = 0.81, p < 0.001).

The hemodynamic parameters improved during the postoperative period as the myocardium recovered. The application of transpulmonary thermodilution was safe and reliable and it added useful information to the conventionally measured pressure values in neonates and infant following open heart surgery. We found lower global enddiastolic volume indices and higher extravascular lung water indices compared to adult ranges, whereas the cardiac indices were the same. Age related and disease specific reference values of the transpulmonary thermodilution parameters are yet to be determined in children.

In ROC analysis, a postoperative NT-proBNP level of 2051 pmol/l was diagnostic for cardiac index (CI) lower than 3 l/min/m2 with 79% sensitivity and 95% specificity (AUC: 0.87 ± 0.06), whereas a postoperative NT-proXNP level of 079 pmol/l was diagnostic for that with 89% sensitivity and 90% specificity (AUC: 0.91 ± 0.05). The length of mechanical ventilation and ICU stay did not correlate with the baseline or the peak natriuretic peptide levels. NT-proBNP and NT-proXNP, but not NT-proANP level at 24 hours after surgery were correlated to the length of mechanical ventilation (r = 0.51, p = 0.015 and r = 0.47, p = 0.027, respectively). The area under the curve (AUC) of NT-proBNP and NT-proXNP at 24 hours after surgery for prolonged mechanical ventilation (> 72h) in ROC analysis was 0.81 ± 0.10 and 0.72 ± 0.11, respectively.

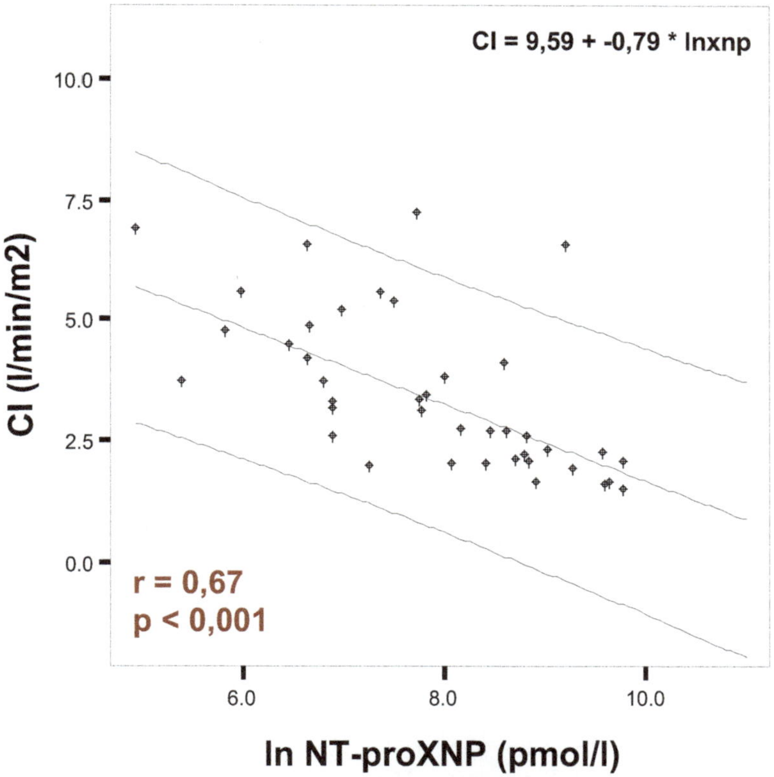

Fig. 3. Relationship between logarithmic transformed NT-proXNP levels and Cardiac index

Conventionally measured parameters such as heart rate, mean arterial pressure and pulse-pressure product exhibited weaker correlations with CI than natriuretic peptide levels. Parameters measured by echocardiography i.e. fractional shortening and calculated pressures of the right ventricle were not correlated to CI. Clinical and laboratory values, except for creatinine level and creatinine clearance, showed no correlation with CI or NT-proXNP. According to our findings, natriuretic peptides and NT-proXNP are indicators of hemodynamic parameters following pediatric cardiac surgery that can only be measured by invasive hemodynamic monitoring.

3.5 Pediatric cardiac population–follow-up period

Pediatric cardiac population follow-up period Pediatric patients with simple cardiac lesions after corrective surgery show a marked reduction in BNP and NT-proBNP levels compared to the preoperative period. The same is true after catheter interventions, like closure of atrial septal defect or closure of ductus arteriosus. In patients with residual defects, like pulmonary stenosis or pulmonary arterial hypertension, serial measurements of BNP or NT-proBNP levels provide a useful, easy and non-invasive tool for follow-up and it can be used for quantification of the disease severity. During the follow-up of cardiac transplant patients rejection can be detected by increase of BNP levels.

4. Conclusion

Natriuretic peptide levels are age dependent and show significant variability according to the type of the cardiac malformation and the actual hemodynamic condition. Recently, age related normal values have been established in the neonatal period and it allows detection of the congental heart disease in different age groups. Right sided hemodynamic ventricular stress is encountered with lower BNP values. Preoperative and postoperative application of natriuretic peptides provides a useful tool for the detection of postoperative complications. The new analyte, NT-proXNP seems to have promising characteristics, because it reflects the cardiac output changes earlier than the BNP, NT-proBNP assay.

5. Acknowledgment

TAMOP TAMOP-4.2.2/B10/1.-2010-0013, who has sponsored the preparation of this chapter.

6. References

Ala-Kopsala M, Ruskoaho H, Leppaluoto J, Seres L, Skoumal R, Tóth M, Horkay F, Vuolteenaho O. (2005) Single assay for amino-terminal fragments of cardiac A- and B-type natriuretic peptides. *Clin Chem* Vol 51 pp 708-18.

Albers S, Mir TS, Hada M, Laer S. (2006)N-terminal probrain natriuretic peptide: normal ranges in the pediatric population including method comparison and interlaboratory variability. *Clin Chem Lab Med* Vol.44 pp 80-85.

Baumgartner H, Bonhoeffer P, De Groot NM, de Haan F, Deanfield JE, Galie N, et al. (2010) ESC Guidelines for the management of grown-up congenital heart disease (new version 2010): the Task Force on the Management of Grown-up Congenital Heart Disease of the European Society of Cardiology (ESC). *Eur Heart J* Vol;31 pp 2915–57.

Berry JG, Askovich B,.Shaddy A, Hawkins J, Cowley CG (2008) Prognostic Value of B-Type Natriuretic Peptide in Surgical Palliation of Children with Single-Ventricle Congenital Heart Disease. *PediatrCardiol*, Vol 29 pp 70–75

Breuer T, Sápi E, Skoumal R, Tóth M, Ala-Kopsala M, Vuolteenaho O, Leppäluoto J, Ruskoaho H, Szatmári A, Székely A. (2007) N-terminal pro-brain natriuretic peptide level inversely correlates with cardiac index after arterial switch operation in neonates. *Pediatric Anesthesia* Vol 17 pp 782-8..

Breuer T, Skoumal R, Horkay F, Merkely B, Ala-Kopsala M, Leppäluoto J, Vuolteenaho O, Ruskoaho H, Tóth M., Székely A. (2010)Strong relationship between NT-proXNP levels and cardiac output following cardiac surgery in neonates and infants. *Acta Anaesthesiologica Scandinavica;* Vol 54 pp 502-9.

Cantinotti M, Vittorini S, Storti S, Prontera C, Murzi M, De Lucia V, et al.(2009) Diagnostic accuracy and clinical relevance of brain natriuretic peptide assay in pediatric patients with congenital heart diseases. J Cardiovasc Med (Hagerstown) Vol 10 pp 706–13

Cantinotti M, Storti S, Parri MS, Prontera C, Murzi B, Clerico A.(2010)Reference intervals for brain natriuretic peptide in healthy newborns and infants measured with an automated immunoassay platform. Clin Chem Lab Med; Vol 48 pp 697–700.

Cantinotti M, Storti S, Ripoli A, Zyw L, Crocetti M, Assanta N, et al. (2010) Diagnostic accuracy of B-type natriuretic hormone for congenital heart disease in the first month of life. Clin Chem Lab Med Vol 48 pp 1333–8.

Cantinotti M, Giovannini S, Murzi B, Clerico A (2011) Diagnostic, prognostic and therapeutic relevance of B-type natriuretic hormone and related peptides in children with congenital heart diseases. *Clin Chem Lab Med*, Vol 49 pp 567-580

Carmona F, Manso PH, Vicente WV, Castro M, Carlotti AP (2008). Risk stratification in neonates and infants submitted to cardiac surgery with cardiopulmonary bypass: a multimarker approach combining inflammatory mediators, N-terminal pro-B-type natriuretic peptide and troponin I. *Cytokine*; Vol 42 pp 317-24.

Clerico A, Recchia FA, Passino C, Emdin M. (2006) Cardiac endocrine function is an essential component of the homeostatic regulation network: physiological and clinical implications. Am J Physiol Heart Circ Physiol; Vol 290 pp H17–29.

Cohen S, Springer C, Avital A, Perles Z, Rein A, Argaman Z, Nir A (2005) Amino-Terminal Pro-Brain-Type Natriuretic Peptide: Heart or Lung Disease in Pediatric Respiratory Distress? *Pediatrics*, Vol 115 pp 1347–1350;

Costello JM, Backer CL, Checchia PA, Mavroudis C, Seipelt RG, Goodman DM. (2005) Effect of cardiopulmonary bypass and surgical intervention on the natriuretic hormone system in children. *J Thorac Cardiovasc Surg*; Vol 130 pp 822-9.

Cowley CG, Bradley JD, Shaddy RE.(2004) B-type natriuretic peptide levels in congenital heart disease. *Pediatr Cardiol*; Vol 25: 336-40.

de Lemos JA, Morrow DA, Bentley JH, et al. (2001) The prognostic value of B-type natriuretic peptide in patients with acute coronary syndromes. N Engl J Med Vol 345 pp 1014– 21.

El-Khuffash A, Slevin M, McNamara P, Molloy EJ (2011) Troponin T, N-terminal pro natriuretic peptide and a patent ductus arteriosus scoring system predict death before discharge or neurodevelopmental outcome at 2 years in preterm infants. *Arch Dis Child Fetal Neonatal Ed*, Vol 96 pp F133–F137

Fried I, Bar-Oz B, Algur N, Fried E, Gavri S, Yatsiv I, Perles Z, Rein A, Zonis Z, Bass R, Nir A (2006) Comparison of N-terminal Pro-B-Type Natriuretic Peptide Levels in Critically Ill Children With Sepsis Versus Acute Left Ventricular Dysfunction. *Pediatrics*, Vol 118 pp e1165

Gerber IL, Stewart PAH, Legget ME, et al (2003) Increased plasma natriuretic peptide levels reflects symptom onset in aortic stenosis. *Circulation*; Vol 107 pp 1884-1890.

Gessler P, Knirsch W, Schmitt B, Russon V, von Eckardstein A (2006) Prognostic value of plasma N-Terminal pro-Brainnatriureticpeptide in children with congenital heart defects and open-heart surgery. *J Pediatr*, Vol 148 pp 372-376

Hall EK, Glatz AC, Quartermain DM, Ravishankar C, Kaufman B, Cohen M, Hanna BD, Goldberg JD (2011) Brain-type natriuretic peptide correlates with right heart pressures in a cross section of pediatric heart transplant patients. *Pediatr Transplant*, Vol 15 pp70-74

Hama N, Itoh H, Shirakami G, Nakagawa O, Suga S, Ogawa Y, Masuda I, Nakanishi K, Yoshimasa T, Hashimoto Y, Yamaguchi M, Hori R, Yasue H, Nakao K. (1995) Rapid ventricular induction of brain natriuretic peptide gene expression in experimental acute myocardial infarction. Circulation; Vol 92 pp 1558-64.

Heise G, Lemmer J, Hübler M, Weng Y, Alexi-Meskishvili V, Böttcher W, Hetzer R, Berger F, Stiller B (2008) Biomarker Responses During Mid-term Mechanical Cardiac Support in Children. *J Heart Lung Transplant*, Vol 27 pp 150–7

Holmgren D, Westerlind A, Lundberg PA, Wåhlander H. (2005) Increased plasma levels of natriuretic peptide type B and A in children with congenital heart defects with left compared with right ventricular volume overload or pressure overload. *Clin Physiol Funct Imaging*; Vol 25 pp 263-9.

Hsu JH, Keller RL, Chikovani O, Cheng H, Hollander SA, Karl TR, Azakie A, Adatia I, Oishi P, Fineman JR. (2007) B-type natriuretic peptide levels predict outcome after neonatal cardiac surgery. *J Thorac Cardiovasc Surg*; Vol 134 pp 939-45.

Hsu JH, Oishi PE, Keller RL, Chikovani O, Karl TR, Azakie A, et al. (2008) Perioperative B-type natriuretic peptide levels predict outcome after bidirectional cavopulmonary anastomosis and total cavopulmonary connection. J Thorac Cardiovasc Surg; Vol 135 pp 746–53

Jenkins KJ (2004) Risk adjustement for congenital heart surgery: the RACHS-1 method. Sem Thorac Cardiovas Surg Pediatr Card Surg Annu, Vol 7 pp 180-184

Joseph L, Nir A, Hammerman C, Goldberg S, Shalom EB, Picard E (2010)N-terminal pro-B-type Natriuretic Peptide as a Marker of Bronchopulmonary Dysplasia in Premature Infants. *Am J Perinatol*, Vol 27 pp 381–386

Kaneko K, Yoshimura K, Ohashi A, Kimata T, Shimo T, Tsuji S (2011) Prediction of the Risk of Coronary Arterial Lesions in Kawasaki Disease by Brain Natriuretic Peptide. *Pediatr Cardiol*, DOI10.1007/s00246-011-9986-8

Kangawa K, Fukuda A, Kubota I, Hayashi Y, Minamitake Y, Matsuo H. (1984)Human atrial natriuretic polypeptides (hANP): purification, structure synthesis and biological activity. J Hypertens Suppl; Vol 2 pp S321-3.

Kato K, Murakimo H, Isozaki O Endocrine J, Thushima T, Takano K (2009) Serum Concentrations of BNP and ANP in patients with thyreotoxicosis. *Endocrine J*, Vol 56 pp 17-27

Knirsch W, Häusermann E, Fasnacht M, Hersberger M, Gessler P, Bauersfeld U (2011) PlasmaB-type natriuretic peptide levels in children with heart disease. ActaPædiatrica ISSN0803–5253

Koch A, Singer M. Normal values of B type natriuretic peptide in infants, children, and adolescents. (2003) *Heart*; Vol 89 pp 875–8.

Koch A, Kitzsteiner T, Zink S, Cesnjevar R, Singer H. Impact of cardiac surgery on plasma levels of B-type natriuretic peptide in children with congenital heart disease (2007). Int J Cardiol; Vol 114 pp 339–44.

Kucher N, Printzen G, Goldhaber SZ. (2003) Prognostic role of brain natriuretic peptide in acute pulmonary embolism. Circulation; Vol 107 pp 2545–2547.

Kunii Y, Kamada M, Ohtsuki S, Araki T, Kataoka K, Kageyama M. (2003) Plasma brain natriuretic peptide and the evaluation of volume overload in infants and children with congenital heart disease. Acta Med Okayama; Vol 57 pp 191–7

Laussen PC, Roth SJ. Fast tracking: efficiently and safely moving patients through the intensive care unit. (2003) *Prog Pediatr Card;* Vol 18 pp 149-158.

Law Y.M., Hoyer A.W., Reller M.D. and Silberbach M., Accuracy of plasma B-type natriuretic peptide to diagnose significant cardiovascular disease in children: the better not pout children! Study (2009), *J Am Coll Cardiol;* Vol 54: pp 1467–1475

Lehot JJ, Villard J, Piriz H, Philbin DM, Carry PY, Gauquelin G, Claustrat B, Sassolas G, Galliot J, Estanove S. (1992) Hemodynamic and hormonal responses to hypothermic and normothermic cardiopulmonary bypass. *J Cardiothorac Vasc Anesth;* Vol 6 pp 132-9.

Lindahl B, Toss H, Siegbahn A, et al. for the FRISC Study Group. (2000) Markers of myocardial damage and inflammation in relation to long-term mortality in unstable coronary artery disease. *N Eng J Med;* Vol 343 pp 1139-1147.

Lowenthal A, Shah A, Bernstein H (2010) Letter by Lowenthal et al Regarding Article,"BNP Levels Predict Outcome in Pediatric Heart Failure Patients: Post Hoc Analysis of the Pediatric Carvedilol Trial". *Circ Heart Fail,* Vol 3: pp e32

Maher KO, Reed H, Cuadrado A, et al. (2008) B-type natriuretic peptide in the emergency diagnosis of critical heart disease in children. *Pediatrics;* Vol 121: pp e1484–8.

Maisel AS, Krishnaswamy P, Nowak RM, et al. (2002) Rapid measurement of B-type natriuretic peptide in the emergency diagnosis of heart failure. *N Eng J Med;* Vol 347 pp 161-167.

Mazurek B, Szydłowski L, Giec-Fuglewicz G, Markiewicz-ŁoskoG (2009) N-terminal Prohormone Brain Natriuretic Peptide-pro BNP Levels in Ventricular Arrhythmias in Children. *Clin.Cardiol,* Vol 32 pp 690–694

Mir TS , Marohn S, Läer S, Eiselt M, Grollmus O, Weil J (2002) Plasma Concentrations of N-Terminal Pro-Brain Natriuretic Peptide in Control Children From the Neonatal to Adolescent Period and in Children With Congestive Heart Failure. *Pediatrics,* Vol 110(6) pp e76.

Mir TS, Haun C, Lilje C, et al. (2006) Utility of N-Terminal Brain Natriuretic Peptide Plasma Concentrations in Comparison to Lactate and Troponin in Children with Congenital Heart Disease Following Open-Heart Surgery. *Pediatr Cardiol.* Vol 27 pp 209-216.

Muta H, Ishii M, Maeno Y, Akagi T, Kato H (2002) Quantitative evaluation of the changes in plasma concentrations of cardiac natriuretic peptide before and after transcatheter closure of atrial septal defect. *Acta Pediatr,* Vol 91 pp 649 652

Nir A, Lindinger A, Rauh M, Bar-Oz B, Laer S, Schwachtgen L, et al. (2009) NT-Pro-B-type natriuretic peptide in infants and children: reference values based on combined data from four studies. *Pediatr Cardiol* Vol 30 pp 3–8.

Paul MA, Backer CL, Binns HJ, Mavroudis C, Webb CL, Yogev R, et al. (2009) B-type natriuretic peptide and heart failure in patients with ventricular septal defect: a pilot study. *Pediatr Cardiol* Vol 30 pp 1094–7

Pietrzak R, Werner B (2009) Usefulness of NT-proBNP in assessment of right ventricular function in children after tetralogy of Fallot correction –apreliminary study. *Kardiol Pol,* Vol 67 pp 378-383

Rauh M, Koch A. (2003) Plasma N-terminal pro-B-type natriuretic peptide concentrations in a control population of infants and children. *Clin Chem;* Vol 49 pp 1563–4.

Ruskoaho H. Cardiac hormones as diagnostic tools in heart failure. (2003) *Endocr Rev* Vol 24 pp 341-56.

Ruskoni P, Ludwig D, Ratnasamy C, Masa R, Harmon WG, Colan SD, Lipshultz S (2010) Serial measurements of serum NT-proBNP as markers of left ventricular systolic function and remodeling in children with heart failure. *Am Heart J*, Vol 160 pp 776-83

Schwachtgen L, Herrmann M, Georg T, Schwarz P, Marx N, Lindinger A (2005). Reference values of NT-proBNP serum concentrations in the umbilical cord blood and in healthy neonates and children. *Z Kardiol* Vol;94 pp 399–404.

Seino Y, Ogawa A, Yasamita T, et al. (2004) Application of NT-proBNP and BNP measurements in cardiac care: a more discerning marker for detection and evaluation of heart failre. *Eur J Heart Fail* ; Vol 6 pp 295-300

Shah A, Feraco AD, Harmon C, Tacy T, Fineman JR, Bernstein HS (2009) Usefulness of Various Plasma Biomarkers for Diagnosis of Heart Failure in Children with Single Ventricle Physiology. *Am J Cardiol*, Vol 104 pp 1280-1284

Shih CY, Sapru A, Oishi P, Azakie A, Karl TR, Harmon C, Asija R, Adatia I, Fineman JR. (2006) Alterations in plasma B-type natriuretic peptide levels after repair of congenital heart defects: a potential perioperative marker. *J Thorac Cardiovasc Surg;* Vol 131 pp 632-8.

Silberbach M, Roberts CT Jr. (2001) Natriuretic peptide signaling: molecular and cellular pathways to growth regulation. *Cell Signal;* Vol 13 pp 221-31.

Soldin SJ, Soldin OP, Boyajian AJ, Taskier MS. (2006) Pediatric brain natriuretic peptide and N-terminal pro-brain natriuretic peptide reference intervals. *Clinica Chimica Acta;* Vol 366 pp 304-308.

Székely A, Breuer T, Sápi E, Székely E, Szatmári A, Tóth M, Hauser B, Gál J. (2010) Transpulmonary thermodilution in neonates undergoing arterial switch surgery. *Pediatric Cardiology;* Vol 32(2) pp 125-30

Tibby SM, Hatherill M, Murdoch IA. (1999) Capillary refill and core-peripheral temperature gap as indicators of haemodynamic status in paediatric intensive care patients. *Arch Dis Child;* Vol 80 pp 163-6.

Tobias JD (2011) B-type Natriuretic Peptide: Diagnostic and Therapeutic Applications in Infants and Children. *J Intensive Care Med*, Vol 26: pp 183-195

Welisch E, Norozi K, Rauch R (2011) N-terminal pro-brain natriuretic peptide level as a screening tool for cardiac involvement in paediatric diseases of extra cardiac origin. *Clin Res Cardiol*, DOI10.1007/s00392-011-0317-0

Wong D, George K, Wilson J, Manlhiot C, McCrindle BW, Adeli K, Kantor PF (2011) Effectiveness of Serial Increases in Amino-Terminal Pro–B-Type Natriuretic Peptide Levels to Indicate the Need for Mechanical Circulatory Support in Children With Acute Decompensated Heart Failure. *Am J Cardiol*, Vol 107 pp 573–578

19

Amyloidosis and Cardiac Surgery

Pavel Zacek and Jan Harrer
Department of Cardiac Surgery, Charles University Prague,
Faculty of Medicine in Hradec Králové,
and University Hospital Hradec Králové
Czech Republic

1. Introduction

Cardiac amyloidosis is a rare and complex pathology resulting in infiltrative restrictive cardiomyopathy and there are only very few clinical pathways through which the diseased amyloidotic heart may be a subject of cardiosurgical intervention. Cardiac surgery may rarely be warranted in very selected cases, and, on the other hand, may be performed mistakenly in misdiagnosed patients with cardiac amyloidosis. In clinical terms, the accumulation of expertise is hampered by the scarcity of its occurrence, heterogeneity of etiological subgroups, late clinical manifestation and polymorphous nature of symptoms.

The term amylon was first coined by Matthias Schleiden, German botanist, in 1838, for waxy starch in plants. In 1842 Karl Rokitansky described amyloidosis in connection with hepatosplenomegaly and Rudolf Virchow used in 1854 iodine for staining of amyloid. Today, more than one and half century later, we recognize amyloidosis as a heterogeneous infiltrative disease in which insoluble protein deposits are accumulated in various organs with deleterious effects on their functional integrity. Kidney, heart, blood vessels, central and peripheral nervous systems, liver, intestines, lungs, eyes, skin or bones may be affected (Cohen 1967).

2. Classification of cardiac amyloidosis

Cardiac amyloidosis is classified with regard to the origin of protein precursors in 6 types: primary (AL), secondary (reactive, AA), senile systemic, hereditary (familial), isolated atrial and hemodialysis-associated amyloidosis. Differentiation between these forms is based on immunohistochemical and genetic testing and implies the patient´s prognosis and therapeutic strategies.

Primary amyloidosis (AL) is the disease of immunoglobulin light-chain proteins produced from plasma cells in multiple myeloma and other plasma cell dyscrasias (Waldenström macroglobulinemia, B-cell lymphoma, a. o.). Its incidence is rare, estimated for 8.9 per million population (Kyle, Linos et al. 1992), however, its clinical course is aggressive with poor prognosis. The median survival without treatment is 13 months and may be prolonged to 17 months with melphalane and prednisone therapy (Kyle, Gertz et al. 1997). Predominant cardiac involvement is the cause of dim course with median life expectancy of 4 months since clinical manifestation of congestive heart failure. Death is attributed to

intractable low cardiac output or fatal arrhytmia. Sudden cardiac death may be preceded by syncope (Chamarthi, Dubrey et al. 1997).
Secondary amyloidosis (AA) is caused by the accumulation of amyloid A fibrils formed from an acute-phase reactant, serum amyloid A protein, in chronic inflammatory diseases like rheumatoid arthritis, familial Mediterranean fever, chronic infections, chronic lung diseases, tuberculosis, and inflammatory bowel disease. The heart seems to be affected less frequently whereas the kidney involvement leads to proteinuria and renal failure. The treatment of the underlying inflammatory process can reverse the disease (Gillmore, Lovat et al. 2001).
Senile systemic amyloidosis is related to liver production of a wild-type transthyretin transport protein (TTR). Amyloid deposits can be found in the heart, aorta, brain, pancreas, lung, liver, kidneys, and other organs. Senile systemic amyloidosis seems to be an age related disease, affecting predominantly men above the age of 70, with age-increasing incidence. Median survival of 75 months indicates less aggressive course of the disease (Cohen 1967; Ng, Connors et al. 2005).
Hereditary (familial) amyloidosis is an autosomal dominant disease in which genetically mutated proteins, namely TTR, form the insoluble deposits. More than 80 transthyretin mutation have been identified as well as mutations in other proteins (fibrinogen Aa, lysozyme, apolipoprotein A-I, and gelsolin) have also been reported (Connors, Richardson et al. 2000). Besides cardiac involvement the other manifestations are peripheral and autonomic polyneuropathy with mainly gastrointestinal symptoms, renal impairment.
Isolated atrial amyloidosis (AANF) is caused by atrial natriuretic peptide secretion in response to atrial dilation in valvular disease and chronic atrial fibrillation as well as in correlation to increasing age. Thin atrial amyloid deposits however do not affect significantly the cardiac performance. Cardiac amyloidosis may also develop in patients receiving long-term dialysis due to accumulation of beta2-microglobulin from chronic uremia (Gorevic, Casey et al. 1985). Amyloid deposits may be found in myocardium, pericardium and valves with minimal clinical impact (Noel, Zingraff et al. 1987).

3. Symptoms and diagnosis

Early diagnosis of cardiac amyloidosis is not easy since its symptoms are polymorphous and do not clearly lead clinicians to think about a rare diagnosis. The dominant pathophysiology is restrictive cardiomyopathy resulting in a diastolic failure. Frequent are arrhythmias, conductions disorders and syncopes. Angina may be present from obstructive intraluminal coronary microangiopathy (Narang, Chopra et al. 1993; Whitaker, Tungekar et al. 2004; Neben-Wittich, Wittich et al. 2005; Tsai, Seldin et al. 2011) which, in usual absence of epicardial coronary stenoses, can be classified as syndrome X - (Yagishita, Tanimoto et al. 2009). Low-voltage QRS amplitudes on ECG ($\leq$ 10 mV in all precordial leads or $\leq$ 5 mV in all limb leads) is a relatively constant finding but not very specific since it may be present also in obesity, emphysema, effusion, hypothyroidism and other clinical conditions (Shah, Inoue et al. 2006). Atrial fibrillation is common.
Besides some indicative information from patient´s history (hematological disorders, chronic inflammatory processes, polyneuropathy) echocardiography, in current clinical practice, has the potential to raise suspicion on cardiac amyloidosis in a given patient. Echocardiography diagnosis of cardiac amyloidosis is based on combination of two dimensional (2D) a Doppler image. In 2D both left and right ventricular wall thickness is

increased. Size of the ventricles remains unchanged while the atria are dilated. Myocardium displays highly abnormal texture described as „granular and sparkling" appearance due to acoustic mismatch between highly reflective amyloid deposits and normal myocardial tissue (Siqueira-Filho, Cunha et al. 1981). Pericardial effusion and signs of pulmonary hypertension are common. Pulsed wave Doppler parameters show diastolic left ventricular dysfunction, typically restrictive pattern, i.e. increased velocity of passive LV filling transmitral E wave and shortening of its deceleration time, shortening of isovolumic relaxation time and inversion of systolic and diastolic pulmonary vein velocity ratio.
Cardiac catheterization can confirm the nonspecific pathophysiology of restrictive cardiomyopathy (elevation of diastolic pressure in both ventricles and right-sided pressure curve with a dip and plateau or square root sign). Normal coronarography despite angina complaints fits the diagnosis of cardiac amyloidosis. Cardiac magnetic resonance imaging enables to visualize in 3D and high-resolution morphologic dimensions of the heart and regional wall motion. Decreased tissue signal intensity along with late subendocardial tissue enhancement by gadolinium can be helpful in differentiating amyloid cardiomyopathy (Maceira, Joshi et al. 2005; Bucciarelli-Ducci, Locca et al. 2007).
Ultimate diagnostic tool, though employed at advanced stage of diagnosis workup, is the biopsy specimen with positive Congo red staining for amyloid. Endomyocardial biopsy, if positive in four samples, gives almost 100% diagnostic sensitivity for amyloidosis. Tissue specimen can also be obtained from rectal submucosa or by abdominal fat aspiration (with sensitivity ranging between 75 - 85%, and 84 - 88%, respectively (Shah, Inoue et al. 2006).
Diagnostic difficulties are obvious: before enough clinical findings are gathered to justify the use of sophisticated and invasive diagnostic tools, the pathway to correct diagnosis may be tedious. Incorporating the possibility of cardiac amyloidosis into clinician´s thinking and careful consideration of all available data and findings is mandatory for obtaining the proper diagnosis fast.

4. Non-surgical treatment

Conservative management of restrictive cardiomyopathy resulting from structural myocardial alteration is limited. Diuretics are used to balance the signs of congestive heart failure, with narrow margin against low-cardiac output. Calcium channel blockers are contraindicated for negative inotropic effect, as well as beta-blockers (Griffiths, Hughes et al. 1982; Gertz, Falk et al. 1985; Gertz, Skinner et al. 1985). Administration of digoxin is risky because of its binding to amyloid fibrils and resulting toxic effects (Rubinow, Skinner et al. 1981). Implantation of permanent pacemaker may be necessitated for conduction disorders, with potential for alleviation of symptoms (Mathew, Olson et al. 1997).
Chemotherapy in AL amyloidosis, based on hematooncology strategy in treatment of multiple myeloma, includes administration of melphalan orally (with prednisone (Skinner, Anderson et al. 1996)) or in dose-intensive intravenous protocol, followed by autologous blood stem cell transplantation (Comenzo, Vosburgh et al. 1998; Moreau, Leblond et al. 1998). The rationale is to reduce or abolish the supply of amyloidogenic monoclonal light chain protein from the plasma cell clone which may facilitate the regression of plasma deposits and improve the quality of life. Alternatively, thalidomide with dexamethasone, or bortezomib may be administered (Charaf, Iskandar et al. 2009). In selected patients, the combined chemotherapy and stem cell transplantation may prolong the survival, however, it carries the risk of increased morbidity and mortality (Saba, Sutton et al. 1999).

5. Cardiac surgery in cardiac amyloidosis

Cardiac surgery, in logical consequence of low prevalence of cardiac amyloidosis, difficult straightforward diagnostics and very limited scope of action due to the nature of the disease, has a relatively small window of experience. Majority of the authors have published anecdotic case reports and only data on transplanted patients accumulate the evidence from small cohorts. Basically, there are three clinical pathways in which a patient with cardiac amyloidosis may be referred for cardiac surgery:

5.1 Amyloidosis misdiagnosed as a coronary artery or heart valve disease

Unsuspected cardiac amyloidosis as a cause of sudden fatal circulatory collapse in the course other cardiological or surgical intervention has been reported rather early (Goldman and Legnami 1966; Lindholm and Wick 1986; Kotani, Hashimoto et al. 2000; Wang and Pollard 2000). Postmortem examination in these case reports usually reveals surprisingly advanced stage of structural damage of the myocardium by amyloid deposits. Striking disparity between the gross morphological alteration and paucity of both clinical signs and diagnostic findings underlines the obvious difficulties of proper management strategies in cardiac amyloidosis.

Fatal response of the amyloidotic myocardium to the insult conveyed by anesthesia, general or cardiac surgery can be explained by concurrence of various pathophysiology mechanisms. Potential dysbalance of circulating volume in reaction to administration of anesthetic drugs cannot be adequately compensated in restrictive cardiomyopathy. Vicious circle is further potentiated by the myocardial inability to increase its contractile performance as well as by diffuse myocardial ischemia and susceptibility to arrhythmias. Standard treatment options, pharmacological support or counterpulsation, usually fail to resolve the circulatory shock.

In recent era of high volume cardiac surgery, the risk of referral of cardiac amyloidosis misdiagnosed for coronary or valve disease for cardiac surgery operation keeps to be present despite current improvements in diagnostic process. Obvious difficulties in proper diagnosis making of cardiac amyloidosis are combined with systemic bias of routine clinical thinking. Patient´s symptoms that are indicative of far more prevalent diagnoses, namely coronary artery disease, prompt to perform coronarography. Though not typical for cardiac amyloidosis, stenoses of epicardial coronary arteries can either be clearly present on coronarography or at least stenoses of some degree may be assumed as a sufficient explanation of angina symptoms. Once labeled as patients with coronary artery disease a routine echocardiography is usually performed with focus on systolic ventricular function and presence of mitral regurgitation. When cardiac hypertrophy is not strikingly present diastolic dysfunction can be easily overlooked or not taken into account.

Fatal outcome of coronary artery bypass grafting in misdiagnosed patients with cardiac amyloidosis has been reported by several authors (Massoudy, Szabo et al. 2003; Massias, Vyssoulis et al. 2006; Zacek, Medilek et al. 2007). In our institutional records (unpublished data) there were four fatal cases of undiagnosed cardiac amyloidosis indicated for coronary surgery (3x) or mitral and tricuspid valve repair (1x) (Fig. 1). In 3 ischemic patients, however, only two had debatable coronary stenoses while the third had a severe left main stenosis. Echocardiography was undiagnostic in all three of them. Postmortem microscopy revealed advanced stage of cardiac amyloidosis also with documented obliterative deposition of amyloid in small coronary vessels (Fig 2). The echocardiography of the patient

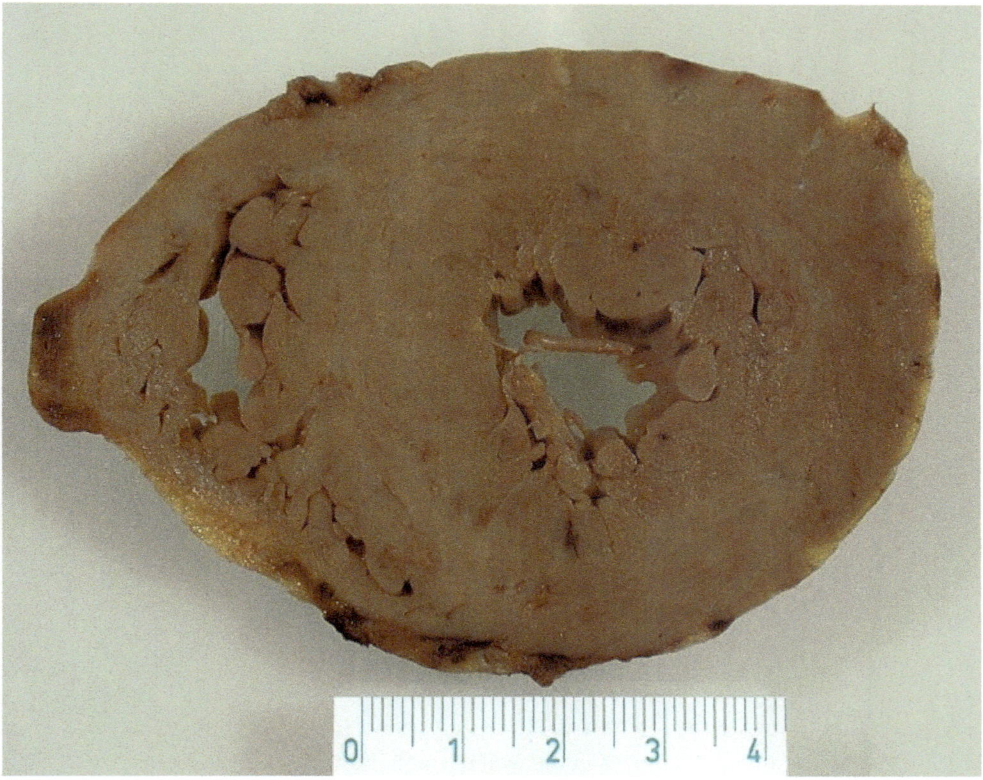

Fig. 1. Marked myocardial hypertrophy 610 g) in 75-year-old patient indicated for coronary artery bypass grafting for hemodynamically significant left main stem stenosis. Type of cardiac amyloidosis not identified (negative for AL, AA and senile amyloidosis). Besides presyncope in patient history no relevant data indicative of possible presence of amyloidosis were traced.

indicated for mitral and tricuspid surgery displayed no clear indications of amyloid restrictive cardiomyopathy even on retrospective reevaluation.

From the published data there is evident lack of constant and specific signs that could reroute in real world the misdiagnosis in process and avoid disastrous and unjustified cardiac operation. Low QRS voltage seems to be very constant but of low specificity. Interestingly, constant is the surgeon´s immediate tactile recognition of rubbery, stiff and nodular surface of myocardium. In obvious absence of diagnostic pattern that can safely indicate the correct diagnosis of cardiac amyloidosis the only advice is, first, meticulously include in consideration all the available data from patient history and examination, and, second, be sensitive for "small discrepancies" between the symptoms and objective findings (e.g., two of our patients had no clear angina but an effort dyspnea and fatigue were taken as an equivalent of this in presence of moderate stenoses on coronarography).

Correct diagnosis of cardiac amyloidosis would prevent disastrous outcome of bypass surgery in case of insignificant involvement of epicardial coronary arteries. Contrary to this, coincidence of severe coronary disease coinciding with amyloid disease will necessitate

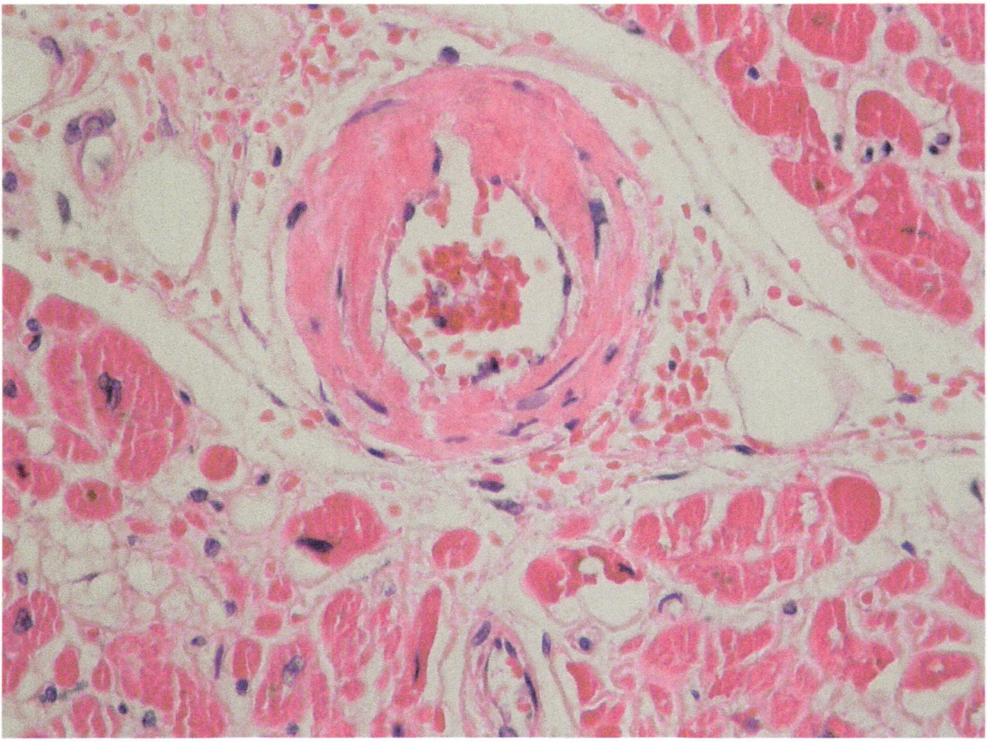

Fig. 2. Obstructive amyloid deposits in the wall of small intramyocardial artery (hematoxyllin-eosin, 400x)

percutaneous coronary intervention even in a difficult topography, instead of a surgery. Severe valve disease in a known cardiac amyloidosis would most probably lead to decision for conservative treatment.

5.2 Planned surgical intervention in correctly diagnosed cardiac amyloidosis

In contradiction to the abovementioned, very few reports describe intentional reconstructive cardiac surgery in patients with diagnosed cardiac amyloidosis. In 1983, Goffin coined a term dystrophic valvular amyloidosis for isolated amyloid deposits in cardiac valves (Goffin 1980). Successful aortic valve replacement was described by Iqbal (Iqbal, Reehana et al. 2006). In two cases, severe mitral regurgitation from papillary muscle or chordae rupture was successfully treated by valve repair and valve replacement (Coisne, Corbi et al. 2003; Nishi, Mitsuno et al. 2008). Obstructive intramural coronary amyloidosis was the speculative explanation for ischemic papillary muscle rupture in the latter case (Coisne, Corbi et al. 2003). Namai replaced successfully both mitral and aortic valve for endocarditis in a 62-year-old patient with multiple myeloma combined with renal amyloidosis (Namai, Sakurai et al. 2010). Uneventful postoperative course in these rare cases indicates that degree and distribution of morphological derangement, and moreover, the resulting functional deficit may vary considerably and therefore cannot be easily estimated prospectively.

5.3 Heart transplantation as ultimate surgical option in amyloid cardiomyopathy

Cardiac transplantation is logically the only substantial surgical treatment option for the heart with profound structural alteration due to the vast deposits of amyloid. From methodological point of view, however, principal concerns involve the operative risk of transplant surgery in patients with multiorgan amyloid disease, and the subsequent risk of recurrent amyloidosis in the transplanted graft. The shortage of donor organs is also difficult to ignore.

The first reports of successful heart transplantation for cardiac amyloidosis are dated back to early 80-ties (Conner, Hosenpud et al. 1988; Hall and Hawkins 1994). Mc Gregor reported in 1998 the Mayo Clinic experience (McGregor, Rodeheffer et al. 1998) of 8 patients but the largest cohort was published by Dubrey in 2004 (Dubrey, Burke et al. 2001; Dubrey, Burke et al. 2004) comprising 24 patients transplanted over the period of 18 years. In AL amyloidosis patients, the survival was 50%, 50%, and 20% at 1, 2, and 5 years in those without subsequent chemotherapy contrary to 71%, 71%, and 36% respectively in 7 AL transplanted patients with additional chemotherapy. Without chemotherapy the median of amyloid recurrence in the graft was 11 months. Survival of the 7 non-AL amyloidosis patients was 86%, 86%, and 64% at 1, 2, and 5 years. Overall 5-year survival of all amyloid patients was 38% in contrast to 67% in patients undergoing heart transplantation for other indications (Dubrey, Burke et al. 2004).

Regardless of the relatively small patient cohorts it can be assumed that the outcome of heart transplantation for AL amyloidosis is significantly worse than in general heart transplant population, namely due to progression of the systemic disease (Shah, Inoue et al. 2006; Luo, Chou et al. 2010).

In some clinical settings, heart transplantation may need to be combined with liver or kidney transplantation (Gillmore, Stangou et al. 2001; Schwartz, Kuiper et al. 2007; Audard, Matignon et al. 2009; Baumgratz, Vila et al. 2009). Liver transplantation should be instrumental or potentially curative in familial amyloidosis for abolishment of the aberrant transthyretin production. Scarcity of reported cases preclude consistent conclusion but it seems that precise knowledge of specific transthyretin mutation subtype may help to differentiate the outcome of transplantation strategy (Sharma, Perri et al. 2003).

6. Conclusion

In conclusion, cardiac amyloidosis is a complex pathology with poor prognosis since the onset of clinical manifestation even at the dawn of modern chemotherapy and stem cell transplantation. Should this disease be addressed by cardiac surgery the only therapeutic option is heart transplantation which, however, still remains to be debatable in view of postoperative results, recurrent amyloid disease of the graft and donor-organ shortage. Intentional cardiosurgical procedure for accompanying cardiac disorders can hardly be advised even in selected patients. On contrary, maximal vigilance has to be maintained to avoid misdiagnosing cardiac surgery for other more frequent cardiac maladies which otherwise can lead to unnecessary operation with fatal outcome.

7. References

Audard, V., M. Matignon, et al. (2009). Successful long-term outcome of the first combined heart and kidney transplant in a patient with systemic Al amyloidosis. *Am J Transplant* Vol 9 No (1): 236-240.

Baumgratz, J. F., J. H. Vila, et al. (2009). Heart transplantation in primary amyloidosis. *Rev Bras Cir Cardiovasc* Vol 24 No (3): 409-412.

Bucciarelli-Ducci, C., D. Locca, et al. (2007). Value of cardiovascular magnetic resonance for determining cardiac involvement in systemic amyloidosis. *Eur Heart J* Vol 28 No (10): 1186.

Cohen, A. S. (1967). Amyloidosis. *N Engl J Med* Vol 277 No (10): 522-530 contd.

Coisne, D., P. Corbi, et al. (2003). Obstructive intramural coronary amyloidosis and papillary muscle rupture. *Heart* Vol 89 No (2): E8.

Comenzo, R. L., E. Vosburgh, et al. (1998). Dose-intensive melphalan with blood stem-cell support for the treatment of AL (amyloid light-chain) amyloidosis: survival and responses in 25 patients. *Blood* Vol 91 No (10): 3662-3670.

Conner, R., J. D. Hosenpud, et al. (1988). Heart transplantation for cardiac amyloidosis: successful one-year outcome despite recurrence of the disease. *J Heart Transplant* Vol 7 No (2): 165-167.

Connors, L. H., A. M. Richardson, et al. (2000). Tabulation of transthyretin (TTR) variants as of 1/1/2000. *Amyloid* Vol 7 No (1): 54-69.

Dubrey, S. W., M. M. Burke, et al. (2004). Cardiac transplantation for amyloid heart disease: the United Kingdom experience. *J Heart Lung Transplant* Vol 23 No (10): 1142-1153.

Dubrey, S. W., M. M. Burke, et al. (2001). Long term results of heart transplantation in patients with amyloid heart disease. *Heart* Vol 85 No (2): 202-207.

Gertz, M. A., R. H. Falk, et al. (1985). Worsening of congestive heart failure in amyloid heart disease treated by calcium channel-blocking agents. *Am J Cardiol* Vol 55 No (13 Pt 1): 1645.

Gertz, M. A., M. Skinner, et al. (1985). Selective binding of nifedipine to amyloid fibrils. *Am J Cardiol* Vol 55 No (13 Pt 1): 1646.

Gillmore, J. D., L. B. Lovat, et al. (2001). Amyloid load and clinical outcome in AA amyloidosis in relation to circulating concentration of serum amyloid A protein. *Lancet* Vol 358 No (9275): 24-29.

Gillmore, J. D., A. J. Stangou, et al. (2001). Clinical and biochemical outcome of hepatorenal transplantation for hereditary systemic amyloidosis associated with apolipoprotein AI Gly26Arg. *Transplantation* Vol 71 No (7): 986-992.

Goffin, Y. (1980). Microscopic amyloid deposits in the heart valves: a common local complication of chronic damage and scarring. *J Clin Pathol* Vol 33 No (3): 262-268.

Goldman, B. S. and F. A. Legnami (1966). Senile cardiac amyloidosis: autopsy finding in a patient dying after implantation of a cardiac pacemaker. *Can Med Assoc J* Vol 94 No (20): 1055-1058.

Gorevic, P. D., T. T. Casey, et al. (1985). Beta-2 microglobulin is an amyloidogenic protein in man. *J Clin Invest* Vol 76 No (6): 2425-2429.

Griffiths, B. E., P. Hughes, et al. (1982). Cardiac amyloidosis with asymmetrical septal hypertrophy and deterioration after nifedipine. *Thorax* Vol 37 No (9): 711-712.

Hall, R. and P. N. Hawkins (1994). Cardiac transplantation for AL amyloidosis. *BMJ* Vol 309 No (6962): 1135-1137.

Chamarthi, B., S. W. Dubrey, et al. (1997). Features and prognosis of exertional syncope in light-chain associated AL cardiac amyloidosis. *Am J Cardiol* Vol 80 No (9): 1242-1245.

Charaf, E., S. B. Iskandar, et al. (2009). Cardiac amyloidosis responding to bortezomib: case report and review of literature. *Curr Cardiol Rev* Vol 5 No (3): 228-236.

Iqbal, S., S. Reehana, et al. (2006). Unique type of isolated cardiac valvular amyloidosis. *J Cardiothorac Surg* Vol 1 No: 38.

Kotani, N., H. Hashimoto, et al. (2000). Fatal perioperative myocardial infarction in four patients with cardiac amyloidosis. *Anesthesiology* Vol 92 No (3): 873-875.

Kyle, R. A., M. A. Gertz, et al. (1997). A trial of three regimens for primary amyloidosis: colchicine alone, melphalan and prednisone, and melphalan, prednisone, and colchicine. *N Engl J Med* Vol 336 No (17): 1202-1207.

Kyle, R. A., A. Linos, et al. (1992). Incidence and natural history of primary systemic amyloidosis in Olmsted County, Minnesota, 1950 through 1989. *Blood* Vol 79 No (7): 1817-1822.

Lindholm, P. F. and M. R. Wick (1986). Isolated cardiac amyloidosis associated with sudden death. *Arch Pathol Lab Med* Vol 110 No (3): 243-245.

Luo, J. M., N. K. Chou, et al. (2010). Heart transplantation in patients with amyloidosis. *Transplant Proc* Vol 42 No (3): 927-929.

Maceira, A. M., J. Joshi, et al. (2005). Cardiovascular magnetic resonance in cardiac amyloidosis. *Circulation* Vol 111 No (2): 186-193.

Massias, S., G. Vyssoulis, et al. (2006). Progressive heart failure in a patient after coronary artery bypass grafting. *Hellenic J Cardiol* Vol 47 No (2): 114-117.

Massoudy, P., A. K. Szabo, et al. (2003). Amyloid of heart and lungs in a patient with low output syndrome after coronary artery bypass grafting. *Herz* Vol 28 No (5): 453-456.

Mathew, V., L. J. Olson, et al. (1997). Symptomatic conduction system disease in cardiac amyloidosis. *Am J Cardiol* Vol 80 No (11): 1491-1492.

McGregor, C., R. Rodeheffer, et al. (1998). Heart transplantation in primary systemic amyloidosis. *J Heart Lung Transplant* Vol 17 No: 51.

Moreau, P., V. Leblond, et al. (1998). Prognostic factors for survival and response after high-dose therapy and autologous stem cell transplantation in systemic AL amyloidosis: a report on 21 patients. *Br J Haematol* Vol 101 No (4): 766-769.

Namai, A., M. Sakurai, et al. (2010). Cardiac surgery in a patient with multiple myeloma combined with renal amyloidosis. *Gen Thorac Cardiovasc Surg* Vol 58 No (7): 341-343.

Narang, R., P. Chopra, et al. (1993). Cardiac amyloidosis presenting as ischemic heart disease. A case report and review of literature. *Cardiology* Vol 82 No (4): 294-300.

Neben-Wittich, M. A., C. M. Wittich, et al. (2005). Obstructive intramural coronary amyloidosis and myocardial ischemia are common in primary amyloidosis. *Am J Med* Vol 118 No (11): 1287.

Ng, B., L. H. Connors, et al. (2005). Senile systemic amyloidosis presenting with heart failure: a comparison with light chain-associated amyloidosis. *Arch Intern Med* Vol 165 No (12): 1425-1429.

Nishi, H., M. Mitsuno, et al. (2008). Severe mitral regurgitation due to cardiac amyloidosis--a rare reason for ruptured chordae. *Interact Cardiovasc Thorac Surg* Vol 7 No (6): 1199-1200.

Noel, L. H., J. Zingraff, et al. (1987). Tissue distribution of dialysis amyloidosis. *Clin Nephrol* Vol 27 No (4): 175-178.

Rubinow, A., M. Skinner, et al. (1981). Digoxin sensitivity in amyloid cardiomyopathy. *Circulation* Vol 63 No (6): 1285-1288.

Saba, N., D. Sutton, et al. (1999). High treatment-related mortality in cardiac amyloid patients undergoing autologous stem cell transplant. *Bone Marrow Transplant* Vol 24 No (8): 853-855.

Shah, K. B., Y. Inoue, et al. (2006). Amyloidosis and the heart: a comprehensive review. *Arch Intern Med* Vol 166 No (17): 1805-1813.

Sharma, P., R. E. Perri, et al. (2003). Outcome of liver transplantation for familial amyloidotic polyneuropathy. *Liver Transpl* Vol 9 No (12): 1273-1280.

Schwartz, B. G., J. J. Kuiper, et al. (2007). Combined cardiac and liver transplantation for the treatment of familial amyloidosis. *Proc (Bayl Univ Med Cent)* Vol 20 No (2): 146-148.

Siqueira-Filho, A. G., C. L. Cunha, et al. (1981). M-mode and two-dimensional echocardiographic features in cardiac amyloidosis. *Circulation* Vol 63 No (1): 188-196.

Skinner, M., J. Anderson, et al. (1996). Treatment of 100 patients with primary amyloidosis: a randomized trial of melphalan, prednisone, and colchicine versus colchicine only. *Am J Med* Vol 100 No (3): 290-298.

Tsai, S. B., D. C. Seldin, et al. (2011). Myocardial infarction with "clean coronaries" caused by amyloid light-chain AL amyloidosis: a case report and literature review. *Amyloid* No.

Wang, M. M. and J. B. Pollard (2000). Postoperative ventricular fibrillation and undiagnosed primary amyloidosis. *Anesthesiology* Vol 92 No (3): 871-872.

Whitaker, D. C., M. F. Tungekar, et al. (2004). Angina with a normal coronary angiogram caused by amyloidosis. *Heart* Vol 90 No (9): e54.

Yagishita, A., S. Tanimoto, et al. (2009). Cardiac amyloidosis presumptively diagnosed as cardiac syndrome X. *Circ J* Vol 73 No (7): 1349-1351.

Zacek, P., K. Medilek, et al. (2007). Cardiac amyloidosis in the cardiosurgical operating room--a rare but fatal trap. *Thorac Cardiovasc Surg* Vol 55 No (2): 65-67.

20

Ivabradine Versus Beta-Blockers in Patients with Conduction Abnormalities or Left Ventricular Dysfunction Undergoing Coronary Artery Bypass Grafting

Luminita Iliuta[1,2] and Roxana Enache[2]
[1]*Department of Cardiac Surgery, "Prof. Dr. C. C. Iliescu" Emergency Institute of Cardiovascular Diseases, Bucharest*
[2]*"Carol Davila" University of Medicine and Pharmacy, Bucharest*
Romania

1. Introduction

Postoperative rhythm disorders are a serious complication of coronary surgery and they are associated with increased morbidity and mortality. Atrial fibrillation is the most common complication after cardiac surgery, with an incidence of 30% after coronary artery bypass grafting (Camm et al.,2010). There are few data about the etiology of atrial fibrillation in this setting, factors such as intraoperative atrial ischemia, pericarditis, and excessive adrenergic stimulation, were incriminated in its occurrence in vulnerable patients (Lucio et al., 2004). The peak incidence of postoperative atrial fibrillation is between postoperative days 2 and 4 (Camm et al.,2010). Although frequently these arrhythmias are benign and transient, patients developing postoperative atrial fibrillation are more likely to have perioperative myocardial infarction, stroke, congestive heart failure, respiratory failure, prolonged hospitalization and intensive coronary unit (ICU) stay and therefore increased economic burden of their care (Lucio et al., 2004; Iliuta et al., 2009; Burgess et al., 2006).

Many clinical trials and multiple meta-analyses evaluated the efficacy of pharmacological and non-pharmacological interventions in prevention of postoperative atrial fibrillation. The meta-analyses and systematic reviews showed that interventions to prevent and/or treat postoperative atrial fibrillation with beta-blockers, sotalol, or amiodarone and, less convincingly, atrial pacing, are favoured with respect to outcome (atrial fibrillation occurence, stroke, and length of hospitalisation) (Burgess et al., 2006; Crzstal et al., 2004). Currently, preoperative or early postoperative administration of beta-blockers is considered a first line choice to prevent atrial fibrillation after coronary artery bypass grafting except in patients with contraindications to beta-blocker therapy (Camm et al.,2010; Eagle et al., 2004). In patients with conduction abnormalities, severe left ventricular dysfunction, active bronchospasm or marked resting bradycardia the use of beta-blockers is difficult and controversial.

The hyperpolarization-activated pacemaker current (If) channel inhibitor ivabradine, which induces heart rate reduction by selective sinus node inhibition, showed improvement of clinical outcomes in patients with stable coronary artery disease and left ventricular systolic dysfunction (Fox et al., 2008) or chronic heart failure (Swedberg et al., 2010). Data regarding

the benefits of ivabradine used postoperatively in patients with conduction abnormalities or left ventricular dysfunction undergoing coronary surgery are scarce.
The main objectives of our study were to compare the efficacy and safety of heart rate lowering agent ivabradine versus beta-blocker metoprolol used perioperatively in patients undergoing coronary artery bypass grafting and having conduction abnormalities (first degree atrioventricular block or bundle branch block) or left ventricular dysfunction and also to determine whether prophylactic therapy with ivabradine can reduce hospital stay and economic costs after cardiac surgery by lowering the risk associated with an increased heart rate.

2. Methods

This trial was an open-label, randomized, clinical trial which enrolled 315 patients undergoing coronary artery bypass grafting with arteries (internal mammary, radial, gastroepiploic) or inverted saphenous veins in a single center (Cardiac Surgery Department of "Prof. Dr. C. C. Iliescu" Emergency Institute of Cardiovascular Diseases, Bucharest, Romania) between January 1st, 2006 and December 31st, 2007. Surgical management and treatment of the patients were based on a common standard protocol.

2.1 Eligibility criteria

Patients included in the clinical trial were patients undergoing elective coronary artery bypass grafting who had conduction abnormalities, left ventricular systolic dysfunction or both.

2.2 Exclusion criteria

Patients non-eligible for the study were patients exhibiting one or more of the following conditions:
1. second and third degree atrioventricular block
2. bradycardia (heart rate less than 50 beats per minute) or conditions associated with increased risk for bradycardia (vagal predominance, sick sinus syndrome)
3. NYHA class IV heart failure
4. cardiogenic shock
5. severe chronic obstructive pulmonary disease or pulmonary impairment
6. known hypersensitivity to beta-blockers or ivabradine
7. active participation in another clinical trial
8. failure to comply with the hospital protocol or absence to follow-up.

Study drop out criteria included the occurrence of adverse events: severe bradycardia, skin reactions, gastrointestinal symptoms, cold extremities. The study protocol was approved by the institute Management and Ethics Committee. All patients included in the trial gave written informed consent for participation in this study.

2.3 Study groups

After inclusion in the study, two days before surgery, patients were randomized in three groups:
1. Group A: 104 patients to receive metoprolol 100 mg once daily;
2. Group B: 106 patients to receive metoprolol 50 mg once daily and ivabradine 5 mg twice daily;
3. Group C: 105 patients to receive ivabradine 5 mg twice daily.

The treatment phase comprised 2 days preoperatively and at least 10 days postoperatively and the patients were followed-up for 30 days after surgery (Fig. 1).

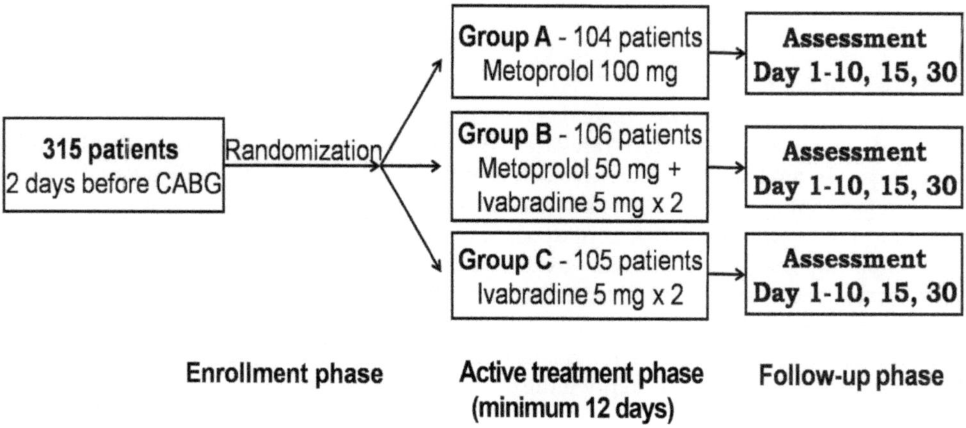

Fig. 1. Study phases and distribution of study population

2.4 Clinical and laboratory assessments

Patients were evaluated at baseline (ie. 2 days before surgery), daily from Day 1 until Day 10 postoperatively, on Day 15, and at the end of the treatment on Day 30 postoperatively. Patients with short in-hospital evolution were evaluated ambulatory.

Clinical parameters included NHYA class, ventricular rhythm, patient compliance, and quality of life.

Laboratory parameters assessed were: usual blood tests (white and red blood cell count, platelet count, hemoglobin, hematocrit, alanine aminotransferase and aspartate aminotransferase, lactate dehydrogenase, blood chemistry), electrocardiogram (ECG) (with the evaluation of rhythm and rate), 24-h ECG Holter monitoring and echocardiographic measurements of the left ventricular dimensions, left ventricular systolic and diastolic performance, left atrium dimensions and compliance (data not shown in the present report).

Cardiac rhythm was continuously monitored in the intensive care unit. During further hospital stay, subsequent ECG tests and a 24-h ECG Holter monitoring was carried out prior to discharge.

Follow-up visits were in Day 15 and in Day 30 postoperatively and included a physical examination and a 15-minutes interview, a resting ECG, an echocardiogram and a 24-h ECG Holter monitoring. Early episodes of heart failure were diagnosed based on clinical signs and symptoms and by transthoracic and transesophageal echocardiography. The presence of bradycardia or second or third degree atrioventricular block was assessed using clinical examination, resting ECG and 24-h ECG Holter monitoring.

2.5 Study endpoints

The efficacy endpoints were 30-days mortality, in-hospital occurrence of atrial fibrillation/arrhythmias, in-hospital occurrence of third degree atrioventricular block and need for pacing, in-hospital worsening heart failure and duration of hospitalization and immobilization. Safety endpoints were occurrence of bradycardia, gastrointestinal complaints, sleep disturbances, and cold extremities. A composite efficacy and safety endpoint including 30-days mortality, in-hospital atrial fibrillation/arrhythmias, in-hospital atrioventricular block/need for pacing, or in-hospital heart failure worsening was also defined.

2.6 Statistical analyses

No sample size assumptions have been made for this trial. Continuous variable are presented as mean ± standard deviation (SD). Categorical variables are displayed as percentages. To analyze the differences between the treatment groups, the Student *t* test was used for the continuous variables and the chi-square test for the categorical variables For each endpoint, a two-sided 95% confidence interval (CI) was calculated and an overall χ^2-test comparing the two treatment groups was used. Also, we performed simple and multivariate, linear and logistic regression analysis and we calculated relative risks and correlation coefficients. For the primary endpoints Kaplan-Meier curves were constructed and log-rank tests were used. All statistical analyses were performed using SYSTAT and SPSS software. A p value <0.05 defined the statistical significance.

3. Results

In the entire study population (315 patients), mean age was 62 ± 8 years, and 65.7% of patients were males. Baseline demographics and clinical characteristics of the three treatment groups are displayed in Table 1. There were no differences in age and gender of patients, presence of left ventricular dysfunction or conduction abnormalities between study groups, systolic blood pressure or mean baseline heart rate. Also, there were no differences between groups in mean number of grafts/patient and grafts type, risk score for atrial arrhythmias and mean duration of treatment.

The percentages of patients with previous episodes of atrial fibrillation were similar in the three groups (18.3% in group A, 19.8% in group B, and 19.1% in group C). There were similar proportions of patients with left ventricular dysfunction and conduction abnormalities (first degree atrioventricular block, complete left bundle branch block, bifascicular and trifascicular block) in the three treatment groups.

The primary efficacy and safety, single and composite endpoints in the treatment groups are shown in Table 2. In-hospital postoperative atrial fibrillation or tachyarrhythmias occurred less frequently with combined therapy (metoprolol and ivabradine) than with metoprolol or ivabradine alone used in the postoperative management of patients with coronary artery bypass grafting (7.6% events in group B versus 11.5% events in group A and 17.1% events in group C, p <0.001). The associated relative risk showed a higher protective value for the occurence of postoperative atrial fibrillation in patients with coronary artery bypass grafting treated with combined therapy compared with metoprolol monotherapy (-2.9 vs. -1.8) (Fig. 2).

In group C the frequency of early postoperative third degree atrioventricular block or need for pacing was lower (2.9%) than in group A (13.5%) and in group B (9.4%) (p <0.0001). The frequency of heart failure worsening was lower in patients treated with ivabradine only (1.9%) or ivabradine combined with metoprolol (6.6%) than in patients receiving only metoprolol (11.5%) (p <0.001) (Table 2). The associated relative risks for early postoperative complete atrioventricular block or need for permanent pacing and for postoperative heart failure worsening were lower in ivabradine-treated groups (Fig. 2).

Characteristic	Group A N = 104	Group B N = 106	Group C N = 105
Age (years)	63 (12)	63 (12)	63 (13)
% female	32.7%	35.9%	34.3%
Weight (kg)	75 (15)	76 (13)	77(14)
Height (cm)	172 (9)	170 (11)	171 (10)
Heart rate/24h	78 (15)	76 (16)	77 (14)
Left ventricular dysfunction	43.3%	43.4%	41.9%
Conduction abnormalities	46.2%	47.2%	46.7%
Systolic blood pressure (mmHg)	152 (22)	150 (28)	153 (23)
Previous episodes of atrial arrhythmias	18.3%	19.8%	19.1%
Hypertension	62.5%	66.0%	64.8%
Diabetes mellitus	28.9%	33.1%	30.5%
Re-intervention (previous coronary artery bypass grafting)	10.6%	12.3%	11.4%

Note. Parameters are expressed as mean values (standard deviation) or percentages. All p values for comparisons between groups were non-significant.

Table 1. Baseline demographics and clinical characteristics of study population by treatment group

Endpoint	Group A N = 104	Group B N = 106	Group C N = 105
30-day mortality, in-hospital atrial fibrillation/arrhythmias	16 (15.4%)	11 (10.4%)	22 (21.0%)
30-day mortality, in-hospital atrial fibrillation/arrhythmias, in-hospital atrioventricular block/need for pacing, or in-hospital heart failure worsening	42 (40.4%)	28 (26.4%)	27 (25.7%)
Death at 30 days	4 (3.8%)	3 (2.8%)	4 (3.8%)
In-hospital atrial fibrillation/arrhythmias	12 (11.5%)	8 (7.6%)	18 (17.1%)
In-hospital 3 degree atrioventricular block/need for pacing	14 (13.5%)	10 (9.4%)	3 (2.9%)
In-hospital heart failure worsening	12 (11.5%)	7 (6.6%)	2 (1.9%)
Hospitalization duration >15 days	12 (11.5%)	10 (9.4%)	9 (8.6%)
Immobilization for >3 days	10 (9.6%)	7 (6.6%)	7 (6.7%)
Sleep disturbances/ gastrointestinal symptoms/ skin reactions	3 (2.9%)	3 (2.8%)	3 (2.9%)

Table 2. Composite and single efficacy and safety endpoints by treatment group

The rates of 30-day mortality were lower in the combined therapy group (2.8%) versus metoprolol or ivabradine monotherapy groups (3.8% in each monotherapy group).

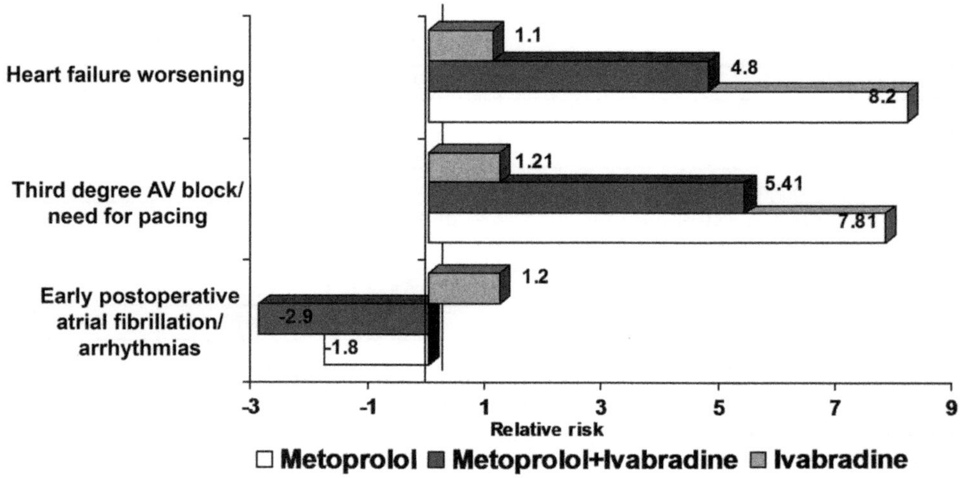

Note. AV, atrioventricular.

Fig. 2. The relative risks of ivabradine and combined therapy with ivabradine and metoprolol versus metoprolol monotherapy for early postoperative atrial fibrillation, complete atrioventricular block/need for pacing and postoperative heart failure worsening.

The overall quality of life was better in ivabradine groups. Ivabradine-treated patients had shortened hospital stay (the mean duration of hospital stay in the group A was 10.2 ± 6.3 days, compared to 8.5 ± 6.8 days in group B and 8.2 ± 6.4 days in group C), and reduced immobilization duration in the immediate postoperative period (2.0 ± 3 days in group A, 1.1 ± 3 days in group B and 1.1 ± 3 days in group C) (Table 2).

The cumulative incidence of non-cardiac side effects (sleep disturbances, gastrointestinal symptoms, and skin reactions) was similar in ivabradine (2.9%), metoprolol (2.9%) or combined ivabradine or metoprolol therapy (2.8%) groups (Table 2).

For the composite efficacy endpoint of 30-day mortality and in-hospital atrial fibrillation/arrhythmias the rates were 10.4% in the combined therapy group, 15.4% in the metoprolol group and 21.0% in the ivabradine monotherapy group. For the composite efficacy and safety endpoint of 30-day mortality, in-hospital atrial fibrillation/arrhythmias, in-hospital atrioventricular block/need for pacing, or in-hospital heart failure worsening, the rates were 25.7% in the ivabradine group, 26.4% in the ivabradine plus metoprolol group and 40.4% in the metoprolol group respectively ($p = 0.0002$) (Table 2), thus showing ivabradine therapy was superior to metoprolol therapy in terms of these composite endopoints. Kaplan Meier curves generated for primary endpoints also showed the superior efficacy and safety in ivabradine groups, either ivabradine monotherapy or combined ivabradine and metoprolol therapy (Fig. 3). Log-rank tests were highly significant from Days 4-5 of treatment period to Day 30.

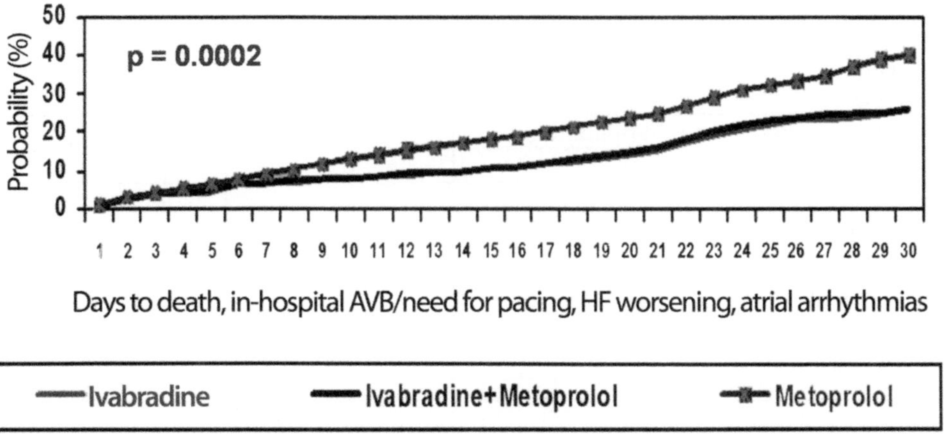

Note. AVB, atrioventricular block, HF, heart failure.

Fig. 3. Kaplan-Meier curves for the composite endpoint of 30-days mortality, in-hospital atrial fibrillation/arrhythmias, in-hospital atrioventricular block/need for pacing, or in-hospital heart failure worsening in the three treatment groups: ivabradine alone versus combined ivabradine plus metoprolol and metoprolol alone

The associated relative risks for the composite efficacy and safety endpoint of 30-day mortality, in-hospital atrial fibrillation/arrhythmias, in-hospital atrioventricular block/need for pacing, or in-hospital heart failure worsening in ivabradine-treated groups (with or without metoprolol) versus metoprolol-treated group in a subgroups analysis according to age, preoperative conduction abnormalities, NYHA class, previous episodes of atrial fibrillation and grafts number and type are shown in Table 3 and illustrated in Fig. 4. Ivabradine therapy (alone or associated to metoprolol) remained superior to metoprolol therapy in terms of the composite efficacy and safety endpoint of of 30-day mortality, in-hospital atrial fibrillation/arrhythmias, in-hospital atrioventricular block/need for pacing, or in-hospital heart failure worsening.

4. Discussion

The present study is, to the best of our knowledge, the first study which evaluated the use of ivabradine for prevention of postoperative atrial fibrillation or other tachyarrhythmias in patients undergoing coronary artery bypass surgery and assessed the efficacy and safety of ivabradine therapy in this setting. Atrial fibrillation is the most common complication which occurs after cardiac surgery, with frequencies ranging from 30% after coronary artery bypass grafting, 40% after valve surgery, and 50% after combined coronary artery bypass grafting/valve surgery (Camm et al., 2010). Development of atrial fibrillation immediately after coronary artery bypass grafting results in longer intensive care unit and hospital stays (Villareal et al., 2004; Tamis & Steinberg, 2000), and a significantly higher (two- to three-fold)

Composite endpoint of 30-days mortality, in-hospital atrial fibrillation/arrhythmias, in-hospital atrioventricular block/need for pacing, or in-hospital heart failure worsening	Relative risk metoprolol group N = 104	Relative risk ivabradine groups (with or without metoprolol) N = 211
Age		
≤70 years	1.5	1.5
>70 years	7.8	4.9
Previous episodes of atrial fibrillation	7.9	5.3
Preoperative conduction abnormalities	8.2	6.3
NYHA class		
NYHA I-II	1.5	1.2
NYHA III-IV	8.7	5.7
Number of grafts		
≥3 grafts	3.9	2.5
2 grafts	1.3	1.2
1 graft	1.2	1.1
Graft type		
Exclusively arterial	6.2	3.8
Exclusively venous	6.7	3.8
Combined venous and arterial	6.3	3.3

Table 3. Relative risks for the composite efficacy and safety endpoint of 30-days mortality, in-hospital atrial fibrillation/arrhythmias, in-hospital atrioventricular block/need for pacing, or in-hospital heart failure worsening in metoprolol versus ivabradine-treated patients

risk of postoperative stroke (Villareal et al., 2004; Reed et al., 1988). Post-operative atrial fibrillation has also been shown to independently predict post-operative delirium and neurocognitive decline (Burgess et al., 2006). Patients at risk for postoperative atrial fibrillation have been identified and include those with chronic obstructive pulmonary disease, proximal right coronary artery disease, prolonged cross-clamp time, atrial ischemia, advanced age, and withdrawal of beta-blockers (Eagle et al., 2004). Withdrawal of beta-blockers before surgery is a significant risk factor for the development of postoperative atrial fibrillation and should be avoided (Camm et al., 2010).

Because of the increased morbidity and mortality risk and of longer hospitalisations (up to five days [Eagle et al., 2004]) associated with the development of atrial fibrillation during the immediate postoperative period and because of the economic burden of these outcomes, prevention of postoperative atrial fibrillation becomes increasingly important. Various meta-analyses and systematic reviews assessed and identified pharmacologic and non-pharmacologic intervention to best prevent and treat postoperative atrial fibrillation.

At present, beta-blockers are the mainstay of therapy for prevention of postoperative atrial fibrillation in cardiac surgery. Both the ACC/AHA 2004 Guideline update for coronary artery bypass graft surgery for and the most recent ESC Guidelines for the management of atrial fibrillation recommend beta-blocker therapy as a class I indication in the prophylactic management of postoperative atrial fibrillation in patients without contraindications to beta-blocker therapy (Camm et al., 2010; Eagle et al., 2004). Studies showed that withdrawal of

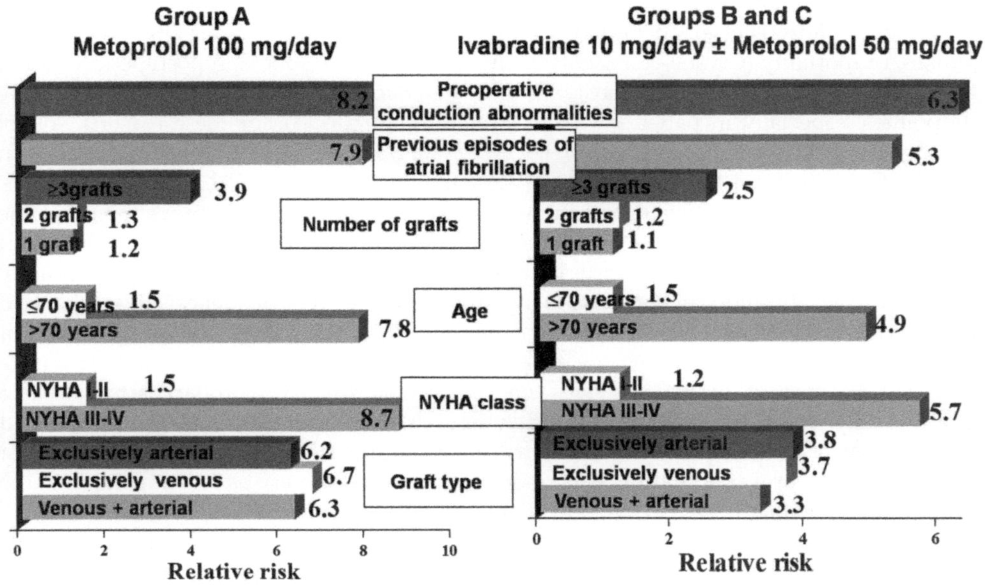

Fig. 4. Relative risks for the composite efficacy and safety endpoint of 30-days mortality, in-hospital atrial fibrillation/arrhythmias, in-hospital atrioventricular block/need for pacing, or in-hospital heart failure worsening in metoprolol versus ivabradine-treated patients in a subgroup analysis according to age, preoperative conduction abnormalities, NYHA class, previous episodes of atrial fibrillation and grafts number and type.

beta-blockers in the perioperative period doubles the incidence of postoperative atrial fibrillation after coronary artery bypass grafting (Eagle et al., 2004). Virtually every study of beta-blockers administered for the purpose of reducing postoperative atrial fibrillation has shown benefit in this regard, even if data regarding improvement of hospital stay or reduction of stroke incidence are still controversial (Iliuta et al., 2009). Most beta-blockers trials have examined the initiation of prophylaxis in the postoperative period. But it seems to be an even greater benefit if beta-blocker therapy is initiated before surgery. That is why the ESC guidelines for the management of atrial fibrillation recommend that treatment should be started at least 1 week before surgery with a beta$_1$-blocker without intrinsic sympathomimetic activity (Camm et al., 2010). The beta-blockers used in studies assessing atrial fibrillation prevention in cardiac surgery were propranolol (Matangyi et al., 1985), atenolol (Lamb et al., 1988), metoprolol (Lucio et al., 2004; Crystal et al., 2004; Kamei et al., 2006; Celik et al., 2009), acebutolol (Daudon et al., 1986), timolol (White et al., 1984), carvedilol (Kamei et al., 2006; Celik et al., 2009), betaxolol (Iliuta et al., 2009), either compared to control or to another beta-blocker.

Another antiarrhythmic agent used for the prevention of atrial fibrillation in cardiac surgery patients is sotalol which was shown to reduce the incidence of postoperative atrial fibrillation (Burgess et al., 2006; Crystal et al., 2004) compared to placebo or to other beta-blocker such as atenolol (Sanjuan et al., 2004), metoprolol (Parikka et al., 1998) or propranolol (Suttorp et al., 1990) but it had no impact on length of hospital stay, risk of strokes, or mortality (Crystal et al., 2004). However, the use of sotalol in postoperative atrial fibrillation is limited because of its significant side effects such as bradycardia and torsade de pointes, especially in patients with electrolyte disturbances. For these reasons, sotalol therapy for atrial fibrillation prevention in cardiac surgery patients is a class IIb indication in the ESC Guidelines for the management of atrial fibrillation (Camm et al., 2010).

Amiodarone and its beneficial effect in postoperative atrial fibrillation prevention was the subject of various studies and meta-analyses. Amiodarone decreased the incidence of postoperative atrial fibrillation (Burgess et al., 2006; Bagshaw et al., 2006) and significantly shortened the duration of hospital stay, and reduced the incidence of stroke and postoperative ventricular tachyarrhythmia (Burgess et al., 2006; Bagshaw et al., 2006), but not postoperative mortality (Bagshaw et al., 2006). The beneficial effects of amiodarone were observed irrespective of patients age, type of cardiac surgery (coronary artery bypass grafting only or valve surgery with or without coronary artery bypass grafting), and preoperative beta-blocker therapy. At present, amiodarone has a class IIa indication for atrial fibrillation prevention in patients undergoing cardiac surgery as recommended in the in the ESC Guidelines for the management of atrial fibrillation (Camm et al., 2010).

Other pharmacologic agents used in clinical study for the prevention of postoperative atrial fibrillation were digoxin, which was not found to be effective for atrial fibrillation prevention (Kowey et al., 1992) or calcium channel blockers, of which non-dihydropyridines significantly reduced supraventricular tachyarrhythmias in a subgroup analysis of a meta-analysis (Wijeysundera et al., 2003). Hypomagnesaemia is an independent risk factor for postoperative atrial fibrillation. A meta-analysis of randomized trials showed that prophylactic i.v. magnesium reduced the probability of postoperative atrial fibrillation (Miller et al., 2005).

From the non-pharmacologic interventions investigated for atrial fibrillation prevention in the postoperative setting, prophylactic atrial pacing reduced the incidence of post-operative atrial fibrillation regardless of the atrial pacing site or pacing algorithm used, (Burgess et al., 2006; Crystal et al., 2004) but results are controversial.

Despite this relative large range of prophylactic interventions for postoperative atrial fibrillation, there are subgroups of patients with conditions that limit the use of beta-blockers or other antiarrhythmic drugs. Among such conditions are cardiac conduction abnormalities or severe left ventricular dysfunction, active bronchospasm. In these patients ivabradine, a selective sinus node inhibitor, could be a viable alternative. Ivabradine is a specific inhibitor of the If current in the sinoatrial node. Consequently, it is a pure heart-rate-lowering agent in patients with sinus rhythm, without affecting blood pressure, myocardial contractility, intracardiac conduction, or ventricular repolarisation.

In BEAUTIFUL study, performed in patients with coronary artery disease and left ventricular systolic dysfunction (left ventricular ejection fraction of less than 40%), even if ivabradine failed to change the primary composite endpoint of cardiovascular death, admission to hospital for acute myocardial infarction, or admission to hospital for new-onset or worsening heart failure in any of the subgroups analysed, in a subgroup of patients with baseline heart rate of 70 bpm or higher it reduced the incidence of endpoints related to coronary artery disease (admission to hospital for fatal and non-fatal acute myocardial infarction) (Fox et al., 2008). Therefore, ivabradine can be used safely to patients with coronary artery disease and impaired left-ventricular systolic function, in conjunction with beta-blockers. Furthermore, a combination of ivabradine with β blockade also improved coronary artery disease outcomes in patients with heart rates of 70 bpm or more (Fox et al., 2008). These results suggest that further lowering of heart rate has beneficial effects on coronary disease outcomes.

In SHIFT study, performed in patients with stable symptomatic chronic heart failure and a left ventricular ejection fraction of 35% or lower, with a resting heart rate of 70 bpm or higher, ivabradine substantially and significantly reduced major risks associated with heart failure when added to optimal standard treatment: cardiovascular death or hospital admission for worsening heart failure (Swedberg et al., 2010).

The results of these two studies supporting the importance of heart rate reduction with ivabradine for improvement of clinical outcomes in heart failure or coronary artery disease with systolic left ventricular dysfunction were the rationale for using ivabradine alone or in combination with metoprolol for prevention of postoperative atrial fibrillation and reduction of subsequent morbidity, mortality and associated economic costs in patients undergoing coronary artery bypass grafting.

In our study, heart rate reduction and prevention of postoperative atrial fibrillation or tachyarrhythmias in the combined therapy group (ivabradine and metoprolol) was proven to be more effective than with metoprolol or ivabradine alone during the immediate postoperative management of patients undergoing coronary artery bypass grafting. Ivabradine-treated patients' quality of life was improved due to shortened hospital stay, reduced immobilization duration in the immediate postoperative period, less atrial or ventricular arrhythmias, less worsening heart failure.

Because postoperative atrial fibrillation is associated with increased morbidity and mortality and longer, more expensive hospital stays, we defined a composite efficacy and safety endpoint of 30-days mortality, in-hospital atrial fibrillation/arrhythmias, in-hospital atrioventricular block/need for pacing, or in-hospital heart failure worsening. Ivabradine and combined therapy (ivabradine and metoprolol) were superior to metoprolol in respect to the composite efficacy and safety endpoints for prevention of atrial fibrillation after coronary artery bypass grafting.

4.1 Study limitations

One limitation of our study is the absence of an washout period. About 85% of patients had preoperative beta-blocker therapy and it was not stopped before the randomization. The practice in our department was to routinely continue preoperative beta-blocker therapy without any pause and changing the active principle according to the study group. Another limitation is the fact that about 30% of the patients with previous episodes of atrial fibrillation received prior to the inclusion in the study an antiarrhythmic agent such as amiodarone or sotalol. These limitations would induce a possible underestimation of some results.

5. Conclusion

In patients treated with ivabradine the quality of life was improved due to shorter hospital stay, less atrial or ventricular arrhythmias, less need for permanent pacing, less worsening heart failure, shortened immobilization during the immediate postoperative period with subsequent improvement in the psychological status, as well as due to lack of significant side effects.

Considering the ivabradine efficacy and safety profile, the heart rate reduction in the early postoperative period after coronary surgery in patients with conduction abnormalities or left ventricular dysfunction with ivabradine therapy emerged as the best treatment in this trial.

Ivabradine should be regarded as an attractive alternative pharmacological strategy for rhythm and heart rate control in the early postoperative period in patients undergoing coronary artery bypass grafting with relative or absolute contraindications to beta-blocker therapy.

6. References

Bagshaw SM, Galbraith PD, Mitchell LB, et al (2006). Prophylactic amiodarone for prevention of atrial fibrillation after cardiac surgery: a meta-analysis. *The Annals of Thoracic Surgery*, Vol.82, No.5, (November 2006), pp. 1927–1937, ISSN 0003-4975

Burgess DC, Kilborn MJ, Keech AC (2006). Interventions for prevention of postoperative atrial fibrillation and its complications after cardiac surgery: a meta-analysis. *European Heart Journal*, Vol.27, No.23, (December 2006), pp. 2846–2857, ISSN 0195-668x

Camm AJ, Kirchhof P, Lip GYH, et al (2010). Guidelines for the management of atrial fibrillation. *European Heart Journal*, Vol.31, No.19, (October 2010), pp. 2369–2429, ISSN 0195-668x

Celik T, Iyisoy A, Jata B, et al (2009). Betablockers for the prevention of atrial fibrillation after coronary artery bypass surgery: carvedilol versus metoprolol. *International Journal of Cardiology*, Vol.135, No.3, (July 2009), pp. 393-396, ISSN 0167-5273

Crystal E, Garfinkle MS, Connolly SS, et al (2004). Interventions for preventing post-operative atrial fibrillation in patients undergoing heart surgery. *Cochrane Database of Systematic Reviews*, No.4, (October 2004), Art. No.CD003611

Crystal E, Thorpe KE, Connolly SJ, et al (2004). Metoprolol prophylaxis against postoperative atrial fibrillation increases length of hospital stay in patients not on preoperative beta blockers: the beta blocker length of stay (BLOS) trial. *Heart*, Vol.90, No.8, (August 2004), pp. 941–942, ISSN 1355-6037

Daudon P, Corcos T, Gandjbakhch I, et al (1986). Prevention of atrial fibrillation or flutter by acebutolol after coronary bypass grafting. *American Journal of Cardiology*, Vol.58, No.10, (November 1986), pp. 933–966, ISSN 0002-9149

Eagle KA, Guyton RA, Davidoff R, et al (2004). ACC/AHA 2004 guideline update for coronary artery bypass graft surgery: a report of the American College of Cardiology/American Heart Association Task Force on Practice Guidelines (Committee to Update the 1999 Guidelines for Coronary Artery Bypass Graft Surgery). *Circulation*, Vol.110, No.14, (October 2004), pp. e340-437, ISSN 0009-7322

Fox K, Ford I, Steg PG, et al; BEAUTIFUL Investigators (2008). Ivabradine for patients with stable coronary artery disease and left-ventricular systolic dysfunction (BEAUTIFUL): a randomised, double-blind, placebo-controlled trial. *Lancet*, Vol.372, No.9641, (September 2008), pp. 807-16, ISSN 0140-6736

Iliuta L, Christodorescu R, Filipescu D, et al (2009). Prevention of perioperative atrial fibrillation with betablockers in coronary surgery: betaxolol versus metoprolol.

Interactive Cardiovascular and Thoracic Surgery, Vol.9, No.1, (July 2009), pp. 89-93, ISSN 1569-9293

Kamei M, Morita S, Hayashi Y, et al (2006). Carvedilol versus metoprolol for the prevention of atrial fibrillation after off-pump coronary bypass surgery: rationale and design of the carvedilol or metoprolol post-revascularization atrial fibrillation controlled trial (COMPACT). Cardiovascular Drugs and Therapy, Vol.20, No.3 (June 2006), pp. 219-227, ISSN 0920-3206

Kowey PR, Taylor JE, Rials SJ, Marinchak RA (1992). Meta-analysis of the effectiveness of prophylactic drug therapy in preventing supraventricular arrhythmia early after coronary artery bypass grafting. *American Journal of Cardiology,* Vol.69, No.9 (April 1992), pp. 963-965, ISSN 0002-9149

Lamb RK, Prabhakar G, Thorpe JA, et al (1988). The use of atenolol in the prevention of supraventricular arrhythmias following coronary artery surgery. *European Heart Journal,* Vol.9, No.1, (January 1988), pp. 32-36, ISSN 0195-668x

Lucio Ede A, Flores A, Blacher C, et al. Effectiveness of metoprolol in preventing atrial fibrillation and flutter in the postoperative period of coronary artery bypass graft surgery. *Arquivos Brasileiros de Cardiologia,* Vol.82, No.1, (January 2004), pp. 42-46; 37-41, ISSN 0066-782X

Matangi MF, Neutze JM, Graham KJ, et al (1985). Arrhythmia prophylaxis after aorta-coronary bypass: the effect of minidose propanolol. *The Journal of Thoracic and Cardiovascular Surgery,* Vol.89, No.3, (March 1985), pp. 439-43, ISSN 0022-5223

Miller S, Crystal E, Garfinkle M, et al (2005). Effects of magnesium on atrial fibrillation after cardiac surgery: a meta-analysis. *Heart,* Vol.91, No.5, (May 2005), pp. 618-623, ISSN 1355-6037

Parikka H, Toivonen L, Heikkila L, et al (1998). Comparison of sotalol and metoprolol in the prevention of atrial fibrillation after coronary artery bypass surgery. *Journal of Cardiovascular Pharmacology,* Vol.31, No.1, (January 1998), pp. 67-73, ISSN 0160-2446

Reed G III, Singer DE, Picard EH, DeSanctis RW (1988). Stroke following coronary-artery bypass surgery. A case-control estimate of the risk from carotid bruits. *New England Journal of Medicine,* Vol.319, No.19 (November 1988), pp. 1246-1250, ISSN 0028-4793

Sanjuan R, Blasco M, Carbonell N, et al (2004). Preoperative use of sotalol versus atenolol for atrial fibrillation after cardiac surgery. *The Annals of Thoracic Surgery,* Vol.77, No. 3 (March 2004), pp. 838-843, ISSN 0003-4975

Suttorp MJ, Kingma JH, Tjon Joe Gin RM, et al (1990). Efficacy and safety of low- and high-dose sotalol versus propranolol in the prevention of supraventricular tachyarrhythmias early after coronary artery bypass operations. *The Journal of Thoracic and Cardiovascular Surgery,* Vol.100, No.6, (December 1990), pp. 921-926, ISSN 0022-5223

Swedberg K, Komajda M, Böhm M, et al; SHIFT Investigators (2010). Ivabradine and outcomes in chronic heart failure (SHIFT): a randomised placebo-controlled study. *Lancet,* Vol.376, No.9744, (September 2010), pp. 875-85, ISSN 0140-6736

Tamis JE, Steinberg JS (2000). Atrial fibrillation independently prolongs hospital stay after coronary artery bypass surgery. *Clinical Cardiology,* Vol.23, No.3, (March 2000), pp. 155-159, ISSN 1932-8737

Villareal RP, Hariharan R, Liu B, et al (2004). Postoperative atrial fibrillation and mortality after coronary artery bypass surgery. *Journal of the American College of Cardiology*, Vol.43, No.5, (March 2004), pp. 742–748, ISSN 0735-1097

White HD, Antman EM, Glynn MA, et al (1984). Efficacy and safety of timolol for prevention of supraventricular tachyarrhythmias after coronary artery bypass surgery. *Circulation*, Vol.70, No.3, (September 1984), pp. 479–484, ISSN 0009-7322

Wijeysundera DN, Beattie WS, Rao V, Karski J (2003). Calcium antagonists reduce cardiovascular complications after cardiac surgery: a meta-analysis. *Journal of the American College of Cardiology*, Vol.41, No.9, (May 2003), pp. 1496–1505, ISSN 0735-1097

Permissions

The contributors of this book come from diverse backgrounds, making this book a truly international effort. This book will bring forth new frontiers with its revolutionizing research information and detailed analysis of the nascent developments around the world.

We would like to thank Assoc. Prof. Cuneyt Narin, MD, for lending his expertise to make the book truly unique. He has played a crucial role in the development of this book. Without his invaluable contribution this book wouldn't have been possible. He has made vital efforts to compile up to date information on the varied aspects of this subject to make this book a valuable addition to the collection of many professionals and students.

This book was conceptualized with the vision of imparting up-to-date information and advanced data in this field. To ensure the same, a matchless editorial board was set up. Every individual on the board went through rigorous rounds of assessment to prove their worth. After which they invested a large part of their time researching and compiling the most relevant data for our readers. Conferences and sessions were held from time to time between the editorial board and the contributing authors to present the data in the most comprehensible form. The editorial team has worked tirelessly to provide valuable and valid information to help people across the globe.

Every chapter published in this book has been scrutinized by our experts. Their significance has been extensively debated. The topics covered herein carry significant findings which will fuel the growth of the discipline. They may even be implemented as practical applications or may be referred to as a beginning point for another development.

The editorial board has been involved in producing this book since its inception. They have spent rigorous hours researching and exploring the diverse topics which have resulted in the successful publishing of this book. They have passed on their knowledge of decades through this book. To expedite this challenging task, the publisher supported the team at every step. A small team of assistant editors was also appointed to further simplify the editing procedure and attain best results for the readers.

Our editorial team has been hand-picked from every corner of the world. Their multi-ethnicity adds dynamic inputs to the discussions which result in innovative outcomes. These outcomes are then further discussed with the researchers and contributors who give their valuable feedback and opinion regarding the same. The feedback is then collaborated with the researches and they are edited in a comprehensive manner to aid the understanding of the subject.

Apart from the editorial board, the designing team has also invested a significant amount of their time in understanding the subject and creating the most relevant covers. They scrutinized every image to scout for the most suitable representation of the subject and create an appropriate cover for the book.

The publishing team has been involved in this book since its early stages. They were actively engaged in every process, be it collecting the data, connecting with the contributors or procuring relevant information. The team has been an ardent support to the editorial, designing and production team. Their endless efforts to recruit the best for this project, has resulted in the accomplishment of this book. They are a veteran in the field of academics and their pool of knowledge is as vast as their experience in printing. Their expertise and guidance has proved useful at every step. Their uncompromising quality standards have made this book an exceptional effort. Their encouragement from time to time has been an inspiration for everyone.

The publisher and the editorial board hope that this book will prove to be a valuable piece of knowledge for researchers, students, practitioners and scholars across the globe.

List of Contributors

Meral Kanbak
Hacettepe University School of Medicine, Department of Anesthesiology and Reanimation, Ankara, Turkey

Filiz Üzümcügil
TCSB Ankara Etlik Zübeyde Hanım Maternity and Women's Health Clinic Teaching and Research Hospital, Department of Anesthesiology and Reanimation, Ankara, Turkey

Mohammad Hamid
Aga Khan University, Pakistan

Maurizio Mangione, Paolo Marcheschi and Stefano Dalmiani
Medical Informatics, Gabriele Monasterio, CNR / Tuscany Region Foundation, Italy

Alessandro Taddei
Medical Informatics, Gabriele Monasterio, CNR / Tuscany Region Foundation, Italy
CNR Institute of Clinical Physiology, G. Pasquinucci Heart Hospital, Massa, Italy

Maria Carmona and Matheus Vane
Discipline of Anesthesiology, University of São Paulo Medical School, São Paulo, Brazil

Luiz Malbouisson
Postoperative ICU, Institute of General Hospital, University of São Paulo Medical School, São Paulo, Brazil

Theofani Antoniou
Onassis Cardiac Surgery Center, Athens, Greece

Kassiani Theodoraki
Areteion University Hospital, University of Athens School of Medicine, Athens, Greece

Thomas Kenny and Martin Ashton-Key
National Specialised Commissioning Team, England

Paul M. H. J. Roekaerts
Department of Intensive Care, The Netherlands

John H. Heijmans
Department of Anaesthesiology, University Hospital Maasticht, Maastricht, The Netherlands

Robert Wagner
Centre for Cardiovascular and Transplant Surgery, St Anne's University Hospital, Masaryk University, Brno, Czech Republic

Yavuz M. Bilgin
Department of Hematology, Erasmus Medical Center Rotterdam, The Netherlands

Martín Martínez Rosas
Physiology Department, National Institute of Cardiology "Ignacio Chavez", Mexico D.F., Mexico

Eduardo Wilfrido Goicoechea-Turcott
Faculty of Medicine, National Autonomous University of Mexico (UNAM), Mexico D.F., Mexico

Pastor Luna Ortiz
Pharmacology Department, National Institute of Cardiology "Ignacio Chavez", Mexico D.F., Mexico

Alberto Salazar and Benito Antón Palma
Laboratory of Molecular Neurobiology, National Institute of Psychiatry "Ramón de la Fuente", Mexico, D.F., Mexico

Philip Johnson and Andrew Westbrook
Department of Anaesthesia, Intensive Care and Pain Medicine, St Vincent's University Hospital, Elm Park, Dublin, Ireland

Marcin Wąsowicz
Department of Anesthesia and Pain Management, Toronto General Hospital, Cardiovascular Intensive Care Unit, Toronto General Hospital, Department of Anesthesia, University of Toronto, Canada

Susanne Maria Picker
Transfusion Medicine, University Hospital of Cologne, Germany

Aaron M. Ranasinghe and Robert S. Bonser
University of Birmingham, Cardiovascular Medicine, School of Clinical and Experimental Medicine, Birmingham, UK
UHB NHS FT, Department of Cardiothoracic Surgery, Edgbaston, Birmingham, UK

Anne Q. N. Nguyen, Alain Deschamps, France Varin, Louis P. Perrault and André Y. Denault
Montreal Heart Institute and Université de Montréal, Canada

Vered Molina-Hazan and Gideon Paret
Department of Pediatric Critical Care, Safra Children's Hospital, Chaim Sheba Medical Center, Tel Hashomer, Affiliated to The Sackler School of Medicine, Tel Aviv University, Tel Aviv, Israel

Sara Ferrando-Martínez
Laboratory of Immunovirology, Infectious Diseases Service, HU Virgen del Rocío, Institute of Biomedicine of Seville (IBiS), Seville, Spain
Laboratory of Molecular Immuno-Biology, HGU Gregorio Marañón, Madrid, Spain

M. Ángeles Muñoz-Fernández
Laboratory of Molecular Immuno-Biology, HGU Gregorio Marañón, Madrid, Spain

Manuel Leal
Laboratory of Immunovirology, Infectious Diseases Service, HU Virgen del Rocío, Institute of Biomedicine of Seville (IBiS), Seville, Spain

Andrea Székely, Tamás Breuer and Béla Merkely
Department of Anesthesiology and Intensive Care, Department of Cardiology, Semmelweis University and Department of Cardiology Gottsegen György, Hungarian Institute of Cardiology, Budapest, Hungary

Pavel Zacek and Jan Harrer
Department of Cardiac Surgery, Charles University Prague, Faculty of Medicine in Hradec Králové and University Hospital Hradec Králové, Czech Republic

Luminita Iliuta
Department of Cardiac Surgery, "Prof. Dr. C. C. Iliescu" Emergency Institute of Cardiovascular Diseases, Bucharest, Romania
"Carol Davila" University of Medicine and Pharmacy, Bucharest, Romania

Roxana Enache
"Carol Davila" University of Medicine and Pharmacy, Bucharest, Romania